Textbook of Violence Assessment and Management

Textbook of Violence Assessment and Management

Edited by

Robert I. Simon, M.D.
Kenneth Tardiff, M.D., M.P.H.

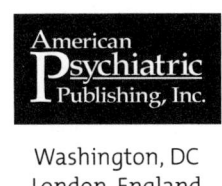

Washington, DC
London, England

Note: The authors have worked to ensure that all information in this book is accurate at the time of publication and consistent with general psychiatric and medical standards, and that information concerning drug dosages, schedules, and routes of administration is accurate at the time of publication and consistent with standards set by the U.S. Food and Drug Administration and the general medical community. As medical research and practice continue to advance, however, therapeutic standards may change. Moreover, specific situations may require a specific therapeutic response not included in this book. For these reasons and because human and mechanical errors sometimes occur, we recommend that readers follow the advice of physicians directly involved in their care or the care of a member of their family.

Books published by American Psychiatric Publishing, Inc., represent the views and opinions of the individual authors and do not necessarily represent the policies and opinions of APPI or the American Psychiatric Association.

To purchase 25–99 copies of this or any other APPI title at a 20% discount, please contact APPI Customer Service at appi@psych.org or 800–368–5777. To purchase 100 or more copies of the same title, please e-mail bulksales@psych.org for a price quote.

Copyright © 2008 American Psychiatric Publishing, Inc.
ALL RIGHTS RESERVED

Manufactured in the United States of America on acid-free paper
12 11 10 09 08   5 4 3 2 1
First Edition

Typeset in Adobe Palatino and The Mix

American Psychiatric Publishing, Inc.
1000 Wilson Boulevard
Arlington, VA 22209–3901
www.appi.org

Library of Congress Cataloging-in-Publication Data
Textbook of violence assessment and management / edited by Robert I. Simon, Kenneth Tardiff. -- 1st ed.
   p. ; cm.
Includes bibliographical references and index.
ISBN 978-1-58562-314-3 (alk. paper)
 1. Dangerously mentally ill. 2. Risk assessment. 3. Violence. I. Simon, Robert I. II. Tardiff, Kenneth, 1944-
 [DNLM: 1. Social Behavior Disorders--diagnosis. 2. Violence--prevention & control. 3. Mentally Ill Persons--psychology. 4. Professional-Patient Relations. 5. Risk Assessment--methods. 6. Social Behavior Disorders--therapy. WM 600 T355 2008]
 RC569.5.V55T47 2008
 616.8582--dc22
                                                                        2008004457

British Library Cataloguing in Publication Data
A CIP record is available from the British Library.

Dedicated to all who are committed to understanding, treating, and preventing violence.

Contents

Contributors xi

Foreword xvii
Paul S. Appelbaum, M.D.

Preface xxi

Acknowledgments xxiii

I
ASSESSMENT PRINCIPLES

1 Clinical Risk Assessment of Violence 3
Kenneth Tardiff, M.D., M.P.H.

2 Structured Risk Assessment of Violence 17
John Monahan, Ph.D.

3 Cultural Competence in Violence Risk Assessment 35
Russell F. Lim, M.D.
Carl C. Bell, M.D.

4 Psychological Testing in Violence Risk Assessment 59
Barry Rosenfeld, Ph.D., A.B.P.P.
Ekaterina Pivovarova, M.A.

II
MENTAL DISORDERS AND CONDITIONS

5 Mood Disorders 77
    Rif S. El-Mallakh, M.D.
    R. Jeannie Roberts, M.D.
    Peggy L. El-Mallakh, Ph.D.

6 Schizophrenia and Delusional Disorder 105
    Martha L. Crowner, M.D.

7 Posttraumatic Stress Disorder 123
    Thomas A. Grieger, M.D., D.F.A.P.A.
    David M. Benedek, M.D., D.F.A.P.A.
    Robert J. Ursano, M.D., D.F.A.P.A.

8 Substance Abuse Disorders 141
    Rodney Burbach, M.D.

9 Personality Disorders 161
    William H. Reid, M.D., M.P.H.
    Stephen A. Thorne, Ph.D.

10 Neurological and Medical Disorders 185
    Karen E. Anderson, M.D.
    Jonathan M. Silver, M.D.

11 Impulsivity and Aggression 211
    Sara T. Wakai, Ph.D.
    Robert L. Trestman, Ph.D., M.D.

III
TREATMENT SETTINGS

12 Outpatient Settings 237
    James C. Beck, M.D., Ph.D.

13 Inpatient Settings 259
    Cameron D. Quanbeck, M.D.
    Barbara E. McDermott, Ph.D.

14 Emergency Services 277
Jean-Pierre Lindenmayer, M.D.
Anzalee Khan, M.S.

IV

TREATMENT AND MANAGEMENT

15 Psychopharmacology and Electroconvulsive
Therapy 301
Leslie Citrome, M.D., M.P.H.

16 Psychotherapeutic Interventions 325
John R. Lion, M.D.

17 Seclusion and Restraint 339
Kenneth Tardiff, M.D., M.P.H.
John R. Lion, M.D.

V

SPECIAL POPULATIONS

18 Children and Adolescents 359
Peter Ash, M.D.

19 The Elderly. 381
Robert Weinstock, M.D.
Stephen Read, M.D.
Gregory B. Leong, M.D.
J. Arturo Silva, M.D.

VI

SPECIAL TOPICS

20 Forensic Issues. 409
Charles L. Scott, M.D.

21 Legal Issues of Prediction, Protection,
and Expertise 429
Daniel W. Shuman, J.D.
Britt Darwin-Looney, J.D.

22 Sexual Violence and the Clinician.....................441
   John M.W. Bradford, M.B.Ch.B., D.P.M.
   Paul Fedoroff, M.D.
   Philip Firestone, Ph.D.

23 Violence Toward Mental Health Professionals........461
   William R. Dubin, M.D.
   Autumn Ning, M.D.

24 Intimate Partner Violence and the Clinician..........483
   Susan Hatters Friedman, M.D.
   Joy E. Stankowski, M.D.
   Sana Loue, Ph.D., J.D., M.P.H.

25 Workplace Violence and the Clinician................501
   Ronald Schouten, M.D., J.D.

26 Vehicular Crashes and the Role of
   Mental Health Clinicians............................521
   Alan R. Felthous, M.D.
   Thomas M. Meuser, Ph.D.
   Thomas Ala, M.D.

27 School Violence.....................................537
   Carl P. Malmquist, M.D., M.S.

28 Clinically-Based Risk Management of
   Potentially Violent Patients........................555
   Robert I. Simon, M.D.

Index...567

Contributors

Thomas Ala, M.D.
Associate Professor of Clinical Neurology, Center for Alzheimer's Disease and Associated Disorders, Southern Illinois University School of Medicine, Springfield, Illinois

Karen E. Anderson, M.D.
Assistant Professor, Psychiatry and Neurology Movement Disorders, University of Maryland School of Medicine, and Director, University of Maryland Huntington's Disease Clinic, Baltimore, Maryland

Paul S. Appelbaum, M.D.
Elizabeth K. Dollard Professor of Psychiatry, Medicine and Law, and Director, Division of Psychiatry, Law and Ethics, Department of Psychiatry, Columbia University College of Physicians and Surgeons, New York, New York

Peter Ash, M.D.
Associate Professor, Department of Psychiatry and Behavioral Sciences, Emory University, Atlanta, Georgia

James C. Beck, M.D., Ph.D.
Professor of Psychiatry, Harvard Medical School; Associate Director, Law and Psychiatry Service, Department of Psychiatry, Massachusetts General Hospital, Boston, Massachusetts

Carl C. Bell, M.D.
President/Chief Executive Officer, Community Mental Health Council and Foundation, Inc.; Professor of Psychiatry and Public Health, University of Illinois at Chicago, Chicago, Illinois

David M. Benedek, M.D., D.F.A.P.A.
Associate Professor, Department of Psychiatry, Uniformed Services University, Bethesda, Maryland

John M.W. Bradford, M.B.Ch.B., D.P.M.
Professor and Head of Division of Forensic Psychiatry, University of Ottawa; Associate Chief, Royal Ottawa Health Care Group, Ottawa, Ontario, Canada

Rodney Burbach, M.D.
Medical Review Officer, U.S. Nuclear Regulatory Commission, Washington, D.C.; Chairman, Department of Family Practice, and former Medical Director, Addiction Treatment Center, Suburban Hospital Bethesda, Maryland; Clinical Instructor, Georgetown University School of Medicine, Washington, D.C.

Leslie Citrome, M.D., M.P.H.
Professor of Psychiatry, New York University School of Medicine, New York, New York; Director, Clinical Research and Evaluation Facility, Nathan S. Kline Institute for Psychiatric Research, Orangeburg, New York

Martha L. Crowner, M.D.
Associate Clinical Professor of Psychiatry, Columbia College of Physicians and Surgeons, New York, New York

Britt Darwin-Looney, J.D.
Praesidium, Inc., Arlington, Texas

William R. Dubin, M.D.
Professor and Vice Chair, Department of Psychiatry, Temple University School of Medicine; Chief Medical Officer, Temple University Hospital-Episcopal Campus, Philadelphia, Pennsylvania

Peggy L. El-Mallakh, Ph.D.
Assistant Professor, Department of Nursing Education, University of Louisville School of Nursing, Louisville, Kentucky

Rif S. El-Mallakh, M.D.
Associate Professor, Director, Mood Disorders Research Program, Department of Psychiatry and Behavioral Sciences, University of Louisville School of Medicine, Louisville, Kentucky

Paul Fedoroff, M.D.
Associate Professor, Division of Forensic Psychiatry, Department of Psychiatry, University of Ottawa; Director of Forensic Research Unit, University of Ottawa Institute of Mental Health Research, Ottawa, Ontario, Canada

Contributors

Alan R. Felthous, M.D.
Professor and Director of Forensic Psychiatry Division, Department of Neurology and Psychiatry, St. Louis University School of Medicine, St. Louis, Missouri

Philip Firestone, Ph.D.
Professor, Department of Psychology, Faculty of Social Sciences, University of Ottawa, Ottawa, Ontario, Canada

Susan Hatters Friedman, M.D.
Senior Instructor in Psychiatry, Case Western Reserve University School of Medicine; forensic psychiatrist, Northcoast Behavioral Healthcare, Cleveland, Ohio

Thomas A. Grieger, M.D., D.F.A.P.A.
Private practice in forensic psychiatry, Falls Church, Virginia

Anzalee Khan, M.S.
Ph.D. candidate, Department of Psychometrics, Fordham University Rose Hill Campus, Bronx, New York

Gregory B. Leong, M.D.
Clinical Professor of Psychiatry, Department of Psychiatry and Behavioral Sciences, University of Washington School of Medicine, Seattle, Washington; psychiatrist, Western State Hospital, Tacoma, Washington

Russell F. Lim, M.D.
Associate Clinical Professor, Department of Psychiatry and Behavioral Sciences, University of California Davis School of Medicine; Staff Psychiatrist and Director of Diversity Education and Training, Adult Psychiatric Support Services Clinic (APSSC) of Sacramento County, Sacramento, California

Jean-Pierre Lindenmayer, M.D.
Director, Psychopharmacology Research Unit, Manhattan Psychiatric Center, Nathan S. Kline Institute for Psychiatric Research; Clinical Professor, Department of Psychiatry, New York University, New York, New York

John R. Lion, M.D.
Clinical Professor of Psychiatry, University of Maryland School of Medicine, Baltimore, Maryland

Sana Loue, Ph.D., J.D., M.P.H.
Professor in Epidemiology and Biostatistics, Case Western Reserve University School of Medicine, Cleveland, Ohio

Carl P. Malmquist, M.D., M.S.
Professor of Social Psychiatry, University of Minnesota, Minneapolis, Minnesota

Barbara E. McDermott, Ph.D.
Associate Professor of Clinical Psychiatry, Department of Psychiatry and Behavioral Sciences, Division of Psychiatry and the Law, University of California, Davis, California

Thomas M. Meuser, Ph.D.
Director of Gerontology, Associate Professor of Social Work and Psychology, University of Missouri, St. Louis, Missouri

John Monahan, Ph.D.
John S. Shannon Distinguished Professor of Law, Professor of Psychology and Psychiatric Medicine, University of Virginia, Charlottesville, Virginia

Autumn Ning, M.D.
Instructor and Assistant Training Director, Department of Psychiatry, Temple University School of Medicine; Medical Director, Crisis Response Center, Temple University Hospital-Episcopal Campus, Philadelphia, Pennsylvania

Ekaterina Pivovarova, M.A.
Doctoral candidate, Department of Psychology, Fordham University, Bronx, New York

Cameron D. Quanbeck, M.D.
Assistant Clinical Professor, Department of Psychiatry and Behavioral Sciences, Division of Psychiatry and the Law, University of California, Davis, California

Stephen Read, M.D.
Clinical Professor of Psychiatry, Department of Psychiatry and Biobehavioral Sciences, University of California, Los Angeles, David Geffen School of Medicine; psychiatrist, Greater Los Angeles Veterans Affairs Health Care System, Los Angeles, California

Contributors

William H. Reid, M.D., M.P.H.
Clinical Professor of Psychiatry, University of Texas Health Science Center, San Antonio, Texas

R. Jeannie Roberts, M.D.
Mood Disorders Research Program; Instructor, Department of Psychiatry and Behavioral Sciences, University of Louisville School of Medicine, Louisville, Kentucky

Barry Rosenfeld, Ph.D., A.B.P.P.
Professor, Department of Psychology, Fordham University, Bronx, New York

Ronald Schouten, M.D., J.D.
Associate Professor of Psychiatry, Harvard Medical School; Director, Law and Psychiatry Service, Massachusetts General Hospital, Boston, Massachusetts

Charles L. Scott, M.D.
Chief, Division of Psychiatry and the Law, Clinical Professor of Psychiatry, and Director, Forensic Psychiatry Fellowship, University of California Davis Medical Center, Sacramento, California

Daniel W. Shuman, J.D.
M.D. Anderson Foundation Endowed Professor of Health Law, Dedman School of Law, Southern Methodist University, Dallas, Texas

Robert I. Simon, M.D.
Clinical Professor of Psychiatry and Director, Program in Psychiatry and Law, Georgetown University School of Medicine, Washington, D.C.

J. Arturo Silva, M.D.
Private practice of psychiatry, San Jose, California

Jonathan M. Silver, M.D.
Clinical Professor of Psychiatry, New York University School of Medicine, New York, New York; Fellow, American Neuropsychiatric Association; Diplomate, Behavioral Neurology and Psychiatry

Joy E. Stankowski, M.D.
Senior Instructor in Psychiatry, Case Western Reserve University School of Medicine; Chief Clinical Officer, Northcoast Behavioral Healthcare, Cleveland, Ohio

Kenneth Tardiff, M.D., M.P.H.
Professor of Psychiatry and Public Health, Department of Psychiatry, Weill Cornell Medical College, New York, New York

Stephen A. Thorne, Ph.D.
Adjunct faculty, St. Edwards University, Austin, Texas

Robert L. Trestman, Ph.D., M.D.
Director, Connecticut Health; Director, Center for Correctional Mental Health Services Research and Professor of Medicine and Psychiatry, University of Connecticut Health Center, Farmington, Connecticut

Robert J. Ursano, M.D., D.F.A.P.A.
Professor and Chairman, Department of Psychiatry, Uniformed Services University, Bethesda, Maryland

Sara T. Wakai, Ph.D.
Assistant Professor, Center for Correctional Mental Health Services Research, Department of Medicine, University of Connecticut Health Center, Farmington, Connecticut

Robert Weinstock, M.D.
Clinical Professor of Psychiatry, Department of Psychiatry and Biobehavioral Sciences, University of California, Los Angeles, David Geffen School of Medicine; psychiatrist, Greater Los Angeles Veterans Affairs Health Care System, Los Angeles, California

Foreword

How is it that clinicians in the mental health system have come to have responsibility for the assessment and management of violence? The answer lies deep in the history of our field. People with serious mental disorders have long been feared for the oddness of their behavior, and in some cases for the occasional acts of violence that may punctuate their lives. Indeed, funding for the first hospital in the colonial United States, the Pennsylvania Hospital in Philadelphia, which opened in 1751, was obtained in part by the promise of having a place to contain the mentally ill, thus diminishing the perceived threat they posed to the populace. From its inception, then, the mental health system has been intimately linked with the prediction and prevention of violence.

One cannot proceed further without noting that the relationship between mental illnesses and violence has been much exaggerated over the years. Epidemiologic and cohort studies taken as a whole suggest some increased risk of violence in persons with major mental disorders. But not all studies support this conclusion, and in any event the contribution of serious mental disorders is dwarfed by the effects of substance abuse (especially alcohol abuse) and personality traits such as psychopathy. The best available estimate suggests that only 3%–5% of the risk for violence in the United States is attributable to mental illnesses, and it has long been clear that people with serious mental illnesses are much more likely to be the victims of violence than its perpetrators.

Nonetheless, mental illness *is* sometimes causally linked with violence, as when patients act on command hallucinations to harm other people or strike out in fear against imagined persecutors. Manic patients in their irritability or depressed patients in their hopelessness may also cause harm to others. All of these conditions and others are exacerbated by the simultaneous use of alcohol and other disinhibiting substances, the abuse of which is more common among people with mental disorders.

As a result, nearly every phase of the mental health evaluation and treatment process may involve the assessment of violence risk and decisions about its management. This includes outpatient screening and intake, inpatient admissions and discharges, and emergency assessments. In addition, clinicians are often called upon to assess violence risk of people with mental illnesses in the criminal justice system, including in court clinics, forensic hospitals, and jails and prisons. Increasingly common diversion programs, such as mental health courts, may also call for clinical assessments of violence risk. Such importance does society confer on these tasks—and such confidence does it have in the ability of clinicians to perform them—that failure to conform to accepted standards of assessment and management may leave clinicians open to the imposition of liability and to no small amount of public opprobrium.

How well do clinicians perform their assigned predictive tasks? Most studies have not been encouraging for long-term predictions of patient violence, and even over shorter time periods, only modest predictive accuracy has been found. (It should be noted, though, that all research on clinical prediction of violence is complicated by the need to intervene to *prevent* violence when its occurrence is thought likely.) The less than impressive data on clinical prediction have led to the development of actuarial prediction instruments, with the hope that they would show better results. These models are based on the standardized collection of information about key variables, to which a predetermined algorithm is then applied. Indeed, studies of the application of these predictive models generally yield accuracies superior to that of unaided clinical judgment. Moreover, this work has stimulated an important reconceptualization of the predictive process, from making dichotomous judgments of the dangerousness of given individual patients to estimating the violence risk *category* to which a patient belongs.

Have we then reached the promised land of violence risk assessment, where reliance on the new actuarial approaches will supplant the admittedly imperfect clinical predictions that have dominated practice? Not quite yet. Whatever virtues the actuarial approach may have—and they clearly include systematizing the assessment and ensuring that important variables are not overlooked—existing instruments, too, are far from perfect. Their accuracy is less than ideal and falls sharply as the base rate of violence in the population being examined drops. In their rigidity, they do not permit consideration of contingent factors that may affect risk (e.g., the patient has a broken leg and will not be walking for the next six weeks). Many models assume that a single set of predictors will apply to all patients, an assumption implausible on its face. Perhaps most important of all, they rely heavily on "static" risk variables, invariant over time (e.g., past history of violence, exposure to abuse as a child). Thus, once labeled "high risk" by one of the actuarial approaches, a patient has only a faint chance to lose that designation.

Foreword

If the promised land is not yet in sight, there is still no question that this is an exciting time for the science and practice of violence risk assessment. Clinicians and researchers are experimenting with ways of combining actuarial and clinical approaches, in the hope of achieving levels of accuracy unattainable with either alone. Behavioral geneticists have begun to identify gene variants that may be implicated in violence risk and have begun to develop initial models of the interactions of these variants with environmental variables. Functional magnetic resonance imaging, positron emission tomography, and other brain scanning techniques are being used to identify neural circuits that may inhibit or facilitate violent acts. With the knowledge being gained, it seems likely that violence risk prediction in the next generation will look very different than it does today.

The same can be said with regard to the present relatively primitive level of management and treatment of violence risk. When violence appears to be causally linked to the symptoms of mental illnesses, our contemporary interventions typically focus on symptom control. Relatively few interventions—anger management programs are one—target the propensity to violence per se. This situation may also improve in the future as advances in the science of violence causation promote the development of more specific interventions. Indeed, we may some day legitimately be able to speak of prevention of violent propensities, rather than management of risk, as clinicians' primary task.

However promising the future, clinicians must address the needs of patients and the demands of society today. Thus the importance of this book, which summarizes in an accessible format the state of the art of violence assessment and management for mental health clinicians. Here, clinical and actuarial approaches to risk assessment are reviewed, the association of violence with specific psychiatric disorders is addressed, and management of violence is considered in depth. The important settings of the home, workplace, school, and healthcare facility are considered, as are the legal and risk management issues of which all clinicians should be aware. As a guide to dealing with violence today this volume is unparalleled, and I commend it to your thoughtful attention.

Paul S. Appelbaum, M.D.
Elizabeth K. Dollard Professor of Psychiatry, Medicine and Law
Director, Division of Psychiatry, Law and Ethics
Department of Psychiatry
Columbia University College of Physicians and Surgeons

Preface

The assessment and management of violent ideations and behaviors is a core competency that clinicians must possess or acquire. It is the rare clinician who does not assess and treat patients at risk for violence. Accordingly, this book leads off with "Assessment Principles." In this important first section, Drs. Tardiff and Monahan present tutorials on the clinical and actuarial risk assessment of violence. Drs. Lim and Bell underscore the importance of clinicians' competence in evaluating individuals for violence who are from different cultures and racial groups. Dr. Rosenfeld and Ms. Pivovarova provide a much-needed review of adjunctive psychological testing in violence risk assessment.

The textbook's 28 chapters address the diversity of clinical settings and situations where psychiatrists and other mental health professionals evaluate, treat, and manage people with violent ideations and behaviors. The different sections of the book address assessment principles, mental disorders and conditions, treatment settings, treatment and management, special populations, and various special topics. Chapter authors combine evidence-based medicine with expert opinion. The chapters include clinical case examples that are integrated into an in-depth discussion. Each chapter ends with a list of key points that underscore the main learning objectives.

We are fortunate to have enlisted distinguished academicians and clinicians to contribute their experiences to this textbook. Some authors have collaborated with junior colleagues to craft up-to-date, cutting-edge chapters. Each chapter was carefully reviewed by the editors. Much latitude was given to the different authors' writing styles and clinical perspectives.

Overlap among chapters is inevitable but useful. Very few people read a textbook from cover to cover. Instead, readers will select chapters of special importance to review in regard to pressing clinical situations or teaching needs.

Violence is endemic and epidemic. Its roots and causes are many and complex. Violence is not a diagnosis, although it can be associated with psychiatric conditions. People arrested for violent acts come under the jurisdiction of law enforcement agencies and the judicial system. Many have mental disorders. Few are seen by psychiatrists. Some offenders are diverted to mental health courts and forensic treatment facilities. Although psychiatrists and other mental health professionals consult with these agencies, their encounters with individuals who behave violently or have violent thoughts usually occur in the treatment of outpatients and inpatients.

For clinicians in the trenches, evaluating and treating patients with violent ideations and behaviors can be anxiety-provoking, frustrating, sometimes dangerous, and occasionally legally fraught. However, the clinician does not have to worry alone. The *Textbook of Violence Assessment and Management* is on call 24 hours a day for expert consultation, just an arm's reach away.

Robert I. Simon, M.D.
Kenneth Tardiff, M.D.

Acknowledgments

This textbook could not have been published without the committed efforts of many individuals. We want to express our gratitude to all the authors for the time and effort they devoted to researching and writing chapters of such high quality. It is their book as much as ours.

We also want to thank Robert E. Hales, M.D., M.B.A., Editor-in-Chief of American Psychiatric Publishing, Inc., and John McDuffie, Editorial Director, for their vision and support for a textbook on violence assessment and management.

Many thanks go to Ms. Tina Coltri-Marshall for her outstanding work in the difficult task of coordinating the entire textbook project among the editors, numerous authors, and American Psychiatric Publishing staff. Special appreciation goes to Ms. Carol A. Westrick for her competence and undaunted work ethic.

This work was funded, in part, by grant DA06534 from the National Institute on Drug Abuse.

—R.I.S., K.T.

Disclosure of Interests

The contributors have declared all forms of support received within the 12 months prior to manuscript submittal that may represent a competing interest in relation to their work published in this volume, as follows:

Carl C. Bell, M.D.: *Consultant,* AstraZeneca

John M. Bradford, M.D.: *Grant support,* Canadian Institute Health Research, Janssen-Ortho; *Speakers' bureau,* Janssen-Ortho, Pfizer

Leslie Citrome, M.D., M.P.H.: *Consultancy, honoraria, or clinical research support,* Abbott Laboratories, AstraZeneca, Barr Laboratories, Bristol-Myers Squibb, Eli Lilly and Company, GlaxoSmithKline, Janssen Pharmaceutica, Jazz Pharmaceuticals, Pfizer

William R. Dubin, M.D.: *Speakers' bureau,* AstraZeneca, Pfizer

The following contributors stated that they had no competing interests during the year preceding manuscript submittal:

Thomas Ala, M.D.; Peter Ash, M.D.; James C. Beck, M.D.; Martha Crowner, M.D.; Peggy L. El-Mallakh, Ph.D., R.N.; Rif S. El-Mallakh, M.D.; Paul Fedoroff, M.D.; Alan R. Felthouse, M.D.; Philip Firestone, Ph.D.; Susan Hatters Friedman, M.D.; Thomas A. Grieger, M.D., D.F.A.P.A.; Anzalee Khan, M.S.; Jean-Pierre Lindenmayer, M.D.; John R. Lion, M.D.; Barbara E. McDermott, Ph.D.; John Monahan, Ph.D.; Autumn Ning, M.D.; Cameron D. Quanbeck, M.D.; William H. Reid, M.D., M.P.H.; R. Jeannie Roberts, M.D.; Charles L. Scott, M.D.; Daniel W. Shuman, J.D.; Jonathan M. Silver, M.D.; Robert I. Simon, M.D.; Kenneth Tardiff, M.D.; Robert L. Trestman, Ph.D., M.D.; Sara T. Wakai, Ph.D.

PART I

Assessment Principles

CHAPTER 1

Clinical Risk Assessment of Violence

Kenneth Tardiff, M.D., M.P.H.

This chapter presents a clinical model for the short-term risk assessment of violence. Assessment of the risk of violence by patients is expected of all clinicians who have a relationship with a patient for evaluation or treatment: psychiatrists, other physicians, psychologists, nurses, social workers, activity therapists, and all other staff members who have responsibilities for patients. The responsibility to assess the risk of violence exists when clinicians evaluate a patient in the emergency department and decide whether to discharge or admit; see a patient in an office setting for the first time and between outpatient visits; admit a patient to a hospital and order a level of observation; and provide other immediate treatment as the patient enters the hospital. It exists during in-hospital diagnosis and treatment, including monitoring the patient and deciding whether seclusion or restraint should be used. It exists in the decision to discharge the patient and in the planning and implementation of care after discharge.

The focus of this chapter is to describe *clinical* methods to evaluate the risk of violence in the short term (within days or a week), because an increased risk of violence should result, as soon as possible, in preventive clinical actions such as change in medication, monitoring, and admitting to or discharge from a hospital. Unlike clinical methods of assessing the risk of violence, actuarial methods of assessing the risk of violence use structured instruments with items that are selected to measure areas thought to be related to the overall risk of violence in an individual. Usually these items are scored and used to predict the long-term risk of violence after discharge from prison or forensic psychiatric treatment facilities. The actuarial method has been applied to psychiatric patients in the long-term prediction of violence; however, this does not assist the clinician in the treatment of a potentially violent patient, because the clinician managing such a patient is primarily interested in the risk of violence in the next few days to a week. A number of researchers have reviewed many instruments that assess the risk of violence by using actuarial methods. They found that greater integration of clinical, dynamic data more relevant to general adult psychiatry is needed in the assessment of the short-term risk of violence (Harris et al. 2004; Kumar and Simpson 2005; Kroner et al. 2005; Mills 2005).

Principles in the Assessment of the Risk of Violence

A well-trained psychiatrist or other mental health professional should be able to assess a patient's short-term violence potential with assessment techniques analogous to those used in the short-term prediction of suicide potential. The time frame for both is several days to a week. Beyond that time, many factors may intervene after the initial decision is made about risk, as in the case of the stabilized schizophrenic patient who stops his or her medication or the abstinent spouse abuser who resumes drinking. As in the assessment of suicide risk, the evaluator focuses on the clinical aspects of the evaluation—namely, psychopathology—but also must take into consideration demographic, historical, and environmental factors that may be related to an increased risk of violence or suicide (Tardiff et al. 2000).

The evaluation of violence potential is analogous to that of suicide potential. Even if the patient does not express thoughts of violence, the clinician should routinely ask the subtle question, "Have you ever lost your temper?" in much the same way as one would check for suicide potential with the question "Have you ever felt that life was not worth living?" If the answer is "yes" in either case, the evaluator should proceed with the evaluation in terms of how, when, and so on, with reference to violence as well as suicide potential.

When making a decision about violence potential, the clinician also should interview family members, police, and other persons with information about the patient and about violent incidents to ensure that the patient is not minimizing his or her dangerousness. It is also important to contact or attempt to contact the patient's current and past therapists

Clinical Risk Assessment of Violence

and review old charts for previous episodes of violence, police and arrest reports, and other available records such as judicial proceedings.

Factors in the Assessment of the Risk of Violence

The model presented in this section describes at least 10 factors that must be evaluated in determining whether a patient poses a short-term risk of violence (Table 1–1). These factors are not scored to produce a global numerical indication of risk, such as 6 out of 10 indicating risk but 4 out of 10 not indicating risk of short-term violence. Rather, information obtained in each area should be synthesized and weighed by the evaluator to form a clinical decision about short-term risk of violence. The clinician must keep in mind that some factors may be more important than others for the individual patient, such as a history of violence with alcohol use or accompanying noncompliance with medication or other aspects of treatment. Even after making a decision about the patient's risk of violence, the clinician must keep in mind that unexpected events can still occur that may provoke violence, such as resumption of alcohol or drug use or a patient's spouse asking for a divorce.

This model represents a consensus among experts that has not been empirically tested but has been used as a standard by myself and other psychiatrists, both in testifying as expert witnesses in a number of malpractice suits and in daily practice.

Appearance of the Patient

The appearance of the patient may prompt further scrutiny of the potential for violence. This applies both to the loud, agitated, angry-

TABLE 1–1. Factors that must be evaluated in the assessment of short-term risk of violence

1. Appearance of the patient
2. Presence of violent ideation and degree of formulation and/or planning
3. Intent to be violent
4. Available means to harm and access to the potential victim
5. Past history of violence and other impulsive behaviors
6. Alcohol or drug use
7. Presence of psychosis
8. Presence of certain personality disorders
9. History of noncompliance with treatment
10. Demographic and socioeconomic characteristics

appearing patient who is impatient and refuses to comply with the usual intake procedures in the emergency department or clinic and to the quiet, guarded patient to whom one must carefully listen to detect subtle violent ideation. Dysarthria, unsteady gait, dilated pupils, tremors, and other signs of acute drug or alcohol intoxication dictate caution and serious consideration of the potential for violence, even though threats of violence may not have been expressed.

Presence of Violent Ideation and Degree of Planning/Formulation

The clinician should begin by assessing whether the patient has thoughts of violence toward other persons. As in the evaluation of suicide ideation, evaluation of violent ideation includes assessment of how well planned the ideation or threat is—that is, the degree of formulation. Relatively speaking, vague threats of killing someone, such as "I'm going to get even with her" or "She'll be sorry to see me," are not as serious as the patient's saying, "I'm going to kill my wife with a gun because she had an affair."

Intent

If a patient has thoughts of harming someone, it is important to explore whether he or she really intends to do something or is just having thoughts of violence. This disclosure may arise during an outpatient treatment session, as an offhand comment on the inpatient unit, or during any other contact with the patient. The patient's mere thought of violence may not be sufficient for the clinician to take actions such as warning someone, changing medication, or hospitalizing the patient. For some patients these thoughts of violence may seem intrusive, alien, and disturbing, and they will say that they do not intend to do anything to carry them out.

Available Means

The availability of a means of inflicting injury or death is important in the assessment of violence potential. If the patient is thinking about getting a gun or already has one, the clinician should obviously take a threat of violence more seriously. The clinician always should ask a potentially violent patient if he or she has or has ready access to a gun. Vigorous efforts should be made to have the patient get rid of the gun or to have it taken from the patient by family members or others. Removal of the gun must be verified by a callback by staff. When guns are removed,

Clinical Risk Assessment of Violence

the potential for homicide is reduced; however, that does not necessarily preclude the patient's attacking the victim in other, less lethal ways.

"Available means" also applies to the physical availability of the potential victim. How easily accessible is he or she to the patient? Does the potential victim live in a secluded place or in a city building without a doorman? Geography is another aspect of availability. A schizophrenic patient who threatens his or her father may be more of an immediate threat if actually living with the father as opposed to living in a different city or state at a distance from him.

Past History of Violence or Impulsive Behaviors

A past history of violence or other impulsive behaviors is often related to future violence. Clinicians should ask about injuries to other persons, destruction of property, suicide attempts, reckless driving, reckless spending, criminal offenses, sexual acting out, and other impulsive behaviors. Past violence increases the risk of future violence by a patient. Episodes of past violence should be "dissected" in a detailed, concrete manner by the clinician. This includes obtaining details as to the time and place of past violence; who was present; who said what to whom; what the patient saw; what the patient remembers; what family members, friends, or staff members remember about the violent episode; why the patient was violent (e.g., because of psychosis); and what could have been done to avoid the violence. Often there is a pattern of escalation of violence, whether it involves the dynamics of a couple in a domestic violence situation or the increasing agitation of a schizophrenic inpatient for whom interactions with other patients have become too intense.

The past history of violence should be treated as any other medical symptom. This includes noting the date of onset, frequency, place, and severity of violence. Severity is measured by degree of injury to the victim, from pushing to punching, causing injuries such as bruises, and onward to more serious injuries such as broken bones, lacerations, internal injuries, or even death. Severity, target, and frequency of violence can be measured by a written instrument such as the Overt Aggression Scale (Yudofsky et al. 1986 ; see Figure 1–1). Information that should be obtained and recorded about past history of violence includes prior psychological testing, imaging, laboratory testing, and other evaluations, as well as past treatment, hospitalizations, and response to treatments.

Alcohol and Drug Use

Alcohol and drug use can exacerbate the psychopathology in other psychiatric disorders and can cause violence in persons with no other

Name of patient _____ Name of rater _____

Sex of patient _____ Date _____ Shift _____

Aggressive behavior *(check all that apply)*

Verbal aggression
___ Makes loud noises, shouts angrily
___ Yells mild personal insults (e.g., "You're stupid")
___ Curses viciously, uses foul language in anger, makes moderate threats to others or self
___ Makes clear threats of violence toward other or self (e.g., "I'm going to kill you") or requests help to control self.

Physical aggression against objects
___ Slams door, scatters clothing, makes a mess
___ Throws objects down, kicks furniture without breaking it, marks the wall
___ Breaks objects, smashes windows
___ Sets fires, throws objects dangerously

Physical aggression against self
___ Picks or scratches skin, hits self, pulls hair (with no or minor head injury only)
___ Bangs head, hits fist into objects, throws self onto floor or into objects (hurts self without serious injury)
___ Small cuts or bruises, minor burns
___ Mutilates self, makes deep cuts, bites that bleed, internal injury, fracture, loss of consciousness, loss of teeth

Physical aggression against other people
___ Makes threatening gestures, swings at people, grabs at clothes
___ Strikes, kicks, pushes, pulls hair (without injury to them)
___ Attacks others, causing mild or moderate physical injury (bruises, sprain, welts)
___ Attacks others, causing severe physical injury (broken bones, deep lacerations, internal injury)

Time incident began _____ Duration _____

Intervention: _____

_____

FIGURE 1–1. The Overt Aggression Scale.

Adapted from Yudofsky et al. 1986.

psychiatric disorder. It is important to recognize that alcohol and many drugs can produce violence through intoxication as well as withdrawal. Heavy use of alcohol and drugs can cause changes in the brain that may lead to chronic impairment and psychiatric symptoms related to violent behavior (Tardiff et al. 2005; Volavka and Tardiff 1999). The ingestion of alcohol can be associated with aggression and violence as a result of disinhibition, particularly in the initial phase of intoxication. Intoxication is accompanied by emotional lability and impaired judgment. In some cases, alcohol withdrawal may lead to delirium, and violence may result from gross disorganization of behavior or as a response to threatening auditory hallucinations or delusional thinking (Bushman 1997; Langevin et al. 1987; McCormick and Smith 1995).

Cocaine, particularly when absorbed through the nasal route, initially produces a feeling of well-being and euphoria. With continued use, particularly when the cocaine is taken intravenously or smoked in the form of crack, the euphoria turns to grandiosity, psychomotor agitation, suspiciousness, and, frequently, violence. Suspiciousness becomes first paranoid ideation and then paranoid delusional thinking. Thus, violence results from delusional thinking as well as from the stimulation effect of cocaine (Denison et al. 1997; Linaker 1994).

Violence may occur during intoxication with a number of hallucinogens, but less commonly than it occurs in phencyclidine (PCP) intoxication. Within 1 hour of oral use (5 minutes if the drug is smoked or taken intravenously), PCP often produces marked violence, impulsivity, unpredictability, and grossly impaired judgment. There also may be delusional thinking or delirium (Convit et al. 1988).

With intense or prolonged amphetamine use, a feeling of well-being and confidence turns to confusion, rambling, incoherence, paranoid ideation, and delusional thinking, which are accompanied by agitation, fighting, and other forms of aggression (Miczek and Tidey 1989).

Inhalants are substances containing hydrocarbons, such as gasoline, glue, paint, and paint thinners, that are used by young children and early adolescents to produce intoxication. Inhalant intoxication may be characterized by belligerence and violence as well as impaired judgment.

Anabolic steroids are used by young men to enhance muscle growth and performance in athletics. Reports and systematic studies have found that after several months of self-administering these drugs, these men become irritable, combative, and violent (Choi et al. 1989; Pope and Katz 1994).

Psychosis

Psychosis is not a diagnosis, but it is a symptom that can be found in a number of disorders, including schizophrenia, delusional disorder, neurological and medical disorders, substance abuse disorders, and mood disorders, especially with mania. These disorders are discussed elsewhere in this book. When psychosis is present, regardless of the disorder, it increases the risk of violence (Anderson and Silver 1999).

Schizophrenic patients can be delusional and can have ideas of persecution. Patients may believe that people are trying to harm them; that the police, the FBI, or other organizations are spying on them; that some unknown mechanism is controlling their minds; or that the therapist is harming them (e.g., through medication). Patients with paranoid delusions in schizophrenia may react to these persecutory delusions by retaliating against the presumed source of the persecution. Patients with other types of schizophrenia may attempt to kill other persons because of some form of psychotic identification with the victim. Hallucinations associated with schizophrenia have been known to result in violent behavior and homicide (Andreasen et al. 1995; Dixon et al. 1991; Modestin and Ammann 1996).

Other aspects of schizophrenia, apart from psychotic processes, can also result in violence. Sudden, unpredictable changes in affect may be associated with anger, aggression, and violent behavior. Some schizophrenic patients are violent because of generalized disorganization of thought and a lack of impulse control accompanied by purposeless excited psychomotor activity (akathisia), or they may inadvertently come into physical contact with other patients, which may lead to fights. Schizophrenic patients also may use violence to attain what they want, to express anger, or to deliberately hurt others.

The psychotic paranoid patient, regardless of diagnosis, poses a problem because his or her delusions may not be obvious or the patient may attempt to hide them. Therefore, the evaluator must listen for subtle clues and should follow up regarding the assessment of violence toward others but must be careful not to confront the patient with insistent questioning about the presence of paranoid delusions (Taylor and Felthous 2006).

A manic patient may become violent as a result of delusional thinking in which the patient believes he or she is being persecuted because of some special attribute. Manic patients usually put all their impulses, including violent ones, into action. A typical situation in which manic patients erupt with violence is when they feel contained and not free to do what they want to do (McElroy et al. 1992).

Personality Disorders

Violence by persons with antisocial personality disorder is often vicious and persistent. They will continue punching, or hitting with objects, beyond what is needed to subdue the other person and win the fight. These patients have no remorse for their actions, and the victim is perceived as deserving the beating. The person with borderline personality disorder can be violent and make suicidal gestures when rejected or feeling rejected by others. The violence and suicide attempts are part of a broader picture of impulsivity and instability of interpersonal relationships. Persons with narcissistic personality can be violent occasionally when angry, such as when they are not given something they think they deserve. The person with paranoid personality rarely attacks those seen as persecutors, but when violence does occur it can be severe, even taking the form of mass murder. The person with intermittent explosive disorder is violent during circumscribed episodes, often with little apparent precipitating cause or out of proportion to any identifiable cause (Bernstein et al. 1993; Gunderson et al. 1991; Hare et al. 1991; Herpertz et al. 1997; Kemperman et al. 1997).

Noncompliance With Treatment

A history of noncompliance with treatment should alert the clinician that the patient is at an increased risk of violent behavior. Noncompliance may be indicated by a history of irregular attendance at scheduled appointments or laboratory and other clinical workups, or by the patient's refusing to take certain medications for a psychiatric or medical disorder or deliberately missing doses of medication. Measuring the patient's blood levels of medication may assist the clinician in monitoring the patient's compliance with the medication. Contact with the patient's family—with the consent of the patient—also may assist in determining whether the patient is taking medication as prescribed. Depot medication, particularly antipsychotic medications for schizophrenia and other psychotic disorders, also can be used to ensure compliance by these patients.

Demographic Characteristics

Demographic characteristics of patients should be considered in the assessment of violence potential. Young persons and men have been found to be at increased risk of violence, as are persons from environments of poverty, familial disruption, or decreased social control in which violence is considered an acceptable means of attaining a goal in the absence of other legitimate means or adequate education. The environment from which the patient comes is thus an important consideration in the determination of violence potential.

Case Examples

Case Example 1

The patient was a 25-year-old single white man with a history of paranoid schizophrenia who was discharged from the military in the 1970s because he developed delusions that he was a spy for the government and had killed people. He was sent to a Veterans Administration (VA) hospital for treatment and was discharged to the clinic for outpatient treatment.

After discharge from the hospital, he still voiced paranoid ideation and the delusion that he was a spy. He was not certain that he had killed people and stated that there was no history of violence. He denied any suicidal or violent ideation when first seen in the clinic. An in-depth, comprehensive assessment of his short-term violence potential was performed at that time. He was given oral haloperidol and continued to attend the clinic on a monthly basis. He was compliant with the medication for years and was seen by a psychiatric resident who updated the initial evaluation of violence and suicide potential monthly under the supervision of an attending psychiatrist.

The patient continued to be delusional about being a spy but denied any suicidal or violent ideation or intent. He lived alone and worked part-time installing carpet for a small business. One day, he slashed and killed his employer with a carpet knife. A lawsuit resulting from this act was filed against the VA.

It was determined that the murder was not predictable and that the patient had been monitored consistently, had received adequate treatment, and had been compliant with medication; the judge consequently ruled in favor of the VA. Although it was not admissible in the court, I read the patient's diary, and he had made no mention of thoughts or intent to kill anyone, including his employer.

Case Example 2

The patient was a 36-year-old single, biracial man with a history of schizoaffective disorder and polysubstance abuse, including cocaine and alcohol. He was brought into the psychiatric emergency department by the police after a physical altercation with a staff member at his residence. He had become verbally aggressive for several weeks and had stopped taking his valproic acid and olanzapine. On the day of the violent episode, he had run into the street, was brought back to the residence, and then threw a chair at a staff member. He had a history of two suicide attempts and had been psychotic on a number of occasions. In the emergency department he de-escalated considerably but made frequent references to people trying to kill him. He was given haloperidol and lorazepam intramuscularly after refusing oral medication and was subsequently able to speak calmly with the psychiatric resident and attending psychiatrist. He was placed in the locked seclusion room and allowed to remain on the gurney. Twenty minutes later, he swung a metal intravenous pole that he had detached from the gurney and broke the camera with which the staff had been monitoring him. The police were called, and three officers in riot gear subdued him. He was put in four-point restraints in seclusion and placed on constant observation with additional intramuscular haloperidol and lorazepam.

This case illustrates a psychotic patient who stopped medications and probably used cocaine and alcohol. He became violent but appeared to calm down with medication in the emergency department. However, once in seclusion with no restraints or close observation, he tore a metal pole from the gurney. He had become a very seriously violent person. Adequate police were called to subdue him as he vigorously swung the pole. Eventually he was properly restrained and put under adequate supervision with additional medication.

Conclusion

This chapter has described violence by patients with a number of psychiatric disorders. Violence differs among psychiatric disorders in terms of frequency, the manner in which it is expressed, and the psychopathology and dynamics that produce it. Violence is seen more frequently by clinicians and is more problematic in antisocial personality, borderline personality, and intermittent explosive disorders; schizophrenia and other psychotic disorders; mania; and alcohol and drug abuse.

A model has been presented here for assessing the potential for violence among patients in the short term (days or a week). This time period is of great relevance in clinical decisions regarding a patient's admission to a hospital, monitoring and treatment in the hospital, and discharge from the hospital; the development of an aftercare plan; and outpatient monitoring of the patient's potential for violence between office visits. The clinician assessing violence potential must rely on as many sources of data as possible, including interviews with the patient, friends and family, police, current and former treaters, and past clinical and other types of records.

Key Points

- Ten factors involved in evaluating a patient's potential for violence are outlined in Table 1–1. In brief, they include appearance, ideation and planning, intent, means and access, past history, alcohol and drug use, presence of psychosis, presence of personality disorder, history of treatment noncompliance, and demographic and socioeconomic characteristics.
- All ten of the factors are weighed by the clinician in the final assessment of whether the patient poses a short-term risk of violence to others.
- If the patient poses a short-term risk of violence, some action is necessary on the part of the evaluator. Action may include changing the treatment plan, hospitalizing the patient, warning the intended victim and/or the police, and other creative maneuvers to prevent the imminent violence by the patient.
- All of the data used to determine whether a patient is at risk for violence must be documented in writing; the thinking process by which the decision was made also must be evident in the written documentation.
- Reassessment of violence potential should be made at short intervals (e.g., from visit to visit or every few days) if the patient is to continue to be treated outside the hospital or other institution.
- In the hospital and emergency department, safety and monitoring of a potentially violent patient are essential, and treatment after discharge must be detailed in writing and arranged in a timely manner.

References

Anderson KE, Silver JM: Neurological and medical diseases and violence, in Medical Management of the Violent Patient: Clinical Assessment and Therapy. Edited by Tardiff K. New York, Marcel Dekker, 1999, pp 87–124

Andreasen NC, Arndt S, Alliger R, et al: Symptoms of schizophrenia: methods, meanings, and mechanisms. Arch Gen Psychiatry 52:341–351, 1995

Bernstein DP, Useda D, Siever LJ: Paranoid personality disorder: a review of its current status. J Personal Disord 7:53–62, 1993

Bushman BJ: Effects of alcohol on human aggression: validity of proposed explanation. Recent Dev Alcohol 13:227–304, 1997

Choi PYL, Parrott AC, Cowan D: High dose anabolic steroids in strength athletes: effects upon hostility and aggression. J Psychopharmacol 3:102–113, 1989

Convit A, Nemes ZC, Volavka J: History of phencyclidine use and repeated assaults in newly admitted young schizophrenic men. Am J Psychiatry 154:1176–1183, 1988
Denison ME, Paredes A, Booth JB: Alcohol and cocaine interactions and aggressive behaviors. Recent Dev Alcohol 13:283–291, 1997
Dixon L, Haas G, Weiden PH, et al: Drug abuse in schizophrenic patients: clinical correlates and reasons for use. Am J Psychiatry 148:224–230, 1991
Gunderson JG, Ronningstam E, Smith LE: Narcissistic personality disorder: a review of data on DSM-III-R descriptions. J Personal Disord 5:167–177, 1991
Hare RD, Hart SD, Harper TJ: Psychopathy and the DSM-IV criteria for antisocial personality disorder. J Abnorm Psychol 100:391–398, 1991
Harris GT, Rice ME, Camilleri JA: Applying a forensic actuarial assessment (the Violence Risk Appraisal Guide) to nonforensic patients. J Interpers Violence 19:1063–1074, 2004
Herpertz S, Gretzer EM, Steinmeyer V, et al: Affective instability and impulsivity in personality disorder. J Affect Disord 44:31–37, 1997
Kemperman I, Russ MJ, Shearin E: Self-injurious behavior and mood regulation in borderline patients. J Personal Disord 11:146–157, 1997
Kroner DG, Mills JF, Reddon JR: A coffee can, factor analysis and prediction of antisocial behavior: the structure of criminal risk. Int J Law Psychiatry 28:360–374, 2005
Kumar S, Simpson AI: Application of risk assessment for violence methods to general adult psychiatry: a selective review of the literature. Aust NZ J Psychiatry 39:328–335, 2005
Langevin R, Ben-Aron G, Wortzman R, et al: Brain damage, diagnosis, and substance abuse among violent offenders. Behav Sci Law 5:77–86, 1987
Linaker OM: Assaultiveness among institutionalized adults with mental retardation. Br J Psychiatry 164:62–78, 1994
McCormick RA, Smith M: Aggression and hostility in the substance abuser: the relationship to abuse patterns, coping style, and relapse trigger. Addict Behav 20:555–564, 1995
McElroy SL, Keck PE, Pope HG, et al: Clinical and research implications of the diagnosis of dysphoric or mixed mania or hypomania. Am J Psychiatry 149:1633–1644, 1992
Miczek KA, Tidey JW: Amphetamines: aggressive and social behavior. NIDA Research Monographs 94:68–79, 1989
Mills JF: Advances in the assessment and prediction of interpersonal violence. J Interpers Violence 20:236–241, 2005
Modestin T, Ammann R: Mental disorders and criminality: male schizophrenia. Schizophr Bull 22:69–82, 1996
Pope HG, Katz DL: Psychiatric and medical effects of anabolic-androgenic steroid use: a controlled study of 160 athletes. Arch Gen Psychiatry 51:375–386, 1994
Tardiff K, Leone AC, Marzuk PM: Suicide risk measures, in Handbook of Psychiatric Measures. Edited by Rush AJ. Washington, DC, American Psychiatric Press, 2000, pp 261–270
Tardiff K, Wallace Z, Tracy M, et al: Drug and alcohol use as determinants of New York City homicide trends from 1990–1998. J Forensic Sci 50:1–5, 2005

Taylor PJ, Felthous AR: Introduction to this issue: international perspectives on delusional disorders and the law. Behav Sci Law 24:235–240, 2006

Volavka J, Tardiff K: Substance abuse and violence, in Medical Management of the Violent Patient: Clinical Assessment of Therapy. Edited by Tardiff K. New York, Marcel Dekker, 1999, pp 153–177

Yudofsky SC, Silver JM, Jackson W: The Overt Aggression Scale for the objective rating of verbal and physical aggression. Am J Psychiatry 143:35–39, 1986

CHAPTER 2

Structured Risk Assessment of Violence

John Monahan, Ph.D.

For more than 50 years it has been commonplace in the behavioral sciences to distinguish "clinical" from "actuarial" methods of risk assessment and to conclude that the advantage in predictive validity lies with the actuarial (Meehl 1954). For example, William Grove and Paul Meehl (1996) located 136 empirical studies comparing clinical and actuarial prediction and found them overwhelmingly to support the superiority of the latter over the former. Their conclusion: "We know of no social science controversy for which the empirical studies are so numerous, varied, and consistent as this one" (p. 318; see also Grove et al. 2000). A more recent comprehensive review disaggregated studies in terms of the type of behavior being predicted and found that "one area in which the statistical method is most clearly superior to the clinical approach is the prediction of violence" (Aegisdottir et al. 2006, p. 368; see also Swets et al. 2000).

There is less consensus, however, on exactly what is meant by "actuarial" risk assessment and how it differs from the "clinical" kind. I argue here that the dichotomous organization of the field of risk assessment may have outlived its usefulness. Risk assessment may be better

---

Case examples reprinted from Monahan J, Steadman HJ, Appelbaum PS, et al.: *Classification of Violence Risk Professional Manual.* Lutz, FL, Psychological Assessment Resources, 2005, pp. 12 and 18. Used with permission.

seen to exist on a continuum of *structure*, with completely unstructured (corresponding to "clinical") risk assessment occupying one end of the continuum, completely structured risk assessment (corresponding to "actuarial") occupying the other, and additional forms of more-than-unstructured-but-less-than-fully-structured risk assessment lying between these poles.

I first consider unstructured violence risk assessment and then describe and illustrate three types of increasingly structured approaches to violence risk assessment. At the outset, however, it is necessary to make three clarifying points. First, it is sometimes incorrectly believed that actuarial prediction eschews all reliance on clinical judgment. For example, Sreenivasan et al. (2000, p. 439) stated, "The actuarial method requires no clinical input, just a translation of the relevant material from the records to calculate the risk score. Indeed, there is no compelling reason for a clinician to be involved." Although the risk factors on a given actuarial tool may and often do include those obtained from records, there is no reason why this needs to be so in order for the risk assessment to be properly called "actuarial." Indeed, "actuarial tables can be constructed that rely entirely on data that must be obtained through clinical judgment (e.g., 'add ego strength score to impulse control score and subtract maternal deprivation score,' etc.)" (Monahan 1981, p. 64). As Hilton et al. (2006, p. 402)—among the strongest proponents of actuarial methods—noted, "because some of the best indicators [of risk] require clinical skill to measure, accurately appraising violence risk is likely to remain a task for the clinician, but the place for clinical judgment is *within* rather than *outside* actuarial tools" (emphasis added; see also Litwack 2001; Westen and Weinberger 2004).

Second, it is sometimes inaccurately claimed that one factor that clearly distinguishes clinical from actuarial prediction is the time frame over which the prediction is valid, with clinical prediction aiming to assess violence risk in the short term (e.g., over days or weeks) and actuarial prediction designed to assess long-term violence risk (e.g., over months or years). It is certainly true that actuarial instruments are sometimes validated over long periods of time (e.g., the Violence Risk Appraisal Guide [VRAG, discussed later in this chapter] was developed using a 7-year follow-up). However, in the seven major empirical studies that form the evidence base for estimating the validity of *clinical* prediction of violence in the community, the follow-up periods varied from 6 months to 5 years, with a median of 3 years (Monahan 2006b). It should also be noted that the most recently developed *structured* violence risk assessment instrument, the Classification of Violence Risk (COVR, discussed later) was validated over a period of only 20 weeks, which is substantially shorter than the validation period used in *any* of the studies of clinical prediction.

The final clarifying point is that clinical and actuarial prediction are not neatly distinguished by the former's exclusive reliance on "dynamic" risk factors and the latter's exclusive reliance on "static" ones. Many appear to believe that clinical prediction, because it emphasizes changeable risk factors, has obvious implications for treatment whereas actuarial prediction, because it uses unchangeable risk factors, has no implications for clinical intervention. It is no doubt true that discussions of changeable risk factors are more often to be found in the literature on clinical than on actuarial prediction. The point is easily overstated, however. Guides to clinical prediction (e.g., Monahan 1981) often stress "static" unchangeable risk factors (e.g., a history of violence, gender), and structured violence risk assessment tools can and do include "dynamic" changeable risk factors that are amenable to clinical treatment (e.g., lack of insight and impulsivity on the HCR-20 [discussed later] and anger control and substance abuse on the COVR) (Monahan and Appelbaum 2000).

Unstructured Violence Risk Assessment

Unstructured risk assessment relies on the subjective judgment of professionally educated people who are experienced at making predictive judgments; in the case of violence, these typically include psychiatrists, psychologists, and social workers. In unstructured assessment, risk factors are selected and measured based on the mental health professional's theoretical orientation and prior clinical experience. What these risk factors are, or how they are measured, might vary from case to case depending on which seem most relevant to the professional doing the assessment. At the conclusion of the assessment, risk factors are combined in an intuitive or holistic manner to generate an overall professional opinion about a given individual's level of violence risk.

Research has not been kind to unstructured violence risk assessment. One early review of studies challenging the predictive accuracy of unstructured risk assessments of violence concluded that "Of those predicted to be dangerous, between 54% and 99% are false positives— people who will not, in fact, commit a violent act" (Monahan 1981, p. 21). Little has transpired in recent decades to increase confidence in the ability of mental health professionals, using their unstructured clinical judgment, to accurately assess risk of violence in the community (Monahan 2007). In the most methodologically sophisticated study on this topic, for example, researchers took as their subjects male and female patients being examined in the acute psychiatric emergency department of a large civil hospital (Lidz et al. 1993). Psychiatrists and nurses were asked to assess the risk of patient violence to others over the next 6-month period. Patients who elicited professional concern regarding future violence were moderately more likely to be violent after discharge (53%) than were patients who had not elicited such concern (36%). In other words, of the patients predicted to be violent by the clinicians, one out of two later committed a violent act, whereas of the patients predicted to be safe by the clinicians, one out of three later committed a violent act. The accuracy of clinical predictions of violence was statistically significant for male patients but not for female ones.

Taken as a whole, as Douglas Mossman (1994, p. 790) has stated, research supports the conclusion that "clinicians are able to distinguish violent from nonviolent patients with a modest, better-than-chance level of accuracy." In recent years, however, the lack of strong empirical support for the validity of unstructured violence risk assessment has motivated clinical researchers to explore alternative forms of risk assessment, ones that disaggregate the process of risk assessment into its component parts and then proceed to *structure* some or all of those components.

Varieties of Structured Violence Risk Assessment

Violence risk assessment might usefully be seen as having three components: selecting and measuring risk factors, combining them, and generating a final risk estimate (Monahan 2006b).

In the first component, *selecting and measuring risk factors*, the mental health professional performing the assessment decides which risk factors to measure and how to measure them. In unstructured risk assessment, as described earlier, risk factors are selected and measured on the basis of the mental health professional's theoretical orientation and prior clinical experience and may vary from case to case as theory or experience dictate. In contrast, in all forms of structured risk assessment, decisions about which risk factors to measure and how to measure them are made in advance, before the risk assessment begins. Explicit rules specify a risk factor's operational definition and quantification. In structured risk assessment, the mental health professional performing the assessment has no discretion regarding the selection or measurement of risk factors: these decisions are "structured" for him or her in advance by the appearance-specified variables, with instructions on how these variables are to be scored on a formal risk assessment instrument.

The second component, *combining risk factors*, involves taking the person's individually measured risk factors (i.e., "scores" on each of the risk factors) and assembling them into a single overarching estimate of violence risk. In unstructured risk assessment, risk factors are assembled in an intuitive or holistic manner to generate a clinical opinion about violence risk. In some forms of structured risk assessment, risk factors are assembled into an estimate of risk by means of a mathematical process specified in advance. That process is usually as simple as adding the scores of the individual risk factors together to yield a total score, but it can involve more complex statistical procedures as well (Banks et al. 2004).

In the third component, *generating a final risk estimate*, the mental health professional responsible for the risk estimate reviews the likelihood of violence produced by the first two components of the risk assessment process. In unstructured risk assessment, because the risk factors are already combined in an intuitive or holistic manner to generate a clinical opinion about violence risk, there is nothing for the clinician to "review." His or her clinical opinion is the clinician's final estimate of violence risk. In structured risk assessment, however, the final risk estimate offered by the clinician may differ from the risk estimate produced by the first two (structured) components of the assessment process, on the basis of additional (unstructured) information the clinician has gathered from interviews, significant others, or available records—information not included on the structured risk assessment instrument. As we will see, some forms of structured risk assessment allow for a final clinical review, whereas others preclude it by structuring even the final risk estimate.

To illustrate these three increasingly structured types of risk assessment, I briefly describe recently available instruments that structure one, two, or all three components of the risk assessment process.

The HCR-20

The "HCR-20," first published in 1995 and revised in 1997, consists of a series of 20 ratings addressing **H**istorical, **C**linical, and **R**isk management factors (Webster et al. 1997). In one study, the HCR-20 was completed for civilly committed patients who were followed for approximately two years after discharge into the community. When the scores were divided into five categories, 11% of the patients scoring in the lowest category were found to have committed or threatened a physically violent act, compared with 40% of the patients in the middle category and 75% of the patients in the highest category (Douglas et al. 1999; see also Douglas et al. 2005).

Selecting and Measuring Risk Factors

The 20 factors on this structured risk assessment tool were not derived from a specific empirical research project. Rather, they represent the authors' judgment of which risk factors have emerged most strongly across many empirical studies of violence risk. The 10 "historical" items on the HCR-20 are 1) previous violence, 2) young age at first violent incident, 3) relationship instability, 4) employment problems, 5) substance use problems, 6) major mental illness, 7) psychopathy, 8) early maladjustment, 9) personality disorder, and 10) prior supervision failure. The five "clinical" items are 11) lack of insight, 12) negative attitudes, 13) active symptoms of major mental illness, 14) impulsivity, and 15) unresponsiveness to treatment. The five "risk management" items are 16) plans lack feasibility, 17) exposure to destabilizers, 18) lack of personal support, 19) noncompliance with remediation attempts, and 20) stress.

Each of the 20 items is measured on a three-point scale according to the certainty that the risk factor is present: A score of 0 equals "no"—the item is definitely absent or does not apply; a score of 1 equals "maybe"—the item is possibly present, or is present only to a limited extent; and a score of 2 equals "yes"—the item definitely is present.

Combining Risk Factors

The HCR-20 structures the process of selecting and measuring risk factors, but for clinical purposes, it does *not* structure the process of combining risk factors to reach an overall estimate of risk. As stated in the professional manual for the HCR-20 (Webster et al. 1997, pp. 21–23):

> For clinical purposes, it makes little sense to sum the number of risk factors present in a given case, and then use fixed, arbitrary cutoffs to classify the individual as low, moderate, or high risk... [It] is both possible and reasonable for an assessor to conclude that an assessee is at high risk for violence based on the presence of a single risk factor—if, for example, that risk factor is "Active Symptoms of Major Mental Illness" and reflects the assessee's stated intent to commit a homicide.... In sum, at present it may be neither possible nor desirable to develop cutoff scores for the determination of summary or final risk judgments in clinical settings.

Generating a Final Estimate of Risk

For clinical purposes the HCR-20 does not structure the process of combining risk factors to reach an overall estimate of risk. Rather, it allows the clinician to combine the 20 measured risk factors in an intuitive manner to yield an overall estimate of risk. Thus there is no need for a "clinical review" of a structured risk estimate, and so none is performed.

The Classification of Violence Risk

The first violence risk assessment software, called the Classification of Violence Risk (COVR), was published in 2005. COVR is an interactive software program designed to estimate the risk that an acute psychiatric patient will be violent toward others over the next several months. The program can measure 40 risk factors. Used on a laptop or desktop computer, COVR guides the evaluator through a brief chart review and a 10-minute interview with the patient and then generates a report that places the patient's violence risk into one of five categories—with a 1% likelihood of violence in the first category, a 26% likelihood of violence in the middle category, and a 76% likelihood of violence in the highest category—including the confidence interval for the given risk estimate.[1]

Selecting and Measuring Risk Factors

The COVR software was constructed from data generated in the MacArthur Violence Risk Assessment Study (Monahan et al. 2001). In this research, more than 1,000 patients in acute civil psychiatric facilities were assessed on 134 potential risk factors for violent behavior. Patients were followed for 20 weeks in the community after discharge from the hospital, and their violence toward others was assessed. The software is capable of assessing those 40 risk factors for violence that emerged as most predictive of violence in the original research, but in any given case assesses only those risk factors necessary to classify the patient's violence risk. Among the risk factors assessed most frequently by the COVR are the seriousness and frequency of prior arrests, young age, male gender, being unemployed, the seriousness and frequency of having been abused as a child, a diagnosis of antisocial personality disorder, the *lack* of a diagnosis of schizophrenia, whether the individual's father used drugs or left the home before the individual was 15 years old, substance abuse, impaired anger control, and violent fantasies.

Combining Risk Factors

To combine risk factors into a preliminary estimate of risk, the COVR relies on "classification tree" methodology. This approach allows many

---

[1] Note that the author of this chapter is one of the owners of COVR.

different combinations of risk factors to classify a person as high or low risk. On the basis of a sequence established by the classification tree, a first question is asked of all persons being assessed. Contingent on the answer to that question, one or another second question is posed, and so on. The classification tree process is repeated until each person is classified into a final risk category. This "interaction" model contrasts with the more typical "main effects" approach to structured risk assessment, such as used by the HCR-20 and the VRAG (discussed later), in which a common set of questions is asked of everyone being assessed.

Generating a Final Estimate of Risk

In the view of its authors, the COVR software is useful in informing, but not replacing, clinical decision making regarding risk assessment. The authors recommend a two-phased violence risk assessment procedure in which a patient is first administered the COVR, and then the preliminary risk estimate generated by the COVR is reviewed by the clinician ultimately responsible for making the risk assessment, in the context of additional information believed to be relevant and gathered from clinical interviews, significant others, and/or available records. The authors of the COVR believed it essential to allow for such a review, for two reasons. The first has to do with possible limits on the generalizability of the validity of the software. For example, is the predictive validity of the COVR generalizable to forensic patients, to people outside the United States, to people who are younger than 18 years old, or to the emergency-department assessments of persons who have not recently been hospitalized? The predictive validity of this instrument may well generalize widely. Yet there comes a point at which the sample to which a structured risk assessment instrument is applied differs so much from the sample on which the instrument was constructed and validated (Monahan et al. 2005b) that one would be hard pressed to castigate the evaluator who took the structured risk estimate as advisory rather than conclusive.

The second reason for allowing clinicians the option to review structured risk estimates is that the clinician may note the presence of rare risk or protective factors in a given case, factors that—precisely because they are rare—will not have been taken into account in the construction of the structured instrument (Appelbaum et al. 2000). In the context of structured instruments for assessing violence risk, the most frequently mentioned rare risk factor is a direct threat—that is, an apparently serious statement of intention to do violence to a named victim (as with the HCR-20).

Case Examples of the Use of the COVR

The COVR manual (Monahan et al. 2005a) gives three case examples of the use of the COVR in clinical practice:

Case Example 1: High Risk

Mr. Smith is a 27-year-old salesman who has been hospitalized for the eighth time with a diagnosis of bipolar disorder. After 5 days in the hospital, he is being considered for discharge. Mr. Smith had been hospitalized for making an aggressive act toward his wife while manic and intoxicated. Because of this, the clinician responsible for the discharge decision requests that the COVR be administered. The next day, a COVR report is given to the responsible clinician that concludes "The likelihood that Mr. Smith will commit a violent act toward another person in the next several months is estimated to be between 65% and 86%, with a best estimate of 76%." The report also lists the risk factors used to produce this estimate.

The clinician, after reviewing the COVR report and all the information in Mr. Smith's hospital chart, interviews Mr. Smith. The interview fails to uncover any unusual protective factors that would call into question the estimate of violence risk that the COVR had produced. Moreover, it is clear that his manic state has not fully resolved. The clinician decides not to discharge Mr. Smith at the current time but rather to continue a course of medication and anger management groups, designed to lower his violence risk, and to recommend that Mr. Smith continue with anger management and intensive substance abuse treatment in the community after discharge. With Mr. Smith's consent, his wife is counseled about her risk if his symptoms recur and he starts drinking again.

Case Example 2: Low Risk

Ms. Jones is a 42-year-old female accountant who has been hospitalized for the first time for several days with a diagnosis of major depression. She is being considered for discharge. An ambiguous threat Ms. Jones made about a coworker had been noted in her hospital chart by a nurse, so the clinician responsible for the discharge decision requests that the COVR be administered. The next day, a COVR report is given to the responsible clinician that concludes "The likelihood that Ms. Jones will commit a violent act toward another person in the next several months is estimated to be between 0% and 2%, with a best estimate of 1%." The report also lists the risk factors used to produce this estimate.

The clinician, after reviewing the COVR report and all the information in Ms. Jones' hospital chart, interviews Ms. Jones. The interview fails to uncover any unusual risk factors that would call into question the estimate of violence risk that the COVR had produced, and Ms. Jones explains the ambiguous comment, which turns out not actually to have been a threat, to the clinician's satisfaction. Because she seems less depressed and is not suicidal, the clinician decides to discharge Ms. Jones at the current time and to follow up with routine care in the community.

Case Example 3: Moderate Risk

Mr. Brown is a 21-year-old security guard who has been hospitalized for several days with a diagnosis of borderline personality disorder with comorbid substance dependence, after getting into a shouting match with his girlfriend and cutting his arms. He is being considered for discharge. Because the chart indicates that Mr. Brown had been involuntarily committed on two prior occasions as "dangerous to others," the clinician responsible for the discharge decision requests that the COVR be administered. The next day, a COVR report is given to the responsible clinician that concludes "The likelihood that Mr. Brown will commit a violent act toward another person in the next several months is estimated to be between 20% and 32%, with a best estimate of 26%." The report also lists the risk factors used to produce this estimate.

The clinician, after reviewing the COVR report and all the information in Mr. Brown's hospital chart, interviews Mr. Brown. During the interview, Mr. Brown states his apparently serious intention to "teach a lesson she'll never forget" to his girlfriend, who has told him that he cannot come back to live with her. He also responds affirmatively to a question about whether he has a firearm in the house. The clinician believes that this clinical information is indicative of a high risk of imminent violence. The clinician decides not to discharge Mr. Brown at the current time but rather to continue a course of medication and psychotherapy designed to lower his violence risk. The clinician also decides to inform Mr. Brown's former girlfriend of the threat.

The Violence Risk Appraisal Guide

The Violence Risk Appraisal Guide (VRAG), first published in 1993, measures 12 risk factors designed to predict violence in mentally ill offenders. In a more recent prospective study with 467 male forensic patients, the VRAG showed impressive predictive validity. Patients were placed into one of nine categories of violence risk: 11% of the patients who scored in the lowest category on the VRAG were later found to commit a new violent act, compared with 42% of the patients in the middle category and 100% of the patients in the highest category (Harris et al. 2002).

Selecting and Measuring Risk Factors

The VRAG was developed from a sample of more than 600 men from a maximum-security hospital in Canada. All had been charged with serious criminal offenses. Approximately 50 predictor variables were coded from institutional files. The criteria used to develop the instrument were any new criminal charge for a violent offense or return to the institution for an act that otherwise would have resulted in a criminal charge for a violent offense. The average time at risk in the community was approximately 7 years after discharge. A series of analyses identified 12 variables for inclusion in the instrument: 1) score on the Hare Psychopathy Checklist–Revised, 2) separation from parents at under age 16, 3) victim injury in index offense, 4) diagnosis of schizophrenia, 5) never married, 6) elementary school maladjustment, 7) female victim in index offense, 8) failure on prior conditional release, 9) property offense history, 10) age at index offense, 11) alcohol abuse history, and 12) diagnosis of personality disorder. For all variables except numbers 3, 4, 7, and 10, the nature of the relationship to subsequent violence was positive (i.e., subjects who injured a victim in the index offense, had received a diagnosis of schizophrenia, chose a female victim for the index offense, or were older were significantly *less* likely to be violent recidivists than other subjects).

Combining Risk Factors

Each of the 12 risk factors measured by the VRAG is statistically weighted, and the weighted scores are summed together to yield an overall estimate of violence risk.

Generating a Final Estimate of Risk

Importantly, the authors of the VRAG (Quinsey et al. 2006) do *not* allow for any clinical review of the structured risk estimate that this instrument produces:

> What we are advising is not the addition of actuarial methods to existing practice, but rather the replacement of existing practice with actuarial methods. This is a different view than we expressed a decade ago, when we advised the practice of adjusting actuarial estimates of risk by up to 10% when there were compelling circumstances to do so.... We no longer think this practice is justifiable: Actuarial methods are too good and clinical judgment is too poor to risk contaminating the former with the latter. (p. 197)

A comparison of unstructured violence risk assessment and the various forms of increasingly structured violence risk assessment is presented in Table 2–1.

Use of Structured Violence Risk Assessment in Clinical Practice

The literature on the incorporation of any form of structured risk assessment into the clinical practice of predicting violence is thin, but all of it

TABLE 2–1. Unstructured and structured methods of violence risk assessment

Method	Number of structured components	Structured selection and measurement of risk factors?	Structured combination of risk factors?	Structured final risk estimate?
Unstructured	0	No	No	No
HCR-20	1	Yes	No	No
COVR	2	Yes	Yes	No
VRAG	3	Yes	Yes	Yes

Note. COVR=Classification of Violence Risk; HCR=Historical, Clinical, and Risk Management; VRAG=Violence Risk Appraisal Guide.

suggests that only a minority of mental health professionals routinely employ some form of structured risk assessment.

Elbogen et al. (2002) surveyed 134 clinicians in Nebraska and asked about the relevance to violence risk assessment of a large number of risk factors. Some of the risk factors were those found on structured risk assessment instruments such as the VRAG, the HCR-20, and the COVR. Others were not research based but rather were variables obtained from interviews with clinicians regarding their beliefs about what predicted violence (e.g., "impulsive behavior while in care"): "results show that nearly every clinician perceived dynamic, behavioral variables to be significantly more relevant than research-based factors.... Behavioral risk factors were perceived as more relevant than research risk factors from the HCR-20 and the VRAG, and from three of the four domains of the MacArthur Risk Assessment Study [i.e., the COVR]" (p. 43).

Tolman and Mullendore (2003) surveyed 93 practitioners of general clinical psychology and 71 diplomates of the American Board of Forensic Psychology from Michigan regarding instruments used in conducting violence risk assessments. They found that the VRAG was used in making violence risk assessments by 27% of the diplomates and by 9% of the general practitioners, and the HCR-20 was used by 31% of the diplomates and 2% of the general practitioners. For diplomates, the VRAG and the HCR-20 were among the top five instruments used to assess violence risk, whereas for the general practitioners, these structured risk assessment instruments were not among the top five instruments used. Rather, general practitioners tended to rely on all-purpose instruments whose relationship to violence risk is either unsubstantiated, such as the Minnesota Multiphasic Personality Inventory–2 (see

Melton et al. 1997), or proven to be invalid, such as the Rorschach (Lilienfeld et al. 2000).

Finally, Lally (2003) surveyed a national sample of 64 diplomates from the American Board of Forensic Psychology regarding the use of various procedures for assessing violence risk. The VRAG was rated as "Acceptable"—but not as "Recommended"—by more than half of the respondents. The HCR-20 was rated by the majority as somewhere between "Acceptable" and "No Opinion."

Although it would appear from these three surveys that most mental health professionals have yet to incorporate structured violence risk assessment tools into their routine clinical or forensic practice, when mental health professionals *do* predicate their risk assessments on the use of a structured instrument, courts uniformly find these risk assessments to be admissible scientific evidence (see Monahan 2006a for a compilation of recent federal and state cases). Not only courts but also legislatures are increasingly coming to look favorably on structured violence risk assessment. In 2003, Virginia became the first jurisdiction to *require* that a named structured violence risk assessment tool, with a cutoff score specified by law, be used to assess violence risk. This was done for the purpose of evaluating candidates for civil commitment as a sexually violent predator. The relevant statute directs the Department of Corrections to identify all prisoners incarcerated for sexually violent offenses "who receive a score of four or more on the Rapid Risk Assessment for Sexual Offender Recidivism or a like score on a comparable, scientifically validated instrument as designated by the Commissioner [of the Department of Mental Health, Mental Retardation, and Substance Abuse Services]" (Va. Code. Ann. § 37.2–903[c] 2005). The Rapid Risk Assessment of Sexual Offender Recidivism (RRASOR) is a completely structured (i.e., actuarial) instrument consisting of four items: 1) number of prior sex offense convictions or charges (from 1 to 6 or more); 2) age at release (25 years or older versus younger than 25); 3) victim gender (only females versus any males); and 4) relationship to victim (only related versus any nonrelated). The latter parenthetical items receive a higher score than the former items. A total score of 4 on the RRASOR corresponds to a 10-year recidivism rate of 48.6%, whereas a score of 5 corresponds to a 73.1% recidivism rate (Hanson 2004). In 2006, this statute was amended by the Virginia legislature to replace the RRASOR with another actuarial tool of somewhat higher predictive validity, the Static-99 (Hanson and Thornton 2000). Only prisoners who score above the specified cutoff score on the structured risk assessment instrument are sent on for a subsequent clinical evaluation of violence risk and "mental abnormality."

Conclusion

In unstructured risk assessment, neither the selection nor the measurement of the risk factors used in the assessment is specified in advance. Therefore, there are no risk factor "scores" that can be combined to yield a quantitative estimate of risk and no need for a clinical review of such an estimate. The three forms of structured risk assessment described here all specify in advance *at least* which risk factors are to be addressed and how those risk factors are to be measured. The HCR-20 structures *only* the choice and measurement of risk factors. The COVR goes on to *also* structure the manner in which the risk factors are combined to yield an estimate of risk, but the COVR allows the clinician to review this estimate in the context of other (unstructured) available information before issuing a final risk estimate. The VRAG, in contrast, is a *completely structured* (i.e., actuarial) risk assessment tool. No clinical review is allowed: the structured risk estimate that is produced when the risk factors are combined is the final product of the risk assessment process.

Although the three specific structured risk assessment tools considered here are the most frequently discussed in the literature, it should be emphasized that they are merely illustrative of a larger group of instruments that—like the HCR-20—structure only the choice and measurement of risk factors (e.g., Kropp and Hart 2000), or—like the COVR—also structure the manner in which the risk factors are combined to yield an overall estimate of risk but allow the clinician to review this structured estimate in the context of other available information (e.g., Hanson 1997), or—like the VRAG—stipulate that the structured risk estimate that is available when the risk factors are combined is the final product of the risk assessment process (Harris et al. 2003).

If structured violence risk assessment is superior to unstructured violence risk assessment, which specific form of structured risk assessment has the highest predictive validity? Should the clinician structure only one component of the risk assessment process (as the HCR-20 does), two components (as the COVR does), or all three components (as the VRAG does)? On this issue, perhaps because some of these instruments are so new, there are many strong opinions but no widespread acceptance of a single view among either researchers or practitioners. Finally, although structured violence risk assessment—of whatever form—appears to be demonstrably superior to unstructured violence risk assessment, and despite the increasing receptivity of courts and legislatures to the use of structured violence risk assessment, only a minority—perhaps only a small minority—of practicing mental health professionals in the United States routinely employ any form of structured violence risk assessment at the latter end of the first decade of the twenty-first century.

Key Points

- To improve the predictive validity of violence risk assessment, the assessment process can fruitfully be disaggregated into its three components: 1) selecting and measuring risk factors, 2) combining risk factors, and 3) generating a final estimate of risk.
- Violence risk assessment instruments recently have been created that structure one, two, or all three of these component parts of the risk assessment process.
- All forms of structured violence risk assessment appear to have greater predictive validity than unstructured ("clinical") violence risk assessment.
- Consensus has not yet been achieved as to which form of structured violence risk assessment has the greatest predictive validity.
- Courts and legislatures are increasingly open to the use of structured violence risk assessment.
- At the present time, relatively few practicing mental health professionals employ any form of structured violence risk assessment.

References

Aegisdottir S, White M, Spengler P, et al: The Meta-Analysis of Clinical Judgment Project: fifty-six years of accumulated research on clinical versus statistical prediction. Couns Psychol 34:341–382, 2006

Appelbaum P, Robbins P, Monahan J: Violence and delusions: data from the MacArthur Violence Risk Assessment Study. Am J Psychiatry 157:566–572, 2000

Banks S, Robbins P, Silver E, et al: A multiple-models approach to violence risk assessment among people with mental disorder. Crim Justice Behav 31:324–340, 2004

Douglas K, Ogloff J, Nicholls T, et al: Assessing risk for violence among psychiatric patients: the HCR-20 violence risk assessment scheme and the Psychopathy Checklist: Screening Version. J Consult Clin Psychol 67:917–930, 1999

Douglas K, Yeomans M, Boer D: Comparative validity analysis of multiple measures of violence risk in a sample of criminal offenders. Crim Justice Behav 32:479–510, 2005

Elbogen E, Mercado C, Scalora M, et al: Perceived relevance of factors for violence risk assessment: a survey of clinicians. International Journal of Forensic Mental Health 1:37–47, 2002

Grove W, Meehl P: Comparative efficiency of informal (subjective, impressionistic) and formal (mechanical, algorithmic) prediction procedures: the clinical–statistical controversy. Psychol Public Policy Law 2:293–323, 1996

Grove W, Zald D, Lebow B, et al: Clinical versus mechanical prediction: a meta-analysis. Psychol Assess 12:19–30, 2000

Hanson R: The Development of a Brief Actuarial Scale for Sexual Offense Recidivism. Ottawa, ON, Canada, Department of the Solicitor General of Canada, 2004

Hanson R, Thornton D: Improving risk assessments for sex offenders: a comparison of three actuarial scales. Law Hum Behav 24:119–136, 2000

Harris G, Rice M, Cormier C: Prospective replication of the Violence Risk Appraisal Guide in predicting violent recidivism among forensic patients. Law Hum Behav 26:377–394, 2002

Harris G, Rice M, Quinsey V, et al: A multi-site comparison of actuarial risk instruments for sex offenders. Psychol Assess 15:413–425, 2003

Hilton N, Harris G, Rice M: Sixty-six years of research on the clinical versus actuarial prediction of violence. Couns Psychol 34:400–409, 2006

Kropp P, Hart S: The Spousal Assault Risk Assessment (SARA) Guide: reliability and validity in adult male offenders. Law Hum Behav 24:101–118, 2000

Lally S: What tests are acceptable for use in forensic evaluations? A survey of experts. Prof Psychol Res Pr 34:491–498, 2003

Lidz C, Mulvey E, Gardner W: The accuracy of predictions of violence to others. JAMA 269:1007–1011, 1993

Lilienfeld S, Wood S, Garb H: The scientific status of projective techniques. Psychological Science in the Public Interest 2: 27–66, 2000

Litwack T: Actuarial versus clinical assessments of dangerousness. Psychol Public Policy Law 7:409–443, 2001

Meehl P: Clinical Versus Statistical Prediction: A Theoretical Analysis and a Review of the Evidence. Minneapolis, University of Minnesota, 1954

Melton G, Petrila J, Poythress N, et al: Psychological Evaluations for the Courts: A Handbook for Mental Health Professionals and Lawyers, 2nd Edition. New York, Guilford, 1997

Monahan J: The Clinical Prediction of Violent Behavior. Washington, DC, Government Printing Office, 1981

Monahan J: A jurisprudence of risk assessment: forecasting harm among prisoners, predators, and patients. Va Law Rev 92:391–435, 2006a

Monahan J: *Tarasoff* at thirty: How developments in science and policy shape the common law. Univ Cincinnati Law Rev 75:497–521, 2006b

Monahan J: The scientific status of research on clinical and actuarial predictions of violence, in Modern Scientific Evidence: The Law and Science of Expert Testimony, Vol 1. Edited by Faigman D, Kaye D, Saks M, et al. St. Paul, MN, West Publishing Company, 2007, pp 120–147

Monahan J, Appelbaum P: Reducing violence risk: diagnostically based clues from the MacArthur Violence Risk Assessment Study, in Effective Prevention of Crime and Violence Among the Mentally Ill. Edited by Hodgins S. Dordrecht, The Netherlands, Kluwer Academic Publishers, 2000, pp 19–34

Monahan J, Steadman H, Silver E, et al: Rethinking Risk Assessment: The MacArthur Study of Mental Disorder and Violence. New York, Oxford University Press, 2001

Monahan J, Steadman H, Appelbaum P, et al: The Classification of Violence Risk. Lutz, FL, Psychological Assessment Resources, 2005a

Monahan J, Steadman H, Robbins P, et al: An actuarial model of violence risk assessment for persons with mental disorders. Psychiatr Serv 56:810–815, 2005b

Mossman D: Assessing predictions of violence: being accurate about accuracy. J Consult Clin Psychol 62:783–792, 1994

Quinsey V, Harris G, Rice M, et al: Violent Offenders: Appraising and Managing Risk, 2nd Edition. Washington, DC, American Psychological Association, 2006

Sreenivasan S, Kirkish P, Garrick T, et al: Actuarial risk assessment models: a review of critical issues related to violence and sex-offender recidivism assessments. J Am Acad Psychiatry Law 28:438–448, 2000

Swets J, Dawes R, Monahan J: Psychological science can improve diagnostic decisions. Psychological Science in the Public Interest 1:1–26, 2000

Tolman A, Mullendore K: Risk evaluations for the courts: is service quality a function of specialization? Prof Psychol Res Pr 34: 225–232, 2003

Va. Code. Ann. § 37.2–903(c) 2005

Webster C, Douglas K, Eaves D, et al: HCR-20: Assessing Risk for Violence (Version 2). Vancouver, BC, Canada, Simon Fraser University, 1997

Westen D, Weinberger J: When clinical description becomes statistical prediction. Am Psychol 59:595–613, 2004

CHAPTER 3

Cultural Competence in Violence Risk Assessment

Russell F. Lim, M.D().

Carl C. Bell, M.D.

The impact of cultural factors on the assessment of the risk of violence is complex and multifactorial. In earlier chapters of this textbook, the assessment of violence potential is dependent on historical information: psychiatric, medical, developmental, social, substance use, family history, and socioeconomic status. Almost all risk factors are affected by culture, including age, gender, mental illness diagnoses, substance abuse, and age at first event of violence. Cultural beliefs about violence and religion vary from group to group. Some groups may feel that wives are supposed to be subservient (e.g., Muslims, Chinese, Vietnamese, Cambodians, Christians) and use that as justification for violence, whereas others strongly adhere to nonviolence. Psychiatric diagnosis is particularly vulnerable to influence by ethnicity; for example, we know that African Americans and Hispanics are overdiagnosed with psychotic disorders and underdiagnosed with bipolar disorder (Adebimpe 1981; Bell and Mehta 1980). Age at first episode of violence also can be inaccurate; for Asian Americans, for example, admitting to a history of violence would be shameful, and the information thus would be suppressed (Yick 1999). Substance abuse is more prevalent in some ethnicities, such as in Native Americans (Substance Abuse and Mental Health Services Administration 2003), but that does not necessarily mean that people of these ethnicities are more prone to violence.

The supplement to the Surgeon General's report on mental health (U.S. Department of Health and Human Services 2001a) "Mental Health: Culture, Race and Ethnicity" acknowledges that because very little published mental health research exists on cultural, racial, and ethnic issues in general—and even less on the issue of violence risk assessment in different cultural, racial, and ethnic groups in varying contexts—discussing cultural sensitivity/competence in violence risk assessment is a challenge.

Recognizing this reality, we must first understand why there is so little creditable information about different cultural, racial, and ethnic groups in mental health literature. For years, the United States has tried to be a "color-blind" melting pot, and the consideration of the dynamics of culture, race, and ethnicity have been selectively ignored by science. Accordingly, when the topic of cultural sensitivity or competence surfaces, individuals become anxious, defensive, and very rigid in their perspectives. "Race constitutes a stubbornly resistant malady in the United States because of 'the color line'—a visible (and invisible) barrier that separates whites from nonwhites" (Pulera 2002, p. 3). The American Psychiatric Association recognized the existence of structural (institutional) racism by asserting that racist policies occur at an organizational or group level and that these policies are embedded in the operating contexts of particular organizations or institutions in such a way that racist assumptions may be difficult to recognize (American Psychiatric Association 2006).

One such assumption is that "one size fits all," and that the standard is European or European American. Of course this is a form of "monocultural ethnocentrism" (Sue and Sue 1999) and is as difficult to recognize for the majority culture in the United States as it is for a fish to recognize water. Recent studies have implicated racism and racial discrimination, both individual and structural, as factors leading to disparities in overall healthcare and mental healthcare, including diagnosis and treatment (U.S. Department of Health and Human Services 2001a). Racially biased attitudes may implicitly affect provider decision making, leading to denial of services for some populations or to inappropriate assessment and diagnosis that in turn leads to ineffective treatment (Miranda et al. 2002; West et al. 2006). In the case of violence risk assessment, this may lead to an overdetermination of the risk of violence. Thus, considering the nation's overall lack of success at appropriately responding to cultural, racial, and ethnic differences, the issue of cultural sensitivity or competence in violence risk assessment and management is extremely sensitive.

Problems in Assessing Violence Risk in People of Color

There are a great many myths and stereotypes related to violence and other symptoms in people of color—that is, people from racial and cultural groups other than European American (Pierce et al. 1999). For example, concerning youth, Dr. Satcher's Surgeon General's Report on Youth Violence noted one myth about youth violence, namely that "African American and Hispanic youths are more likely to become involved in violence than other racial or ethnic groups" (U.S. Department of Health and Human Services 2001b, p. 5). However, the fact is that race and ethnicity have little bearing on the overall proportions of racial and ethnic groups that engage in nonfatal violent behavior (U.S. Department of Health and Human Services 2001b). Furthermore, although African American and Hispanic youths have higher homicide rates than European American youths, these differences drop out when variables of socioeconomic status are controlled (Hollinger et al. 1994; Sampson et al. 1997).

Dr. Satcher's report on youth violence also noted that risk factors can predict the likelihood of future violence. Accordingly, these factors are useful in identifying vulnerable populations that may benefit from intervention efforts. However, risk *markers* such as race and ethnicity are frequently confused with risk *factors*. The distinction is that risk markers have no causal relation to violence (U.S. Department of Health and Human Services 2001b). Finally, Dr. Satcher's report noted that "no single risk factor or combination of factors can predict violence with unerring accuracy" (U.S. Department of Health and Human Services 2001b, p. 77). The reasons why this is true can be summed up in the maxim "risk factors are not predictive factors due to protective factors" (Bell 2007, p. 14).

In studies of violence risk assessment, the findings in adults parallel the findings in youths with regard to issues of culture, race, and ethnicity. The ethnic groups at greatest risk for interpersonal violence are American Indian/Alaskan Native women and men, African American women, and Hispanic women, at 25% risk (Tjaden and Thoennes 2000). Statistics from 2002 show that the death rate due to homicide per 100,000 was 4.1 for Caucasians, 39.6 for African Americans, 11.1 for American Indians and Native Alaskans, 5.2 for Asians and Pacific Islanders, and 17.5 for Hispanic Americans (Keppel et al. 2002). In 2001, arrests for aggravated assault show 99.6 per 100,000 for Caucasians, 320 for African Americans, 144.6 for Americans Indians and Native Alaskans, and 37.5 for Asians and Pacific Islanders. Hispanics were not listed as a separate ethnic group (Tseng et al. 2004). Suicide, anger/revenge, and mass murder stemming from domestic or romantic conflict are the chief forms of violence in the European-American community (Petee et al. 1997). Serial killing has been stereotypically linked to European Americans; however, a recent article by Walsh (2005) showed that this type of homicide by African Americans has been underreported. Thus, being a minority—with the exception of being Asian American—was associated with being a victim of a violent attack. The distinction must be made that being associated with something does not necessarily predict it, hence the distinction of a *risk marker* not being a *risk factor* because there has been no causal link proven. Furthermore, although it is true that there are racial and ethnic differences in homicide rates, these differences drop out when variables of socioeconomic status are controlled (Bell 2002). Socioeconomic inequality, not race, facilitates higher rates of violence among ethnic minority groups (Johnson 2000).

Demographic factors associated with increased risk for violence in adults are race and ethnicity; however, because these risk factors "tend to dissipate when other factors are taken into account statistically" (Hucker 2004), it is likely that in adults, race and ethnicity are also actually risk *markers* and not risk *factors*, as was seen in adolescents. This finding is supported by the MacArthur Violence Risk Assessment Study (Steadman et al. 1998), which found that although there was an overall association between race and violence, African Americans and European Americans who lived in comparably disadvantaged neighborhoods had the same rates of violence.

A common stereotype is that people of color (e.g., African Americans) are more dangerous than people without color (i.e., perceived European Americans). Another variation of this effect is the finding that minority children are more frequently evaluated and reported as victims of child abuse, according to Lane et al. (2002), which shows a reporting bias and does not necessarily indicate that minorities are more likely to be abusive toward their children. Clinician biases are also seen in increased rates of seclusion and restraint of African Americans compared with whites in the psychiatric inpatient ward (Flaherty and Meagher 1980) and in the more and larger doses of oral and injectable antipsychotic medications given to African American patients than to similar white patients by psychiatric clinicians in psychiatric emergency and inpatient services (Primm 2006). Flaherty and Meagher (1980) speculated that "the stereotype of the black male made the staff feel and act as if blacks were more dangerous, prompting more restrictive measures" (p. 681). Flaherty and Meagher's study also found that black patients were less likely to be referred to recreational and occupational therapy, whereas these services were routinely ordered for whites on the unit. The physicians on the unit reported that they ordered these therapies routinely unless a patient was too dangerous or psychotic to participate.

The reasons for the overdetermination of dangerousness in people of color have been poorly studied, and the few studies examining this issue tend to be dated. Flaherty and Meagher (1980) found that all-white inpatient treatment teams spent less time discussing black patient issues compared with white patient issues. Adebimpe (1981) and others (Gross et al. 1969) have observed similar low allocations of time on black patient issues and attribute part of this problem to the social and cultural distance between the patient and clinician. Adebimpe (1981) cited differences in vocabulary, modes of communication, value systems, and expression of distress and a breakdown in rapport as factors that increase diagnostic errors. Jones and Gray (1985) stated that "white psychiatrists seem to have more difficulty relating to black male patients than to [black] female patients" (p. 25) and hypothesized that this may be because white psychiatrists expect black men to be threatening (i.e., they adhere to a common societal negative stereotype of black men). Although these important studies are classic, they are from a time when experimental design and statistical methodology were less sophisticated, and modern studies should be performed to expand upon and update these findings.

The following two cases illustrate how an individual's or clinician's cultural experiences and assumptions can influence violent behavior and the risk assessment of violent behavior.

Case Example 1:
Racism and Oppression in a Hawaiian Man

A 35-year-old biracial Caucasian and Hawaiian man was imprisoned after being convicted of killing his ex-wife's father, a Portuguese American man who had disapproved of his daughter's marrying someone who was not Portuguese. The patient had murdered the victim by punching him to death. The patient was an amateur boxer and at the time of the killing was using cocaine and complaining that he was in danger from others. He was eventually released after the completion of his prison sentence and placed in a board and care for persons with mental disorders and substance abuse disorders. He lived there with other men belonging to various ethnic groups and would get into fights when a roommate would call him by a racial slur.

According to the HCR-20 (Historical, Clinical, and Risk Management) Survey, this patient had many risk factors, including substance abuse, a mental disorder (substance-induced delusional disorder), and a previous history of violence. Because he belonged to a group that had been taken advantage of by previous explorers of Hawaii, decimated by imported diseases, and overthrown from power in 1893, he had a sense of disempowerment. Likewise, his cultural institutions were dismantled by missionaries and foreign businessmen. He felt a sense of shame about his Hawaiian identity because he felt powerless and unable to be an effective part of society (Schultz-Ross 1997).

In response to the resident's violence, the staff of the board and care facility started a group that emphasized the understanding of Hawaiian culture. His individual work focused on his owning his nonviolence, as opposed to his seeing it as obedience to orders that he resented. The intervention was intended to increase his sense of self-respect and thus reduce his levels of shame. Another intervention would have been to target improvement of interpersonal relationships; for example, *hooponopono*, an indigenous mental health intervention, might have been more effective (Rezentes 1996).

Case Example 2:
Racism, Transference, and Countertransference

A male Caucasian patient was to be evaluated at a prison for a psychiatric disorder. He was 6 feet tall, heavy, and muscular. His voice was loud, and he spoke with a heavy Southern accent. He glared angrily at anyone who came near. His psychiatrist, a thin, 5-foot-tall African American wearing glasses, began to question the patient, but he refused to answer, saying, "Not to you!" The patient was a devout Christian and read the Bible daily. He had been convicted of murdering an elderly Caucasian woman by tackling her, lifting her up in the air, and dropping her on the sidewalk. He was convinced that she meant him harm and felt no remorse for his actions. He also believed that the correctional officers meant him harm.

Eventually, the patient agreed to speak with the psychiatrist. Initially the patient distrusted him because of his race, but the larger reason was because the physician was employed by the prison. Although the patient's racism could have been the reason he did not want to speak to his doctor, his reluctance was eventually found to be driven by paranoia (Schultz-Ross 1997).

Given this background, how confident can we be as psychiatrists in assessing the risk of violence in psychiatric patients? Tardiff (1998) stated that psychiatrists are fairly reliable assessors, but the influence of the ethnicity of the patient and the evaluator was not examined. Our position is that knowing some cultural information about patients—such as any differing cultural norms, religious beliefs, and experiences with racism—and knowing our own stereotypic biases will improve psychiatric diagnosis and improve the therapeutic alliance so that the potential for violence is much reduced.

Interpersonal Violence

Interpersonal violence is defined as a pattern of assaultive and coercive behaviors, including physical, sexual, and psychological attacks as well as economic coercion. The assessment of IPV is somewhat different from risk assessments done in psychiatric hospitals, clinics, and prisons. The person being evaluated is usually the victim and may or may not volunteer that he or she is being abused. Culture and religion also affect the assessment and management of this potentially violent situation.

Intimate partner violence (IPV) is a form of interpersonal violence between two people who are intimate, including spouses, couples, and partners. The term was developed to replace *wife abuse* or *spousal abuse* in order to include gay partners. Within the women's movement, IPV usually refers to violence toward women; the term is also used in reference to gay female relationships.

IPV is pervasive, with one in four women in the United States experiencing abuse during their lifetime (Tjaden and Thoennes 2000). In 2002, the World Health Organization identified domestic violence as a serious public health problem, with victims experiencing more operative procedures, visits to doctors, and hospital stays than nonvictims. Domestic violence not only causes acute injuries but also has been linked to serious health consequences such as chronic pain, abdominal complaints, sexually transmitted infections, unwanted pregnancies, depression, posttraumatic stress disorder, miscarriages, and premature labor (Krug et al. 2002). Unfortunately, many victims suffer in silence and receive no assistance for their abusive situation. Healthcare and mental healthcare professionals play a crucial role in identifying victims because these professionals have regular opportunities to ask their patients about domestic violence, regardless of the reason for the medical visit. Patients should be routinely screened for domestic violence by directly asking about domestic violence, regardless of symptoms, injuries, or reason for the visit (Mayor's Office to Combat Domestic Violence 2003). In the latter part of this chapter, we discuss some culturally specific information useful in the assessment and prevention of IPV.

Case Example 3:
Domestic Violence in a Puerto Rican Woman

Ms. A, a 30-year-old Puerto Rican woman from New York, married an Argentinean man she met in college. She was a second-generation

Puerto Rican American woman born to immigrant parents in the lower middle class, whereas her husband was wealthy and belonged to the aristocracy. They had moved to Los Angeles to be near the husband's older brother. Ms. A's husband began to drink and would beat her when he was intoxicated. She asked her husband to stop his behavior, and he would apologize and agree not to hit her anymore, but it continued to happen. She eventually asked her brother-in-law for advice, but he said that she must be doing something wrong. Her feeling after this conversation was that the brother-in-law did not approve of her. She became pregnant, and after the birth of their first child, the beatings intensified. Ms. A filed for divorce and moved back to New York to live with her family. Her family was not supportive of her because they felt that divorce was wrong. After several years, she remarried to a Puerto Rican man. He also began to beat her several years after they married. She remained silent about the abuse for 3 years, but she eventually went to a counseling center. Separation was suggested, but she adamantly refused. Her husband left her for several months, and she allowed him to move back in.

This case demonstrates the powerful influence of family support. Ms. A would rather risk being physically hurt than bear the brunt of her family's disapproval and suffer their withdrawal of support (Schultz-Ross 1997).

Critical Concepts: Culturally Appropriate Assessment

Culture can be defined as a set of meanings, norms, beliefs, and values shared by a group of people. These beliefs and values are taught, reinforced, and reproduced to the next generation. Culture refers to a system of meanings in which words, behaviors, events, and symbols have attached meanings that are agreed upon by the members within the cultural group. Thus, an individual's culture shapes how he or she makes sense of the social and natural world. Finally, culture includes both the subjective components of human behavior (the shared ideas and meanings that exist within the minds of individuals within a group) as well as the objective components (the observable behaviors and interactions of these individuals).

One's culture shapes what symptoms one expresses and how they are expressed (Mezzich et al. 2000), and it influences the meaning that one attributes to symptoms and how one interacts with the healthcare system. Culture also influences what a society regards as appropriate or inappropriate behavior, and it thus exerts a powerful influence on an individual's potentially violent behavior. War, with its sociocultural upheaval and association with posttraumatic stress disorder, is one example of how cultural-historical events can cause or contribute to psychopathology (Du and Lu 1997; Kirmayer 2001). Likewise, culture can also exert a protective influence on mental health. Traditional healing approaches and spiritual/religious interventions may also provide meaningful benefits to patients (Ton and Lim 2006), as may interventions that are culturally syntonic.

Culturally competent care involves combining general culture-specific knowledge with specific information from the patient and being aware of biases that either the clinician or the patient may bring to the evaluation. Because individuals can belong to more than one cultural group, they may not comply with the norms of their stated cultural group and may in fact emphasize some cultural values of that group and deemphasize others.

The DSM-IV-TR Outline for Cultural Formulation

The publication of DSM-IV and its text revision, DSM-IV-TR (American Psychiatric Association 1994, 2000) represented a turning point in the application of cultural psychiatry principles with the introduction of the Outline for Cultural Formulation (OCF; DSM-IV-TR Appendix I). The OCF gives clinicians a framework for assessing the impact of culture on the diagnosis and treatment of psychiatric illness (Table 3–1). Because culture plays such a crucial role in all aspects of mental health and illness, it is important to incorporate cultural assessment as part of any intervention. The culturally competent clinician seeks to acquire knowledge about the cultural groups of his or her patients. Although such knowledge is essential, a framework to organize and make sense of the information is extremely helpful. However, the clinician inevitably will encounter many patients who are affiliated with cultural groups of which the clinician has inadequate knowledge. Furthermore, patients may not fully engage in all the beliefs and practices of a given cultural group.

The first part of the DSM-IV-TR OCF describes how the individual sees him- or herself and relationships to others. Clinicians should be aware that cultural identity is multidimensional and can have many different aspects, such as country of origin, language spoken, religious beliefs, identified ethnicity, sexual orientation, marital status, and so on. The patient's cultural identity is constructed during the interview but can be completed in greater detail during the social and developmental history.

Part two of the formulation has to do with the patient's beliefs about his or her illness. The clinician asks what the patient thinks is causing the problem and what the patient would do to solve it. In the case of

TABLE 3–1. DSM-IV-TR outline for cultural formulation

A. Cultural identity of the individual
B. Cultural explanations of the individual's illness
C. Cultural factors related to psychosocial environment and levels of functioning
D. Cultural elements of the relationship between the individual and the clinician
E. Overall cultural assessment for diagnosis and care

Source. American Psychiatric Association 2000.

violent behavior, this question would relate to the reasons behind and justification for such behavior. Part three of the formulation concerns stressors and supports and includes an extended family assessment regarding the family's influence on the patient as well as the role that religion plays in the patient's life. Part four is an examination done by the clinician to assess what role the clinician's and patient's ethnicities are playing in the interaction. (As in Case 2 above, there could be transference on the patient's part and countertransference from the evaluator's perspective, leading to fear on the evaluator's part and to aggression from the patient.) Part five assembles the previous four parts to make a formulation that informs treatment, such as the cultural history in Case 1 above, leading to a culturally appropriate treatment plan.

DSM-IV-TR also includes culture-bound syndromes, such as *amok*, *boufée delirante*, *pibloktoq*, and *zar*. Although these can provide an explanation of violent behavior, they are seen in cultures not often encountered in daily clinical practice. These syndromes are included in Table 3–2 for reference. Using the DSM-IV-TR OCF in concert with a cultural consultant or someone familiar with a particular culture's beliefs, values, and norms to help understand individuals' beliefs about their behavior, their family relationships, and their religious beliefs will yield much more useful information for the assessment and management of violence.

Culturally Appropriate Assessment in the Psychiatric Setting

In clinical settings, a potentially violent situation occurs when an individual who has a history of violence, but is not currently threatening to become violent, is being interviewed. In this situation there is a lot of time to assess the patient's risk for violence and to plan how to respond to the violence if it does become urgent or emergent. All patients, regardless of cultural, racial, or ethnic origin, should be assessed for the

Cultural Competence in Violence Risk Assessment | 45

TABLE 3–2. DSM-IV-TR culture-bound syndromes that involve violence or aggression

Amok: A dissociative episode characterized by a period of brooding followed by an outburst of violent, aggressive, or homicidal behavior directed at people and objects. The episode tends to be precipitated by a perceived slight or insult and seems to be prevalent only among males. The episode is often accompanied by persecutory ideas, automatism, amnesia, exhaustion, and a return to premorbid state following the episode. Some instances of amok may occur during a brief psychotic episode or constitute the onset or an exacerbation of a chronic psychotic process. The original reports that used this term were from Malaysia. A similar behavior pattern is found in Laos, Philippines, Polynesia (*cafard* or *cathard*), Papua New Guinea, and Puerto Rico (*mal de pelea*), and among the Navajo (*iich'aa*).

Bouffée delirante: A syndrome observed in West Africa and Haiti. This French term refers to a sudden outburst of agitated and aggressive behavior, marked confusion, and psychomotor excitement. It may sometimes be accompanied by visual and auditory hallucinations or paranoid ideation. These episodes may resemble an episode of brief psychotic disorder.

Pibloktoq: An abrupt dissociative episode accompanied by extreme excitement of up to 30 minutes' duration and frequently followed by convulsive seizures and coma lasting up to 12 hours. This is observed primarily in arctic and subarctic Eskimo communities, although regional variations in name exist. The individual may be withdrawn or mildly irritable for a period of hours or days before the attack and will typically report complete amnesia for the attack. During the attack, the individual may tear off his or her clothing, break furniture, shout obscenities, eat feces, flee from protective shelters, or perform other irrational or dangerous acts.

Zar: A general term applied in Ethiopia, Somalia, Egypt, Sudan, Iran, and other North African and Middle Eastern societies to the experience of spirits possessing an individual. Persons possessed by a spirit may experience dissociative episodes that may include shouting, laughing, hitting the head against a wall, singing, or weeping. Individuals may show apathy and withdrawal, refusing to eat or carry out daily tasks, or may develop a long-term relationship with the possessing spirit. Such behavior is not considered pathological locally.

Source. American Psychiatric Association 2000.

risk for violence. Assessing for potential violence is a serious undertaking and, if possible, should not be rushed. Furthermore, repeated risk assessments for violence should occur in the same way that repeated risk assessments for suicide occur. Time permitting, these assessments should involve a prolonged clinical assessment and a thorough review of the individual's documented history from every possible source, including legal records and discussions with family, friends, witnesses, attorneys, and victims (Johnson 2000). Occasional use of screening instruments such as the HCR-20 may be helpful in the clinical assessment. *The single strongest predictive factor* for the assessment of violence risk is a history of violence. It is vital that the evaluator assess whether the patient has had singular or repetitive episodes of violence and whether these episodes have been planned or impulsive. Assessment of the outcome of the patient's violent episodes (whether they lead to harm to others, harm to property, harm to self, or no physical or emotional harm) and comparison of these episodes with the norms of the patient's cultural group is also important.

When assessing an individual for future violence, one must distinguish between a clinically oriented assessment and a statistically based assessment. A clinical assessment is based on an evaluator's skill, experience, and knowledge. A statistical assessment is an actuarial prediction based on statistical models and the use of risk factor instruments. In any setting, an actuarial assessment is more accurate than a clinical assessment. Ideally, psychiatrists performing violence risk assessment should be aware of their cultural, racial, and ethnic stereotypes and prejudices, and ethically, they should take these biases into account during their assessment. Here is where the OCF of DSM-IV-TR could be helpful, but in our personal experience we find it is underused.

When assessing patients of different cultural, racial, and ethnic backgrounds who may be potentially violent, it is important not to micro-insult or micro-aggress against the patient in the process of the evaluation (Bell et al. 2006). For example, for a younger white male psychiatrist to call an elderly black male patient by his first name may be perceived by the patient as a subtle insult. Equally insulting is asking a person of color for his or her Medicaid card instead of asking how he or she plans to pay for the service (Bell et al. 2006). It is also important to be culturally sensitive to how some people of color perceive and respond to dominance or authority. For example, because of African Americans' concerns about racism, asking an African American to submit to a search for weapons upon entering a clinical setting such as an emergency department or inpatient unit may be mistaken for discrimination instead of standard operating procedure. This may also be true of visible security presence in a clinical setting. Probably one of the most culturally insensitive acts of the majority culture against people of color is the denial of the existence of racism, which frequently happens when a person of color raises the issue of racism or is being victimized by a racial stereotype—a common experience for people of color. One example of stereotyping is the presumption of guilt and criminal intent when people of color are singled out by police for questioning (e.g., the traffic stop for "driving while Black or Hispanic"). This is their reality.

Culturally Appropriate Assessment in Interpersonal Violence

We now focus on specific cultural knowledge that will help in the assessment of patients who may be subject to IPV but who come to the psychiatrist's office for another reason. There is much more in the literature about the assessment of IPV in ethnic minorities than there is about the risk assessment of ethnic minorities for violent behavior. The following case illustrates how a culturally competent clinician may use cultural knowledge and norms to properly assess a patient for IPV.

Case Example 4: A Pregnant Pakistani Adolescent

Sheryl comes in for her first visit to a psychiatrist. She is 17 years old and has been married to her 19-year-old husband for 3 months. He answers most of the questions for her and states that she is depressed and does nothing around the house. The husband refuses to leave the room when asked to do so. Nevertheless, the psychiatrist insists, and the husband leaves the room. Sheryl never makes eye contact with the physician. When the psychiatrist assesses her for IPV, she denies it. When asked if her husband controls what she does, she states, "Of course he does. He is my husband."

Knowing nothing further about the patient than the stated case, we would be alarmed by the overly controlling partner and the patient's lack of eye contact. We know, however, that she emigrated from Pakistan and is Muslim. The culturally specific information that we would find helpful in this situation is that generally, Muslim women expect to be married and expect that the marriage will be arranged. A study by Hassouneh-Phillips (2001) showed that American Muslim women view marriage as a means to achieving personal and spiritual happiness. They also believe that good wives are obedient, because the Qur'an states that men have more strength so their duty is to protect and support their women (Mayor's Office to Combat Domestic Violence 2003).

As mentioned earlier, culture influences how people view and perceive abuse; whether they seek help, how they communicate their experiences; and from whom they are likely to seek assistance. Cultural factors may serve as barriers to treatment, such as an extended family structure in which a family elder supports the abuse, or a church leader who advises the woman to go back to her husband. The clinician should communicate with each patient as an individual, without expecting generalized reactions from their respective cultural groups.

IPV is more common in cultures in which women are considered to be inferior. African Americans tend to use violence as a resource of control to compensate for a lack of other resources such as money, respect, power, prestige, or knowledge (Weil and Lee 2004). Before going on to more specific cultural information, we would like to discuss an approach to using such information. Table 3–3, presents a "culturally competent assessment A–E" for incorporating cultural knowledge with the patient evaluation. A is for Assumptions, and cultural assessment involves looking at our own cultural assumptions. B is for the Beliefs of the group being evaluated, as in knowing and understanding those beliefs. C signifies that effective Communication can be a bridge between the belief systems of the evaluator and the patient. D, for Diversity, allows us to understand how patients' individual experiences make them different from others in their cultural group. E is for Education—what a clinician needs in order to understand how other groups differ from our own—and for Ethics and how they are changed by differing cultural beliefs (Thompson 2005). With this A–E mnemonic as a backdrop, we present some culture-specific information about cultural groups found in the literature to see how culture influences their experience of IPV.

Somalis

Pan et al. (2006) conducted interviews in San Diego, California, with members of the Somali, Latino, and Vietnamese communities. They found that Somali community members felt that physical violence was an unacceptable means of conflict resolution. However, IPV is viewed as an acceptable means of maintaining the patriarchal structure of the Somali family. The major sources of conflict within the family were changes in gender roles and responsibilities since resettling in the United States. The power dynamic in the family was reversed when families came to the United States because government aid checks were issued to the Somali women, not the men. Thus, Somali men reported feelings of helplessness and uselessness because they have lost their role as the breadwinner for the family, and many try to regain control through violence.

Somali women are responsible for maintaining harmony within the family by supporting their husband, obeying his wishes, and not upsetting or angering him. IPV perpetrated by the husband can be justified in situations in which the wife defied the husband's wishes. Somali men view this as the husband's right to "teach his wife a lesson." Interestingly enough, there is no term for IPV in the Somali language. Both genders report that it is a commonly held belief among women that if a husband does not beat his wife, it means he does not love her. Most Somalis are

TABLE 3–3. Culturally competent assessment A–E

A	Assumptions	The act of taking for granted or supposing that a concept or idea is true.
B	Beliefs	Shared concepts about how a group operates.
C	Communication	Two-way sharing of information that results in an understanding between the sender and the receiver.
D	Diversity	The way in which people actually differ (regardless of other people's assumptions or beliefs) and the effect those differences have on their response to healthcare and to the practitioner.
E	Education, Ethics	Gaining knowledge about a diverse group and understanding that ethical issues may be viewed differently by different groups.

Source. Adapted from Thompson 2005.

Muslims, and Islamic traditions are thought to reduce tension in families and thus reduce the incidence of domestic violence. Hassouneh-Phillips (2001) reported that renegotiated Islamic marriage contracts did not stop IPV, nor did consulting with the Imam. However, Potter (2007) reported that in one case, consulting with religious leaders resulted in the removal of the husband from the home. As in many non-Western cultures, family members and community elders are frequently called upon as a resource for resolving conflict between spouses. Traditionally, the wife consults with the men in her family, who then talk to the husband. However, Somali women in the United States do not have access to this type of family support because they are refugees fleeing a lengthy civil war. During the resettlement process, refugees receive information about American laws related to IPV, and women are told to call the police to report violence in the home. However, this can be counterproductive to their marriage because involving outsiders in family matters is deemed "Americanized" and is an appropriate reason to seek a divorce. Somali community members report that men can divorce their wives if they become "too Americanized." Thus, many Somali women are trapped in violent situations with no culturally viable means of resolving the problem.

Asian Americans

In assessing any Asian culture, it may be useful to know that Asians value the importance of the family over the individual. They believe in conflict avoidance and that personal problems such as marital issues should remain private so as not to shame and dishonor the family and cause a loss of face. Before marriage, a woman follows and obeys her father; after marriage, she follows and obeys the husband; and after the death of her husband, she follows and obeys the son (Xu et al. 2001).

Yoshioka and Dang (2000) did a survey of Asian American families about their attitudes toward family violence. The men had the highest score in support of male privilege. They believed that a man has the right to discipline his wife, that he should be able to have sex whenever he wants it, that he is the ruler of his home, and that some wives deserve beatings. It is a sign of weakness to ask for help, and family members would discourage the disclosure of problems and would make excuses for the abuser. Asian Americans' respect for their elders would result in pressure not to report (see Table 3–4 for a list of barriers to reporting IPV). Violence was justified if the wife had an extramarital affair, lost emotional control, or made a financial decision without consulting the husband. Older respondents and men were more tolerant toward the use of force to resolve family conflict (Yick and Agbayani-Siewart 1997).

Vietnamese

The Vietnamese community in San Diego (Pan et al. 2006), as do many non-Western ethnic communities, sees domestic violence as a family matter. Sharing information about the family with outsiders is viewed as inappropriate. Violence, ignoring problems, and seeking outside assistance (court, counselors, police) are cited as unacceptable ways of resolving conflict, which creates a trap, because the victim cannot involve outsiders to resolve his or her problems with violence. Shame is a major barrier to accessing services. The responsibility for maintaining peace and family harmony falls on the woman, who accomplishes this task by obeying her husband's wishes and attending to the needs of her husband, much like what was seen in Somali families. Strong family ties and respect for family members are cited as ways of promoting harmony in the family. Acceptable strategies for conflict resolution include soliciting and listening to the advice of parents and elders or discussing problems in a peaceful manner. The primary stressors for IPV were economic. Bui and Morash (1999) stated that "for Vietnamese Americans, women's economic contributions could not reduce husbands' dominant positions and violence, but economic hardship could prevent abused women from leaving an abusive relationship " (p. 790). Vietnamese participants reported that sending money to family members in Vietnam or sponsoring family members to the United States are major sources of tension. In addition, they repeatedly identified excessive gambling as a cause of tension within the family. Both men and women

TABLE 3–4. Barriers to culturally appropriate interpersonal violence assessment in Asian American patients

Institutional
  Monolingual worker
  Immigration status
  Welfare policy
  Refugee resettlement
  Racism and homophobia
  Lack of health insurance, training, child care, and affordable housing
  Nonadaptive systems

Cultural
  Values/Beliefs
  Isolation
  Shame
  Other kinds of relationships (i.e., same gender or interracial)
  Community
  Religion and spirituality
  No support from community or family

Individual
  Values around shame
  Low self-esteem/self-confidence
  Inability to speak English
  Lack of cultural fluency
  Age
  Lack of marketable skills
  Status
  Socialization patterns
  Not knowing resources and law

Source. This material was reprinted and/or adapted from the Family Violence Prevention Fund's publication entitled "(Un)heard Voices: Domestic Violence in the Asian American Community" (2007). The report was authored by Sujata Warrier, Ph.D. Production was made possible by a grant from the Violence Against Women Office, Office of Justice Programs, U.S. Department of Justice.

gamble, and many spend their families' income either in the casinos or in underground gambling rings.

Cambodians

Weil and Lee (2004) described cultural factors that increase the risk of IPV for Cambodian women. The cultural expectations of the wife are that she will obey and respect the husband, not be sexually promiscuous before or after marriage, and accept the problems of the marriage. Women are blamed for problems regardless of fault, and in fact, the cultural belief is that the woman must have done something wrong to deserve such punishment. A contributing factor is that most women were physically abused by their parents before their marriages. Women do not have the right to divorce or leave a husband who is hitting them and cannot have their husbands arrested for violent acts against the family.

Latinos

In the Latino community, family harmony is supported by following family traditions and celebrations and helping each other. Physical violence and verbal aggression are considered unacceptable ways of resolving conflict. Open communication between family members and leaving potentially volatile situations are viewed as acceptable ways of resolving conflict. Gender roles in this community appear to be slowly changing as families adjust to living in the United States; men are starting to recognize that women may have more to contribute to the family than the domestic tasks of cooking, house cleaning, and childcare.

Latina women are asking for more equitable distribution of labor and decision making in the household; however, they are still responsible for the vast majority of housework and childcare. Adolescent girls reported frustration about the amount of responsibility they held in the household compared with their brothers. The frequently mentioned causes of tension in the family were economics, immigration status, and substance use. Women from the Latino community reported that the threat of deportation due to their undocumented status is often used as a means of controlling them and ensuring that they do not leave abusive situations. For example, women reported that men often say that if their wives call the police, they will be deported. When compared with the Somali and Vietnamese communities, the Latino community appears to be more aware of the availability of domestic violence intervention services but has a limited understanding of how to use the services and how to work with service providers. Significant barriers to access are language and cultural differences, fear of deportation, and the inability to effectively use identified services (Pan et al. 2006).

African Americans

African American families have a legacy of racism and stereotypes that works against both members of the married couple. Black men, like most men, may experience entitlement dysfunction when they see that they are being fitted into a gender role stereotype. They are often seen as menacing, so they have been legitimized by this stereotype to be intimidating and controlling. African American women have an image of having much sexual, social, physical, and economic power. They can also be seen as invulnerable, insensitive, stoic, and in need of domestication and control. Victims of IPV feel shame about their inability to have a perfect family. Those who have darker complexions, tall physiques, are overweight, fight back, or have a mental illness are thought to deserve abuse (Bell and Mattis 2000). Some African American adolescent women are coerced into intimate relationships with older African American males and may be labeled as morally suspect or hypersexual. Financial pressures may make leaving an abusive relationship seemingly impossible, because the single mother and her children would end up homeless (Bell and Mattis 2000). Finally, Richie (1996) noted that many African American women who are being battered by their partners or sons are reluctant to report violence out of fear of contributing to the victimization of African American men.

Potter (2007) found that many African American women seek support from religious leaders when trying to deal with IPV, and many are not supported for reporting the violence or for wanting to leave their husbands. The victim is often sent back to the perpetrator with the mandate that they "should work things out" because Ephesians 5:21–33 states "submit yourselves unto your own husbands, as unto the Lord. For the husband is the head of the wife, even as Christ is the head of the church.... Therefore as the church is subject unto Christ, so let the wives be to their own husbands in everything."

Key Points

- The culturally appropriate assessment of the risk of violence is vital in developing effective interventions that are culturally congruent.
- As the United States becomes more ethnically diverse every year, the likelihood increases that our patients will be from cultures with which we are unfamiliar.
- A violence risk assessment of culturally diverse patients requires the clinician to become familiar with basic norms about violence, coping strategies and behaviors, gender roles, and the roles of spirituality and religion in the patient's culture.

- Frameworks such as the DSM-IV-TR OCF or the "culturally appropriate assessment A–E" mnemonic outlined in this chapter may prove helpful in organizing the assessment of violence risk in culturally diverse patients.
- Ultimately, the clinician has the responsibility not to stereotype patients either diagnostically or as "more prone to violence" when the data do not support that linkage.
- More research needs to be done so that clinicians may further understand the links between ethnicity, socioeconomic status, and the risk of violent behavior.

References

Adebimpe VR: Overview: white norms and psychiatric diagnosis of black patients. Am J Psychiatry 138:279–285, 1981

American Psychiatric Association: Diagnostic and Statistical Manual of Mental Disorders, 4th Edition. Washington, DC, American Psychiatric Association, 1994

American Psychiatric Association: Diagnostic and Statistical Manual of Mental Disorders, 4th Edition, Text Revision. Washington, DC, American Psychiatric Association, 2000

American Psychiatric Association: Resolution Against Racism and Racial Discrimination and Their Adverse Impacts on Mental Health: Position Statement, July 2006. Available at http://www.psych.org/edu/other_res/lib_archives/archives/200603.pdf. Accessed February 9, 2007

Bell CC: Violence prevention 101: implications for policy development, in Perspectives on Crime and Justice 2000–2001 Lecture Series, Vol V. Washington, DC, National Institute of Justice, March 2002, pp 65–93. Available at http://www.ncjrs.gov/pdffiles1/nij/187100.pdf. Accessed February 10, 2007

Bell CC: Prevention is the future. Clinical Psychiatry News 35:14, 2007

Bell CC, Mattis J: The importance of cultural competence in ministering to African American victims of domestic violence. Violence Against Women 6:515–532, 2000

Bell CC, Mehta H: The misdiagnosis of black patients with manic depressive illness. J Natl Med Assoc 72:141–145, 1980

Bell CC, Dove HW, Williamson JL: Challenges and obstacles in treating mentally ill black patients. Psychiatric Times 23:48-49, 2006. Available at http://giftfromwithin.org/html/challenge.html. Accessed December 16, 2007

Bui HN, Morash M: Domestic violence in the Vietnamese immigrant community: an exploratory study. Violence Against Women 5:769–795, 1999

Du N, Lu F: Assessment and treatment of posttraumatic stress disorder among Asians, in Working With Asian Americans. Edited by Lee E. New York, Guilford, 1997, pp 275–294

Flaherty JA, Meagher R: Measuring racial bias in inpatient treatment. Am J Psychiatry 137:679–682, 1980

Gross H, Herbert MR, Kantterud GL, et al: The effects of race and sex on the variation of diagnosis and disposition in a psychiatric emergency room. J Nerv Ment Dis 148:638–642, 1969
Hassouneh-Phillips D: Marriage is half faith and the rest is fear of Allah. Violence Against Women 7:927–946, 2001
Hollinger PC, Offer D, Barter JT, et al: Suicide and Homicide Among Adolescents. New York, Guilford, 1994
Hucker S: Psychiatric Aspects of Risk Assessment, 2004. Available at http://www.violence-risk.com/risk/assessment.htm. Accessed February 10, 2007
Johnson B: Assessing the risk for violence, in Psychiatric Aspects on Violence: Understanding Causes and Issues in Prevention and Treatment. Edited by Bell CC. San Francisco, CA, Jossey-Bass, 2000, pp 33–36
Jones BE, Gray BA: Black and white psychiatrists: therapy with blacks. J Natl Med Assoc 77:19–25, 1985
Keppel KG, Pearcy JN, Wagener DK: Trends in Racial and Ethnic-Specific Rates for the Health Status Indicators: United States, 1990–98. (Healthy People 2000 Statistical Notes No 23, pp 1–12). Rockville, MD, U.S. Department of Health and Human Services, 2002
Kirmayer LJ: Cultural variations in the clinical presentation of depression and anxiety: implications for diagnosis and treatment. J Clin Psychiatry 62 (suppl):22–28, 2001
Krug EG, Dahlberg LL, Mercy JA, et al: World Report on Violence and Health. Geneva, Switzerland, World Health Organization, 2002
Lane WG, Rubin DM, Monteith R, et al: Racial differences in the evaluation of pediatric fractures for physical abuse. JAMA 288:13:1603–1609, 2002
Mayor's Office to Combat Domestic Violence: Medical Providers' Guide to Managing the Care of Domestic Violence Patients Within a Cultural Context, August 2003. Available at http://www.nyc.gov/html/ocdv/downloads/pdf/providers_dv_guide.pdf. Accessed March 25, 2007
Mezzich JE, Otero AA, Lee S: International psychiatric diagnosis, in Comprehensive Textbook of Psychiatry, 7th Edition. Edited by Kaplan HI, Sadock BJ. Baltimore, MD, Williams & Wilkins, 2000, pp 839–853
Miranda J, Lawson W, Escobar J: Ethnic minorities. Ment Health Serv Res 4:231–237, 2002
Pan A, Daley S, Rivera LM, et al: Understanding the role of culture in domestic violence: the Ahimsa Project for Safe Families. J Immigr Minor Health 8:35–43, 2006
Petee TA, Padgett KG, York TS: Debunking the stereotype: an examination of mass murder in public places. Homicide Studies 1:317–337, 1997
Pierce CM, Earls FJ, Kleinman A: Race and culture in psychiatry, in The Harvard Guide to Psychiatry. Edited by Nicholi AR. Cambridge, MA, Belknap Press, 1999, pp 735–743
Potter H: Battered black women's use of religious services and spirituality for assistance in leaving abusive relationships. Violence Against Women 13:262–284, 2007
Primm AB: The assessment of African American patients, in Clinical Manual of Cultural Psychiatry. Edited by Lim RF. Washington, DC, American Psychiatric Publishing, 2006, pp 35–68

Pulera DJ: Visible Differences: Why Race Will Matter to Americans in the Twenty-First Century. New York, Continuum International Publishing, 2002

Rezentes WC: Ka Lama Kukui Native Hawaiian Psychology: An Introduction. Honolulu, HI, A'Alii Books, 1996

Richie B: Compelled to Crime: The Gender Entrapment of Black Battered Women. New York, Routledge, 1996

Sampson RJ, Raudenbush SW, Earls F: Neighborhoods and violent crime: a multilevel study of collective efficacy. Science 277:918–924, 1997

Schultz-Ross RA: Violent behavior, in Culture and Psychopathology. Edited by Tseng WS, Strelzer J. New York, Brunner/Mazel, 1997, pp 173–189

Steadman H, Mulvey E, Monahan J, et al: Violence by people discharged from acute psychiatric inpatient facilities and by others in the same neighborhoods. Arch Gen Psychiatry 55:393–401, 1998

Substance Abuse and Mental Health Services Administration: Results from the 2002 National Survey on Drug Use and Health: National Findings, 2003. Available at http://www.oas.samhsa.gov/nhsda/2k2nsduh/Results/2k2Results.htm. Accessed April 15, 2007

Sue DW, Sue D: Counseling the Culturally Different: Theory and Practice, 3rd Edition. New York, Wiley, 1999

Tardiff K: Prediction of violence in patients. Journal of Practical Psychology and Behavioral Health 4:12–19, 1998

Thompson R: Intimate partner violence: a culturally sensitive approach. Adv Nurse Pract 13:57–59, 2005

Tjaden P, Thoennes N: Full Report of the Prevalence, Incidence, and Consequences of Violence Against Women: Findings from the National Violence Against Women Survey (Report No NCJ 183781). Washington, DC, U.S. Department of Justice, 2000

Ton H, Lim, RF: The assessment of culturally diverse individuals, in Clinical Manual of Cultural Psychiatry. Edited by Lim RF. Washington, DC, American Psychiatric Publishing, 2006, pp 3–31

Tseng WS, Matthews D, Elwyn TS: Cultural Competence in Forensic Mental Health. New York, Brunner-Rutledge, 2004

U.S. Department of Health and Human Services: Culture, Race, and Ethnicity: A Supplement to Mental Health: A Report of the Surgeon General. Rockville, MD, U.S. Department of Health and Human Services, Public Health Service, Office of the Surgeon General, 2001a

U.S. Department of Health and Human Services: Youth Violence: A Report of the Surgeon General. Rockville, MD, U.S. Department of Health and Human Services, 2001b

Walsh A: African Americans and serial killing in the media: the myth and the reality. Homicide Studies 9:271–291, 2005

Warrier S: Unheard voices: domestic violence in the Asian American community. Family Violence Prevention Fund, 2007. Available at http://www.endabuse.org/programs/immigrant/files/UnheardVoices.pdf. Accessed March 3, 2007

Weil JM, Lee HH: Cultural Considerations in understanding family violence among Asian American Pacific Islander families. J Comm Health Nurs 21:217–227, 2004

West JC, Herbeck DM, Bell CC, et al: Race/Ethnicity among psychiatric patients: variations in diagnostic and clinical characteristics reported by practicing clinicians. Focus 4:48, 2006

Xu X, Campbell JC, Zhu F: Intimate partner violence against Chinese women: the past, present, and future. Trauma Violence Abuse 2:296–315, 2001

Yick AG: Domestic violence in the Chinese American community: cultural taboos and barriers. Family Violence and Sexual Assault Bulletin 15:16–23, 1999

Yick AG, Agbayani-Siewart P: Perception of domestic violence in a Chinese American Community. J Interpers Violence 12:832–897, 1997

Yoshioka MR, Dang Q: Asian family violence: a study of the Cambodian, Chinese, Korean, South Asian, and Vietnamese communities in Massachusetts. Boston, MA, Asian Task Force Against Domestic Violence, 2000

CHAPTER 4

Psychological Testing in Violence Risk Assessment

Barry Rosenfeld, Ph.D., A.B.P.P.

Ekaterina Pivovarova, M.A.

In recent years, the research and clinical literature on risk assessment has focused almost exclusively on the development and validation of structured assessment techniques. Yet despite the increased attention to actuarial risk assessment (discussed in Chapter 2 by Monahan), most practicing clinicians rely on unstructured or structured professional judgment, essentially conducting a clinical evaluation and reaching a conclusion about violence risk. A recent survey of board certified forensic psychologists indicated that very few of those surveyed routinely use formal risk assessment measures (Archer et al. 2006). Instead, forensic evaluators continue to incorporate specialized psychological testing to address important elements of an individual's violence risk.

Even among ardent supporters of actuarial risk assessment, psychological testing and measurement can often play an invaluable role (e.g., in quantifying psychopathy or identifying excessive defensiveness). Although the specific tests and techniques that are used necessarily vary depending on patient history, evaluation setting, and the nature of the violence in question (e.g., sexual, domestic), there are a number of instruments that are sufficiently common to be critical for any thorough risk assessment. However, these measures should not be considered a replacement for systematic approaches to risk assessment (i.e., "structured professional judgment" instruments) but rather an adjunctive method to inform the clinical evaluation process.

A comprehensive review of all psychological tests that may be used or useful in violence risk assessment is beyond the scope of this chapter. Instead, we present a brief review of clinical factors and commonly used measures that should be considered when evaluating risk of violence. In addition, we address some of the variations and specialized instruments that may be useful with special populations such as sexual offenders, although it is not possible to address adequately all settings and populations (for example, death penalty evaluations and suicide risk assessments are not discussed). Finally, in this chapter we focus chiefly on risk *assessment*, but it should be noted that the identification of risk *management* strategies is an equally important aspect of violence risk assessment. Many of the measures described here might be used to help monitor violence risk or response to treatment as part of an ongoing risk management approach. The following case example highlights many of the assessment issues discussed in this chapter.

Case Example

Assessing Violence Risk in a Criminal Defendant

For the past several months, Shawn, a 23-year-old medical student, had been dating one of his medical school classmates, Veronica. As the relationship evolved, Shawn became increasingly jealous, accusing Veronica of flirting with one of their professors and eventually demanding that she confess to her infidelity. Veronica ended the relationship shortly after this confrontation, but Shawn continued to initiate contact with Veronica after class despite her repeated insistence that they had nothing more to discuss. One day Shawn arrived at Veronica's apartment unannounced, demanding she let him in to talk about their relationship. Veronica refused to allow him into the apartment and told Shawn she would call the police if he continued to harass her. Soon afterward Veronica began receiving telephone calls in the night; the caller typically would hang up without speaking, but occasionally she heard a man's voice on the phone calling her insulting names. Several days later Veronica thought she saw Shawn sitting in a car parked across the street from her apartment. She telephoned the police, who confronted Shawn and, on searching his car, discovered a camera, a stun gun, a large knife, and a pair of handcuffs. However, because Shawn had not actually assaulted Veronica, the charges of harassment and stalking carried a relatively modest penalty. Nevertheless, the court referred Shawn for a mental health evaluation, requesting an evaluation of his mental state and violence risk as well as recommendations for what treatment, if any, was necessary.

Psychological Testing in Violence Risk Assessment

Evaluating Violence Risk

As is evident from the preceding case example, not all violence risk assessments occur in "typical" mental health or criminal justice settings. In fact, some of the most challenging evaluations concern atypical situations or individuals. Because certain measures may have been shown to be more adequate for particular populations, context plays a critical role in determining what psychological instruments may be useful in violence risk assessment.

Clinicians engage in violence risk assessments both in civil and criminal settings. Risk assessment in a civil context generally focuses on whether an individual should be placed in a psychiatric institution or forcibly medicated over his or her objection. Questions about violence risk in criminal settings, on the other hand, typically arise in the context of parole and sentencing decisions, where risk of future violence and criminal behavior are important considerations. In general, violence risk assessment in a criminal context is concerned with longer-term risks rather than the acute risk of violence necessary for involuntary psychiatric hospitalization, but this dichotomy is not always clear-cut (e.g., sex offender commitment hearings, although civil in nature, arise after a criminal conviction and involve long-term violence risk assessments). In short, a critical issue in evaluating violence risk is determining the time frame of concern (short-term versus long-term predictions).

Once the context and nature of the risk assessment question are clear, decisions can be made as to which procedures and instruments might be useful. Some of these instruments are useful because they include elements of a structured or actuarial risk assessment (e.g., psychopathy), whereas others may directly address critical elements of the individual's clinical or risk profile (e.g., psychosis or substance abuse).

Psychopathy

Psychopathy is probably the most well established and widely known risk factor for future violence, cutting across most contexts and populations. The term *psychopathy* has been used to describe the subset of individuals who engage in violent and criminal behavior, show no remorse for their actions or empathy for their victims, and yet maintain a superficial veneer of sociability and poise. A thorough review of the psychopathy literature could easily fill several volumes. For the purpose of violence risk assessment, it is probably sufficient to note that this construct comprises a central element of both clinical and actuarial (as well as structured professional judgment) approaches to risk assessment.

The central "measure" of psychopathy for the past two decades has been Hare's Psychopathy Checklist (PCL) and its subsequent revision (PCL-R; Hare 1991). The PCL was developed to measure the core concepts of psychopathy and has been extensively validated in forensic mental health research. Not only is the PCL-R considered by many to be a critical element of any violence risk assessment, it is also incorporated into many of the empirically supported actuarial risk assessment measures (e.g., the HCR-20 [Historical, Clinical, and Risk Management] and Violence Risk Appraisal Guide). However, the PCL-R is not a psychological "test," per se, but rather a clinical rating scale. The measure consists of 20 items that are evaluated by a trained clinician on the basis of clinical interview, official records, and third-party information. Each item is scored on a scale of 0–2, with 0 indicating that the item does not apply, 1 indicating that the item applies "somewhat," and 2 indicating that the item clearly applies to the individual. Scores are typically evaluated against published normative data, either by identifying the individual's level of psychopathy (e.g., percentile relative to typical criminal offenders or forensic psychiatric patients) or by identifying those individuals who score above the threshold used to identify "psychopathy" (i.e., greater than 30). Although considerable research has focused on elucidating a factor structure for this measure, most clinicians rely on the total score for evaluating violence risk.

However, despite its importance in violence risk assessment, the PCL-R has a number of limitations that are rarely acknowledged by mental health evaluators. For example, although research studies typically demonstrate a high degree of interrater reliability across different clinicians, individual evaluators may not have received comparable training. Thus, the accuracy of PCL-R ratings will vary considerably across clinicians, and contradictory PCL estimates are not uncommon.

In addition, mental health evaluators may be confused about the different versions of the PCL that exist, at times using measures incorrectly. For example, Hare and Hart developed a screening version of the PCL for use in research settings where identification of "probable" psychopaths may be useful (Hart et al. 1995). Yet many clinicians utilize this briefer instrument in clinical evaluations, seemingly unaware of the different purpose and validation data that pertain to the screening version (e.g., a higher rate of "false positives": incorrect classifications of nonpsychopathic offenders as psychopathic). Likewise, the PCL has been adapted for adolescents (the PCL-YV, or Youth Version; Forth et al. 2003), although the validity of this measure for violence risk assessment is far less convincing than for the PCL-R.

The utility of the PCL for evaluating violence risk in women is also far less clear than its utility in men, because the construct of psychopathy has been less often explored in women offenders. The few studies that have examined the use of the PCL-R in women have failed to clarify whether this instrument is equally useful in women. Finally, cross-cultural research on the construct and measurement of psychopathy is still in a relatively nascent stage. Although a growing number of studies have supported the utility of the PCL in other countries and settings, and considerable research has analyzed the cross-racial validity of the PCL in North American offenders (e.g., comparing Caucasian and African American samples), this research has largely been restricted to Western, highly developed countries (e.g., Sweden, the Netherlands, the United Kingdom). In fact, little evidence exists to support (or contradict) the utility of the PCL as an aid for evaluating violence risk in non-Western cultures. Hence, considerable caution is warranted when utilizing this measure in violence risk assessment with individuals who fall outside the primary validation sample (North American males in prison). In the vignette described earlier, for example, the PCL-R would likely lead to an unrealistically low estimate of violence risk, largely because of Shawn's high-achieving background and lack of childhood behavior problems or other serious antisocial behaviors.

General Personality Assessment

Although psychopathy may be one of the most powerful violence risk factors, the assessment of an individual's violence risk often requires a broader, more comprehensive approach to personality assessment. The most common approach to personality assessment in forensic settings is the use of broad-based self-report inventories such as the Minnesota Multiphasic Personality Inventory–2 (MMPI-2; Butcher et al. 1989), the Personality Assessment Inventory (PAI; Morey 1991), and the Millon Clinical Multiaxial Inventory–3 (MCMI-III; Millon 1994). As is discussed later, not only can these measures provide important information along a number of different personality dimensions but also, and perhaps more importantly, they can inform the evaluator about the individual's approach to testing (i.e., the presence of defensiveness or symptom exaggeration).

The latter element of objective personality measures—the assessment of test-taking style—is a critical component of psychological evaluations of violence risk. Because many individuals are motivated to mask the true extent of their psychological difficulties, the mental health evaluator engaged in violence risk assessment must consider the possibility that the individual being evaluated has not been honest in reporting his or her history, symptoms, behaviors, or thoughts. Hence, a thorough assessment of test-taking style is typically critical to any violence risk assessment, particularly when the individual's self-report will make up a significant component of the evaluation (which is often, but not necessarily, the case). Although several instruments (e.g., MMPI-2, MCMI-III, PAI) include scales that assess defensiveness, there is little dispute that the MMPI-2 is the best-validated measure for evaluating test-taking style. Of course, the presence of defensiveness does not correspond to an elevated risk of violence, but it does suggest that the individual's denial, lack of insight or awareness, or deliberate minimization of symptoms likely results in inaccurate (unrealistic) test results and self-report. It is worth noting that although these instruments also include multiple scales and indices to evaluate symptom exaggeration (malingering), this pattern is rarely observed in the evaluation of violence risk because little motive exists for exaggerating the severity of one's symptoms. Furthermore, for the sake of brevity, the discussion that follows focuses primarily on the MMPI-2, with the acknowledgement that similar scales and interpretations may be available from other measures.

Assuming that the individual has responded honestly to the MMPI-2, interpretation of the Clinical and Supplementary scales of the instrument can be helpful in identifying general aggressive tendencies. It should, of course, be noted that the presence of a "profile" that is linked to an elevated risk of violence is by no means sufficient to conclude that an individual is at high risk for violence. Nevertheless, a personality style associated with an elevated risk of violence may provide one indicator of possible violence risk. Likewise, evidence of a psychotic disorder, which in itself may not correspond to an elevated risk of violence, could provide important data in cases where the individual's history or clinical presentation suggests delusional beliefs of a threatening or paranoid nature, as in the vignette previously described.

The scenario of paranoid delusions notwithstanding, the MMPI-2 profile most commonly associated with violence is the 3–4/4–3 profile. This profile has been described as indicative of poorly controlled anger and hostility, although more recent research on these scales and this code type has been equivocal. In addition, the Overcontrolled Hostility Scale, which was developed to identify individuals who engaged in severe acts of violence that seemed disproportionate to the provocation, has also been used to explain seemingly extreme violent incidents by individuals who had little prior history of violence, although most authors caution against using this scale as a *predictive* measure because it was developed using retrospective analyses (Greene 2000).

A number of other MMPI-2 subscales exist that are both less controversial and less widely studied than the Overcontrolled Hostility Scale. For example, a number of subscales have been developed specifically for the Psychopathic Deviance Scale (Scale 4) that break down elevations on this clinical scale into smaller, content-based subdivisions. The five subscales developed by Harris and Lingoes are Familial Discord, Authority Conflict, Social Imperturbability, Social Alienation, and Self Alienation (Harris R, Lingoes J: Subscales for the Minnesota Multiphasic Personality Inventory. San Francisco, CA, The Langley Porter Clinic, unpublished manuscript, 1955). Although some of these subscales (e.g., Social and Self Alienation) are less intuitively relevant to violence risk, Osberg and Poland (2001) found modest correlations ($r=0.36$) between Authority Conflict and Self Alienation and future criminal behavior among a sample of inmates who were eventually released. In fact, these subscales provided considerable incremental validity beyond the larger scale. Thus, although relatively little research has applied these subscales to violence risk assessment, particularly in prospective studies, they may provide a useful element of MMPI-2 interpretation in risk assessment settings.

The PAI, another widely used, multi-scale, objective personality inventory, has also been used in violence risk assessment. The PAI not only includes several scales intended to measure aggressive tendencies (Aggressive Attitude, Verbal Aggression, and Physical Aggression), but also includes a summary index intended to quantify violence potential. Unfortunately, despite this scale's potential, relatively little research has supported its use as a risk assessment tool (Morey and Quigley 2002). Likewise, the PAI Correctional Report includes an "Institutional Risk Circumplex" intended to help evaluate the offender's likelihood of engaging in violent behavior within a prison setting, although at present this index too has little empirical support for its utility (Edens and Ruiz 2005).

Finally, the MCMI-III includes subscales for Antisocial Personality Disorder along with scales tapping Sadistic and Negativistic (oppositional) personality traits (Millon 1994). Although elevations on these scales, either in isolation or in combination with other scales, are often interpreted as indicating aggressive tendencies, relatively little research has addressed—let alone supported—these interpretations. In short, although multi-scale inventories such as the MMPI-2, PAI, and MCMI-III have considerable potential and are frequently utilized in violence risk assessment, empirical support for many of the indices and interpretations is extremely limited, and the need for caution in making any conclusions regarding violence risk cannot be overemphasized.

What About the Rorschach?

Despite growing questions about the reliability and validity of the Rorschach, even using the widely taught Exner scoring system (Lillienfeld et al. 2000), many mental health clinicians continue to use or consider using the Rorschach test in violence risk assessment (Archer et al. 2006). Although it might be tempting to declare unequivocally that this practice is unwarranted, there may be particular settings and individuals for whom this measure provides useful information. As noted earlier, defensiveness and denial of psychological difficulties are particularly common phenomena in violence risk assessment, and thus psychological tests that might be less susceptible to that defensiveness are clearly desirable. However, the potential and reality are often far apart when analyzing the utility of projective tests such as the Rorschach.

A number of researchers have attempted to identify scores or determinants on projective testing that might indicate an elevated risk of violence (Gacano and Meloy 1994; Greco and Cornell 1992), although this limited literature has yet to result in any reliable and valid indices that consistently correspond to a heightened risk of violence. For example, Gacano and Meloy (1994) described a series of "supplemental aggression ratings" for the Rorschach that have been used in several studies, with occasional significant associations with a history of violence or sadistic personality traits. However, support for these indices has been extremely limited and largely inconsistent. Researchers have occasionally reported significant associations with one or more of these variables, but research has yet to demonstrate a consistent pattern of findings suggestive of clear concurrent—let alone predictive—validity.

However, the failure to identify Rorschach indices that correspond to heightened risk of violence does not necessarily render the measure clinically useless. In fact, even ardent critics of the Rorschach acknowledge the potential utility of this measure for identifying psychotic thinking. Particularly in cases in which the risk for future violence appears intertwined with psychotic symptoms (e.g., delusional beliefs of a threatening nature), the Rorschach may help the evaluator identify the presence of psychosis even in the context of an individual's defensiveness or denial of symptoms. Of course, identifying *indicators* of psychosis does not necessarily—or even usually—correspond to heightened risk of violence; however, it may provide useful data to inform the evaluating clinician. Thus, in these limited circumstances, the Rorschach test may provide incremental utility over other, more frequently utilized assessment techniques. In fact, in the vignette described earlier, the Rorschach might represent a useful technique for evaluating the extent to which Shawn's jealousy and seemingly irrational behavior represent the emergence of a psychotic disorder rather than more chronic aggressive tendencies (i.e., psychopathy).

Measures That Address Specific Personality Characteristics

In addition to broad constructs (such as psychopathy) and broad measures of personality functioning (such as the MMPI-2 and PAI), a number of specific personality characteristics have potential relevance in violence risk assessment, including anger, hostility, impulsivity, and aggression. Although multiple measures exist for each of these characteristics (some of which are briefly described later), their utility is clearly contingent on honest responses, because self-report measures are particularly vulnerable to distorted responses. Although some evaluators may rely on the measures described, considerable caution must be exercised unless convincing evidence exists to support the accuracy and honesty of the respondent. Hence, these measures are much more frequently utilized in risk assessment research than in clinical practice. Moreover, the research literature addressing predictors of violence has generated conflicting findings regarding the salience of personality traits that may predispose an individual to violence.

One of the personality characteristics that has received considerable attention as a potential risk factor for violence is *anger*. Several measures of anger exist, including the Novaco Anger Scale (Novaco 1994), the State/Trait Anger Expression Inventory (Spielberger 1988), and the Anger subscale of the Aggression Questionnaire (Buss and Perry 1992). Most of these measures conceptualize anger as a personality trait, with the assumption that individuals who have either excessive anger or difficulty modulating the expression of their anger will be more prone to violent behaviors. For example, the Novaco Anger Scale was designed to evaluate responses to situations that are intended to provoke anger. Initial research demonstrated strong reliability—both internal consistency and test-retest (critical to the conceptualization of anger as a character trait)—as well as strong associations with violent behavior across a number of different populations (e.g., incarcerated felons, domestic violence offenders, and psychiatric patients). In fact, the MacArthur Risk Assessment Study of violence committed by psychiatric patients during and after release into the community found strong support for the Novaco scale as a predictor of future violence (Monahan et al. 2001). Other measures of anger, however, have had far less empirical support, typically being used only in correlational or retrospective studies with little evidence to support their predictive validity. Nevertheless, the findings from the MacArthur study provide some support for the hypothesis that elevated levels of anger are associated with an increased risk of violence.

A closely related construct, *hostility*, has received far less support. In fact, measures of hostility (e.g., the Cook-Medley Hostility Inventory, the Hostility subscale of the Aggression Questionnaire) have rarely been used in prospective research (Buss and Perry 1992; Cook and Medley 1954). Indeed, the distinction between hostility and anger is not altogether clear, and considerable overlap exists between the two constructs. Some theorists conceptualize anger as a largely cognitive process (and therefore one that can be directed at inanimate objects as well as humans), whereas they see hostility as more interpersonal in nature, but correlations between measures of anger and hostility are usually quite high (e.g., greater than 0.7). Thus, the distinction between these constructs for the purposes of violence risk assessment may be largely semantic.

Distinguishing the construct of *aggression* from anger and hostility is equally complex and is further complicated by the lack of a singular accepted definition of aggression. In fact, many theorists have described aggression in purely behavioral terms, essentially relegating this term to a milder version of violence. For example, Leonard Berkowitz (1993), an eminent social psychologist, described *aggression* as "any form of behavior that is intended to injure someone physically or psychologically" (p. 3). Thus, measures of aggression such as the Aggression Questionnaire typically elicit information regarding the frequency of verbal and physical aggression (e.g., "If somebody hits me, I hit back"). Although elevations on this scale are often associated, for obvious reasons, with a history of violence, the utility of this scale for identifying violence potential among individuals without a clear history is less apparent.

A final personality characteristic that has received growing empirical support as a risk factor for future violence is *impulsivity*. Although frequently studied by neurologists and biologists, impulsivity has only occasionally been studied as a risk factor for human violence (and it is one of the items on the PCL-R). In fact, Barratt (1994) proposed that impulsive aggression may often be due to an underlying biological predisposition he termed *behavioral disinhibition*. Barratt conceptualized impulsivity as comprising three factors—motor, cognitive, and nonplanning—and he developed the Barratt Impulsivity Scale (now in its eleventh revision) to measure these three dimensions of impulsivity. Although the Barratt scale was not intended to aid in violence risk assessment, the MacArthur Risk Assessment Study found strong evidence for the predictive validity of the measure in identifying psychiatric patients at elevated risk of future violence. Thus, although still relatively understudied, this measure of impulsivity may have some utility in violence risk assessment.

Other Measures of Potential Relevance in Violence Risk Assessment

The importance of substance abuse in violence risk assessment, whether in isolation or in conjunction with a major mental disorder, cannot be overstated. Although considerable variability across drugs and drug users exists, there is little dispute that active substance abuse represents a significant risk factor for future violence. Thus, measures of substance abuse such as the Substance Abuse Subtle Screening Inventory (SASSI, now in its third revision; Miller et al. 1988) have obvious appeal as a supplement to any violence risk assessment. Not only does the SASSI help identify individuals with both current and potential risk of substance abuse, but this measure also includes a scale intended to measure defensive responding. Although research supporting the SASSI has not addressed its utility in violence risk assessment, it nevertheless may help address a potentially important risk factor. For example, in the case vignette presented at the beginning of this chapter, the evaluation of substance abuse as a potential contributing factor, perhaps in conjunction with the evidence of an emerging psychotic disorder, not only might help improve the assessment of Shawn's potential for future violence, but also may provide invaluable information for developing a risk management strategy to help reduce the risk of future violence.

As noted earlier, defensiveness is a paramount concern in violence risk assessment. Although scales to assess defensiveness are embedded within a number of broader measures, clinicians who are not inclined to use these measures, whether due to time constraints or other considerations, may find it helpful to use a measure specifically intended to evaluate defensiveness. The most widely used and well validated measure of defensiveness is the Paulhus Deception Scales (PDS, formerly called the Balanced Inventory of Desirable Responding) (Paulhus 1998). The PDS is a 40-item self-report measure designed to assess two types of socially desirable responding: impression management and self-deception. Numerous studies have demonstrated strong reliability and concurrent validity of this measure, with strong correlations with other measures of defensiveness. Thus, high scores on this scale may help identify individuals for whom self-report may be unreliable and may even facilitate distinguishing between individuals who are deliberately attempting to distort their presentation (the Impression Management subscale) and those who lack insight and rely excessively on denial (the Self-Deceptive Enhancement subscale). However, little research has utilized the PDS prospectively in violence risk assessment, and thus questions arise as to the incremental validity of this scale in the assessment process.

Assessing the Risk of Sexual Violence

Sexual offenders are a unique population of offenders that warrant additional consideration during the risk assessment process. Not only are most sexual offenses violent in nature, but the risk factors associated with sexual offending (or re-offending) are often quite different from those associated with nonsexual violence (Hanson and Bussiere 1998). Particularly given the emergence of Sexually Violent Predator (SVP) commitment statutes, the need for sexual violence risk assessments has consistently grown in recent decades. Although the emergence of SVP statutes has resulted in the development of numerous actuarial risk assessment instruments specifically designed for sex offender evaluations, structured professional judgment instruments are also widely used. However, both approaches rely heavily on static risk factors (e.g., nature of prior sexual offenses, age of victim), leaving clinicians with little ability to differentiate among large groups of offenders or, more importantly, to monitor change or improvement. Dynamic risk factors, which are better represented in structured professional judgment instruments, include the presence of deviant sexual urges, attitudes tolerant of sexual assault, and cognitive distortions (Craig et al. 2005). Identifying methods for evaluating these risk factors represents a critical step in the clinician's risk assessment process.

One particularly controversial technique to aid in evaluating sex offenders is the penile plethysmograph (PPG), a method of quantifying physiological arousal to deviant sexual imagery (Murphy et al. 1991). Despite its invasive nature and the discomfort most mental health evaluators experience at the thought of utilizing this technique, the PPG is considered to be the most well established laboratory method of assessing sexual deviance and represents one of the strongest predictors of sexual offense recidivism, typically surpassing actuarial risk assessment techniques (Hanson and Bussiere 1998; Laws et al. 2000). In general, the PPG is used with either visual or auditory stimuli of various types of sexual content (e.g., violent, consensual, or nonconsensual sex), which are presented to the individual in order to determine relative

Psychological Testing in Violence Risk Assessment | 71

arousal patterns. However, despite its frequent use in sex offender treatment settings, this technique has a number of significant limitations, including the relatively modest research literature supporting its predictive validity. Questions also exist regarding the potential impact of anxiety, sexual abstinence, and conscious repression of arousal on the relative arousal ratio on the PPG. Furthermore, clinicians are likely to encounter privacy and ethical issues in using this highly intrusive instrument, particularly when the risk assessment has been mandated and true consent is not obtained.

In response to the limitations of the PPG, Gene Abel, one of the leading researchers on treatment of sexual offenders, developed an alternative approach to evaluating deviant sexual arousal, the Abel Assessment of Sexual Interest (AASI; Abel et al. 1998). The AASI, designed to be a less invasive measure than the PPG, is composed of three parts: the individual's subjective rating of sexual interest, a measure of Visual Reaction Time (VRT) in response to sexual stimuli, and a questionnaire designed to elicit attitudes and cognitions thought to correspond to sexual offending. However, the key component of the AASI is the measure of VRT, which records the amount of time the individual examines visual stimuli presented on the computer screen. This measure hinges on the assumption that sexual offenders who spend relatively more time viewing images that depict sexually deviant material are likely to have greater arousal to these stimuli and are therefore more likely to reoffend than individuals who spend relatively little time viewing sexually deviant images. In addition, by comparing viewing patterns for multiple possible types of paraphilic interest, the AASI may help differentiate the specific nature of an individual's deviant arousal, helping guide treatment and risk management strategies.

However, relatively little research has examined either the AASI in general or the VRT in particular. Abel et al. (2004) found some support for the utility of the VRT in identifying child molesters, but virtually no research has addressed the validity of this measure in other populations of sex offenders. Moreover, the effectiveness of the VRT in differentiating different subgroups of sex offenders (e.g., pedophiles versus adult rapists) or identifying offenders with a high likelihood of re-offending is not clear. As discussed earlier, the self-report sections of the AASI are also clearly vulnerable to the biased responding that occurs so often in violence risk assessment (and even more so among sex offender evaluations, given the negative ramifications of admitting deviant sexual arousal). However, despite the limited research on its validity, the AASI holds some promise as a potential aid to violence risk assessment for sexual offenders. That said, at present it is clear that the AASI does not yet have the requisite empirical support necessary to be considered a measure of risk of future sexual violence.

Conclusion

The importance of accurate violence risk assessment cannot be overstated, because the potential ramifications of errors can be devastating. Fortunately, a growing number of psychological tests and techniques can assist the clinician performing such evaluations. In the case example presented earlier, psychological testing might help to illuminate many potentially critical violence risk factors such as psychosis, impulsivity, and anger management issues and substance abuse. For example, a Rorschach Inkblot test might be useful to evaluate the possibility of an underlying psychosis that might account for Shawn's jealousy. In addition, personality tests such as the MMPI and SASSI could provide useful information regarding the extent of Shawn's substance abuse that might help explain his increasingly problematic behavior (which, given his status as a medical student, likely reflects a significant change from his baseline) and provide an alternative avenue for intervention. In addition, such measures would provide information regarding the validity of Shawn's self-report through an evaluation of his response style (i.e., the presence or absence of defensiveness). Finally, evaluating impulsivity and anger through either self-report (e.g., the Barratt or Novaco scales) or clinical ratings (as elicited by the PCL) would help clarify the extent to which Shawn's recent behavior actually reflects a change in, rather than a continuation of, long-standing personality characteristics. A finding of changed behavior might support the hypothesis that Shawn's behavior is the result of an emerging mental disorder that is potentially (likely) treatable, with specific treatment recommendations being guided by the nature of the disorder. A determination that Shawn's behavior is a manifestation of long-standing personality characteristics would highlight the need to more closely examine his past behavior as an indication of his current violence risk (which may be less relevant in the context of an emerging mental disorder).

This chapter outlines a number of different psychological assessment techniques that may be useful supplements to a clinical evaluation of violence risk. Whether the clinician uses an actuarial approach, a structured professional judgment approach, or an unstructured clinical evaluation, accurate determination of violence risk requires careful assessment of the risk factors that have been identified in the research literature. Although the scope and comprehensiveness of the measures described in this chapter vary widely—as does their validity in risk assessment settings—mental health evaluators have multiple options available to them beyond the simple actuarial checklists often utilized. Thorough risk assessment and risk management requires a comprehensive assessment of a wide range of behaviors and cognitions in order to minimize the risk of errors, both of omission or commission.

Key Points

- Psychological testing can be a valuable supplement to any risk assessment approach.
- Evaluating defensiveness is critical, particularly when self-report is relied on.
- Assessing underlying psychosis, sexual deviance, or substance abuse can help identify important risk-enhancing symptoms.
- Formal assessment of psychopathy can bolster any risk assessment method.
- Limitations exist regarding validity of assessment in populations other than Western, English-speaking adults.

References

Abel GG, Huffman J, Warberg B, et al: Visual reaction time and plethysmography as measures of sexual interest in child molesters. Sex Abuse 10:81–95, 1998

Abel GG, Jordan A, Rouleau JL, et al: Use of visual reaction time to assess male adolescents who molest children. Sex Abuse 16:255–265, 2004

Archer RP, Buffington-Vollum JK, Stredny RV, et al: A survey of psychological test use patterns among forensic psychologists. J Personal Assess 87:84–94, 2006

Barratt ES: Impulsiveness and anger, in Violence and Mental Disorders: Developments in Risk Assessment. Edited by Monahan J, Steadman HJ. Chicago, IL, University of Chicago Press, 1994

Berkowitz L: Aggression. New York, McGraw-Hill, 1993

Buss AH, Perry M: The Aggression Questionnaire. J Pers Soc Psychol 63:452–459, 1992

Butcher JN, Dahlstrom WG, Graham JR, et al: Minnesota Multiphasic Personality Inventory-2: Manual for Administration and Scoring. Minneapolis, University of Minnesota Press, 1989

Cook SS, Medley DM: Proposed hostility and pharisaic-virtue scores for the MMPI. J Appl Psychol 38:414–418, 1954

Craig LA, Browne KD, Stringer I, et al: Sexual recidivism: a review of static, dynamic and actuarial predictors. J Sex Aggress 11:65–84, 2005

Edens JF, Ruiz MA: Personality Assessment Inventory Interpretive Report for Correctional Settings (PAI-CS). Odessa, FL, Psychological Assessment Resources, 2005

Forth AE, Kosson DS, Hare RD: The Hare Psychopathy Checklist: Youth Version. North Tonawanda, NY, Multi-Health Systems, 2003

Gacano CB, Meloy JR: The Rorschach Assessment of Aggressive and Psychopathic Personalities. Mahwah, NJ, Lawrence Erlbaum, 1994

Greco C, Cornell D: Rorschach object relations of adolescents who committed homicide. J Pers Assess 59:574–583, 1992

Greene RL: The MMPI-2: An Interpretive Manual, 2nd Edition. Boston, MA, Allyn & Bacon, 2000

Hanson RK, Bussiere MT: Predicting relapse: a meta-analysis of sexual offender recidivism studies. J Consult Clin Psychol 66:348–362, 1998

Hare RD: The Hare Psychopathy Checklist–Revised, 2nd Edition. North Tonawanda, NY, Multi-Health Systems, 1991

Hart SD, Cox D, Hare RD: The Hare Psychopathy Checklist: Screening Version. North Tonawanda, NY, Multi-Health Systems, 1995

Laws DR, Hanson RK, Osborn CA, et al: Classification of child molesters by plethysmographic assessment of sexual arousal and a self-report measure of sexual preference. J Interpers Violence 15:1297–1312, 2000

Lillienfeld SO, Wood JM, Garb HN: The scientific status of projective techniques. Psychological Science in the Public Interest 1:27–66, 2000

Miller FG, Roberts J, Brooks MK, et al: SASSI-3: Substance Abuse Subtle Screening Inventory, 3rd Edition. Springville, IN, SASSI Institute, 1988

Millon T: The Millon Clinical Multiaxial Inventory–III Manual. Minneapolis, MN, National Computer Systems, 1994

Monahan J, Steadman H, Silver E, et al: Rethinking Risk Assessment: The MacArthur Study of Mental Disorder and Violence. New York, Oxford University Press, 2001

Morey LC: Personality Assessment Inventory Professional Manual. Odessa, FL, Psychological Assessment Resources, 1991

Morey LC, Quigley BD: The use of the Personality Assessment Inventory (PAI) in assessing offenders. Int J Offender Ther Comp Criminol 46:333–349, 2002

Murphy WD, Haynes MR, Worley PJ: Assessment of adult sexual interest, in Clinical Approaches to Sex Offenders and Their Victims. Edited by Hollin CR, Howells H. Chichester, UK, Wiley, 1991

Novaco RW: Anger as a risk factor for violence among mentally disordered, in Violence and Mental Disorders: Developments in Risk Assessment. Edited by Monahan J, Steadman HJ. Chicago, IL, University of Chicago Press, 1994

Osberg TM, Poland DL: Validity of the MMPI-2 Basic and Harris-Lingoes subscales in a forensic sample. J Clin Psychol 87:1369–1380, 2001

Paulhus DL: Paulhus Deception Scales. Toronto, ON, Canada, Multi-Health Systems, 1998

Spielberger C: State-Trait Anger Expression Inventory Professional Manual. Odessa, FL, Psychological Assessment Resources, 1988

PART II
Mental Disorders and Conditions

CHAPTER 5

Mood Disorders

Rif S. El-Mallakh, M.D.
R. Jeannie Roberts, M.D.
Peggy L. El-Mallakh, Ph.D.

Mood disturbances and violence are intimately related in a variety of ways. Violence may play a role in the development of subsequent mood disorders and can exacerbate or perpetuate existing mood disorders. Alternatively, violence may be a consequence or correlate of a mood disturbance. In addition, several biological, social, and psychological factors that are associated with violence and aggression frequently co-exist with mood disturbances, so that co-occurring violence and mood disturbances are frequently seen in individuals or systems. In these situations, violence can be directed toward self, others, or property.

Violence in the Genesis of Mood Disturbances

Exposure to violence is a major predictor of subsequent depressive symptoms. This has been repeatedly documented in a wide range of studies.

Passive Exposure

Witness to Domestic Violence

Early life experiences can affect both the biology and behavior of an individual. For example, abuse or neglect of young individuals will influence the development of mood disorders and problem behaviors later in life. Miller (2005) reported that childhood abuse and exposure to trauma may be linked to increased production and secretion of cortisol and epinephrine, which have been linked to depression and anxiety. Research also suggests that infants exposed to domestic violence between their parents can exhibit signs of trauma and some behavioral problems, such as aggression (Bogat et al. 2006; Whitaker et al. 2006). However, Bogat et al. (2006) suggested that passive exposure to parental violence does not alter an infant's temperament.

As children grow older, passive exposure to violence between their parents can have more dramatic effects. As many as 10%–24% of children may be exposed to intimate partner violence (IPV) between their parents or to other family violence (Martin et al. 2006; Silverstein et al. 2006). Martin et al. (2006) maintained that exposure to violence occurs prior to age 11 in 80% of families with IPV. If community violence is included, the rate of adolescents who have witnessed violence may be as high as 40% (Hanson et al. 2006). Prevalence rates of depression and anxiety are increased in adolescents and young adults (ages 13–21) who experience passive exposure to IPV (Hindin and Gultiano 2006; Martin et al. 2006). Young women may be at greater risk than young men (Hindin and Gultiano 2006). In addition, Hazen et al. (2006) reported that problem behaviors increase in children ages 4–14 years who experience passive exposure to IPV in the home. Behavioral problems span both internalizing (e.g., depression, low self-esteem) and externalizing problems (e.g., aggression, acting out) (Hazen et al. 2006). These effects are independent of maternal depression (Hazen et al. 2006; Martin et al. 2006). This is an important observation, because maternal depression is associated with an increase in adolescent depression and school dysfunction but not an increase in problematic behavior (Peiponen et al. 2006; Silverstein et al. 2006). Sternberg et al. (2006) found that exposure to family violence in older children, ages 10–16 years, also increased subsequent depression and behavioral problems; this effect was greater for girls than boys.

Parental Substance Abuse

Parental substance abuse can result in both direct and indirect problems for children. At the very least, children of substance-abusing parents are neglected. However, more frequently, substance abuse is associated with a variety of factors that independently or in combination can be quite harmful. These include domestic violence and several forms of abuse, including verbal, emotional, physical, and sexual abuse. Parental substance abuse is associated with an increased risk of depression, aggression, behavioral problems, and substance abuse in the children (Edwards et al. 2006; Hanson et al. 2006; Peiponen et al. 2006; Sher et al. 2005; Whitaker et al. 2006).

Direct Abuse or Neglect

Childhood abuse and neglect are clearly associated with a substantial increase in the risk for subsequent depression and maladaptive behaviors (Cukor and McGinn 2006; Reigstad et al. 2006; Widom et al. 2007). This is true in all cultures in which it has been studied (Afifi 2006).

Verbal and Emotional Abuse

The experience of verbal abuse during childhood (e.g., "You are stupid") increases depression, anger, and hostility in young adults (Sachs-Ericsson et al. 2006; Teicher et al. 2006). Verbal and emotional abuse influence the development of self-concept and lead to a self-critical style of cognitive processing that contributes to low self-esteem (Cukor and McGinn 2006; Sachs-Ericsson et al. 2006). This impaired self-image may be one of the underlying phenomena that increase the risk of subsequent sexual victimization as a young adult (Rich et al. 2005).

Physical Abuse

Physical abuse may be a major contributing factor in the development of violence in later life (Huizinga et al. 2006). Physical abuse is also pivotal in the development of depression in youth and on into adulthood (Cukor and McGinn 2006; Reigstad et al. 2006; Widom et al. 2007; Wright et al. 2004). Physical abuse may occur in either the home environment or in school. Bullying is a form of verbal and physical violence that can have major impact on development. The odds of experiencing social problems and depression with suicidal ideation and attempts are 3.9 times higher among victims of bullying compared with nonvictims (Brunstein Klomek et al. 2007; Kim et al. 2006). Furthermore, bullying behaviors have been linked to mood disturbances. The odds of bullies developing social problems, depression, and suicidality are 1.8 times higher compared with people who are not bullies, and bullies who are also targets of other bullies are 4.9 times as likely to develop social problems (Brunstein Klomek et al. 2007; Kim et al. 2006). High-profile school shooters such as those at Columbine High School or Virginia Tech had been bullied by classmates.

Sexual Abuse

Sexual abuse of children is associated with a wide variety of physical and psychological sequelae, many of which are lifelong. Early sexual abuse is associated with a significant increase in depression in both males and females (Conway et al. 2004; Gladstone et al. 2004; Martin et al. 2004; Peleikis et al. 2005). The risk of subsequent suicide attempts is 15 times higher in boys who experience early sexual abuse compared with nonabused boys (Martin et al. 2004); among women, suicide ideation is 4.5 times higher (Masho et al. 2005). The consequences of childhood sexual abuse include greater severity of depressive illness in adult patients over age 50 (Gamble et al. 2006; McGuigan and Middlemiss 2005). Adult women who have experienced childhood sexual abuse are more likely to be victims of violence (Gladstone et al. 2004) and other forms of trauma, including sexual assault (Banyard et al. 2002; Rich et al. 2005). Sexual abuse perpetrated by adult women can be just as harmful as sexual abuse perpetrated by men (Denov 2004).

Adult Assault

After personality development is complete, adult assaults (sexual or physical) can increase the likelihood of the development of mood disturbances (Johansen et al. 2006). Consequences of being a victim of assault include depression, anxiety disorders, and substance abuse; these can persist for decades (Acierno et al. 2007).

Intimate Partner Violence

Intimate partner violence, perhaps the most common type of violence in our society, is pervasive throughout several socioeconomic classes and ethnic groups. Thirty percent of African American women seeking medical care in a large public hospital reported severe IPV (Paranjape et al. 2007), and 54% of women attending a rural family practice clinic reported IPV (Coker et al. 2005). Researchers have estimated that 10%–24% of representative samples of children may be exposed to IPV (Martin et al. 2006; Silverstein et al. 2006). In addition, 13% of middle-class women also have experienced IPV (Anderson et al. 2002). Exposure to IPV is associated with a significant increase in the risk for both depression and posttraumatic stress disorder (PTSD; Avdibegovic and Sinanovic 2006; Bonomi et al. 2006; Houry et al. 2006; Lipsky et al. 2005; Paranjape et al. 2007; Varma et al. 2006) as well as more medical problems, reduced functioning, and increased medical disability (Bonomi et al. 2006; Coker et al. 2005). Depression risk is almost 6 times higher in women who are victims of IPV compared with those who are not, and PTSD is 9.4 times higher (Houry et al. 2006). Sexual IPV is specifically associated with an increase in depression and suicide ideation (Pico-Alfonso et al. 2006); Houry et al. (2006) have observed that suicidal ideation in women who have experienced IPV is 17.5 times higher compared with women who have not experienced IPV. However, depression frequently predates the episodes of IPV, and the presence of depression in young women actually increases the likelihood of dating-violence (Foshee et al. 2004; Rivera-Rivera et al. 2006). African American women may be at particular risk for mood disturbances due to high rates of IPV; 18% also abuse alcohol, which can worsen prognosis (Paranjape et al. 2007). Women in abusive relationships have a great need for emotional support (Theran et al. 2006), and African American women appear to obtain much support through spirituality and affiliation with religious institutions (Mitchell et al. 2006; Watlington and Murphy 2006).

Community Violence, War, and Terrorism

Although violence at a personal level is a major factor in the development of mood disturbances, violence at the community level also contributes to subsequent depression, suicidal ideation, and suicide attempts. For example, community violence can increase the risk of depressive symptoms in adolescents, particularly girls (Goldstein et al. 2007; Hammack et al. 2004).

Terrorists count on the psychological impact of indirect violence to achieve their aims. After the September 11, 2001, attacks in New York and Washington, D.C., and the March 11, 2004, attack in Madrid, Spain, there was an increase in the prevalence rates of major depression (9.4% prevalence in New York City and 8% in Madrid, compared with 6.4% in population-based surveys [Kessler et al. 2006]) and, to a lesser degree, PTSD (Miguel-Tobal et al. 2006; Person et al. 2006). This increase was also associated with a 49% increase in suicide attempts along the East coast of the United States after the September 11 attacks (Starkman 2006).

Gaylord (2006) has estimated that 10%–17% of combat veterans will experience psychiatric problems, including PTSD and depression. These disorders may last for long periods of time after the end of hostilities (Fiedler et al. 2006). However, among civilians who are trapped in war zones or are direct targets of attacks or abuse, rates of PTSD have been estimated at almost 33%, and rates of depression are approximately 41% (Hashemian et al. 2006; Loncar et al. 2006).

Treatment Approaches

Pharmacological approaches to treatment are geared toward treating the depression and PTSD that may be associated with past or current exposure to violence. In addition, researchers have investigated the effectiveness of various forms of psychotherapy in the treatment of depression and PTSD resulting from exposure to violence; these include supportive therapy, cognitive-behavioral therapy, and forgiveness therapy (Deblinger et al. 2006; Reed and Enright 2006). Focused therapies such as cognitive-behavioral or forgiveness therapy appear to be more effective than unfocused supportive therapy (Deblinger et al. 2006; Reed and Enright 2006). Forgiveness therapy has been central to national attempts at healing past abuse, such as the South African Truth and Reconciliation Commission (Potter 2006). Adult treatment for childhood abuse is effective in reducing symptoms and dysfunction (Martsolf and Draucker 2005). The approach for women involved in IPV depends on the timing of the abuse. Women in a current abusive relationship benefit more from emotional support, whereas women with past abuse require practical support (Theran et al. 2006).

Prevention is a critically important focus for those at risk for developing violence-related mood disturbances. Identification of children at greatest risk due to violence or substance abuse in their families, and provision of appropriate support to prevent depression, aggression, substance abuse, and future victimization, would be the ideal approach (Sternberg et al. 2006). Past abuse predicts future abuse; policymakers can use this knowledge to direct appropriate resources toward prevention of future abuse among those at risk.

Case Example 1

Ms. A is a 36-year-old woman who presented to the emergency psychiatric service with a complaint of worsening depression and suicidal ideation. She had a previous psychiatric history of recurrent major depression since adolescence, PTSD, and prescription benzodiazepine abuse. She was not currently in treatment but had been treated in the past with psychotherapy and a variety of antidepressant, anxiolytic, and antipsychotic medications. She had had three previous hospitalizations, all associated with suicide attempts. The current episode began when her boyfriend, with whom she lived, had become more abusive. He had attempted to strangle her and had then raped her after an argument about his alcohol abuse. She reported a remote history of childhood emotional abuse by an alcoholic father prior to her parents' divorce and sexual molestation by her mother's boyfriend when she was 13 years old.

Ms. A was admitted to a crisis stabilization unit for 10 days, started on an antidepressant (sertraline, 100 mg/day), and engaged in supportive and insight-oriented psychotherapy. After discharge she engaged in outpatient psychotherapy and pharmacotherapy. She continued to complain of anxiety, and due to her history of benzodiazepine abuse, gabapentin was started and increased to 1,200 mg three times daily. She reconciled with her abusive boyfriend after he stopped using alcohol. However, the relationship remained tumultuous, and he relapsed into alcohol abuse again soon after the reconciliation. As the chaos in the relationship increased, the patient dropped out of treatment and was lost to follow-up.

This case illustrates many of the relationships among violence, victimization, and mood disturbance. Early verbal and emotional abuse led to Ms. A's low self-esteem. Early sexual abuse contributed to her role as a victim. These early experiences contributed to early-onset depression and worsening of these symptoms in adulthood. Similarly, they allowed Ms. A to be tolerant of her role as victim and allow herself to return to, and remain within, an emotionally, physically, and sexually abusive relationship. The severity of the ongoing depressive and anxiety symptoms had previously led the patient to prescription benzodiazepine abuse. Despite participation in both psychotherapy and pharmacotherapy, she returned to her previous maladaptive behaviors.

Summary

Aggression and depression are intimately related. Early exposure to aggression, either as a witness or as a victim, increases the likelihood of depression, the chronicity of depression, and the likelihood of becoming a perpetrator of future aggression. Similarly, early abuse increases the risk of subsequent victimization and chronic depression.

Mood Disorders in the Genesis of Violence

As noted earlier, violence and aggression are associated with subsequent onset of mood and anxiety symptoms as well as full depressive and posttraumatic stress disorders. However, mood disorders have also been identified as a precursor to the onset of aggression. The presence of a mood disorder increases the likelihood of an individual's being a victim of violence (Brunstein Klomek et al. 2007; Lehrer et al. 2006) and a perpetuator of violence (Brunstein Klomek et al. 2007).

Depression in adolescents is one of the major predictors of aggression, violence (a more extreme form of aggression) (Blitstein et al. 2005; Teicher et al. 2006), or oppositional and delinquent behaviors (Rowe et al. 2006). Major depressive disorder and bipolar disorder are both associated with an increase in irritability, aggression, and potential violence against others and self (Grunebaum et al. 2006; Knox et al. 2000; Najt et al. 2007; North et al. 1994; Schuepbach et al. 2006). Bipolar illness, in particular, may be associated with aggression due to the nature of its core symptoms of irritability, lability, grandiosity, and paranoia (Feldmann 2001; Swann 1999).

Patients with bipolar disorder who were admitted involuntarily to an inpatient unit were more likely to have comorbid substance abuse and up to three times more likely to be aggressive after admission (Barlow et al. 2000; Schuepbach et al. 2006). An analysis of 576 consecutive admissions for mania suggested that acute mania may have four distinct phenomenological subtypes: pure, aggressive, psychotic, and depressive (mixed) mania (Sato et al. 2002). When a patient's illness recurs, the profile of symptoms, including aggression, remains relatively consistent (Cassidy et al. 2002), supporting the clinical notion that there is a high association between past and future violence. The increase in aggression associated with mania is associated with an increase in legal problems. Whereas patients with schizophrenia or schizoaffective illnesses are more likely to be arrested (Grossman et al. 1995), patients with bipolar disorder are more likely than those with unipolar depression to have legal problems (Calabrese et al. 2006). At the time of their arrest, a large number of bipolar subjects were manic (74.2% of the 66 subjects studied) and/or psychotic (59%) (Quanbeck et al. 2004). Many of these patients had already come to the attention of the healthcare system and had recently been discharged from an inpatient unit but had not attended their outpatient follow-up (Quanbeck et al. 2004). This may explain why bipolar subjects are overrepresented among sex offenders, with approximately 35% of sex offenders having a bipolar disorder (usually with comorbid antisocial personality disorder or substance abuse) (Dunsieth et al. 2004; McElroy et al. 1999).

However, aggression can also occur during depressive episodes. In bipolar patients, aggression can be a relatively common presentation of agitated depression (Maj et al. 2003). Aggression is also common in unipolar depression (Posternak and Zimmerman 2002). A syndrome of high irritability and other hypomanic symptoms in unipolar depressed patients has been labeled *mixed depression* (Sato et al. 2005) and may be associated with significant aggression (Sato et al. 2005).

The effect of antidepressant medications in the treatment of aggression is unclear. Antidepressant treatment has been variously reported to increase and decrease aggression (Bond 2005; Goedhard et al. 2006; Healy et al. 2006; Mitchell 2005). If there is an anti-aggression effect of antidepressants, it is weak (Goedhard et al. 2006). An increase in aggression associated with antidepressant use may possibly occur exclusively in individuals with bipolar disorder or occult bipolar disorder—that is, those in whom an episode of mania has not yet occurred.

Antipsychotic medications or mood stabilizers are generally used to treat aggression (Afaq et al. 2002; Barzman et al. 2006). Valproate is perhaps one of the best studied agents and has been found to be superior

Mood Disorders

to other antiepileptics such as topiramate (Gobbi et al. 2006) or oxcarbazepine (MacMillan et al. 2006) A meta-analysis of controlled trials suggests that the effect of these interventions is generally small (Goedhard et al. 2006). Dopamine antagonist antipsychotic medications may be minimally better than serotonin-dopamine antagonist medications (Goedhard et al. 2006). Effective pharmacological treatment approaches to reduce aggression and violence in those with mood disturbances are greatly needed.

Case Example 2

Mr. B was a 34-year-old white man with a history of bipolar disorder. He reported that he experienced frequent "mood swings." He described these as brief periods (minutes to hours) in which he quickly lost his temper. During these periods, he could become aggressive toward strangers or toward significant others to whom he was emotionally attached. He reported frequent fights and previous arrests for assault. Mr. B also had a history of significant alcohol and marijuana abuse, which he minimized. He denied that his marijuana use was a problem and stated that it helped him calm down. He also did not view his alcohol abuse as a problem because he did not "drink every day" and maintained that he could quit "at any time." On questioning, he reported episodes of reduced sleep, reduced need for sleep, increased irritability, increased rapid thoughts and distractibility, and increased involvement in multiple problematic behaviors. These periods lasted 4–5 days and occurred three or four times annually. He also reported periods of depression that were generally brief, lasting only 2 weeks, during which he also manifested irritability, loss of interest, loss of pleasure, low self-esteem, increased frustration, and suicidal ideation. He reported that he had used both alcohol and marijuana during these episodes. He had no periods of significant sobriety. A tentative diagnosis of type II bipolar disorder was made, along with intermittent explosive disorder and alcohol and marijuana abuse. Mr. B was offered treatment with divalproex and psychotherapy and was encouraged to attend treatment for substance abuse. He never sought out substance abuse treatment and never stopped using marijuana, but he had brief periods in which he stopped using alcohol. These periods of abstinence from alcohol generally lasted less than 1 month. His compliance with divalproex and psychotherapy was very poor. He continued to have periods of depression and impulsive rage, and he continued to abuse alcohol and marijuana. Two years after his initial presentation, Mr. B committed suicide with a self-inflicted gunshot wound.

Mr. B's case illustrates typical characteristics of a difficult patient with comorbid mood disorder and substance abuse. Unlike Ms. A, Mr. B had not experienced extreme adversity. His aggressive behavior was common and usually directed at others. His depression was probably made worse by his substance use. Marijuana users frequently believe that marijuana use is calming and reduces aggression (Arendt et al. 2007); however, marijuana use is specifically associated with an increase in violence (Maremmani et al. 2004). Ultimately, Mr. B directed the aggression against himself.

Summary

Aggression is common in individuals who are experiencing an episode of mania, and there may be a subtype of mania in which aggression is the core feature. Aggression may also be common in unipolar major depression. The effect of antidepressants on aggression is unclear. If there is an anti-aggression effect of these agents, it is weak. Most commonly, the mood-stabilizing antiepileptic medications and antipsychotic medications are used to treat aggression, but their anti-aggression effect appears to be weak.

Mood Disorders and Violence Toward the Self

Deliberate Self-Harm

Violence can be directed toward the self as an act of nonsuicidal self-harm. Tuisku et al. (2006) defined *self-harm* as "direct, socially unaccepted, repetitive behavior that causes minor to moderate physical injury." Deliberate self-harm (DSH) "appears to reflect an externalizing response in an isolated individual who has commonly been exposed to earlier deprivational experiences" (Parker et al. 2005). Risk factors for DSH include early onset of mood symptoms, recent diagnosis, young age, family history of suicide, and comorbid disorders, especially anxiety disorders and substance abuse (particularly alcohol). It is important to make the distinction between DSH and suicidal intent; whereas DSH is self-directed injury without any suicidal intent and frequently with the goal of reducing anxiety or dysphoria, suicide is a self-destructive act with a specific intent to end one's life. Despite this distinction, it remains a fact that individuals with DSH also have a higher risk for subsequent suicide (Groholt et al. 2000).

Deliberate Self-Harm and Depression

Although DSH is almost always associated with dysphoria, it is not always associated with the syndrome of depression. DSH can occur in the setting of depression associated with both bipolar disorder and unipolar major depressive disorder. Haw et al. (2001) looked at a cohort of

Mood Disorders

106 patients who presented to a hospital following an episode of DSH and found that 92% of these patients had a psychiatric diagnosis and that the most common diagnosis was affective disorder (72% using ICD-10 criteria).

As stated earlier (see "Violence in the Genesis of Mood Disturbances"), early adverse life events have a major impact on subsequent mood states. Similarly, early adversity is a major correlate of subsequent DSH behaviors (Gladstone et al. 2004; Parker et al. 2005). Gladstone et al. (2004) examined DSH behaviors, personality characteristics, and childhood variables, including parental styles and childhood sexual/physical abuse, among 125 women with depressive disorders. Findings indicated that participants who were victims of childhood sexual assaults were more likely to engage in DSH as adults (Gladstone et al. 2004). In addition, respondents who were victims of childhood sexual abuse became depressed earlier in life than nonabused control subjects (Gladstone et al. 2004).

Adolescents with DSH generally have less severe depressive symptoms than individuals with suicidal ideation but more severe symptoms than those without any history of self-injurious ideation. In a community sample, adolescents who have a history of self-harm reported more depressive symptoms than those without a self-harm history (Muehlenkamp and Gutierrez 2004). In a study of 218 adolescents, ages 13–19, who were receiving outpatient treatment for a depressive mood disorder, adolescents who had DSH behavior had less severe depressive symptoms than those with suicidal ideation or suicide attempts (Tuisku et al. 2006). Similarly, among adults, the degree of seriousness of a self-injurious act was associated with depression and intent. In a study of 49 prisoners in Germany, measures of depression and hopelessness were both highly correlated with suicidal intent and lethality; less lethal methods were not correlated with depression (Lohner and Konrad 2006). Impulsive acts of self-harm were rarely associated with depression (Lohner and Konrad 2006).

DSH behaviors are not fixed over the lifetime. For example, 70% of 132 adolescents who had deliberately poisoned themselves and who were followed up for 6 years stopped the self-harm behaviors within 3 years of the index event (Harrington et al. 2006). DSH continued into adulthood mainly among those with psychiatric disorders. Only 56% of these study participants had a psychiatric disorder, and the most common psychiatric diagnosis was depression (Harrington et al. 2006). DSH behaviors may appear *de novo* in the elderly. Lamprecht et al. (2005) looked at older people presenting to an acute hospital with an episode of DSH. Sexual distribution among males and females was equal.

Only 37% had a major depressive illness at the time of the DSH assessment, but 21% of the males had no psychiatric diagnoses at the time of the DSH (Lamprecht et al. 2005).

In young adults, the lack of depression in subjects with DSH has also been noted. Among 1,986 high-functioning military recruits (62% male), only 10% of those with a history of DSH reported depressive symptoms on the Beck Depression Inventory (Klonsky et al. 2003). Peers viewed self-harmers as having strange and intense emotions and a heightened sensitivity to interpersonal rejection (Klonsky et al. 2003).

Given that DSH may not necessarily be associated with depression, why does it occur? Tzemou and Birchwood (2007) examined dysfunctional thinking patterns and intrusive memories in patients diagnosed with both unipolar depressive and bipolar mood disorders. They recruited 49 participants diagnosed with major depression or manic or hypomanic episodes. Twenty healthy control subjects were also recruited from the same areas in Central England. Compared with the healthy controls, dysfunctional attitudes were abnormal in the mood-disordered groups when ill (Tzemou and Birchwood 2007). Interestingly, whereas dysfunctional attitudes resolved in bipolar subjects as they became euthymic, they persisted into euthymia for those diagnosed with unipolar major depression (Tzemou and Birchwood 2007).

Deliberate Self-Harm and Bipolar Illness

Intentional self-harm in mania is rare and is probably related to the depressed mood that can occur during manic episodes (Ostacher and Eidelman 2006). However, DSH is more common during bipolar depressions than it is in unipolar depressive illness (Parker et al. 2005). Parker et al. (2005) reported that across samples of depressed individuals, more individuals with bipolar disorder tended to report DSH behaviors compared with those with unipolar depression. Smith et al. (2005) examined the prevalence rates of bipolar disorders and major depression among 87 young adults with recurrent depression; 83.9% of study respondents met criteria for major depressive disorder, and 16.1% met criteria for a DSM-IV-TR–defined (American Psychiatric Association 2000) bipolar disorder. The authors reported that among the respondents diagnosed with major depression, 45.7% had a history of DSH and 13.0% had a history of a previous suicide attempt. Of the 14 respondents diagnosed with bipolar disorder, 71.4% had DSH and 28.6% had a history of deliberate self-harm.

One of the best-known occurrences of DSH was that performed by the Dutch artist Vincent van Gogh (1853–1890), who had bipolar disorder (Jamison 1993). On Christmas Eve in 1888, van Gogh cut off his own earlobe with a razor blade as he was apparently attempting to attack an acquaintance. Following this episode of self-harm, van Gogh exhibited alternating states of "madness and lucidity" and received treatment in an asylum in Saint-Remy. Two months after his discharge from the asylum, he committed suicide by shooting himself "for the good of all" (Van Gogh Gallery 2007).

Mood Disorders and Suicide

Suicide, the act of ending one's life, is the most dramatic form of self-harm. Epidemiological research indicates that in 2004, 31,484 individuals in the United States died from suicide or self-inflicted injury (10.8 per 100,000 population; Centers for Disease Control and Prevention 2006). Extensive research has examined risk factors for suicide, and several studies have identified a history of prior suicide attempts as a very strong predictor of suicide risk (American Psychiatric Association 2003; Borges et al. 2006; Gaynes et al. 2004). Certain sociodemographic characteristics have also been associated with high suicide risk. These include male gender, European American ethnicity, and advanced age. However, the National Comorbidity Survey Replication Study found that low-income, "non-Hispanic Black" (p. 1750) ethnicity and age younger than 45 years were significant correlates of suicide ideation (Borges et al. 2006). Additional risk factors include the presence of a psychiatric disorder (particularly depression), alcohol abuse, physical and sexual abuse, and a family history of suicide (Gaynes et al. 2004). Psychiatric disorders may be present in up to 90% of those who commit suicide (American Psychiatric Association 2003). Divorced, separated, or widowed individuals have a higher risk of suicide (American Psychiatric Association 2003). Conversely, high-conflict or violent marriages may increase the risk for suicide among married individuals (American Psychiatric Association 2003).

Unipolar Depression and Suicide

Numerous studies have identified depression as a significant risk factor for suicide. This contributes to mortality rates associated with depression that are approximately 20 times higher than the general population (American Psychiatric Association 2003). The fraction of people who have committed suicide that were depressed at the time of their death has been estimated to range from 15% (Rich et al. 1986) to 97.5% (Sinclair et al. 2005). However, most studies, including those based on psychological autopsies, estimate a rate of 30%–34% (Arato et al. 1988; Foster et al.

1999; Henriksson et al. 1993). The fraction of adolescent suicides that involve depression may be slightly higher, at 43% (Brent et al. 1993).

Comorbid psychiatric conditions may additionally increase the risk for suicide. Paramount among these is co-occurring substance use, which accounts for some 45% of completed suicides (Rich et al. 1986). Additionally, aggression (Dervic et al. 2006; Keilp et al. 2006) and Cluster B personality disorders (Dervic et al. 2006) are associated with suicide attempts in depressed individuals with a history of childhood sexual abuse.

A decline in depression and hopelessness was associated with a decline in suicidal ideation in 198 people diagnosed with major depression (Sokero et al. 2006). There is a close correlation between the increased use of antidepressants and an observed decline in overall suicide rate (Gibbons et al. 2006; Korkeila et al. 2007), but this trend may have begun prior to the introduction of antidepressants (Safer and Zito 2007). Antidepressants may have no effect on suicide ideation (Hammad et al. 2006) or may actually increase the risk of suicide attempts among depressed adults (Tiihonen et al. 2006) and suicide ideation among adolescents (Bridge et al. 2007; Dubicka et al. 2006), but they may reduce completed suicides (Tiihonen et al. 2006). The U.S. Food and Drug Administration has placed a warning on all antidepressants that they may increase suicidal ideation in adolescents (Kuehn 2007). Although lithium is rarely used in major depressive disorder, it appears to have an antisuicide effect similar to that seen in bipolar illness (Guzzetta et al. 2007).

Bipolar Disorder and Suicide

Lifetime prevalence of all bipolar disorders is approximately 2%; bipolar type I disorder has an incidence rate of 0.8% compared with 1.2% for bipolar II disorder. Suicide risk is high in bipolar disorder. Angst and Preisig (1995) followed up 406 patients for 36 years; their findings indicated that 11% committed suicide regardless of whether they were diagnosed with type I or type II disorder. Other estimates approach 19% (Ostacher and Eidelman 2006). This risk appears higher than in unipolar major depression. Chen and Dilsaver (1996) examined data from the Epidemiologic Catchment Area study to estimate lifetime rates of suicide attempts in mood disorders; findings indicated that 29.2% of respondents with bipolar disorder attempted suicide compared with 15.9% of those with unipolar depressive disorder.

Additionally, when subjects with bipolar disorder attempt suicide, the lethality of that attempt may be greater. Among 2,395 hospital admissions of patients with unipolar depression and bipolar disorder, subjects with bipolar disorder had a higher incidence of more lethal suicide attempts (Raja and Azzoni 2004). The odds of completed suicide in those with bipolar disorder is 2.0 times higher compared with those with unipolar depression (Raja and Azzoni 2004). However, prevalence rates of suicide may be inflated, because researchers typically focus on hospitalized patients and those who have received treatment from a mental health provider. This self-selected population may be more ill compared with those who receive treatment from primary care providers or those who do not receive any psychiatric treatment.

Risk for suicide is highest during a depressive episode of bipolar disorder. Isometsa et al. (1994) found that among patients diagnosed with bipolar disorder, 80% of completed suicides occurred during a depressive episode. Mortality from suicide in persons with bipolar depression may be 30 times that of normal control subjects (Ostacher and Eidelman 2006). However, suicidal ideation and suicide completions may occur during the mixed (Dilsaver et al. 1994) or even manic phase (Cassidy and Carroll 2001). Rapid cycling also carries a higher likelihood for more serious suicide attempts but not an increase in completed suicides compared with other types of episodes (42% vs. 27%; MacKinnon et al. 2003).

Suicide risk is highest in newly diagnosed bipolar patients. Fagiolini et al. (2004) found that among 104 patients with bipolar disorder, 50% attempted suicide within 7.5 years of the initial onset of the illness (either mania or depression). In these young bipolar patients, suicide rarely occurs during episodes of mania.

Lithium appears to have a clear effect on reducing completed suicide in bipolar patients, with a fivefold reduction in relative risk (Baldessarini et al. 2006; Tondo et al. 2001). More impressively, lithium reduces nonsuicidal DSH and nonpsychiatric mortality in bipolar patients (Cipriani et al. 2005).

Case Example 3

Mr. C was a 66-year-old married white man with a lifelong history of alcohol abuse and depression. He had been treated intermittently with antidepressants but never persisted in psychiatric treatment for more than 3 months. He had had a chaotic relationship with his wife of 44 years and had been verbally and physically abusive. For unknown reasons, in the setting of ongoing alcohol abuse, he shot and killed his wife and then killed himself.

Suicide and homicide are ultimately two sides of the same coin. Individuals who commit suicide are more likely to have a history of violence. In enmeshed relationships, homicide-suicide is frequently seen as the only solution.

Summary

DSH behaviors frequently occur independently of suicide and should be considered separate phenomena. However, individuals who engage in DSH are at a higher risk of subsequent suicide. Subjects who engage in DSH behavior have generally experienced early abuse. Both major depression and bipolar illness are significant risk factors for completed suicides. Bipolar disorder carries a much higher risk for completed suicide than does major depression. Comorbid disorders, particularly substance abuse, increase the suicide risk. Antidepressants may increase suicide ideation but do not appear to increase completed suicides and may reduce the severity of suicide attempts. Lithium has a clear antisuicide effect in both bipolar illness and unipolar major depression.

The Biology of Aggression in Mood Disorders

There are many biological associations between mood symptoms and aggression or violence. These include increased aggression with increased cytokine activity (Zalcman and Siegel 2006), catecholamine metabolism (Volavka et al. 2004), testosterone (Pope et al. 2000), and hypothalamic-pituitary-adrenal axis dysfunction (Malkesman et al. 2006; Shea et al. 2005). However, the most consistent findings are associations with the serotonergic system.

Among the many findings associated with serotonergic dysfunction in aggression, platelet serotonin 2A receptor (5-HT$_{2A}$) binding was increased in subjects with trait aggression (Lauterbach et al. 2006). Prefrontal cortical 5-HT$_{2A}$ binding was also increased in aggressive suicidal patients (Oquendo et al. 2006). Similarly, relative increases in plasma tryptophan levels (a precursor to serotonin) are associated with increased aggression and hostility (Lauterbach et al. 2006; Suarez and Krishnan 2006). Lower cerebrospinal fluid 5-hydroxyindoleacetic acid concentration was independently associated with severity of lifetime aggressivity and a history of a higher-lethality suicide attempt and may be part of the diathesis for these behaviors. The dopamine and norepinephrine systems do not appear to be as significantly involved in suicidal acts, aggression, or depression (Placidi et al. 2002). However, the most compelling findings regarding the involvement of serotonin in both mood disturbance and violence is found in the serotonin transporter polymorphisms.

Mood Disorders

Several recent studies have investigated the role of polymorphisms in the serotonin reuptake pump or the serotonin transporter gene (*5HTTLPR*). A common polymorphism of this gene is a deletion in the area of the gene that regulates its transcription into messenger RNA and ultimate translation into expressed protein—the promoter region. Individuals with this deletion, called the short or "s" allele, express fewer serotonin transporters. Individuals who are homozygous for the "s" allele (*ss*) are more likely to develop depression (odds ratio, 1.5–179; Cervilla et al. 2006) and depression after a traumatic event (Caspi et al. 2003; Kaufman et al. 2004). Thus, the observed link between early life adversity, or later life trauma, and subsequent depression, is related, at least in part, to having the *ss* genotype (Caspi et al. 2003; Kaufman et al. 2004). Although stressful life events or extreme adversity are clearly associated with subsequent depression, adversity is quite potent in inducing depression in subjects with the *ss* genotype, such that the dosage of adversity required to produce depression is much lower in individuals homozygous for the short form of *5HTTLPR* (Cervilla et al. 2007). Several studies have also found that the *ss* genotype is also associated with subclinical depressive symptoms in individuals without depression (Gonda and Bagdy 2006; Gonda et al. 2005, 2006).

The *ss* genotype of *5HTTLPR* is also associated with aggression. In a case control study of conduct disorder with or without aggression, it was found that the *ss* genotype was strongly associated with aggression but not conduct disorder without aggression (Sakai et al. 2006). A positron emission tomography study of *5HTTLPR* density found that reduced transporter density is associated with impulsive aggression (Frankle et al. 2005). Although this study did not examine the genotype of the study subjects, it found that the phenotype that is expected with the *ss* genotype is associated with aggression (Frankle et al. 2005). Among schizophrenic patients who attempted suicide, the *ss* genotype of *5HTTLPR* was associated with violent suicide attempts but was not associated with nonviolent suicide attempts or with nonattempters (Bayle et al. 2003)

Key Points

- Early exposure to aggression, either as a witness or as a victim, increases the likelihood of future depression, the severity and chronicity of future depressions, and the likelihood of perpetrating future aggression.

- Early abuse increases the likelihood of subsequent victimization.
- Early sexual abuse increases the likelihood of subsequent sexual victimization.
- Substance abuse increases the risk for perpetrating violence, becoming a victim of violence, and depression related to exposure to violence. Conversely, exposure to violence increases the risk of subsequent substance abuse.
- Aggression is common in individuals who are experiencing an episode of mania. There may be a subtype of mania in which aggression is the core feature.
- Aggression may also be common in unipolar major depression.
- The effect of antidepressants on aggression is unclear. If there is an anti-aggression effect, it is weak.
- Mood-stabilizing antiepileptic and antipsychotic medications are used to treat aggression independent of diagnosis, but again, any anti-aggression effect is weak.
- There are many biological markers for associated aggression and mood disturbance.
- The serotonin system appears to be implicated in the interface of aggression and mood disturbance.
- A genetic polymorphism in the serotonin transporter is strongly associated with depression after adversity and is also associated with aggression in depressed and nondepressed subjects.
- Deliberate self-harm (DSH) behaviors frequently occur independently of suicide and should be considered separate phenomena. However, acts of DSH increase risk for subsequent suicide.
- DSH behavior is associated with early abuse.
- DSH behavior is usually associated with dysphoria but not necessarily with depression.
- Both major depression and bipolar illness are significant risk factors for completed suicides. Bipolar disorder carries a much higher risk for completed suicide than does major depression.
- Comorbid disorders, such as substance use, increase suicide risk.
- Antidepressants may increase suicide ideation but do not appear to increase completed suicides and may reduce the severity of suicide attempts.
- Lithium has a clear antisuicide effect in both bipolar illness and unipolar major depression.

References

Acierno R, Lawyer SR, Rheingold A, et al: Current psychopathology in previously assaulted older adults. J Interpers Violence 22:250–258, 2007

Afaq I, Riaz J, Sedky K, et al: Divalproex as a calmative adjunct for aggressive schizophrenic patients. J Ky Med Assoc 100:17–22, 2002

Afifi M: Depression in adolescents: gender differences in Oman and Egypt. East Mediterr Health J 12:61–71, 2006

American Psychiatric Association: Diagnostic and Statistical Manual of Mental Disorders, 4th Edition, Text Revision. Washington, DC, American Psychiatric Association, 2000

American Psychiatric Association: Practice guideline for the assessment and treatment of patients with suicidal behaviors. Am J Psychiatry 160(suppl): 1–60, 2003

Anderson C, Roux G, Pruitt A: Prenatal depression, violence, substance use, and perception of support in pregnant middle-class women. J Perinat Educ 11:14–21, 2002

Angst J, Preisig M: Outcome of a clinical cohort of unipolar, bipolar and schizoaffective patients: results of a prospective study from 1959 to 1985. Schweiz Archiv Neurol Psychiatry 146:17–23, 1995

Arato M, Demeter E, Rihmer Z, et al: Retrospective psychiatric assessment of 200 suicides in Budapest. Acta Psychiatr Scand 77:454–456, 1988

Arendt M, Rosenberg R, Fjordback L, et al: Testing the self-medication hypothesis of depression and aggression in cannabis-dependent subjects. Psychol Med 37:935–945, 2007

Avdibegovic E, Sinanovic O: Consequences of domestic violence on women's mental health in Bosnia and Herzegovina. Croat Med J 47:730–741, 2006

Baldessarini RJ, Tondo L, Davis P, et al: Decreased risk of suicides and attempts during long-term lithium treatment: a meta-analytic review. Bipolar Disord 8:625–639, 2006

Banyard VL, Williams LM, Siegel JA: Re-traumatization among adult women sexually abuse in childhood: exploratory analyses in a prospective study. J Child Sex Abuse 11:19–48, 2002

Barlow K, Grenyer B, Ilkiw-Lavalle O: Prevalence and precipitants of aggression in psychiatric inpatient units. Aust NZ J Psychiatry 34:967–974, 2000

Barzman DH, DelBello MP, Adler CM, et al: The efficacy and tolerability of quetiapine versus divalproex for the treatment of impulsivity and reactive aggression in adolescents with co-occurring bipolar disorder and disruptive behavior disorder(s). J Child Adolesc Psychopharmacol 16:666–670, 2006

Bayle FJ, Leroy S, Gourion D, et al: 5HTTLPR polymorphism in schizophrenic patients: further support for association with violent suicide attempts. Am J Med Genet B Neuropsychiatr Genet 119:12–17, 2003

Blitstein JL, Murray DM, Lytle LA, et al: Predictors of violent behavior in an early adolescent cohort: similarities and differences across genders. Health Educ Behav 32:175–194, 2005

Bogat GA, DeJonghe E, Levendosky AA, et al: Trauma symptoms among infants exposed to intimate partner violence. Child Abuse Negl 30:109–125, 2006

Bond AJ: Antidepressant treatments and human aggression. Eur J Pharmacol 526:218–225, 2005

Bonomi AE, Thompson RS, Anderson M, et al: Intimate partner violence and women's physical, mental, and social functioning. Am J Prev Med 30:458–466, 2006

Borges G, Angst J, Nock MK, et al: A risk index for 12-month suicide attempts in the National Comorbidity Survey Replication (NCS-R). Psychol Med 36:1747–1757, 2006

Brent DA, Perper JA, Moritz G, et al: Psychiatric risk factors for adolescent suicide: a case-control study. J Am Acad Child Adolesc Psychiatry 32:521–529, 1993

Bridge JA, Iyengar S, Salary CB, et al: Clinical response and risk of reported suicidal ideation and suicide attempts in pediatric antidepressant treatment: a meta-analysis of randomized controlled trials. JAMA 297:1683–1696, 2007

Brunstein Klomek A, Marrocco F, Kleinman M, et al: Bullying, depression, and suicidality in adolescents. J Am Acad Child Adolesc Psychiatry 46:40–49, 2007

Calabrese JR, Muzina DJ, Kemp DE, et al: Predictors of bipolar disorder risk among patients currently treated for major depression. MedGenMed 8:38, 2006

Caspi A, Sugden K, Moffitt TE, et al: Influence of life stress on depression: moderation by a polymorphism in the 5-HTT gene. Science 301:291–293, 2003

Cassidy F, Carroll BJ: Frequencies of signs and symptoms in mixed and pure episodes of mania: implications for the study of manic episodes. Prog Neuropsychopharmacol Biol Psychiatry 25:659–665, 2001

Cassidy F, Ahearn EP, Carroll BJ: Symptom profile consistency in recurrent manic episodes. Compr Psychiatry 43:179–181, 2002

Centers for Disease Control and Prevention: Homicides and Suicides: National Violent Death Reporting System, United States, 2003–2004. MMWR Morb Mortal Wkly Rep 55:721–724, 2006 [Erratum in: MMWR Morb Mortal Wkly Rep 55:1074–1075, 2006]

Cervilla JA, Rivera M, Molina E, et al: The 5-HTTLPR s/s genotype at the serotonin transporter gene (SLC6A4) increases the risk for depression in a large cohort of primary care attendees: the PREDICT-gene study. Am J Med Genet B Neuropsychiatr Genet 141:912–917, 2006

Cervilla JA, Molina E, Rivera M, et al: The risk for depression conferred by stressful life events is modified by variation at the serotonin transporter 5HTTLPR genotype: evidence from the Spanish PREDICT-Gene cohort. Mol Psychiatry 12:748–755, 2007

Chen YW, Dilsaver SC: Lifetime rates of suicide attempts among subjects with bipolar and unipolar disorders relative to subjects with other Axis I disorders. Biol Psychiatry 39:896–899, 1996

Cipriani A, Pretty H, Hawton K, et al: Lithium in the prevention of suicidal behavior and all cause mortality in patients with mood disorders: a systematic review of randomized trials. Am J Psychiatry 162:1805–1819, 2005

Coker AL, Smith PH, Fadden MK: Intimate partner violence and disabilities among women attending family practice clinics. J Womens Health (Larchmt) 14:829–838, 2005

Conway M, Mendelson M, Glannopoulos C, et al: Childhood and adult sexual abuse, rumination on sadness, and dysphoria. Child Abuse Negl 28:393–410, 2004

Cukor D, McGinn LK: History of child abuse and severity of adult depression: the mediating role of cognitive schema. J Child Sex Abuse 15:19–34, 2006

Deblinger E, Mannarino AP, Cohen JA, et al: A follow-up study of a multisite, randomized, controlled trial for children with sexual abuse-related PTSD symptoms. J Am Acad Child Adolesc Psychiatry 45:1474–1484, 2006

Denov MS: The long-term effects of child sexual abuse by female perpetrators: a qualitative study of male and female victims. J Interpers Violence 19:1137–1156, 2004

Dervic K, Grunebaum MF, Burke AK, et al: Protective factors against suicidal behavior in depressed adults reporting childhood abuse. J Nerv Ment Dis 194:971–974, 2006

Dilsaver SC, Chen YW, Swann AC, et al: Suicidality in patients with pure and depressive mania. Am J Psychiatry 151:1312–1315, 1994

Dubicka B, Hadley S, Roberts C: Suicidal behaviour in youths with depression treated with new generation antidepressants: meta analysis. Br J Psychiatry 189:393–398, 2006

Dunsieth NW Jr, Nelson EB, Brusman-Lovins LA, et al: Psychiatric and legal features of 113 men convicted of sexual offenses. J Clin Psychiatry 65:293–300, 2004

Edwards EP, Elden RD, Colder C, et al: The development of aggression in 18 and 48 month old children of alcoholic parents. J Abnorm Child Psychol 34:409–423, 2006

Fagiolini A, Kupfer DJ, Rucci P, et al: Suicide attempts and ideation in patients with bipolar I disorder. J Clin Psychiatry 65:509–514, 2004

Feldmann TB: Bipolar disorder and violence. Psychiatr Q 72:119–129, 2001

Fiedler N, Ozakinci G, Hallman W, et al: Military deployment to the Gulf War as a risk factor for psychiatric illness among U.S. troops. Br J Psychiatry 188:453–459, 2006

Foshee VA, Benefield TS, Ennett ST, et al: Longitudinal predictors of serious physical and sexual violence victimization during adolescence. Prev Med 39:1007–1016, 2004

Foster T, Gillespie K, McClelland R, et al: Risk factors for suicide independent of DSM-III-R Axis I disorder. Br J Psychiatry 175:175–179, 1999

Frankle WG, Lombardo I, New AS, et al: Brain serotonin transporter distribution in subjects with impulsive aggressivity: a positron emission study with [11C]McN 5652. Am J Psychiatry 162:915–923, 2005

Gamble SA, Talbot NL, Duberstein PR, et al: Childhood sexual abuse and depressive symptom severity: the role of neuroticism. J Nerv Ment Dis 194:382–385, 2006

Gaylord KM: The psychosocial effects of combat: the frequently unseen injury. Crit Care Nurs Clin North Am 18:349–357, 2006

Gaynes BN, West SL, Ford CA, et al: Screening for suicide risk in adults: a summary of the evidence for the U.S. Preventive Services Task Force. Ann Intern Med 140:822–835, 2004

Gibbons RD, Hur K, Bhaumik DK, et al: The relationship between antidepressant prescription rates and rate of early adolescent suicide. Am J Psychiatry 163:1898–1904, 2006

Gladstone GL, Parker GB, Mitchell PB, et al: Implications of childhood trauma for depressed women: an analysis of pathways from childhood sexual abuse to deliberate self-harm and revictimization. Am J Psychiatry 161:1417–1425, 2004

Gobbi G, Gaudreau PO, Leblanc N: Efficacy of topiramate, valproate, and their combination on aggression/agitation behavior in patients with psychosis. J Clin Psychopharmacol 26:467–473, 2006

Goedhard LE, Stolker JJ, Heerdink ER, et al: Pharmacotherapy for the treatment of aggressive behavior in general adult psychiatry: a systematic review. J Clin Psychiatry 67:1013–1024, 2006

Goldstein AL, Walton MA, Cunningham RM, et al: Violence and substance use as risk factors for depressive symptoms among adolescents in an urban emergency department. J Adolesc Health 40:276–279, 2007

Gonda X, Bagdy G: Relationship between serotonin transporter gene 5HTTLPR polymorphism and the symptoms of neuroticism in healthy population. Psychiatr Hung 21:379–385, 2006

Gonda X, Juhasz G, Laszik A, et al: Subthreshold depression is linked to the functional polymorphism of the 5HT transporter gene. J Affect Disord 87:291–297, 2005

Gonda X, Rihmer Z, Zsombok T, et al: The 5HTTLPR polymorphism of the serotonin transporter gene is associated with affective temperaments as measured by TEMPS-A. J Affect Disord 91:125–131, 2006

Groholt B, Ekeberg O, Haldorsen T: Adolescents hospitalised with deliberate self-harm: the significance of an intention to die. Eur Child Adolesc Psychiatry 9:244–254, 2000

Grossman LS, Haywood TW, Cavanaugh JL, et al: State psychiatric hospital patients with past arrests for violent crimes. Psychiatr Serv 46:790–795, 1995

Grunebaum MF, Galfalvy HC, Nichols CM, et al: Aggression and substance abuse in bipolar disorder. Bipolar Disord 8:496–502, 2006

Guzzetta F, Tondo L, Centorrino F, et al: Lithium treatment reduces suicide risk in recurrent major depressive disorder. J Clin Psychiatry 68:380–383, 2007

Hammack PL, Richards MH, Lug Z, et al: Social support factors as moderators of community violence exposure among inner-city African American young adolescents. J Clin Child Adolesc Psychol 33:450–462, 2004

Hammad TA, Laughren TP, Racoosin JA: Suicide rates in short-term randomized controlled trials of newer antidepressants. J Clin Psychopharmacol 26:203–207, 2006

Hanson RF, Self-Brown S, Fricker-Ethal A, et al: Relations among parental substance use, violence exposure and mental health: the national survey of adolescents. Addict Behav 31:1988–2001, 2006

Harrington R, Pickles A, Aglan A, et al: Early adult outcomes of adolescents who deliberately poisoned themselves. J Am Acad Child Adolesc Psychiatry 45:337–345, 2006

Hashemian F, Khoshnood K, Desai MM, et al: Anxiety, depression, and posttraumatic stress in Iranian survivors of chemical warfare. JAMA 296:560–566, 2006

Haw C, Hawton K, Houston K, et al: Psychiatric and personality disorders in deliberate self-harm patients. Br J Psychiatry 178:48–54, 2001

Hazen AL, Connelly CD, Kelleher KJ, et al: Female caregivers' experiences with intimate partner violence and behavioral problems in children investigated as victims of maltreatment. Pediatrics 117:99–109, 2006

Healy D, Herxheimer A, Menkes DB: Antidepressants and violence: problems at the interface of medicine and law. PLoS Med 3:e372, 2006

Henriksson MM, Aro HM, Marttunen MJ, et al: Mental disorders and comorbidity in suicide. Am J Psychiatry 150:935–940, 1993

Hindin MJ, Gultiano S: Associations between witnessing parental domestic violence and experiencing depressive symptoms in Filipino adolescents. Am J Public Health 96:660–663, 2006

Houry D, Kemball R, Rhodes KV, et al: Intimate partner violence and mental health symptoms in African American female ED patients. Am J Emerg Med 24:444–450, 2006

Huizinga D, Haberstick BC, Smolen A, et al: Childhood maltreatment, subsequent antisocial behavior, and the role of monoamine oxidase A genotypes. Biol Psychiatry 60:677–683, 2006

Isometsa ET, Henriksson MM, Aro HM, et al: Suicide in bipolar disorder in Finland. Am J Psychiatry 151:1020–1024, 1994

Jamison KR: Touched with Fire: Manic-Depressive Illness and the Artistic Temperament. New York, Free Press, 1993

Johansen VA, Wahl AK, Eilertsen DE, et al: Acute psychological reactions in assault victims of non-domestic violence peritraumatic dissociation, posttraumatic stress disorder, anxiety and depression. Nord J Psychiatry 60:452–462, 2006

Kaufman J, Yang BZ, Douglas-Palumberi H, et al: Social supports and serotonin transporter gene moderate depression in maltreated children. Proc Natl Acad Sci USA 101:17316–17321, 2004

Keilp JG, Gorlyn M, Oquendo MA, et al: Aggressiveness, not impulsiveness or hostility, distinguishes suicide attempters with major depression. Psychol Med 36:1779–1788, 2006

Kessler RC, Akiskal HS, Ames M, et al: Prevalence and effects of mood disorders on work performance in a nationally representative sample of U.S. workers. Am J Psychiatry 163:1561–1568, 2006

Kim YS, Leventhal BL, Koh YJ, et al: School bullying and youth violence: causes or consequences of psychopathologic behavior? Arch Gen Psychiatry 63:1035–1041, 2006

Klonsky ED, Oltmanns TF, Turkheimer E: Deliberate self-harm in a nonclinical population: prevalence and psychological correlates. Am J Psychiatry 160:1501–1508, 2003

Knox M, King C, Hanna GL, et al: Aggressive behavior in clinically depressed adolescents. J Am Acad Child Adolesc Psychiatry 39:611–618, 2000

Korkeila J, Salminen JK, Hiekkanen H, et al: Use of antidepressants and suicide rate in Finland: an ecological study. J Clin Psychiatry 68:505–511, 2007

Kuehn BM: FDA panel seeks to balance risks in warnings for antidepressants. JAMA 297:573–574, 2007

Lamprecht HC, Pakrasi S, Gash A, et al: Deliberate self-harm in older people revisited. Int J Geriatr Psychiatry 20:1090–1096, 2005

Lauterbach E, Brunner J, Hawelleck B, et al: Platelet 5-HT2A receptor binding and tryptophan availability are not associated with recent history of suicide attempts but with personality traits characteristic for suicidal behavior. J Affect Disord 91:57–62, 2006

Lehrer JA, Buka S, Gortmaker S, et al: Depressive symptomatology as a predictor of exposure to intimate partner violence among U.S. female adolescents and young adults. Arch Pediatr Adolesc Med 160:270–276, 2006

Lipsky S, Field CA, Caetano R, et al: Posttraumatic stress disorder symptomatology and comorbid depressive symptoms among abused women referred from emergency department care. Violence Vict 20:645–659, 2005

Lohner J, Konrad N: Deliberate self-harm and suicide attempt in custody: distinguishing features in male inmates' self-injurious behavior. Int J Law Psychiatry 29:370–385, 2006

Loncar M, Medved V, Jovanovic N, et al: Psychological consequences of rape on women in 1991–1995 war in Croatia and Bosnia and Herzegovina. Croat Med J 47:67–75, 2006

MacKinnon DF, Zandi PP, Gershon E, et al: Rapid switching of mood in families with multiple cases of bipolar disorder. Arch Gen Psychiatry 60:921–928, 2003

MacMillan CM, Korndorfer SR, Rao S, et al: A comparison of divalproex and oxcarbazepine in aggressive youth with bipolar disorder. J Psychiatr Pract 12:214–222, 2006

Maj M, Pirozzi R, Magliano L, et al: Agitated depression in bipolar I disorder: prevalence, phenomenology, and outcome. Am J Psychiatry 160:2134–2140, 2003

Malkesman O, Maayan R, Weizman A, et al: Aggressive behavior and HPA axis hormones after social isolation in adult rats of two different genetic animal models for depression. Behav Brain Res 175:408–414, 2006

Maremmani I, Lazzeri A, Pacini M, et al: Diagnostic and symptomatological features in chronic psychotic patients according to cannabis use status. J Psychoactive Drugs 36:235–241, 2004

Martin G, Bergen HA, Richardson AS, et al: Sexual abuse and suicidality: gender differences in a large community sample of adolescents. Child Abuse Negl 28:491–503, 2004

Martin J, Langley J, Millchamp J: Domestic violence as witnessed by New Zealand children. N Z Med J 119:U1817, 2006

Martsolf DS, Draucker CB: Psychotherapy approaches for adult survivors of childhood sexual abuse: an integrative review of outcomes research. Issues Ment Health Nurs 26:801–825, 2005

Masho SW, Odor RK, Adera T: Sexual assault in Virginia: a population-based study. Womens Health Issues 15:157–166, 2005

McElroy SL, Soutullo CA, Taylor P Jr, et al: Psychiatric features of 36 men convicted of sexual offenses. J Clin Psychiatry 60:414–420, 1999

McGuigan WM, Middlemiss W: Sexual abuse in childhood and interpersonal violence in adulthood: a cumulative impact on depressive symptoms in women. J Interpers Violence 20:1271–1287, 2005

Miguel-Tobal JJ, Cano-Vindel A, Gonzalez-Ordi H, et al: PTSD and depression after the Madrid March 11 train bombings. J Trauma Stress 19:69–80, 2006

Miller MC: The biology of child maltreatment. Harv Ment Health Lett 21:1–3, 2005
Mitchell MD, Hargrove GL, Collins MH, et al: Coping variables that mediate the relations between intimate partner violence and mental health outcomes among low-income, African American women. J Clin Psychol 62:1503–1520, 2006
Mitchell PJ: Antidepressant treatment and rodent aggressive behavior. Eur J Pharmacol 526:147–162, 2005
Muehlenkamp JJ, Gutierrez PM: An investigation of differences between self-injurious behavior and suicide attempts in a sample of adolescents. Suicide Life Threat Behav 34:12–23, 2004
Najt P, Perez J, Sanches M, et al: Impulsivity and bipolar disorder. Eur Neuropsychopharmacol 17:313–320, 2007
North CS, Smith EM, Spitznagel EL: Violence and the homeless: an epidemiologic study of victimization and aggression. J Trauma Stress 7:95–110, 1994
Oquendo MA, Russo SA, Underwood MD, et al: Higher postmortem prefrontal 5-HT2A receptor binding correlates with lifetime aggression in suicide. Biol Psychiatry 59:235–243, 2006
Ostacher MJ, Eidelman P: Suicide in bipolar depression, in Bipolar Depression: A Comprehensive Guide. Edited by El-Mallakh RS, Ghaemi SN. Washington, DC, American Psychiatric Publishing, 2006, pp 117–144
Paranjape A, Heron S, Thompson M, et al: Are alcohol problems linked with an increase in depressive symptoms in abused, inner-city African American women? Womens Health Issues 17:37–43, 2007
Parker G, Malhi G, Mitchell P, et al: Self-harming in depressed patients: pattern analysis. Aust NZ J Psychiatry 39:899–906, 2005
Peiponen S, Laukkanen E, Korhonen V, et al: The association of parental alcohol abuse and depression with severe emotional and behavioral problems in adolescents: a clinical study. Int J Soc Psychiatry 52:395–407, 2006
Peleikis DE, Mykletun A, Dahl AA: Long-term social status and intimate relationship in women with childhood sexual abuse who got outpatient psychotherapy for anxiety disorder and depression. Nord J Psychiatry 59:31–38, 2005
Person C, Tracy M, Galea S: Risk factors for depression after a disaster. J Nerv Ment Dis 194:659–666, 2006
Pico-Alfonso MA, Garcia-Linares MI, Celda-Navarro N, et al: The impact of physical, psychological and sexual intimate male partner violence on women's mental health: depressive symptoms, posttraumatic stress disorder, state anxiety, and suicide. J Womens Health (Larchmt) 15:599–611, 2006
Placidi GP, Oquendo MA, Malone KM, et al: Aggressivity, suicide attempts, and depression: relationship to cerebrospinal fluid monoamine metabolite levels. Biol Psychiatry 52:375–376, 2002
Pope HG Jr, Kouri EM, Hudson JI: Effects of supraphysiologic doses of testosterone on mood and aggression in normal men: a randomized controlled trial. Arch Gen Psychiatry 57:133–140, 2000
Posternak MA, Zimmerman M: Anger and aggression in psychiatric outpatients. J Clin Psychiatry 63:665–672, 2002
Potter NN: Trauma, Truth and Reconciliation: Healing Damaged Relationships. New York, Oxford University Press, 2006

Quanbeck CD, Stone DC, Scott CL, et al: Clinical and legal correlates of inmates with bipolar disorder at time of criminal arrest. J Clin Psychiatry 65:198–203, 2004

Raja M, Azzoni A: Suicide attempts: differences between unipolar and bipolar patients and among groups with different lethality risk. J Affect Disord 82:437–442, 2004

Reed GL, Enright RD: The effects of forgiveness therapy on depression, anxiety, and posttraumatic stress for women after spousal emotional abuse. J Consult Clin Psychol 74:920–929, 2006

Reigstad B, Jorgensen K, Wichstrom L: Diagnosed and self-reported childhood abuse in national and regional samples of child and adolescent psychiatric patients: prevalences and correlates. Nord J Psychiatry 60:58–66, 2006

Rich CL, Young D, Fowler RC: San Diego suicide study: young vs. old subjects. Arch Gen Psychiatry 43:577–582, 1986

Rich CL, Gidycz CA, Warkentin JB, et al: Child and adolescent abuse and subsequent victimization: a prospective study. Child Abuse Negl 29:1373–1394, 2005

Rivera-Rivera L, Allen B, Rodriguez-Ortega G, et al: Dating violence and associations with depression and risk behaviors: female students in Morelos, Mexico. Salud Publica Max 48(suppl):S288–S296, 2006

Rowe R, Maughan B, Eley TC: Links between antisocial behavior and depressed mood: the role of life events and attributional style. J Abnorm Child Psychol 34:293–302, 2006

Sachs-Ericsson N, Verona E, Joiner T, et al: Parental verbal abuse and the mediating role of self-criticism in adult internalizing disorders. J Affect Disord 93:71–78, 2006

Safer DJ, Zito JM: Do antidepressants reduce suicide rates? Public Health 121:274–277, 2007

Sakai JT, Young SE, Stallings MC, et al: Case control and within-family tests for an association between conduct disorder and 5HTTLPR. Am J Med Genet B Neuropsychiatr Genet 141:825–832, 2006

Sato T, Bottlender R, Kleindienst N, et al: Syndromes and phenomenological subtypes underlying acute mania: a factor analytic study of 576 manic patients. Am J Psychiatry 159:968–974, 2002

Sato T, Bottlender R, Kleindienst N, et al: Irritable psychomotor elation in depressed inpatients: a factor validation of mixed depression. J Affect Disord 84:187–196, 2005

Schuepbach D, Goetz I, Boeker H, et al: Voluntary vs. involuntary hospital admission in acute mania of bipolar disorder: results from the Swiss sample of the EMBLEM study. J Affect Disord 90:57–61, 2006

Shea A, Walsh C, Macmillan H, et al: Child maltreatment and HPA axis dysregulation: relationship to major depressive disorder and post traumatic stress disorder in females. Psychoneuroendocrinology 30:162–178, 2005

Sher L, Oquendo MA, Conason AH, et al: Clinical features of depressed patients with or without a family history of alcoholism. Acta Psychiatr Scand 112:266–271, 2005

Silverstein M, Augustyn M, Cabral H, et al: Maternal depression and violence exposure: double jeopardy for child school functioning. Pediatrics 118:792–800, 2006

Sinclair JMA, Harriss L, Baldwin DS, et al: Suicide in depressive disorders: a retrospective case-control study of 127 suicides. J Affect Disord 87:107–113, 2005

Smith DJ, Harrison N, Muir W, et al: The high prevalence of bipolar spectrum disorders in young adults with recurrent depression: toward an innovative diagnostic framework. J Affect Disord 84:167–178, 2005

Sokero P, Eerola M, Rytsälä H, et al: Decline in suicidal ideation among patients with MDD is preceded by decline in depression and hopelessness. J Affect Disord 95:95–102, 2006

Starkman MN: The terrorist attacks of September 11, 2001, as psychological toxin: increase in suicide attempts. J Nerv Ment Dis 194:547–550, 2006

Sternberg KJ, Lamb ME, Guterman E, et al: Effects of early and later family violence on children's behavior problems and depression: a longitudinal, multi-informant perspective. Child Abuse Negl 30:283–306, 2006

Suarez EC, Krishnan KR: The relation of free plasma tryptophan to anger, hostility, and aggression in a nonpatient sample of adult men and women. Ann Behav Med 31:254–260, 2006

Swann AC: Treatment of aggression in patients with bipolar disorder. J Clin Psychiatry 60(suppl):25–28, 1999

Teicher MH, Samson JA, Polcari A, et al: Sticks, stones, and hurtful words: relative effects of various forms of childhood maltreatment. Am J Psychiatry 163:993–1000, 2006

Theran SA, Sullivan CM, Bogat GA, et al: Abusive partners and ex-partners: understanding the effects of relationship to the abuser on women's wellbeing. Violence Against Women 12:950–969, 2006

Tiihonen J, Lonnqvist J, Wahlbeck K, et al: Antidepressants and the risk of suicide, attempted suicide, and overall mortality in a nationwide cohort. Arch Gen Psychiatry 63:1358–1367, 2006

Tondo L, Hennen J, Baldessarini RJ: Lower suicide risk with long-term lithium treatment in major affective illness: a meta-analysis. Acta Psychiatr Scand 104:163–172, 2001

Tuisku V, Pelkonen M, Karlsson L, et al: Suicidal ideation, deliberate self-harm behavior and suicide attempts among adolescent outpatients with depressive mood disorders and comorbid Axis I disorders. Eur Child Adolesc Psychiatry 15:199–206, 2006

Tzemou E, Birchwood M: A prospective study of dysfunctional thinking and the regulation of negative intrusive memories in bipolar 1 disorder: implications for affect regulation theory. Psychol Med 37:689–698, 2007

Van Gogh Gallery: Vincent van Gogh: Biography. Available at http://www.vangoghgallery.com. Accessed March 2007

Varma D, Chandra PS, Thomas T, et al: Intimate partner violence and sexual coercion among pregnant women in India: relationship with depression and post-traumatic stress disorder. J Affect Disord 102:227–235, 2006

Volavka J, Bilder R, Nolan K: Catecholamines and aggression: the role of COMT and MAO polymorphisms. Ann NY Acad Sci 1036:393–398, 2004

Watlington CG, Murphy CM: The roles of religion and spirituality among African American survivors of domestic violence. J Clin Psychol 62:837–857, 2006

Whitaker RC, Orzol SE, Kahn RS: Maternal mental health, substance use, and domestic violence in the year after delivery and subsequent behavior problems in children at age 3 years. Arch Gen Psychiatry 63:551–560, 2006

Widom CS, DuMont K, Czaja SJ: A prospective investigation of major depressive disorder and comorbidity in abused and neglected children grown up. Arch Gen Psychiatry 64:49–56, 2007

Wright J, Friedrich W, Cinq-Mars C, et al: Self-destructive and delinquent behaviors of adolescent female victims of child sexual abuse: rates and covariates in clinical and nonclinical samples. Violence Vict 19:627–643, 2004

Zalcman SS, Siegel A: The neurobiology of aggression and rage: role of cytokines. Brain Behav Immun 20:507–514, 2006

CHAPTER 6

Schizophrenia and Delusional Disorder

Martha L. Crowner, M.D.

In this chapter I discuss assessment and management of acutely violent patients with primary psychotic disorders. Most studies of violent patients are of diagnostically mixed populations that include a large proportion diagnosed with schizophrenia, reflecting clinical populations. I highlight studies of groups of adults with schizophrenia but also discuss studies of mixed groups. Some aspects of assessment and much of management can apply to all severely mentally ill adults. Diagnoses are often imprecise, especially in large community surveys, in which patients are often identified by their predominant symptoms rather than diagnosis. There is little literature to guide discussions of violence in patients with delusional disorder, but these patients are similar to those with chronic schizophrenia, with prominent positive symptoms and low levels of negative symptoms.

My discussion of management of violence primarily covers environmental and interpersonal strategies to prevent violence. Pharmacological management is discussed at length in Chapter 15.

Violence Assessment

The first step in assessing a violent incident is to find out exactly what happened. Ask who did what to whom. The term *violent*, like *aggression*, *agitation*, and *assaultiveness*, is often used quite loosely and imprecisely, sometimes when a patient is simply loud and belligerent. If there was physical contact, learn whether the incident was serious and if so, how serious. Were any weapons involved? Was anyone injured? If so, how badly?

After it is clear that all are safe, interview the victim, assailant, and others present at the time of the incident. Attempt to learn what happened between assailant and victim before the assault. Attempt to identify and piece together the often complex interactions among assailant, victim, external circumstances, and symptoms of illness. Many factors may explain violence in people with psychosis *besides* psychosis and other psychopathology: environmental factors; cultural, interpersonal, and attitudinal factors; and other, unknown factors. Aggression is a universal human drive, the expression of which is shaped by social norms and external contingencies. In some circumstances the expression of aggression in assault can be adaptive.

When assessing violent patients, be especially alert to risk factors that can be changed. These include certain types of psychopathology, substance abuse, treatment nonadherence, and medical comorbidities. Substance abuse is more common in outpatients, but clever and determined inpatients can obtain alcohol and substances of abuse. Medical conditions are not commonly associated with violence but are potentially life threatening and reversible. For example, a woman with diabetes was referred to a unit for violent patients because she had been belligerent and was shoving others. Nurses on the unit saw her stumbling and intermittently confused. Review of medication history revealed a recent increase in insulin dosing, and blood sugar monitoring revealed intermittent hypoglycemia.

Rates of Violence in Community Samples With Psychotic Illness and With No Detected Psychiatric Illness

Violence occurs at low rates in the general population and at moderately higher rates in adults with psychotic illness. In a large survey of about 10,000 adults in the United States, the Epidemiologic Catchment Area survey (Swanson et al. 1990), subjects were classed as violent if they admitted to one of five behaviors within the previous 12 months: physical abuse of a child, physical fighting, physical fighting while intoxicated, fighting with a spouse or partner, and fighting with a weapon. Two percent of those with no disorder had been violent in the previous 12 months. The rate for those with schizophrenia was 13%, whereas for those with major depression it was 12%, for adults who abused cannabis, 19%, and for those who abused alcohol, 25%. Trained nonclinicians administered the Diagnostic Interview Schedule, based on DSM-III (American Psychiatric Association 1980), to arrive at Axis I diagnoses. When a person met criteria for more than one diagnosis, he or she was counted in both categories. Those with more diagnoses were more likely to be violent. In logistic regression analysis, male gender, youth, poverty, substance abuse, and major mental illness all predicted violence, as did the interaction between substance abuse and major mental illness.

Other investigators have had similar findings: a low base rate of violence and a moderate rate in adults with psychotic illness. A large Israeli survey (Stueve and Link 1997) found a 7% rate of violence in the previous 5 years in adults ages 24–33 without identified psychiatric illness and a 21% rate in adults with psychotic or bipolar disorders. They also found higher rates in those with comorbid substance abuse (39%) and very high rates (93%) in those with psychotic or bipolar disorders comorbid with antisocial personality, with or without substance abuse. The relationship between violence and psychotic and bipolar disorders was significant after controlling for substance abuse, antisocial personality disorder, and demographic characteristics. Investigators asked if respondents had been in a physical fight within the previous 5 years or had a weapon in hand during a fight.

Diagnoses of psychosis obtained in large community samples such as these may agree poorly with clinical diagnoses, but these studies give a general idea of comparative rates of violence across diagnoses and with comorbidity. Community samples have the advantage of avoiding the sampling bias that can occur in studies of hospitalized patients (i.e., that many of these subjects are hospitalized because they have been violent).

Association of Symptoms of Mental Illness and Violence

In a study of a diagnostically mixed population (Monahan et al. 2001), and in surveys of large community samples (Arseneault et al. 2000; Link et al. 1998), paranoia or suspiciousness has been associated with assaultiveness. Link et al. (1998) identified a relationship between paranoia, delusions of control and thought insertion (known as threat/control override), and past history of violence in both psychiatrically ill and control subjects. Arseneault et al. (2000) concluded that violence in subjects with schizophrenia was partly explained by excessive perceptions of threat.

A study of 1,410 patients in treatment for schizophrenia, a substudy of the National Institute of Mental Health Clinical Antipsychotic Trials of Intervention Effectiveness (the CATIE project; Swanson et al. 2006), explored the association of violence and symptoms. Serious violence was associated with hostility (odds ratio [OR] 1.65), suspiciousness and persecutory delusions (OR 1.46), hallucinations (OR 1.43), grandiosity (OR 1.31), and excitement (OR 1.30). Delusional thinking alone was not associated with serious violence, but when it occurred with suspiciousness and persecutory delusions, it was highly associated (OR 2.9). Negative symptoms were associated with a decreased risk of serious violence. High levels of positive symptoms with high levels of negative symptoms were not associated with increased risk of serious violence, but high levels of positive symptoms with low levels of negative symptoms were (OR 3.05).

Serious violence was defined as assault with a lethal weapon or a threat with a lethal weapon, assault resulting in injury, or sexual assault. Minor violence was defined as simple assault without a weapon. This study omitted patients in their first episode and patients with treatment-resistant illness. Violence was detected by self-report and family collateral history. Of 1,410 subjects, 15.5% reported minor violence during the previous 6 months and 3.6% reported serious violence. Childhood conduct problems, younger age, and a history of arrests were associated with serious violence. Younger age, living with family, and not feeling listened to by family were associated with minor violence. Together, all variables considered in this study did not explain more than about 18% of the variance in minor and serious violence, suggesting they had little explanatory power. Other factors, tested in other investigations or not yet hypothesized, could be more powerfully linked to violence.

Students and psychiatric residents are routinely taught to ask whether patients experience command hallucinations to harm others. Command hallucinations would seem to be an obvious risk, but experienced clinicians know of many patients who have never been known to comply with hallucinated commands. Reported rates of compliance vary widely. These differences may be partly due to differences in populations studied, because some investigators study only patients with schizophrenia and others study diagnostically mixed groups. Investigators also consider different time frames between command hallucinations and violence. For example, some ask patients if they have ever been violent in response to commands, whereas others ask if patients have been violent in the past year. Differences may be due to failure to consider response sets in self-report data. For example, in some groups, especially forensic populations, patients may be motivated to over-report commands. All studies are retrospective and subject to recall bias.

Schizophrenia and Delusional Disorder | 109

Nevertheless, it is clear that some patients with schizophrenia act aggressively in response to command hallucinations. British investigators have taken a different approach and describe factors associated with compliance to commands. In their review, Braham et al. (2004) noted that most patients with command hallucinations hear harmless commands and that dangerous commands have been associated with less compliance. Factors associated with compliance are perceived benevolence, power, and familiarity of the voice. A delusion congruent with a command hallucination can also make compliance more likely.

In a forensic setting, Taylor (1985) found that the crimes of a group of men motivated by delusions were more serious than crimes of other psychotic men. Investigators conducted lengthy interviews of psychotic and nonpsychotic male prisoners remanded for violent and nonviolent crimes in order to deduce reasons for offending. In the psychotic group, delusions were fairly common precipitants of crimes, but in nonpsychotic men, motives such as panic, self-defense, jealousy, and immediate retaliation were more likely to be associated with serious violence. Although half of the psychotic men in this sample claimed some of the same nonpsychotic motives for their crimes, such as panic, self-defense, immediate retaliation, material gain, and accident, the author wrote that these explanations had psychotic underpinnings. Taylor suggested that psychotic symptoms may frustrate men so they lose self-control and tolerance of others; in this way she proposed an indirect mechanism—that is, irritability or reactivity—through which psychotic symptoms can lead to assault.

Studies of inpatients differ from community samples. Inpatient states associated with assault include paranoia, strong affect, confusion, hyperarousal, and frustration. Hyperarousal and frustration can result from tense, unpredictable, chaotic environments. Certain symptoms may be more predictive of violence in recently hospitalized than in chronically hospitalized patients. In newly admitted inpatients, positive psychotic symptoms and irritability are predictive of violence, but in long-term, chronically psychotic patients, motor excitement, anger, low frustration tolerance, difficulty in delaying gratification (Kay et al. 1988), hostility, suspiciousness, and irritability (Krakowski et al. 1999) are more predictive.

Reactive Versus Instrumental Classification of Assaults

An important goal of interviews after an assault is to determine whether the event can be characterized as reactive or instrumental. In animals and unselected populations of humans, assault can be broadly and crudely classed into these two groups. Reactive events are impulsive, affective, or explosive, whereas instrumental events are coercive, predatory, or psychopathic (Eichelman 1990). This dichotomy is an oversimplification, because motives are often mixed, but it can be useful in treatment planning for mentally ill people. Investigators believe that reactive aggression is more treatable than instrumental aggression (Campbell et al. 1978, 1982, 1984, 1995; Sheard et al. 1976).

In reactive fights, assailants react out of strong emotion. For example, in a study in which we asked assailants to explain their behavior (Crowner et al. 1995), one said, "I couldn't help it. She made me lose face. She keeps insulting me in front of others. I just did it." Another said, "I was upset. She just ticked me off when she hit me with the ping-pong racket. I'm going to kill her if she hits me again." Another said, "I was so angry with him, the way he plays games before he takes his medication. We always have to suffer because he plays those games. We can't get our cigarettes on time. I pushed him to one side so I could get my medication. I didn't think he'd fall."

Instrumental assaults have a concrete goal. For example, a patient-assailant explained, "He didn't want me to have any of his food or candy. He just has to do what I say." Another said, "He sat on my chair [the chair where this man habitually sat] after I stood up to take my medication. I asked him to get up from my chair but he pretended not to hear me, so I lifted up my chair."

Assailants express reasons that have both reactive and instrumental aspects when they say they assaulted someone to make him or her stop a noxious behavior. One said, "He started it. He was bothering me and bothering me. I just have to hit him to make him stop. He instigated it. It's not my fault. I think I broke his nose, but it was not my fault." Another said, "He's always cursing and harassing me. I woke up one morning and just couldn't take it anymore. I just wanted to make him stop, let him know I was in a bad mood that day." A third patient said, "I wanted him to stop bothering the patients. He was bothering another patient. I just wanted to help. I am a fair guy, and I don't like others being bullied."

Research Attempts to Classify Inpatient Assaults

Are the assaults of patients with psychotic illness similar to those of other humans in that they can be classed as coercive or reactive? Or do their motivations usually result from delusions and hallucinations? Nolan et al. (2003) classified inpatient assaults as due to psychosis, impulsivity, or psychopathy. They classed an assault as psychotic or possibly psychotic according to assailant explanation and rater judgments. Assaults due to psychopathy were characterized by planning, lack of remorse, and predatory gain. They characterized reactive assaults as those with an immediate victim provocation, for example, an order to do something or a denial of a request, and without advance planning or predatory gain. Subjects were inpatients at a state hospital on a special unit for violent patients. Investigators interviewed victims, assailants, and witnesses, using a checklist to determine presence or absence of planning, predatory gain, remorse, and victim provocation.

Seventy percent of assailants carried a chart diagnosis of schizophrenia or schizoaffective illness. Of 55 assaults, 20% were judged to be psychotic or possibly psychotic. Eighty percent were judged to be related to psychopathy, poor impulse control, or uncertain factors. Victim provocation was the motive most frequently cited by assailants, but victims rarely agreed they had been provocative.

A more recent study (Quanbeck et al. 2007) made a similar attempt among chronically assaultive patients in a long-term psychiatric hospital in California. Most patients had a primary psychotic disorder. Fifty-seven percent of the patients had been committed under forensic laws. Using record review, the authors classified 839 assaults made by 88 individuals as psychotic, impulsive, or organized. In psychotic assaults there was no provocation or rational motive, and the assailant cited a delusion or hallucination as a motive. Impulsive events were characterized by an immediate provocation. The assailant was pacing, angry, yelling or threatening, could not be calmed, had no obvious secondary gain, and expressed remorse after the incident. Organized assaults were characterized by planning, little or no provocation, little warning, an external goal or social motive such as asserting dominance, and no agitation before the incident. The investigators found that 17% of assaults were psychotic, 54% were impulsive, and 29% were organized. Forensic patients committed more organized assaults, although this result was a nonsignificant trend only.

Videotape Recording of Inpatient Assaults

We installed a video camera system in the dayroom of an inpatient unit for persistently violent patients (Crowner et al. 2005), a room where the patients spent most of their waking hours, in order to study assaults and their precipitants. This allowed detailed, replicable characterization of events. We tested the hypothesis that assault does not come "out of the blue," as assault motivated by psychosis is often described, but can be predicted by immediate antecedent behaviors in victim and assailant. In victims these immediate antecedents could be seen as provocations. Assailants who respond to victim provocation could be seen as reactive.

We detected 155 assaults between 59 patients. Individual patients were often involved in multiple events. Fifty-six additional patients were present on the ward during the study period but were never involved in assaults. Of the group of 59, 56% carried a diagnosis of schizophrenia.

Many of the incidents did not seem serious. To better define this impression, we classed events into seriousness categories based on target of blows (head or remainder of body), staff intervention, and perceived forcefulness of blows. The categories were "play," "warn," and "hurt" (Crowner et al. 1994). Twenty-one of 155 events were classed as "play" assaults. In 76 assaults, patients seemed to be trying to hurt each other. Fifty-seven events had intermediate seriousness, in which patients did not seem to be playful or rageful but to be annoyed and trying to communicate a warning to the victim. One assault could not be classified.

In the 5 minutes before assaults, we found certain threatening and intrusive behaviors, or cues, in both victims and assailants (Crowner et al. 2005). The threatening behaviors were fist shaking, pointing, yelling and arguing, bumping, shoving, and pushing. The intrusive behaviors were following, touching, or moving very close, to within approximately 6 inches. These behaviors could be directed toward the other member of the victim-assailant dyad or toward other people in the area. We found these behaviors before 60% of assaults. In contrast, cues were present in 10% of control periods. When we counted cues, we found more than 10 times as many before assaults compared with control periods. These results remained highly significant after play assaults were dropped from analysis.

When we looked at all assaults, we found threatening and intrusive cues were significantly more numerous in victims than in assailants. Before the events of intermediate severity ("warn" assaults), there were significantly more assailant intrusive cues and more victim-threatening and intrusive cues. These assaults were more likely than others to have any victim cue or any victim intrusive cue.

Many of assaults we detected on camera have been little studied or noted by other investigators. As described in this section, we discovered a series of interactions between patients who were soon afterward involved in assaults, and between them and others on the ward. More serious assaults had fewer victim cues than assaults of intermediate severity. In serious assaults, assailants seemed intensely emotional. Intermediate assaults seemed to have a communicative function in which assailants were telling victims to stop or back off.

Summary of Assessment of Violence

Assault can be understood in many ways. The reactive/instrumental/psychotic classes can be useful but may overlap and blend into each other. Assault can be motivated by reactivity and psychosis. Psychotic patients can react in paranoid and irritable ways to external events rather than solely to internal states. Assault can be motivated by reactivity and a wish to coerce or by psychopathy when it is an acceptable means to make someone else do something such as stop "bothering" the person. Assault can be done in anger or as an attempt to communicate. Motivations expressed by patients cannot always be taken at face value. Reasons patients give can be the same as those given by nonpsychotic people, but as Taylor (1985) concluded, they may have "psychotic underpinnings."

Violence Management

General Principles

Inpatient management of violent patients is truly a team effort, requiring consensus and collaboration with all disciplines, particularly—but not exclusively—nursing. Psychiatrists have a legal and professional responsibility to lead this team by managing group dynamics and by guiding treatment decisions. Assaultive patients very often stir up intensely emotional conflicts within groups of staff members and between patient and professionals. Management decisions should be guided by data, an empathetic engagement with the patient, and calm. Staff are obliged to make all possible efforts to preserve patient dignity and protect patient safety. To balance our obligations to patients with our obligations to the safety of staff demands astute judgment and unusual skill.

The treatment team should have established guidelines for identifying potentially dangerous situations and for choosing interventions to prevent escalation of threatening behaviors. Criteria for intramuscular medication given without patient consent and for seclusion and restraint should be clear, concrete, and accepted by the entire ward staff. Management strategies vary according to local custom; staff will usually turn to what they have done before and what seems to have worked. However, interventions should be the least restrictive necessary to ensure safety and should be based on available data. Restraint and seclusion should be interventions of last resort, because patients find them traumatic and humiliating and because these interventions often lead to injuries of patients and staff. Use of restraint and seclusion is reviewed in this volume (Chapter 17) and also by Bernay and Elverson (2000).

Pharmacological management of violent adults with schizophrenia is discussed at length elsewhere in this volume (see Chapter 15). I only mention briefly a few points here. Medication adherence is often key. The physician must attempt to establish an alliance with the patient, however tenuous, and delicately balance adverse and beneficial effects. Court-ordered treatment may be necessary. When it is clear that the patient is taking medication, and it is not effective after an adequate trial, clozapine can be helpful. Many have documented clozapine's benefits for violent patients, but Krakowski et al. (2006) completed a study directly comparing haloperidol, olanzapine, and clozapine in the treatment of assaultive patients with schizophrenia and schizoaffective disorder. They found that clozapine was more efficacious than olanzapine, and olanzapine was more efficacious than haloperidol. The antiaggressive effects seemed to be above and beyond the antipsychotic and sedative effects of the medications.

Predicting Who Is Likely to Become Violent

The best management of violence is prevention. Use the predictors discussed earlier and past behavior to identify patients who are likely to become violent. The best predictor of future behavior is past behavior. Learn the circumstance of past assault—for example, if the patient assaulted staff members or fellow patients when denied discharge or when being placed in seclusion close to the time of admission. This information can be difficult to obtain reliably from patients alone, so detailed past records are helpful. Circumstances associated with assault may be avoided in the future or at least anticipated with watchfulness and caution.

Designing and Managing Physical Space to Prevent Violence

Assault prevention is an effort of all clinical and even managerial staff. Reactive assaults can be prevented by minimizing potential provocations. Coercive assaults can be prevented by minimizing factors that lead to victimization.

Ward design and furnishing is part of violence prevention. Wards should be designed to optimize patient observation. Staff should observe for heated arguments, threats, and intrusive behaviors and intervene quickly. Eliminate potential weapons such as chairs that can be

Schizophrenia and Delusional Disorder

easily thrown and blood pressure cuffs set in heavy metal posts on wheels. Eliminate places where weapons can be hidden, such as dropped ceilings made of fiberboard squares that can easily be lifted. Safeguard individual patient privacy with barriers in bathrooms, showers, and bedrooms so personal intrusions and reactive, paranoid assaults are less likely. Safeguard personal possessions to decrease thefts. Patients should have secure lockers with functional locks. Valuables such as cash and cigarettes may be best held by staff.

Physical closeness and threats can predict assault. This has practical significance for management of space between patients, for example in lines, elevators, dining rooms, and dayrooms. Avoid crowding, bumping, shoving, and pushing. Do not require patients to wait in lines for medications or meals. In a large psychiatric hospital, patients were escorted daily to off-ward programming. So that escorts could make fewer trips, patients were packed shoulder to shoulder and elbow to belly into elevators; in this setting, angry shouts and shoving were common. Shouts and shoving could easily lead to fistfights in a small enclosed space. This is an excellent example of what not to do.

Managing Interpersonal Interactions to Prevent Violence

Staff should strive to provide a predictable, orderly, safe, and respectful environment. When patients feel threatened or unsafe, they are more likely to be assaultive. Hospital staff members should avoid behavior that could be seen as threatening; always remain calm and nonconfrontational, and never yell. Coercion should be minimal and in the interests of patient safety, not staff convenience. Expectations should be simple, clear, and rational. Rules that are complicated or inconsistent can be confusing and seem hostile. A punitive approach is also usually seen as hostile or aggressive. Swanson et al. (2006) found that patients who felt listened to most of the time were less likely to be violent than those who did not feel listened to. This could certainly apply to patients who feel listened to by hospital staff.

Hospital staff members bear a responsibility to protect patients from victimization by other patients through bullying and theft. This can be done through vigilant observation and means to secure patient property. When staff cannot provide justice, patients provide their own version, often through violence.

Because threatening and intrusive behaviors may often precede assault, staff should observe patients for these and intervene. These behaviors occur in both parties in assaults, so interventions can target potential victims as well as assailants. Psychiatrists should note these behaviors and consider whether they are manifestations of illness that could be treated. For example, a white man with mania was often the target of assaults by fellow patients who were African American. This was a mystery until he was seen and heard edging in on one and muttering racial epithets. When he was more aggressively treated with lithium, he sat for extended periods and was not assaulted.

In the community, targets of assaults are likely to be family members, rather than fellow patients or staff members, and are more likely to be involved in relationships with the assailant marked by mutual hostility and financial dependence (Estroff et al. 1998). Family members should attempt to disentangle themselves from such relationships, decreasing hostility and patients' financial dependence.

Case Examples

The following is an example of a very serious assault; this type of assault is rare and is not part of the studies discussed earlier, except perhaps Taylor's (1985). It illustrates that psychotic factors, particularly delusional thinking, can be forgotten, suppressed, or repressed while nonpsychotic motivations are expressed.

Case Example 1

Mr. A was 48 years old when he was released on parole and committed to a psychiatric hospital after serving a 12-year sentence for killing his common-law wife with a kitchen knife. He related that she started a fight with him over a coat, which she said he did not hang up properly. As she came at him with a large fork, he stabbed her. "She got like that," he said. He denied he was drinking or using illicit substances at the time of the crime. After the crime, he turned himself in at the local precinct.

As he lay in bed in prison, he would occasionally see and hear his wife and long for her. "Don't cry over spilt milk? I still cry over spilt milk," he said. "That saying is wrong."

Records of a psychiatric admission 4 years before the crime revealed that he had gone to his wife's workplace with a knife because he wanted to break the spell he believed she had cast over him. He also believed she was controlling his mind. Of this admission Mr. A had few memories. He could only recall, "They say I was hearing voices." When reminded of the documented circumstances of his previous admission, he became visibly disturbed and said at that time he was acting a fool and was ill.

The following case illustrates the connections among paranoia, irritability, and assaultiveness, as well as treatment recommendations.

Case Example 2

Mr. B was a man in his twenties with a diagnosis of chronic schizophrenia and mild mental retardation. He had been continuously hospitalized for at least 5 years. On the ward he was constantly irritable and paranoid, especially about the food he was served, believing it was deliberately contaminated with crack cocaine or cyanide. He also worried that he was losing weight and that his body was changing in various ways.

Mr. B was seen daily, and he frequently would present a complaint. He asked to see an ophthalmologist for poor near vision and a podiatrist for burning feet and dry skin. He asked to sleep in an open seclusion room because his room was too hot. He refused breakfast, saying he had a cold that he could feel in his chest and head. He asked for cough syrup and to stay in bed. He said he did not get his oral antipsychotic medication and that he could not live without it. Later the same day he complained his mind was exploding because of medication, asked for a decreased dose, and said he needed none.

This patient could be mollified or put off sometimes, but never convinced or brought around. He wanted to explain that all the violent incidents he had been involved in were not his fault. After a few weeks of such complaints, he punched another patient in the head because, as he related, he was upset that he had not received a kosher diet. Fifteen minutes later while passing in the hall, his victim hit Mr. B, and Mr. B became enraged. Staff members tried at length to calm him down, but he hit one in the face.

After it became clear that Mr. B was ingesting little of his medication consistently, a court order for fluphenazine decanoate was obtained. As a result he had increased attention span, better ability to express himself verbally, fewer paranoid and somatic complaints, and much less assaultiveness.

The following case illustrates an assault apparently resulting from physical closeness between two men and paranoia in an environment that was threatening and disorderly and where the assailant did not feel listened to. The patient told of another assault that was reactive, but his reactivity was likely due to his psychotic symptoms. It might also be called antisocial, because he believed he did the right thing in beating another man. A psychiatrist wrote that Mr. C's actions were driven by his personality structure and that he was not agitated or paranoid. This inpatient psychiatrist released him to a shelter the day after Mr. C had beaten another patient with a chair and his fists. In so doing, the psychiatrist may not have appreciated that treatment might prevent future assaults.

Case Example 3

Mr. C was sent to a hospital emergency department after he punched another man at the shelter where he was living. The other man, who was much larger, subsequently punched Mr. C in the eye, causing an orbital fracture. Once he was admitted to the psychiatric unit, Mr. C. expressed a desire to stay at least 6 months because it was a nice environment, unlike the shelter, which he called a "dog-eat-dog world" where other residents stole and counselors ignored him. He explained that he punched the man because he thought he was playing around behind his back, trying to harm him. He realized he was mistaken and, in his own language, "paranoid," but he acknowledged that he had felt nervous with other people behind his back as long as he could recall. In the previous 2 years, he had heard voices telling him he was nothing and was going to be nothing.

He recalled another assault during a previous hospitalization in which he hit another patient with a chair. He said that in this case he was not paranoid but in his "natural senses" and "did right." The other man had been yelling and cursing at him in a violent, hostile voice to get off the phone. Mr. C. became angry and hit him because he felt disrespected, as though the man were telling him he was worthless.

On the psychiatric unit he was tapered off valproate and ziprasidone and started on gradually increasing doses of olanzapine. Perhaps more importantly, he was assigned a private room and allowed to stay there whenever he pleased, by himself, even at meals. Within 3 weeks he started venturing out to take part in group activities. Soon he was seen chatting with his fellow patients, and his grooming and dress improved. He was quiet, watchful, never threatening, and never involved in physical fights. Mr. C was usually abrupt with his psychiatrist but accepted all treatments offered. He was thankful when offered transfer to a state hospital because he believed transfer would offer him a chance to leave the shelter system and obtain Social Security.

Key Points

- Large community surveys find rates of violent behavior in adults with schizophrenia are somewhat higher than in adults with no diagnosed psychiatric illness but are lower than in groups with substance abuse disorders.

- Serious violence in a large group of patients with schizophrenia has been associated with hostility, suspiciousness, persecutory delusions, hallucinations, grandiosity, and excitement.

- Negative symptoms were associated with a decreased risk of serious violence in this same large group. High levels of positive symptoms with high levels of negative symptoms were not linked to increased risk of serious violence, but high levels of positive symptoms with low levels of negative symptoms were.

Schizophrenia and Delusional Disorder

- Psychopathology and historical factors explain only a small amount of the differences in rates of violence between patients with schizophrenia.
- Assaults occur in an interpersonal context and rarely "out of the blue." They can be understood as reactive, coercive, or arising out of psychosis—or, more likely, some combination of these.
- Assaults are often preceded by identifiable behaviors in both the patient who hits and the patient who gets hit: namely, threatening behaviors (e.g., arguing and fist shaking) and intrusive behaviors (e.g., getting very close).
- Assault can be less likely if staff observe patients closely and maintain an orderly, predictable, and respectful milieu.
- Inpatient management of violent patients is a team effort requiring consensus and collaboration with all disciplines.
- Management decisions should be guided by data and vigorous efforts to preserve patient dignity and protect patient and staff safety. Interventions should be the least restrictive necessary to ensure safety.
- Clozapine has been shown to be more efficacious than olanzapine, and olanzapine to be more efficacious than haloperidol, in controlling assaultiveness in inpatients with schizophrenia and schizoaffective illness. The antiaggressive effects of these drugs seem to be above and beyond the antipsychotic and sedative effects.
- The best management is prevention. Violence may be prevented by identifying patients likely to become violent on the basis of known predictors or past behavior. Violence may be prevented by foresighted design of physical space and by providing a safe, predictable milieu.
- Physical closeness and threats can predict assault. Avoid situations that lead to patient crowding, bumping, shoving, and pushing.
- Family members should try to disentangle themselves from relationships with patients marked by mutual hostility and patients' financial dependence.

References

American Psychiatric Association: Diagnostic and Statistical Manual of Mental Disorders, 3rd Edition. Washington, DC, American Psychiatric Association, 1980

Arseneault L, Moffitt TE, Caspi A, et al: Mental disorders and violence in a total birth cohort. Arch Gen Psychiatry 57:979–986, 2000

Bernay LJ, Elverson DJ: Managing acutely violent inpatients, in Understanding and Treating Violent Psychiatric Patients. Edited by Crowner ML. Washington, DC, American Psychiatric Press, 2000, pp 49–68

Braham LG, Trower P, Birchwood M: Acting on command hallucinations and dangerous behavior: a critique of the major findings in the last decade. Clin Psychol Rev 24:513–528, 2004

Campbell M, Schulman D, Rapoport JL: The current status of lithium therapy in child and adolescent psychiatry. J Am Acad Child Psychiatry 17:717–720, 1978

Campbell M, Cohen IL, Small AM: Drugs in aggressive behavior. J Am Acad Child Psychiatry 21:107–117, 1982

Campbell M, Small AM, Green WH, et al: Behavioral efficacy of haloperidol and lithium carbonate: a comparison in hospitalized aggressive children with conduct disorder. Arch Gen Psychiatry 41:650–656, 1984

Campbell M, Adams PB, Small AM, et al: Lithium in hospitalized aggressive children with conduct disorder: a double-blind and placebo-controlled study. J Am Acad Child Adolesc Psychiatry 34:445–453, 1995

Crowner ML, Stepcic F, Peric G, et al: Typology of patient-patient assaults detected by videocameras. Am J Psychiatry 151:1669–1672, 1994

Crowner M, Peric G, Stepcic F, et al: Psychiatric patients' explanations for assaults. Psychiatr Serv 46:614–615, 1995

Crowner ML, Peric G, Stepcic F, et al: Assailant and victim behaviors immediately preceding inpatient assault. Psychiatr Q 76:243–256, 2005

Eichelman BS: Neurochemical and psychopharmacologic aspects of aggressive behavior. Annu Rev Med 41:149–158, 1990

Estroff SE, Swanson JW, Lachiocotte WS, et al: Risk reconsidered: targets of violence in the social networks of people with serious psychiatric disorders. Soc Psychiatry Psychiatr Epidemiol 33:S95–S101, 1998

Kay SR, Wolkenfeld F, Murrill LM: Profiles of aggression among psychiatric patients, II: covariates and predictors. J Nerv Ment Dis 176:547–555, 1988

Krakowski M, Czobor P, Chou JC: Course of violence in patients with schizophrenia: relationship to clinical symptoms. Schizophr Bull 25:505–517, 1999

Krakowski M, Czobor P, Citrome L, et al: Atypical antipsychotic agents in the treatment of violent patients with schizophrenia and schizoaffective disorder. Arch Gen Psychiatry 63:622–629, 2006

Link BG, Stueve A, Phelan J: Psychotic symptoms and violent behaviors: probing the components of "threat/control-override" symptoms. Soc Psychiatry Psychiatr Epidemiol 33:S55–S60, 1998

Monahan J, Steadman H, Silver E, et al: Rethinking Risk Assessment: The Macarthur Study of Mental Disorder and Violence. New York, Oxford University Press, 2001

Nolan KA, Czobor, P, Biman R, et al: Characteristics of assaultive behavior among psychiatric inpatients. Psychiatr Serv 54:1012–1016, 2003

Quanbeck CD, McDermott BE, Lam J, et al: Categorization of aggressive acts committed by chronically assaultive state hospital patients. Psychiatr Serv 58:521–528, 2007

Sheard MH, Marini JL, Bridges CI, et al: The effect of lithium on impulsive aggressive behavior in man. Am J Psychiatry 133:1409–1413, 1976

Stueve A, Link BG: Violence and psychiatric disorders: results from an epidemiological study of young adults in Israel. Psychiatr Q 68:327–342, 1997

Swanson JW, Holzer CE, Ganju VK, et al: Violence and psychiatric disorder in the community: evidence from the Epidemiologic Catchment Area surveys. Hosp Community Psychiatry 41:761–770, 1990

Swanson JW, Swartz M, Van Dorn RA, et al: A national study of violent behavior in persons with schizophrenia. Arch Gen Psychiatry 63:490–499, 2006

Taylor PJ: Motives for offending among violent and psychotic men. Br J Psychiatry 147:491–498, 1985

CHAPTER 7

Posttraumatic Stress Disorder

Thomas A. Grieger, M.D., D.F.A.P.A.
David M. Benedek, M.D., D.F.A.P.A.
Robert J. Ursano, M.D., D.F.A.P.A.

Posttraumatic stress disorder (PTSD) is classified as an anxiety disorder and is defined by exposure to a severe traumatic event and the presence of a cluster of symptoms (American Psychiatric Association 2000). Individuals must have experienced, witnessed, or learned of an event that involved death, injury, or threat to physical integrity and reacted to that event with intense fear, helplessness, or horror. To meet diagnostic criteria, traumatically exposed persons must also have symptoms of re-experiencing the event, avoidance of reminders of the event or numbing of responsiveness, and increased symptoms of arousal or vigilance. The symptom pattern must be present for more than 1 month and result in clinically significant distress or impairment of functioning.

PTSD was first formally recognized by the psychiatric community in 1980 (American Psychiatric Association 1980). During and after the war in Vietnam, clinicians observed that a substantial portion of soldiers were experiencing protracted problems with readjustment into civilian society due to symptoms related to their wartime experiences. A core constellation of psychiatric symptoms became the basis for diagnostic criteria for PTSD, but other difficulties were also observed. Among these were intermittent acts of aggression or violence. Other symptoms associated with PTSD, but not required for the diagnosis, include impaired interpersonal relationships, impaired affect modulation, self-destructive and impulsive behaviors, feelings of constant threat, and changes in personality characteristics. The American Psychiatric Association's practice guidelines note that some individuals with PTSD have an increased expectation of danger that results in an "anticipatory bias" in their perception of their environment and increased readiness for "flight, fight, or freeze" responses (Ursano et al. 2004). This increased readiness for aggression may take the form of a reduced ability to tolerate mild or moderate slights, resulting in acts that are disproportionate to the degree of provocation. Other psychiatric conditions commonly comorbid with PTSD include major depression, substance abuse disorders, and other anxiety disorders (American Psychiatric Association 2000).

Almost all studies of aggression and violence in patients with PTSD have been conducted among combat veterans from the Vietnam era. Violence in patients who develop PTSD in response to sexual assaults, physical assaults, motor vehicle crashes, acts of terrorism, or exposure to natural and manmade disasters has not been well studied. In contrast to other patients with PTSD (e.g., those whose PTSD results from a motor vehicle accident or an isolated sexual assault), war veterans during combat will have experienced extended periods of heightened vigilance and arousal lasting weeks to months and extreme and repeated interpersonal violence. Exposures include being shot at by enemy forces, killing enemy forces, and sometimes being responsible for the wounding or death of noncombatants. Under certain wartime conditions, some may also witness or participate in repeated non-warfare acts of abusive violence or killing of prisoners or civilians (Laufer et al. 1984). Some civilian law enforcement officers may also have similar, but less repeated, exposures.

Veterans with PTSD demonstrate higher levels of anger, problems with anger regulation, increased levels of criminality, increased levels of violence, and greater potential for serious acts of violence when compared with other patient populations. Domains of anger problems include inaccurate perception and processing of environmental cues, heightened physiological and emotional activation, and behavioral inclinations to act in antagonistic or confrontational ways (Chemtob et al. 1997). Patients with regulatory deficits in all three domains display anger and aggression that has been labeled a "ball of rage" (Chemtob et al. 1997).

Although the literature on violence and PTSD is extensive, findings between studies have shown multiple possible explanations for this association and leave open many questions. Are those exposed to serious personal threat more likely to have come from troubled backgrounds prior to the trauma? Does exposure to violence lead to future acts of violence directly, or is it mediated through the development of PTSD? What is the role of comorbid substance use and violence?

Perhaps due to the complex number of pathways to violence, models to predict future acts of violence among veterans with PTSD have not shown useful predictive value. Among one group of veterans with PTSD, demographic variables, exposure to atrocities, severity of PTSD symptoms, severity of drug and alcohol problems, past violent behaviors, past suicidal behaviors, and prior treatment information were used in an attempt to develop such a model (Hartl et al. 2005). Only prior violence history was useful in predicting postdischarge violence; PTSD and depression severity were both poor predictors of high- and low-risk group membership.

Although no precise model exists for predicting violence among patients with PTSD, there are identified risk factors for future violence that can be the focus for management and treatment. Research during the past three decades has examined multiple risk factors in an effort to determine which seem most strongly associated with the violence in patients with PTSD.

Risk Factors for Violence or Aggression

Childhood traumas, level of combat exposure, PTSD symptoms and severity, number of combat roles, exposure to atrocities, and preservice antisocial behaviors have all been examined in relationship to later antisocial behavior and violence. The studies often used different measures, controlled for different potentially contributing variables, and sometimes had conflicting findings. When examined together, preservice antisocial behavior and level of combat exposure were associated with postservice antisocial behavior, including incidents of violence, other nonviolent illegal behaviors, occupational problems, and nonviolent interpersonal problems (Resnick et al. 1989). Number of combat roles, subjective stress in combat, number of specific stress exposures, and total PTSD symptom severity have all been associated with postservice assault and weapons charges (Wilson and Zigelbaum 1983). Among participants in the National Vietnam Veterans Readjustment Study (NVVRS; Kulka et al. 1990), male veterans with PTSD reported an average of 13.3 acts of violence in the preceding year compared with 3.5 acts of violence in those without PTSD. They were also 1.5 times more likely to have been arrested or jailed and 3 times as likely to have been convicted of a felony crime. In another analysis of the NVVRS data, premilitary behaviors and experiences and postservice PTSD were both associated with postservice antisocial behavior (Fontana and Rosenheck 2005).

Compared with other psychiatric inpatients, veterans hospitalized with severe PTSD were seven times more likely to have engaged in one of more acts of violence in the 4 months prior to hospitalization, six times more likely to have destroyed property, six times more likely to have threatened others without a weapon, four times more likely to have engaged in physical fights, and three times more likely to have made threats with a weapon (McFall et al. 1999). Severity of PTSD symptoms was also associated with increased risk to make threats of violence without a weapon, engage in physical fights, and make threats with a weapon. Among veteran psychiatric inpatients with any diagnosis, veterans with combat exposure were more likely to engage in assaults or assault-related behavior during hospital admission than veterans without such experiences (Yesavage 1983).

Premilitary problems, exposure to war zone atrocities, and postwar problems were common among veterans with PTSD (Hiley-Young et al. 1995). One-third of veterans reported childhood physical abuse and approximately one-half endorsed one or more significant adolescent behavioral problems. Eighty-six percent endorsed witnessing abusive war zone violence, and 91% both witnessed and participated in abusive violence (hurting, killing, or mutilating Vietnamese). Postmilitary problems included violence toward their spouse (58%), violence toward others (71%), drug problems (62%), and alcohol problems (73%). Interestingly, no association between premilitary factors and postmilitary violence or criminal behavior was found. Participation in killing during war was associated with postmilitary violence toward others and toward spouses.

One of the few studies that examined the association between PTSD and violence in individuals who developed PTSD as a consequence of mostly non-wartime experiences was conducted in a population of 1,140 incarcerated male felons (Collins and Bailey 1990). Prison arrest records indicated that 14% were currently incarcerated for acts of expressive violence (homicide, rape, or aggravated assault). Only 2.3% of the sample met study criteria for presence of PTSD. Of those, 31% reported combat trauma. Although most inmates did not meet criteria for the disorder, 795 (70%) endorsed at least one of nine symptoms of PTSD. When demographic variables, antisocial characteristics, and substance abuse were controlled for, those who met criteria for the diagnosis of PTSD were 4.58 times more likely to be currently incarcerated for homicide, rape, or assault and were 6.75 times more likely to have been arrested for violence within the past year. Among those who did not meet full criteria for PTSD, the presence of each additional symptom of PTSD increased risk of current incarceration for a violent crime (odds ratio [OR] 1.22) and for arrest for violence in the past year (OR 1.26). Of those arrested for a violent crime who endorsed at least one symptom of PTSD ($N=80$), most reported the PTSD symptoms began 1 or more years prior to the arrest. This suggested that the presence of the symptoms may have contributed to the commission of the crime.

Family Violence

Patients with PTSD may direct aggression toward intimate partners. On the Standard Family Violence Index (throwing something at someone, pushing, grabbing, shoving, slapping, kicking, biting, hitting, beating up, threatening with a gun or knife, or using a gun or knife on someone), veterans with PTSD endorsed an average of 22 such acts in the past year (Beckham et al. 1997). In contrast, combat veterans without PTSD endorsed an average of 0.2 such acts in the past year. Socioeconomic status, aggressive responding, and PTSD severity were associated with increased violence. Yet another study found that presence of PTSD may mediate the effect of combat exposure on later intimate partner violence (Orcutt et al. 2003). Among multiple studies of Vietnam-era veterans, past-year partner violence rates range from 13% to 58%, with higher rates generally seen among inpatients with substance dependence, PTSD, or other psychiatric disorders (Marshall et al. 2005). PTSD severity was also correlated with partner abuse severity. Partner physical abuse has also been associated with interactions of alcohol consumption (frequency and amounts) and severity of hyperarousal symptoms (Savarese et al. 2001). Higher rates of depression and drug abuse are seen in veterans who had engaged in partner violence (Taft et al. 2005).

In a study of veterans with either PTSD or depression, but not both conditions, those in each group endorsed similar rates of partner violence (roughly 80%) and severe partner violence (roughly 40%) during the past year (Sherman et al. 2006). Compared with control couples in which the veteran did not currently meet criteria for a serious psychiatric illness, those with either depression or PTSD were twice as likely to endorse any act of partner violence and four times as likely to endorse an act of severe partner violence. The study did not include veterans with comorbid depression and PTSD, so it did not assess the relationship of comorbid illness and partner violence.

Firearm Ownership and Firearms Behaviors

Possession of firearms or presence of firearms within the household may increase the risk of potential serious violence toward others or may elevate the risk of a successful suicide act. Compared with veterans with substance use problems, veterans with PTSD reported owning more than four times as many total firearms (mean, 3.2 vs. 0.72), more than five times as many handguns (mean, 1.6 vs. 0.28), and five times as many rifles or shotguns (mean, 4.3 vs. 0.86). Interestingly, there was no difference in overall gun ownership between the two groups prior to military service (mean, 1.69 vs. 1.68) (Freeman and Roca 2001). Twenty-two percent endorsed aiming a gun at a family member; 21% endorsed firing a gun within their house; 39% endorsed firing a gun to protect home, self, or family; and 54% endorsed holding a loaded gun with suicide in mind. In a separate study, 33% of the PTSD group endorsed carrying a gun on their person at least some of the time, and 33% endorsed killing or mutilating an animal "in a fit of rage" (not while hunting) (Freeman et al. 2003). Both studies were conducted among clinical samples of veterans with chronic combat-related PTSD. The combination of firearm-related aggressive acts and the presence of numerous firearms in homes of veterans with PTSD suggest a strong potential for lethal violence against others or successful suicide.

Suicide

Patients with PTSD are also at increased risk of suicide or suicide attempts. Comorbidity of PTSD and other psychiatric conditions is common, and a substantial portion of patients with PTSD are diagnosed with three or more other conditions (Brady et al. 2000a). The most commonly comorbid conditions are depressive disorders, substance use disorders, and other anxiety disorders, all of which are associated with an increased risk of suicide. In one study, patients with comorbid depression and PTSD were at increased risk of suicide attempts compared with patients with only depression (Oquendo et al. 2003). In a second study, the presence of Cluster B personality disorders (paranoid, narcissistic, borderline, or antisocial personality) in addition to PTSD and depression further increased the risk of suicide attempts (Oquendo et al. 2005). In both of these studies, the majority of subjects were non-veteran women.

Subthreshold PTSD can also develop after exposure to traumatic events. Individuals not meeting full diagnostic criteria for the disorder experience comparable levels of impairment and suicidality when compared with patients who meet full criteria for the disorder (Zlotnick et al. 2002). In one large national screening study, roughly one in four subjects reported at least one PTSD symptom of at least 1 month's duration (Marshall et al. 2001b). Functional impairment, number of comorbid disorders, presence of a depressive disorder, and current suicidal ideation increased linearly and statistically with each increasing additional PTSD symptom. Individuals with subthreshold PTSD were at greater risk of suicidal ideation even after controlling for the presence of a depressive disorder. These studies highlight the importance of screening all patients with a history of trauma for presence of PTSD symptoms that may increase risk of suicide or suicide attempts.

Assessment and Management of Posttraumatic Stress Disorder and Violence

There are numerous guidelines for the assessment and clinical management of PTSD (National Center for PTSD 2004; Ursano et al. 2004; VA/DOD Clinical Practice Guideline Working Group 2004). All guidelines suggest that management should be prioritized according to the degree to which each symptom or behavior is causing distress or loss of function or may affect future safety. A high percentage of patients with PTSD experience comorbid conditions such as depression or substance abuse. Such comorbid conditions must also be evaluated and may need to be addressed first, because they may be the source of greatest risk for morbidity or future dangerousness.

Knowing the nature of the events leading to the development of PTSD is of key importance in assessing potential future dangerousness. Combat exposures and direct interpersonal violence, such as physical assault, appear much more likely to lead to PTSD-associated violence than traumas such as motor vehicle crashes or natural disasters. Areas to inquire about when assessing combat veterans or others who have experienced extreme acts of interpersonal violence are outlined in Table 7–1. Patients should be asked to elaborate on the details, frequency, and duration of each endorsed experience.

As with all psychiatric evaluations, patients with PTSD should be questioned about present suicidal ideation and past suicidal behaviors. High rates of comorbid depression, substance use disorders, and tendency toward firearm ownership all increase the risk of suicide as well as the risk of harm to others. Each of these areas should be carefully assessed in both acute and chronic care settings. Because spouses are often the most available target of violence, patients should be asked about patterns of interaction and conflict resolution within relationships. If their responses are guarded or inconsistent, it may be necessary to

TABLE 7–1. Violence risk factor assessment in the evaluation of patients with posttraumatic stress disorder

Have you been the victim of a violent sexual or physical assault?
  —How many times have you been assaulted?
  —Did the assault(s) involve the use of a weapon?

Have you been in combat?
  —Have you killed or wounded another in combat?
  —Did you participate in or observe killing, mutilation, or torture of civilians?

Are there specific settings or events that cause you to become irritable or "on guard"?

Have you been involved in a physical altercation within the past 6 months?

Do you own a firearm?
  —Do you keep it loaded?
  —Do you carry a firearm on your person or keep one "at arm's length"?
  —Have you ever pointed a firearm at another person as a warning or threat?

contact family members for corroborating information. If spousal abuse is active and severe, court protective orders or other protective actions may be needed until other solutions can be developed.

If patients endorse angry or hostile attitudes or are the victims of violent interpersonal assault they should be asked about their own history of violent acts. Frequency, severity, and time duration since most recent episode should be obtained. Potential screening questions and follow-up elaboration questions are provided in Table 7–2. For each past act of violence, patients should be questioned about the specific events leading up to the incident; specific provocation by the target of their violence; whether alcohol or drugs were involved; and how their current situation, condition, attitudes, and recent behaviors differ from those present at the time of the prior act. If current conditions closely parallel those present at the time of past acts of violence, specific behavioral "trigger avoidance" or "emotional defusing" plans should be developed and rehearsed in the clinician's office. Shortened intervals between treatment sessions, warnings to individuals specifically at risk, and possibly hospitalization or other protective interventions should also be considered. In all instances, the treatment record should reflect the components of the risk assessment and management decision process.

Clinicians should always be vigilant for their own safety. In emergency department settings, agitated, intoxicated patients with PTSD

TABLE 7–2. Acts of aggression inventory: "In the past year, have you..."

Event inventory
1. Been involved in a physical or verbal altercation with a stranger?
2. Been involved in a physical or verbal altercation with an acquaintance?
3. Been involved in a physical or verbal altercation with a spouse or relative?
4. Hit, kicked, or otherwise harmed or killed an animal in anger?
5. Damaged property as a consequence of being angry?
6. Contemplated or attempted suicide?

For each positive response:
    a. Were you under the influence of alcohol or drugs at the time?
    b. Did you have in your possession a firearm, knife, or other weapon?
    c. Did you use or consider using the weapon?
    d. When was the last time such an incident occurred?
    e. What were the specific circumstances that led up to the event?
    f. What was the outcome of the event?
    g. How did it end?
    h. Did you feel your behavior was appropriate under the circumstances?
    i. Would you likely respond the same way in a similar situation?
    j. How commonly would you encounter similar situations?

may need to be relocated to quieter and less distracting settings. Personal belongings and clothing should be checked for firearms or other weapons. All personnel should be trained in emergency response and restraint techniques. Hospitalized patients with PTSD should be carefully assessed for potential violence prior to discharge. Follow-up visits should be scheduled to occur shortly after discharge, preferably with a provider known to the patient. Family members should be educated on signs of pending violent behavior and given direction on methods for obtaining an emergent reevaluation or engaging other safety plans (such as leaving the home or calling police) if they perceive a threat of violence.

Shoenfeld et al. (2004) provided an overview of pharmacological treatments for PTSD. Most studies of treatment for PTSD have been in non-veteran populations and have not examined the specific efficacy of these agents on symptoms of aggression or irritability. The selective serotonin reuptake inhibitors (SSRIs) have been shown to be effective, well tolerated, and safe in treatment of non–combat-related PTSD. Sertraline was effective during the 12-week acute and 24-week continuation stages of treatment, with improvements seen in intrusive symptoms, avoidance symptoms, and arousal symptoms (Brady et al. 2000b; Davidson et al. 2001b; Londborg et al. 2001). The mean dosage at completion was roughly 150 mg/day. Further ongoing treatment was also effective in preventing relapse of PTSD (Davidson et al. 2001a), and study participants reported improvements in quality of life and functional measures. Participants who discontinued the drug had a worsening of symptoms and a decline in quality of life (Rapaport et al. 2002). Roughly 80% of the participants in these trials were women, and only about 5% had PTSD as a consequence of combat experiences, so the degree of benefit of sertraline in combat veteran populations is not known.

Similar response rates and improvements in symptoms and function were seen in controlled studies of paroxetine versus placebo in the treatment of PTSD (Marshall et al. 2001a). The efficacy of 20 mg/day was comparable with that seen using 40 mg/day. The majority of participants were women, and only 5%–7% had PTSD as a consequence of combat exposure. In one study examining the efficacy of fluoxetine in treatment of PTSD, the majority of the participants were men (80%), and more than half had PTSD from combat experience or other wartime exposures (Martenyi et al. 2002). Dosages in the range of 60 mg/day reduced symptoms; however, the response was not as robust as in other SSRI studies. The investigators did not attempt to analyze the effect of trauma type on treatment response.

Recent studies have shown efficacy for prazosin (an α_1 receptor–blocking antihypertensive medication) in reducing nightmares, improving sleep quality, reducing psychological responses to trauma cues, and improving global clinical status (Daly et al. 2005; Raskind et al. 2006; Taylor et al. 2006). These results suggest that prazosin might also be of benefit in reducing irritability and aggressive behavior. Many case and case series reports also suggest the use of other antidepressants, mood stabilizers, and atypical antipsychotic medications for augmentation treatment of refractory PTSD symptoms, including anger and irritability, that may be tied to potential acts of violence (Friedman 2006; Schoenfeld et al. 2004).

Among available psychotherapeutic choices, cognitive-behavioral treatments have been shown to be most effective in treating patients with PTSD (Ursano et al. 2004). Within this class of treatments, both prolonged exposure therapy (guided imagery of the events and in vivo experiences) and cognitive therapy or cognitive processing therapy (correction of distorted perceptions or appraisal of events) have been shown to have benefit in trauma survivors. As with most clinical trials of PTSD treatments, the early studies have mostly involved women with sexual assault histories or other single-event traumas rather than PTSD arising from combat.

Case Example 1

A 39-year-old Drug Enforcement Agency (DEA) officer was medically retired 2 years ago after he had been shot in the face at close range during a drug raid. During his 15 years with the agency he had seen multiple shootings and had observed fellow officers killed in the line of duty. During covert assignment in South America he had seen drug smugglers torture, kill, and mutilate the bodies of rival gangs. In the past 5 years he had had frequent nightmares with themes of killing and pervasive danger, from which he awakened sweating and shaking. He became progressively withdrawn, ultimately divorced his wife of 10 years, and no longer visited or spoke with family members. He was constantly vigilant of his environment and startled at the sound of loud noises. He presently has frequent suicidal ideation but relates no history of acts of self-harm. He has a concealed weapons permit and carries a concealed handgun on his person whenever he leaves his apartment. He experienced some improvement in his depressed mood, lack of pleasure, and poor sleep after being started on sertraline by his primary care physician 4 months ago. He has nightmares nearly every night and has gradually increased his alcohol use to a pint of vodka per night, consuming it between 4:00 and 11:00 P.M. Some mornings he has little recollection of his activities the prior evening. He was referred to an outpatient practice by his primary care physician.

Initial management should consist of a detailed history of trauma events, current symptoms of PTSD, and presence of other comorbid conditions including depression, history of alcohol use, and drug use. The immediate focus is on safety for the patient and others. Past violent acts and firearm-related behaviors should also be explored. Heavy alcohol use, presence of a firearm, loss of social supports, and suicidal ideation all add to risk. Establishment of rapport and trust may be difficult in an individual who would typically avoid mental health professionals because of career concerns. He will also not likely agree to relinquish his firearm. Because of the potentially depressive effects and disinhibition caused by heavy alcohol use, this is the first area of treatment. He is at risk for complicated withdrawal, so a careful withdrawal history must be obtained and inpatient detoxification should be considered. If he is a safe candidate for outpatient withdrawal, he should be monitored daily for the first week after discontinuation and provided benzodiazepines to ease the symptoms and prevent seizures. Benzodiazepines would also assist with his sleep disturbance acutely, but they should not be used for maintenance treatment. A trial of prazosin should be considered to reduce the frequency and severity of nightmares, and his sertraline dosage may need to be titrated to ensure optimal response. Cognitive-behavioral therapy should be initiated to examine the accuracy of his perception of threats, establish future goals and direction, identify "triggers" for possible aggressive acts and develop alternative response choices, and reestablish communication and social supports. To assist with abstinence from alcohol and to establish lifestyle changes, referral to a self-help group such as Alcoholics Anonymous may be useful.

Case Example 2

A 42-year-old career law enforcement officer was referred by his employee assistance program provider for an evaluation of possible PTSD and medication treatment. During his career, the officer had seen multiple partners wounded in the line of duty and had been shot at on three occasions. One of these shootings resulted in a minor wound. He had recently been reprimanded for excessive use of physical force during an arrest, when he repeatedly struck a suspected drug dealer with his baton in response to verbally abusive statements. He has loud, verbally abusive fights with his wife, but these have not escalated to physical violence. On his screening questionnaire, he reported "sleep problems" and "anger control issues" as his primary concerns. He is on no medications and has no prior psychiatric treatment.

On the basis of his history of exposures, this patient may have at least some symptoms of PTSD. A careful trauma history should be gathered and a thorough review conducted for symptoms of PTSD, depression, substance use, and violent acts toward self and others. If substance use is not a significant problem it would be best to focus on the patient's stated problems initially to help cement a therapeutic relationship. To reduce the potential for disinhibition in this potentially aggressive patient, non-γ-aminobutyric acid (GABA) medications such as trazodone or ramelteon may be preferable to benzodiazepines or sleep agents such as zolpidem. If significant symptoms of PTSD or depression are present, an SSRI medication may be helpful for those conditions and may also resolve sleep problems. Anger control issues would be best managed with cognitive-behavioral therapy focused on themes and situations likely to cause anger and on developing alternative response patterns for such situations. At least one appointment with the patient's spouse would also be beneficial to obtain collateral information about her observations of the patient in comparison with his recollections. The need for ongoing couples therapy could then also be assessed. Informal peer counseling with another senior officer may also be available through the department. This setting could assist the pa-

Posttraumatic Stress Disorder | 135

tient in further expanding his repertoire of response patterns in anger-provoking situations.

Case Example 3

A 26-year-old married National Guard sergeant had completed two tours in Iraq (20 months total) and had just been released from active duty to resume his civilian employment. He was self-referred to an outpatient clinic with symptoms of intrusion, avoidance, emotional numbing, hypervigilance, and arousal. Like many of his friends from the war, he carries a loaded pistol in his car and sometimes on his person, "because I feel naked and vulnerable without it." He does not hold a concealed weapons permit. The patient's wife is concerned that whenever the patient is around persons who appear to be of Western Asian origin he becomes notably agitated and overly reactive to any movement on their part. At times she has feared that he would draw his pistol and use it. This behavior is worse on days following nightmares with themes pertaining to the war. The patient drank heavily when he first returned from deployment but cut back when his wife threatened to leave him.

The initial assessment should include a detailed trauma history with information specific to each incident and the patient's emotional reactions to each incident. All prior acts of violence by the patient should also be reviewed with regard to the situation, persons involved, and outcomes. Because the patient cannot legally carry a concealed weapon, this behavior should be carefully explored with him in terms of his knowledge of the law and likely consequences of breaking it, the risks and benefits of being armed under such circumstances, the reality of perceived threat conditions, and alternative means of self-protection. As part of weekly cognitive-behavioral sessions, he should review incidents of encounters with persons of Western Asian heritage, the exact nature of the situation, his observations, his appraisal of the situation, alternative explanations of the situation, his behavioral responses, and the outcome of any such interactions. The goal would be to develop a more realistic appraisal of threat in relatively safe civilian settings. His wife should be enlisted as a collaborator in the therapy process to assist in calming the patient in circumstances of perceived threat and to provide her observations of his behavior to the therapist as treatment progresses. One of the SSRI medications may be beneficial in reducing the symptoms of intrusion, avoidance, numbing, and hypervigilance/arousal. Prazosin may also be helpful in reducing the frequency and severity of nightmares.

Case Example 4

A 23-year-old active-duty Army sergeant presented to the clinic at the urging of his wife. She has requested a divorce—and then recanted her request—on three occasions since his return from a year-long tour in Afghanistan 3 weeks ago. The sergeant notes that he believes his wife "fell in with the wrong crowd" while he was deployed and "stayed out late partying and messing with drugs." She has acknowledged being unfaithful on one occasion. She told the sergeant she quickly broke things off with the man (whom the sergeant knows), but she continues to makes excuses to spend time away from home. The sergeant believes she is either continuing to see this man or is using drugs with her new friends. She usually leaves the house after an argument about household responsibilities. The sergeant reports he has been excessively irritable and angry because she "isn't keeping the house up like she did before I left. She's more concerned about her friends than about me." He further reports that he becomes filled with desperation when he thinks of his wife leaving him. He acknowledges that he has punched walls and kicked a door after her abrupt departures, but he has neither threatened nor assaulted his wife. He explains that she is the "only girl that ever loved me, so I could never hurt her," but he acknowledges that when he thinks of her with that other guy he gets so angry he sees "flashes of me just choking him—or maybe her, and I can't get those out of my head for 10 or 20 minutes until I turn the radio up loud and smoke a cigarette."

He reports initial insomnia and restlessness, particularly when his wife rejects his sexual advances. His sleep is further interrupted by nightmares related to his experience in Afghanistan. He has become socially withdrawn, noting that "I don't want to go out with my wife's friends because they all know what she's been up to while I've been away—and they don't know what I've been through anyway." He denies appetite, weight, energy, or concentration changes or any suicidal thoughts. He notes "I was depressed [at age 11] when my parents divorced. I talked to a counselor every week for 6 months back then, and I took Prozac—but I don't feel that way now." He was raised by his mother after she divorced his physically abusive father. He had very few friends (no close friends and no girlfriends) and preferred to be alone. There is no history of alcohol or illicit substance use. He joined the military immediately after high school and had been successful in special operations training. He married his wife in a courthouse ceremony after a brief courtship, "mostly so that she could get away from her parents and get benefits while I was deployed." During deployment he thought frequently about the life they would have together upon his return. Now he becomes "just so angry inside" when he recognizes that these dreams may not be realized.

This case highlights the potential complications of current psychosocial circumstances and chronic patterns of coping to the management of a potentially violent patient. The soldier reports some symptoms of PTSD, but the feelings of abandonment precipitated by his wife's action, more so than his PTSD symptoms, may prove to be the triggers of interpersonal violence. Further quantification of current PTSD and depressive symptoms is important. However, clarification of his wife's desires with regard to continuing the marriage, and efforts to help the service member reframe the implications of his wife's abrupt departures (whether they reflect that she merely needs time alone or that she truly wants to end the marriage) may prove more useful in reducing anger. A more detailed exploration of the extent of injurious ideation toward his wife's boyfriend is also warranted. Marital therapy may help both the service member and his spouse clarify their present levels of commitment to the relationship. A past history of response to supportive psychotherapy and SSRIs for depression suggests that medication management and supportive therapy might assist the service member in understanding the intensity of his feelings of abandonment, more effectively expressing his frustrations, and identifying alternative coping mechanisms. Careful monitoring in therapy and the development of rapport may facilitate more intensive care (e.g., day treatment or hospitalization) should the psychosocial situation deteriorate.

Key Points

- In contrast to patients who developed PTSD after a single-event trauma, PTSD patients who underwent repeated threats to life from multiple sources and observed repeated acts of violence toward others over long periods are more likely to show heightened vigilance and possibly aggressive or violent behavior in future settings.

- Further research is clearly necessary on therapeutic interventions targeting combat-related PTSD and PTSD-related violence and aggression. The recommended treatments for PTSD, though supported by reasonable evidence in general, have not been well validated in combat veteran populations—those most likely to feel aggression and display violence as a result of their experiences and illness. Furthermore, no controlled studies exist on the effects of treatments on reducing aggression or violence in patients with PTSD.

- For combat veterans with PTSD, present knowledge and clinical experience suggest that assessment and management of aggression and violence should include the use of pharmacological and psychotherapeutic treatments with demonstrated efficacy in other (i.e., noncombat) PTSD patients.

- Effective management also requires treatment of other comorbid conditions and the development of a hierarchy of problems and interventions.

References

American Psychiatric Association: Diagnostic and Statistical Manual of Mental Disorders, 3rd Edition. Washington, DC, American Psychiatric Association, 1980

American Psychiatric Association: Diagnostic and Statistical Manual of Mental Disorders, 4th Edition, Text Revision. Washington, DC, American Psychiatric Association, 2000

Beckham JC, Feldman ME, Kirby AC, et al: Interpersonal violence and its correlates in Vietnam veterans with chronic posttraumatic stress disorder. J Clin Psychol 53:859–869, 1997

Brady K, Killeen TK, Brewerton T, et al: Comorbidity of psychiatric disorders and posttraumatic stress disorder. J Clin Psychiatry 61(suppl):22–32, 2000a

Brady K, Pearlstein T, Asnis GM, et al: Efficacy and safety of sertraline treatment of posttraumatic stress disorder: a randomized controlled trial. JAMA 283:1837–1844, 2000b

Chemtob CM, Novaco RW, Hamada RS, et al: Anger regulation deficits in combat-related posttraumatic stress disorder. J Trauma Stress 10:17–36, 1997

Collins JJ, Bailey SL: Traumatic stress disorder and violent behavior. J Trauma Stress 3:203–220, 1990

Daly CM, Doyle ME, Radkind M, et al: Clinical case series: the use of prazosin for combat-related recurrent nightmares among Operation Iraqi Freedom combat veterans. Mil Med 170:513–515, 2005

Davidson J, Pearlstein T, Londborg P, et al: Efficacy of sertraline in preventing relapse of posttraumatic stress disorder: results of a 28-week double-blind, placebo-controlled study. Am J Psychiatry 158:1974–1981, 2001a

Davidson JR, Rothbaum BO, van der Kolk BA, et al: Multicenter, double-blind comparison of sertraline and placebo in the treatment of posttraumatic stress disorder. Arch Gen Psychiatry 58:485–492, 2001b

Fontana A, Rosenheck R: The role of war-zone trauma and PTSD in the etiology of antisocial behavior. J Nerv Ment Dis 193:203–209, 2005

Freeman TW, Roca V: Gun use, attitudes toward violence, and aggression among combat veterans with chronic posttraumatic stress disorder. J Nerv Ment Dis 189:317–320, 2001

Freeman TW, Roca V, Kimbrell T: A survey of gun collection and use among three groups of veteran patients admitted to veterans affairs hospital treatment programs. South Med J 96:240–243, 2003

Friedman MJ: Posttraumatic stress disorder among military returnees from Afghanistan and Iraq. Am J Psychiatry 163:586–593, 2006

Hartl TL, Rosen C, Drescher KD, et al: Predicting high-risk behaviors in veterans with posttraumatic stress disorder. J Nerv Ment Dis 193:464–472, 2005

Hiley-Young B, Blake DD, Abueg FR, et al: Warzone violence in Vietnam: an examination of premilitary, military, and postmilitary factors in PTSD inpatients. J Trauma Stress 8:125–141, 1995

Kulka RA, Schlenger WE, Fairbank J, et al: The prevalence of other postwar readjustment problems, in Trauma and the Vietnam War Generation: Report of the National Vietnam Veterans Readjustment Study. New York, Brunner-Mazel, 1990, pp 139–188

Laufer RS, Gallops MS, Frey-Wouters E: War stress and trauma: the Vietnam veteran experience. J Health Soc Behav 25:65–85, 1984

Londborg PD, Hegel MT, Goldstein S, et al: Sertraline treatment of posttraumatic stress disorder: results of 24 weeks of open-label continuation treatment. J Clin Psychiatry 62:325–331, 2001

Marshall AD, Panuzio J, Taft CT: Intimate partner violence among military veterans and active duty servicemen. Clin Psychol Rev 25:862–876, 2005

Marshall RD, Beebe KL, Oldham M, et al: Efficacy and safety of paroxetine treatment for chronic PTSD: a fixed-dose, placebo-controlled study. Am J Psychiatry 158:1982–1988, 2001a

Marshall RD, Olfson F, Hellman C, et al: Comorbidity, impairment, and suicidality in subthreshold PTSD. Am J Psychiatry 158:1467–1473, 2001b

Martenyi F, Brown EB, Zhang H, et al: Fluoxetine versus placebo in posttraumatic stress disorder. J Clin Psychiatry 63:199–206, 2002

McFall M, Fontana A, Raskind M, et al: Analysis of violent behavior in Vietnam combat veteran psychiatric inpatients with posttraumatic stress disorder. J Trauma Stress 12:501–517, 1999

National Center for PTSD: The Iraq War Clinicians Guide, 2nd Edition. Washington, DC, Veterans Administration, 2004. Available at http://www.ncptsd.va.gov/ncmain/ncdocs/manuals/iraq_clinician_guide_v2.pdf. Accessed January 16, 2007

Oquendo MA, Friend JM, Halberstam B, et al: Association of comorbid posttraumatic stress disorder and major depression with greater risk for suicidal behavior. Am J Psychiatry 160:580–582, 2003

Oquendo M, Brent DA, Birmaher B, et al: Posttraumatic stress disorder comorbid with major depression: factors mediating the association with suicidal behavior. Am J Psychiatry 162:560–566, 2005

Orcutt HK, King LA, King DW: Male-perpetrated violence among Vietnam veteran couples: relationships with veteran's early life characteristics, trauma history, and PTSD symptomatology. J Trauma Stress 16:381–390, 2003

Rapaport MH, Endicott J, Clary CM: Posttraumatic stress disorder and quality of life: results across 64 weeks of sertraline treatment. J Clin Psychiatry 63:59–65, 2002

Raskind MA, Peskind ER, Hoff DJ, et al: A parallel group placebo controlled study of prazosin for trauma nightmares and sleep disturbance in combat veterans with post-traumatic stress disorder. Biol Psychiatry 61:928–934, 2006

Resnick HS, Foy DW, Donahoe CP, et al: Antisocial behavior and post-traumatic stress disorder in Vietnam veterans. J Clin Psychol 45:860–866, 1989

Savarese VW, Suvak MK, King LA, et al: Relationships among alcohol use, hyperarousal, and marital abuse and violence in Vietnam veterans. J Trauma Stress 14:717–732, 2001

Schoenfeld FB, Marmar CR, Neylan TC: Current concepts in pharmacotherapy for posttraumatic stress disorder. Psychiatr Serv 55:519–531, 2004

Sherman MD, Sautter F, Jackson MH, et al: Domestic violence in veterans with posttraumatic stress disorder who seek couples therapy. J Marital Fam Ther 32:479–490, 2006

Taft CT, Pless AP, Stalans LJ, et al: Risk factors for partner violence among a national sample of combat veterans. J Consult Clin Psychol 73:151–159, 2005

Taylor FB, Lowe K, Thompson C, et al: Daytime prazosin reduces psychological distress to trauma specific cues in civilian trauma posttraumatic stress disorder. Biol Psychiatry 59:577–581, 2006

Ursano RJ, Bell C, Eth S, et al: Practice guideline for the treatment of patients with acute stress disorder and posttraumatic stress disorder. Am J Psychiatry 161(suppl):3–31, 2004

VA/DOD Clinical Practice Guideline Working Group: Management of Post-Traumatic Stress. Washington, DC, Department of Veterans Affairs and Department of Defense, 2004. Available at http://www.oqp.med.va.gov/cpg/PTSD/PTSD_base.htm. Accessed January 16, 2007

Wilson JP, Zigelbaum SD: The Vietnam veteran on trial: the relation of posttraumatic stress disorder to criminal behavior. Behav Sci Law 1:69–83, 1983

Yesavage JA: Differential effects of Vietnam combat experiences vs. criminality on dangerous behavior by Vietnam veterans with schizophrenia. J Nerv Ment Dis 171:382–384, 1983

Zlotnick C, Franklin CL, Zimmerman M: Does "subthreshold" posttraumatic stress disorder have any clinical relevance? Compr Psychiatry 43:413–419, 2002

CHAPTER 8

Substance Abuse Disorders

Rodney Burbach, M.D.

> And Noah began to be an husbandman, and he planted a vineyard: And he drank of the wine, and was drunken; and he was uncovered within his tent.
>
> *Genesis 9:20–21, King James Version*

> For U.S. Troops at War, Liquor Is Spur to Crime
>
> *The New York Times, March 13, 2007*

From Biblical times through the present, we have known that alcohol is often associated with out-of-control behavior and violence. Alone among abused chemicals, only alcohol directly and commonly increases aggression (Roth 1994). With illegal drugs, in contrast, the associated violence is more often due to drug commerce: conflicts between distributors, arguments and robberies between buyers and sellers, or stealing to raise drug money (Roth 1994). Alcohol sedates the frontal regions of the brain, the regions necessary for more judicious, thoughtful decisions. Almost one-third of American adults drink at levels that increase their risk for physical, mental health, or social problems (National Institute on Alcohol Abuse and Alcoholism [NIAAA] 2004).

Most instances of substance-related violence happen at times and places with no physician in attendance (homes, the street, bars, clubs, discos) (Macdonald et al 1999; Steadman et al 1998). Yet we as clinicians can reduce that type of violence by identifying and treating substance abuse. As Volavka (2002) has noted, alcohol-dependent persons "are not at an increased risk for offending as long as they are sober. Of course, such persons are by definition at a very high risk for not staying sober" (p. 206).

Alcohol and Violence

Case Example 1

In recovery from alcoholism and tortured by guilt, Alex returned to the scene of a bar fight that he had been involved in many months before. He learned the day after the fight that the man he hit had died, and he moved on. Now he returned, but no one remembered him or the man who had died. They were both just passing through.

In a comprehensive study of homicide offenders in Northern Sweden, Lindqvist (1986) found that 66% of the offenders were intoxicated at the time of the killing. A Scandinavian study showed that, in comparisons across countries and over time, a change of 1 liter in annual per capita alcohol consumption was associated with a 2%–10% change in criminal violence (Alcohol and Public Health Research Unit [New Zealand], n.d.). Moderate intoxication can combine with feeling a loss of control in personal relationships, being in a crowded space, and being ineptly refused service to bring on violence. Saying "I was drunk at the time" is a familiar way of avoiding responsibility (Alcohol and Public Health Research Unit [New Zealand], n.d.). Volavka (2002) reported that in short-term experiments, low doses of alcohol "elicit or facilitate" aggression but high doses reduce it (p. 197).

Although alcohol and drugs often play an essential role in violence, many other factors can contribute to violent behavior. Various authors have emphasized the importance of culture and context. In addition, specific factors can include a history of alcoholism, psychological disorders, sleep deprivation, and physical conditions such as temporal lobe dysfunction and hypoglycemia (Benson et al. 2001). Lipsey et al. (1997) described causality in terms of "an alcohol–person–situation interaction," arguing that "alcohol consumption increases the probability of violent behavior only in some persons in some situations" (p. 247). One such scenario is described below.

Case Example 2

Bert and his wife were arguing about their financial problems. Because of his angry, intoxicated outburst, his wife called the police, who came and left. His wife then left the house, taking their child with her. Bert drank

Substance Abuse Disorders | 143

through that night. The next day he called his boss, saying he did not feel well, and he continued to drink. That evening the police pounded on his door to serve a warrant. He called 911, telling the operator that he did not know what was going on, but that he had a gun and he was defending his home. The police placed a cordon around the house.

Three mechanisms have been proposed to explain the link between alcohol and violence: potentiation, inhibition, and disorganization (Pihl and Lemarquand 1998). Thanks to the work of Anna Rose Childress, Ph.D., and others, we have a much better understanding of the physiological effect of alcohol and drugs that tilts the balance between the limbic system ("GO!") and the frontal lobes ("STOP!") ("HBO: Addiction" 2007). The limbic circuits respond quickly and strongly to danger, food, and sex. The frontal brain regions, also vital to the welfare of our species, make us stop and think, bringing in memories and experiences that should influence our behavior. Adolescents have not yet fully developed the circuits needed for the prefrontal cortex to regulate the limbic system, and in addition, their amygdalas are more active.

The relations between rape and alcohol use have been summarized as follows:

> Conservative estimates of sexual assault prevalence suggest that 25% of American women have experienced sexual assault, including rape. Approximately one-half of those cases involve alcohol consumption by the perpetrator, victim, or both. Alcohol contributes to sexual assault through multiple pathways, often exacerbating existing risk factors. Beliefs about alcohol's effects on sexual and aggressive behavior, stereotypes about drinking women, and alcohol's effects on cognitive and motor skills contribute to alcohol-involved sexual assault. (Abbey et al. 2001, p. 43)

Date rape is an important kind of violence to which alcohol contributes. This type of assault in a college setting has been characterized in this way by Koss (1988):

> Among college students, a typical sexual assault occurs on a date, at either the man's or the woman's home, and is preceded by consensual kissing. The assault involves a single assailant who uses no weapon, but twists the woman's arm or holds her down. The woman believes she has clearly emphasized her nonconsent, and tries to resist by reasoning or by physically struggling. (pp. 242–250)

Presley et al. (1998) found that 1.2%–1.5% of college students had tried to commit suicide during the past 12 months due to drinking or drug use. Lower minimum-age drinking laws are associated with higher youth suicide rates (National Institute of Mental Health, n.d.). Particular risk factors include being American Indian or Alaskan Native (National Institute of Mental Health, n.d.). People dependent on substances are more likely to have financial and social problems, to be depressed, to be impulsive, and to engage in high-risk behaviors that result in self-harm (National Institute of Mental Health, n.d.). An impulsive personality is associated with heavier drinking and with violence (Gelles 1985).

Maltreatment of children is another form of violence closely associated with alcohol use.

Case Example 3

Many years after the event, late in therapy, Carla shared her most painful, secret guilt. She had never told anyone this before. As a young mother deserted by her husband, she felt overwhelmed by the needs of their infant. While drinking and intoxicated, when bathing the child, she had knocked a radio from the edge of the tub into the water, thinking it might electrocute the child. The child was not harmed.

The World Health Organization (WHO) has found a strong link between child maltreatment and alcohol abuse. Thirty-five percent of parental child abusers had consumed alcohol or drugs at the time of the incident (U.S. Department of Justice 2001). Risk factors include being young, poor, unemployed, and socially isolated (Krug et al. 2002). WHO suggests a range of prevention strategies, including family support, parenting training, screening for child maltreatment, and services for victims (World Health Organization, n.d.).

> "Shush, be still, be still, no breath. Off just shut off. Find the ceiling's corner and hide in it."
> "There's no fucking safe place no matter what they say. Don't matter what 'they' say."
> "How long do I have to be 5 years old anyway."
> "Be still, be gone, hold onto the quiet numb solitude."
>
> —Notes written by Martha, an adult woman physician, early in her recovery from alcoholism, dealing with the physical and sexual abuse she experienced in childhood (quoted with her permission)

Abused children, when grown up, have an increased risk of alcoholism. However, the evidence for the linkage of childhood abuse to adult alcoholism is stronger for women than for men (Widom and Hiller-Sturmhofel 2001).

> "Thought I had killed my mother. I went outside. She was peeing in the bushes. She came in. I hit her in the head, I was so angry. She was passed out upstairs. I put a feather in front of her nose. She was still breathing."

> —A woman, in recovery from alcoholism, speaking of her early adolescent relationship with her mother, who had severe alcoholism

Vulnerable adults also can be victims of alcohol-related abuse. In the United States, 44% of male and 14% of female abusers of elders were dependent on alcohol or drugs, as were 7% of the victims (Greenberg et al. 1990). Individuals with alcoholism may be financially dependent on older relatives (Bradshaw and Spencer 1999) and may neglect their responsibilities to them (Department of Social Development [South Africa] 2001).

Drinking alcohol exerts a major influence on intimate partner violence. In studying a group of 109 couples in which the women were participating in a study on therapies for women with alcoholism, Drapkin et al. (2005) found that 61% reported some violence and 27% reported severe violence (kicking, biting, hitting). Generally, men are thought to be more violent than women. But Drapkin and colleagues found that in 27% of the couples they studied, men and women contributed equally to the violence. In couples with a disparity in violence, the more violent person was more likely to be the woman than the man (23% vs. 11%). Overall, the women in this study were more likely than the men to be verbally aggressive and psychologically coercive. Among the women in this study, more intensive drinking was associated with more severe violence or verbal aggression (Drapkin et al. 2005). Following up on a random sample of 1,635 U.S. couples, Ramisetty-Mikler and Caetano (2005) found that female-on-male violence predicted marital separation but that heavy drinking by women reduced the risk of separation.

A 1995 national survey found that 23% of black couples, 17% of Hispanic couples, and 11.5% of white couples reported an incident of male-to-female violence in the 12 months preceding. The corresponding rates of female-to-male violence were 30%, 21%, and 15%, respectively, in each instance higher than male-to-female violence. At the time of violence against their partners, 30%–40% of the men and 27%–34% of the women were drinking. The higher prevalence of intimate partner violence among ethnic minorities seems to be related to individual risk factors, the environment, and the type of relationship between the partners (Caetano et al. 2000). The social-structural theory emphasizes poverty, undereducation, high unemployment, and racial discrimination as contributors to increased violence. Another explanation posits a subculture of violence in which some groups in society accept violence as a means of resolving conflicts (Gelles 1985).

Drinking may reduce fear in victims, making them more willing to participate in a dangerous quarrel, and may make them less able to respond appropriately to threats. The likelihood of aggression between two people is "greatest when both are intoxicated, intermediate when one person is intoxicated, and least probable when both are sober" (Murdoch et al. 1990). The diaries of men attending a batterer intervention program revealed that they were 20 times more likely to attack their partner on heavy drinking days, as compared to non-drinking days (Fals-Stewart 2003).

In gang life, alcohol and violence affirm masculinity and male togetherness. Being on the street is the natural social arena for many minority and working-class male adolescents. The entry to life on the street is through a gang. A new member's passing through initiation is celebrated by drunkenness. Gang members may leave alcohol at the gravesite of a dead member to symbolize their unity (Hunt and Laidler 2001).

Alcohol and Suicide

Hayward et al. (1992) found that alcohol was involved in 36% of suicides. In 46% of suicide attempts, the alcohol had been ingested within the previous 2 hours (Merrill et al. 1992).

Case Example 4

For 10 years, Dan was hypomanic and very successful. "People were patting me on the back, telling me how amazing I was." Sometimes he felt an "electric buzz" that he would try to force down with alcohol. Then he began to have financial losses, depression, and conflicts with his wife. "All the brain power I had when I was manic turned against me. I couldn't come up with a good reason not to kill myself." He waited until 11:00 P.M. so that there wouldn't be any children on the road, then got drunk at a local bar and drove his car into a tree at high speed. He survived, with mild, persistent brain injury.

Case Example 5

Evan was a young man with a strong sense of right and wrong who had intense feelings about justice and injustice. He bitterly criticized himself for various deficiencies, including having failed several college courses. He found a reason to live in a several-years' relationship with a young woman who was also troubled and struggling, but then she left and began sending him e-mails accusing him of sexual insensitivity in their relationship. He purchased a .38 revolver, got drunk, and killed himself. First he left money for his roommates for the month's rent, and he left a message on his therapist's answering machine, thanking her for trying to help him. Evan feared he didn't have the courage to kill himself. With alcoholic intoxication, he found the courage.

Cocaine, Methamphetamine, and Violence

The effects of stimulants in animals vary, depending on the animal species and the primate's social position in the group. Low doses may occasion aggression, with higher doses having the opposite effect (Volavka 2002, p. 210)

Cocaine and methamphetamine are known to induce paranoia in people with no history of psychotic illness.

Case Example 6

The sister of one of my patients phoned me, saying she was concerned that her own husband "might have a little problem with cocaine." As we spoke, this woman's husband was standing in their living room, shotgun at his side, peering through the blinds.

Marzuk et al. (1995) studied the relationship between cocaine use and fatal injuries in New York City in 1990–1992. Of the 14,843 New Yorkers who died from homicides, suicides, accidents, and drug overdoses (the medical examiner's laboratory analyzed blood or urine autopsy specimens for about 85% of cases), benzoylecgonine, a cocaine metabolite with a serum half-life of up to 48 hours, was present in 27% of the cases. Cocaine itself, with a serum half-life of 1.5 hours, was present in 18% of cases. About one-third of these fatalities were from accidental overdose; the other two-thirds were from violence or trauma (Marzuk et al. 1995).

Spunt et al. (1990) found that cocaine-related violent events in women most often were a direct, pharmacologic effect of cocaine. In contrast, in white males, cocaine-related violence was committed primarily to obtain money to buy drugs, and in black males, cocaine-related violence was predominantly associated with drug marketing and sales.

Case Example 7

I saw a young man in the hospital who had a bullet in his right arm. When trying to buy cocaine from a drug dealer, he had folded over a $10 bill, trying to fool the dealer into thinking he was paying two $10 bills.

Opioids and Violence

In experiments, ex-abusers given moderate doses of methadone became friendly and "mellow" (Volavka et al. 1974). The irritability and dysphoria of opiate withdrawal may motivate opiate addicts to rob or steal for money. Prostitutes in opiate withdrawal robbed their clients rather then just providing sex (Goldstein 1985).

PCP and Violence

The disruption of sensory input by phencyclidine (PCP) can produce unpredictable and exaggerated reactions to the environment (Zukin et al. 2005). However, those who are violent under the influence of PCP usually have a history of psychosis or antisocial behavior (Roth 1994).

Cannabis and Violence

In most animal experiments, cannabis extracts reduced aggression and increased flight and submission (Miczek 1987). Adolescent delinquents reported that cannabis made them calm and reduced assaultiveness (Tinklenberg et al. 1976). Volavka et al. (1971) and others have conducted numerous experiments studying the effects of cannabis use and have not seen aggression or violence.

Mental Disorders, Substance Abuse, and Violence

Personality disorder, substance abuse, and neurologic impairment can all contribute to violence.

Antisocial personality disorder is a risk factor for developing problem drinking and often develops a few years before the drinking (Bahlmann et al. 2002). Cloninger et al. (1981) describe a subtype of alcoholism that develops early (usually before age 25), is strongly inherited from father to son, has many features of antisocial behavior, and is associated with abnormal serotonin metabolism (Virkkunen and Linnoila 1990). Ondansetron (a selective 5-HT_3 antagonist) reduces drinking in patients with early-onset alcoholism (Johnson et al. 2000).

The general public has a great fear of violence due to mental illness. For example, 81% of the public believes that children with major depression are more likely to be dangerous to themselves or others (Pescosolido et al. 2007).

The National Institute of Mental Health's Epidemiologic Catchment Area (ECA) study found that patients with serious mental illness (schizophrenia, major depression, bipolar disorder) reported a lifetime prevalence of violence of 16%, as compared to 7% among people without mental illness (Swanson 1994). Because serious mental illness is relatively rare, however, it contributes only 3%–5% to society's risk for violence (Friedman 2006).

The increased lifetime prevalence of violence in people with serious mental illness is strongly influenced by their propensity to abuse alcohol and drugs. Having a mental disorder doubles the risk of alcohol abuse, and it increases the risk of drug abuse by four times (Regier et al. 1990). People with no mental disorder who abuse alcohol or drugs are nearly seven times as likely to report violent behavior as are those who do not abuse alcohol or drugs (Friedman 2006).

Steadman et al. (1998) followed 1,136 patients with various psychiatric disorders for 50 weeks after their discharge from inpatient care. The control group was 519 people living in the same neighborhoods. There was no increased risk of violence among the non–substance abusing mentally ill persons. Substance abuse increased the risk among both patients and those in the control group. Substance abuse in combination with a personality disorder produced the highest risk of violence.

In adults with psychotic illness or major mood disorder, violence independently correlates with several risk factors: substance abuse, a history of having been a victim of violence, homelessness, and poor mental health. The 1-year rate of violent behavior for persons with none or only one of these risk factors was 2%, a prevalence close to the ECA's estimate for the general population. It appears, then, that in people with serious mental illness, violence "probably results from multiple risk factors in several domains" (Friedman 2006, p. 2066).

Delusions that someone is trying to harm one and delusions that outside forces control one's mind are both associated with violence. A study of delusional, violent patients found that 83.5% had a history of substance abuse (Beck 2004).

Brain damage (head injury) changes a person's response to alcohol. Less alcohol produces more effect (Finger and Stein 1982), and alcohol is more likely to make the person feel paranoid and inferior (Langevin et al. 1987), setting the stage for violence.

Addiction

Dackis and O'Brien (2005) have characterized addiction as "a disease of brain reward centers that ensure the survival of organisms and species." They describe the mechanism as follows:

> Given their function, reward centers have evolved the ability to grip attention, dominate motivation and compel behavior directed toward survival goals, even in the presence of danger and despite our belief that we are generally rational beings. By activating and dysregulating endogenous reward centers, addictive drugs essentially hijack brain circuits that exert considerable dominance over rational thought, leading to pro-

gressive loss of control over drug intake in the face of medical, interpersonal, occupational and legal hazards. There is even evidence that denial, once thought to be purely "psychological," may be associated with drug-induced dysfunction of the prefrontal cortex. (Dackis and O'Brien 2005, p. 1431)

The case of a well-educated professional man illustrates these dysfunctional processes.

Case Example 8

Frank was a talented physician who could often get a year or two of recovery from his addiction to opiates. That was enough stability to permit him to work and use his medical skills, although not in patient care. In relapse, he returned to the place where he customarily bought drugs, even though he had been robbed there with a knife at his throat only the night before. Several months later, he died alone in a motel room in another state, probably of an overdose.

Interestingly, a cynomolgus monkey that loses social rank undergoes a reduction in dopamine D_2 receptors and is more likely to self-administer cocaine. If that monkey is placed with a different group of monkeys, among which he has higher social standing, he will have an increase of D_2 receptors (Czoty et al. 2004). Could this physiology explain some of the drug abuse among underprivileged groups?

Modafinil may improve impulse control in addicted patients and help them feel better (Dackis 2005), as illustrated in the following case example.

Case Example 9

Geoff, always falling far short of the expectations of his successful father, began using marijuana in early adolescence and later began using cocaine. Geoff's father understood these drug use–related failures as willful misbehavior and tried to discipline him, sometimes physically. Geoff cooperated superficially with the treatment program his parents had tricked him into attending. "Bunch of crap, just sit down and talk. Didn't get anything out of it. Just listen to people's problems." He planned to "get my life sorted out. Just become a social user. Not completely stop." He continued to smoke marijuana while in the treatment program.

After his completion of that treatment program, Geoff's plans to be a "social user" of cocaine quickly and disastrously crashed. He took his second treatment program much more seriously, understanding that he could not safely use marijuana, either. Modafinil seemed to free him of craving for cocaine and probably also helped his attention-deficit/hyperactivity disorder.

Identifying Addiction

For many years, literature and Hollywood have dramatized (sometimes accurately) the lives of alcoholics and drug addicts. The "Decade of the Brain" has now flowered into a moving, scientifically based mass media production, Home Box Office's series *Addiction* (sponsored by the Robert Wood Johnson Foundation, the National Institute on Alcohol Abuse and Alcoholism, and the National Institute on Drug Abuse), which began March 15, 2007. A superb collection of resources can be accessed, and a DVD of the series can be purchased, at the series Web site (http://www.hbo.com/addiction).

Only 10% of patients with alcoholism receive assessment and referral to treatment from their primary care physicians (McGlynn et al. 2003). For physicians, the National Institute on Alcohol Abuse and Alcoholism (NIAAA, 2005) has released an updated version of *Helping Patients Who Drink Too Much: A Clinician's Guide*. "Too much" is defined as five or more drinks in a day for a man, four or more drinks in a day for a woman. (A standard drink is equivalent to 12 ounces of beer, 5 ounces of wine, or 1.5 ounces of 80-proof spirits.)

The single question "How often in the past year have you had five or more drinks [four for a woman] in a day?" can serve to screen for alcohol-related problems (Dawson et al. 2005). As an alternative to the single question during the clinical interview, the guide suggests screening by the written self-report AUDIT—the Alcohol Use Disorders Identification Test.

For persons who screen positive for alcohol-related problems, the next step is to assess the severity and extent of the problems, using a list of symptoms derived from DSM-IV-TR (American Psychiatric Association 2000). The NIAAA's guide provides additional resources and treatment templates.

About 30% of the U.S. population have what is called "at-risk drinking" (National Institute on Alcohol Abuse and Alcoholism 2005), "heavy drinking," or "unhealthy alcohol use" (Saitz 2005). These levels of use do not meet criteria for substance abuse (a substance-related failure to perform obligations at work, school, or home; use in hazardous situations; or recurrent legal or social problems—often associated with antisocial personality disorder). Nor do they meet criteria for substance dependence (a loss of control of use of the substance; a life focused on getting and using the substance).

Often, "at-risk" heavy drinkers who do not meet the criteria for abuse or dependence can voluntarily reduce their alcohol consumption and can benefit from learning that their consumption is greatly above the norm. Habitually they associate with other people who drink heavily, and they conclude, incorrectly, that such a level of consumption is common. The NIAAA guide *Helping Patients Who Drink Too Much* provides a useful comparison and a template for strategies for cutting down.

Treating Addiction

For many years, 12-Step recovery groups have counseled separating from "people, places, and things" associated with drug or alcohol use. Science has now shown that even years into recovery, environmental cues can powerfully induce relapse (Grusser et al. 2004).

"Evidence-Based" strategies to help patients reduce the risk of relapse (Witkiewitz and Marlatt 2007) include the following:

1. Understanding relapse as a process and event, and learning how to identify early warning signs
2. Identifying high-risk situations and developing coping responses
3. Enhancing communications skills, improving interpersonal relationships, and developing a constructive social network
4. Managing negative emotional states
5. Identifying and managing cravings and the "cues" that precede cravings
6. Identifying and challenging cognitive distortions

Pharmacological treatments for addiction, an obvious corollary to our understanding of addiction physiology, are demonstrably useful and are underused. *Helping Patients Who Drink Too Much* succinctly reviews medications approved by the U.S. Food and Drug Administration for the treatment of alcoholism and makes suggestions for their use.

Naltrexone, an opioid-blocking medication, reduces alcohol craving. Volpicelli et al. (1992) and others (O'Malley et al. 1992) have found that naltrexone most consistently helps people with alcoholism drink less often and in less quantity, forestalling the worst consequences of a relapse. Compared with normal subjects, patients with a genetic vulnerability for alcoholism have low β-endorphin levels, with increased β-endorphin release and pleasure after drinking alcohol (Gianoulakis et al. 1996). Naltrexone, an opioid-blocking agent, reduces that response, especially in persons with the G allele form of the gene coding the mu-opioid receptor, the *OPRM1* gene (Ray and Hutchison 2007). However, Krystal et al. (2001) found that naltrexone was not effective overall in Veterans Affairs patients with chronic, severe alcoholism.

Substance Abuse Disorders | 153

Acamprosate, the newest medication certified by the U.S. Food and Drug Administration to treat alcoholism, alters γ-aminobutyric acid and N-methyl D-aspartate systems (Rammes et al. 2001) and also reduces alcohol craving and relapse. It may help people who feel like drinking because of withdrawal.

Case Example 10

Helen has 50 years of happy marriage, a graduate degree, and a close relationship with her adult children. However, more than once, she was intoxicated when she arrived to provide transportation for her grandchildren. Understandably fearful, Helen's children would not let her take the grandchildren, even when she was sober. Acamprosate seemed to make her recovery more comfortable. (She was also taking antidepressant medication.) Although three times daily is the suggested dosing schedule, Helen had loose stools if she took acamprosate more than twice a day. With participation in 12-Step recovery, she stayed sober and regained the trust of her children.

Although some well-done, randomly controlled trials have found statistical efficacy for naltrexone and for acamprosate, other well-conducted trials have not. Project Combine (Anton et al. 2006) randomly assigned 1,383 patients to one of eight groups, to receive medical management plus pills. Four groups received naltrexone, or acamprosate, or both naltrexone and acamprosate, or placebo. Four other groups received one of these medication regimes plus a "combined behavioral intervention" (CBI). A ninth group received CBI and no pills. Acamprosate showed no evidence of efficacy, with or without CBI. Patients receiving medical management with naltrexone, or with CBI, or with both, showed improvement. No combination showed better efficacy than medical management plus naltrexone or medical management plus CBI. Medical management plus placebo had a greater effect, during treatment, than CBI.

Normally, the liver metabolizes alcohol to acetaldehyde and then to harmless acetic acid. The first of these two steps is the rate-limiting step, the "bottleneck" of this two-step metabolic chain. Disulfiram (available for 60 years) inhibits the liver enzyme of the second step, acetaldehyde dehydrogenase. Because acetaldehyde (which is toxic) is metabolized more slowly, blood levels increase (5–10 times higher) and the person becomes ill, experiencing flushing, throbbing of the head and neck, nausea, vomiting, and shortness of breath. However, with present-day dosage (250 mg daily), people in good health are not in medical danger. As one can predict from the physiological mechanism, the severity of the alcohol–disulfiram reaction depends on the quantity of alcohol ingested. For example, the reaction from the small amount of alcohol that may be ingested from a vinegar salad dressing (or absorbed from hair spray or deodorant) is not severe. Some persons with robust acetaldehyde dehydrogenase require an increased disulfiram dose.

In 1986, R.K. Fuller and colleagues, in a carefully done, controlled, blinded study, concluded that disulfiram "may help reduce drinking frequency after relapse" but "does not enhance counseling in aiding alcoholic patients to sustain continuous abstinence or delay the resumption of drinking" (Fuller et al. 1986, p. 1449).

Disulfiram can be useful for those patients who, although committed to not drinking, cannot trust themselves to abstain, especially early in recovery. Because acetaldehyde dehydrogenase requires as long as 2 weeks to regenerate after cessation of disulfiram, taking disulfiram once daily settles for that day the internal discussion, "Will I drink today?" Disulfiram can be used episodically for protection during business trips or vacation.

Case Example 11

Jerome is a distinguished professional, respected by his colleagues, elected by them to chair an organization representing their interests. However, at a lecture, he appeared intoxicated on stage. He could go for weeks without drinking, but if he had a break in his schedule on a nice day, he might step outside for a bit, and his favorite bar was just down the block, across the street. Seldom could he pass it without going in. Disulfiram gave him long-term sobriety.

Interestingly, disulfiram may be useful in treating cocaine addiction through its inhibition of dopamine-β-hydroxylase (DBH), increasing brain dopamine levels and thus producing an unpleasant sense of hyperstimulaton and discomfort in cocaine users. It is particularly effective for patients who are not also abusing alcohol (Carroll et al. 2004). Current studies are looking at the effectiveness of disulfiram for treating cocaine-dependent individuals with different DBH genetic variants.

Topiramate seems to reduce appetitive behavior generally, including overeating; it is one of the few psychotropic medications that tends to reduce, rather than increase, weight (McElroy et al. 2003), alcohol drinking and craving (Johnson et al. 2003), and cocaine use (Kampman et al. 2004). Unfortunately, it often produces fatigue and cognitive dulling (Salinsky et al. 2005).

Leaving aside the very important maintenance treatment of opioid dependence (i.e., methadone, buprenorphine), our key addiction treatments focus on psychologically influencing the emotions and thoughts

Substance Abuse Disorders | 155

of our patients. We are a social species. Meeting with other people who also are recovering from addiction, people who have had similar experiences, people who come to know us and are not angry at us (as families often are at the addicted person), people who seem to be decent people other than the aberration of their alcohol- and drug-related behaviors, people who are succeeding at recovery—all this powerfully encourages and motivates. Learning that addiction is a disease, with powerful genetic and environmental antecedents, not simply a hopeless moral failing, can lift demoralizing guilt and lend credibility to strategies for managing the disease, as we do with other chronic diseases. Patients learn these strategies from other recovering people, from counselors, and from therapists. Although it is not the focus of this chapter, treating comorbid psychiatric illness, and influencing destructive life circumstances, can be vitally important.

Project MATCH disappointed many high hopes by not confirming 10 hypothesized treatment-effective "matches" between treatment type and type of patient with alcoholism. The one "match" was between patients with low psychiatric severity and 12-Step facilitation therapy. NIAAA Director Enoch Gordis remarked that these findings "challenge the notion that patient–treatment matching is necessary in alcoholism treatment" (National Institute on Alcohol Abuse and Alcoholism 1996).

Although it is hard to study 12-Step programs in a rigorous scientific manner, clinicians who treat addiction have long respected 12-Step recovery. Dr. George E. Vaillant made a major scientific contribution, publishing in 1983 (with a revised edition in 1995) *The Natural History of Alcoholism,* a prospective study of more than 700 individuals followed for more than 40 years. Vaillant wrote that "multiple studies that collectively involved a thousand or more individuals, suggest that good clinical outcomes are significantly correlated with frequency of attendance at Alcoholics Anonymous (AA) meetings, with having a sponsor, with engaging in Twelve-Step work and with chairing meetings" (Vaillant 2005, p. 433, citing Emrick 1993). Dr. Vaillant (2005) observes that Project MATCH found, during its first year, that AA alone was as effective as the two most effective professional alternatives: cognitive-behavioral and motivational enhancement therapies.

Key Points

- Alcohol and other drugs of addiction, interacting with personality and circumstances, often increase the likelihood of violence.
- Alcohol is the most widely used of addictive chemicals, and it is the chemical most likely to induce aggression; therefore it has the largest role in violence.
- Patients often do not volunteer information about their drinking or drug use. Every patient should be asked at least the single screening question: How often in the past year have you had five or more drinks in a day? (four or more drinks for a woman). Even a single such day is reason for further evaluation.
- Addictions treatment is effective. It should be tailored to each patient, using supportive therapies (12-Step meetings, individual therapy), counseling and cognitive-behavioral therapies, and pharmacotherapy.

References

Abbey A, Zawacki T, Buck PO, et al: Alcohol and sexual assault. Alcohol Res Health 25:43–51, 2001

Alcohol and Public Health Research Unit: Alcohol and violence: What's the connection? n.d. Available at: http://www.aphru.ac.nz/hot/violence.htm. Accessed March 6, 2007

American Psychiatric Association: Diagnostic and Statistical Manual of Mental Disorders, 4th Edition, Text Revision. Washington, DC, American Psychiatric Association, 2000

Anton RF, O'Malley SS, Ciraulo DA, et al: Combined pharmacotherapies and behavioral interventions for alcohol dependence. JAMA 295:2003–2017, 2006

Bahlmann M, Preuss UW, Soyka M: Chronological relationship between antisocial personality disorder and alcohol dependence. Eur Addict Res 8:195–200, 2002

Beck JC: Delusions, substance abuse, and serious violence. J Am Acad Psychiatry Law 32:169–172, 2004

Benson BL, Rasmussen DW, Zimmerman PR: The Impact of Alcohol Control Policies on the Incidence of Violent Crime. Final report submitted to National Institute of Justice, Grant No. 99-IJ-CX-0041. 2001. Available from NCJRS (NCJ 191199). Available at http://www.ncjrs.gov/pdffiles1/nij/grants/191199.pdf. Accessed July 1, 2007

Bradshaw D, Spencer C: The role of alcohol in elder abuse cases, in Elder Abuse Work: Best Practice in Britain and Canada. Edited by Pritchard J. London, Jessica Kingsley, 1999, pp 332–353

Caetano R, Cunradi CB, Clark CL, et al: Intimate partner violence and drinking patterns among white, black, and Hispanic couples in the U.S. J Subst Abuse 11:123–138, 2000

Carroll KM, Fenton L, Ball S, et al: Efficacy of disulfiram and cognitive behavior therapy in cocaine-dependent outpatients. Arch Gen Psychiatry 61:264–272, 2004

Cloninger CR, Bohman M, Sigvardsson S: Inheritance of alcohol abuse: cross-fostering analysis of adopted men. Arch Gen Psychiatry 38:861–868,1981

Czoty PW, Morgan D, Shannon EE, et al: Characterization of dopamine D1 and D2 receptor function in socially housed cynomolgus monkeys self-administering cocaine. Psychopharmacology (Berl) 174:381–388, 2004

Dackis C: Drug Des Discov 2:79–86, 2005

Dackis C, O'Brien C: Neurobiology of addiction: treatment and public policy ramifications. Nat Neurosci 8:1431–1436, 2005

Dawson DA, Grant BF, Li TK: Quantifying the risks associated with exceeding recommended drinking limits. Alcohol Clin Exp Res 29:902–908, 2005

Department of Social Development: Mothers and fathers of the nation: the forgotten people: the Ministerial report on abuse, neglect and ill-treatment of older persons. South Africa, Department of Social Development, 2001. Available at www.info.gov.za/documents/subjectdocs/subject/social.htm. Accessed March 10, 2007

Drapkin ML, McCrady BS, Swingle JM, et al: Exploring bi-directional couple violence in a clinical sample of female alcoholics. J Stud Alcohol 66:213–219, 2005

Emrick CD, Tonigan JS, Little L: Alcoholics Anonymous: What is currently known? In Research in Alcoholics Anonymous: Opportunities and Alternatives. Edited by McCready VX, Miller WR. Piscataway, NJ, Rutgers Center for Alcohol Studies, 1993, pp 41–76

Fals-Stewart W: The occurrence of partner physical aggression on days of alcohol consumption: a longitudinal diary study. J Consult Clin Psychol 71:45–52, 2003

Finger S, Stein DF: Brain Damage and Recovery. New York, Academic Press, 1982

Friedman RA: Violence and mental illness: how strong is the link? N Engl J Med 355:2064–2066, 2006

Fuller RK, Branchey L, Brightwell DR, et al: Disulfiram treatment of alcoholism: a Veterans Administration cooperative study. JAMA 256:1449–1455, 1986

Gelles RJ: Family violence. Annu Rev Sociol 11:347–367, 1985

Gianoulakis C, Krishnan B, Thavundayil J: Enhanced sensitivity of pituitary beta-endorphin to ethanol in subjects at high risk of alcoholism. Arch Gen Psychiatry 53:250–257, 1996 [Erratum published in 53:555, 1996]

Goldstein PJ: The drugs/violence nexus: a tripartite conceptual framework. J Drug Issues 15:493–506, 1985

Greenberg JR, McKibben M, Raymond JA: Dependent adult children and elder abuse. J Elder Abuse Negl 2:73–86, 1990

Grusser SM, Wrase J, Klein S, et al: Cue-induced activation of the striatum and medial prefrontal cortex is associated with subsequent relapse in abstinent alcoholics. Psychopharmacology (Berl) 175:296–302, 2004

Hayward L, Zubrick SR, Silburn S: Blood alcohol levels in suicide cases. J Epidemiol Community Health 46:256–260, 1992

HBO: Addiction (television series). Home Box Office, 2007. Materials and DVD available at http://www.hbo.com/addiction. Accessed April 22, 2007

Hunt GP, Laidler KJ: Alcohol and violence in the lives of gang members. Alcohol Res Health 25:66–71, 2001

Johnson BA, Ait-Daoud N, Bowden CL, et al: Oral topiramate for treatment of alcohol dependence: a randomized controlled trial. Lancet 17:1677–1685, 2003

Johnson BA, Roache JD, Javors MA, et al: Ondansetron for reduction of drinking among biologically predisposed alcoholic patients. JAMA 284:963–971, 2000

Kampman KM, Pettinati H, Lynch KG, et al: A pilot trial of topiramate for the treatment of cocaine dependence. Drug Alcohol Depend 75:233–240, 2004

Koss MP: Hidden rape: sexual aggression and victimization in a national sample of students in higher education, in Rape and Sexual Assault, Vol 2. Edited by Burgess AW. New York, Garland, 1988, pp 3–25

Krug EG, Dahlberg LL, Mercy JA, et al (eds): World Report on Violence and Health. Geneva, World Heath Organization, 2002

Krystal JH, Cramer JA, Krol WF, et al: Naltrexone in the treatment of alcohol dependence. N Engl J Med 345:1734–1739, 2001

Langevin R, Ben-Aron M, Wortzman G, et al: Brain damage, diagnosis, and substance abuse among violent offenders. Behav Sci Law 5:77–94, 1987

Lindqvist P: Criminal homicide in northern Sweden 1970–1981: alcohol intoxication, alcohol abuse and mental disease. Int J Law Psychiatry 8:19–37, 1986

Lipsey MW, Wilson DB, Cohen MA, et al: Is there a causal relationship between alcohol use and violence? A synthesis of evidence. In Recent Developments in Alcoholism, Vol 13: Alcoholism and Violence. Edited by Galanter M. New York, Plenum, 1997

Macdonald S, Wells S, Giesbrecht N, et al: Demographic and substance use factors related to violent and accidental injuries: results from an emergency room study. Drug Alcohol Depend 55:53–61, 1999

Marzuk PM, Tardiff K, Leon AC, et al: Fatal injuries after cocaine use as a leading cause of death among young adults in New York City. N Engl J Med 332:1753–1757, 1995

McElroy SL, Arnold LM, Shapira NA, et al: Topiramate in the treatment of binge eating disorder associated with obesity: a randomized, placebo-controlled trial. Am J Psychiatry 160:255–261, 2003

McGlynn EA, Asch SM, Adams J, et al: The quality of health care delivered to adults in the United States. N Engl J Med 348:2635–2645, 2003

Merrill J, Milker G, Owens J, et al: Alcohol and attempted suicide. Addiction 87:83–89, 1992

Miczek KA: The Pharmacology of Aggression, in Handbook of Psychopharmacology, Vol 19. Edited by Iversen LL, Iversen SD, Snyder SH. New York, Plenum, 1987, p 257

Murdoch D, Pihl RO, Ross D: Alcohol and crimes of violence: present issues. Int J Addict 25:1065–1081, 1990

National Institute on Alcohol Abuse and Alcoholism [NIAAA]: NIAAA reports Project MATCH main findings. Dec. 17, 1996. Available at http://www.niaaa.nih.gov/NewsEvents/NewsReleases/match.htm. Accessed March 10, 2007

National Institute on Alcohol Abuse and Alcoholism. Unpublished data from the 2001–2002 National Epidemiologic Survey on Alcohol and Related Conditions. 2004. Psychiatr Serv 58:424, 2007

National Institute on Alcohol Abuse and Alcoholism: Helping Patients Who Drink Too Much: A Clinician's Guide, Updated 2005 Edition. Available at http://www.niaaa.nih.gov/guide

National Institute of Mental Health: Suicide Prevention. Available at http://www.nimh.nih.gov/health/topics/suicide-prevention/index.shtml. Accessed March 31, 2007

O'Malley SS, Jaffe AJ, Change G, et al: Naltrexone and coping skills therapy for alcohol dependence: a controlled study. Arch Gen Psychiatry 49:881–887, 1992

Pescosolido BA, Fettes DL, Martin JK, et al: Perceived dangerousness of children with mental health problems and support for coerced treatment. Psychiatr Serv 58:619–625, 2007

Pihl RO, Lemarquand D: Serotonin and aggression in the alcohol-aggression relationship. Alcohol Alcohol 33:55–65, 1998

Presley CA, Leichliter JS, Meilman PW: Alcohol and Drugs on American College Campuses: A Report to College Presidents: Third in a Series, 1995, 1996, 1997. Carbondale, Core Institute, Southern Illinois University, 1998

Ramisetty-Mikler S, Caetano R: Alcohol use and intimate partner violence as predictors of separation among U.S. couples: a longitudinal model. J Stud Alcohol 66:205–212, 2005

Rammes G, Mahal B, Putzke J, et al: The anti-craving compound acamprosate acts as a weak NMDA-receptor antagonist, but modulates NMDA-receptor subunit expression similar to memantine and MK-801. Neuropharmacology 40:749–776, 2001

Ray LA, Hutchison KE: Effects of naltrexone on alcohol sensitivity and genetic moderators of medication response. Arch Gen Psychiatry 64:1069–1077, 2007

Regier DA, Farmer ME, Rae DS, et al: Comorbidity of mental disorders with alcohol and other drug abuse. JAMA 264:2511–2518, 1990

Roth JA: Psychoactive Substances and Violence. Washington, DC, National Institute of Justice, 1994

Saitz R: Clinical practice: unhealthy alcohol use. N Engl J Med 352:596–607, 2005

Salinsky MC, Storzbach D, Spencer DC, et al: Effects of topiramate and gabapentin on cognitive abilities in healthy volunteers. Neurology 64:792–798, 2005

Spunt BJ, Goldstein PJ, Bellucci PA, et al: Race/ethnicity and gender differences in the drugs-violence relationship. J Psychoactive Drugs 22:293–303, 1990

Steadman HJ, Mulvey EP, Monahan J, et al: Violence by people discharged from acute psychiatric inpatient facilities and by others in the same neighborhoods. Arch Gen Psychiatry 55:393–401, 1998

Swanson JW: Mental disorder, substance abuse, and community violence: an epidemiological approach, in Violence and Mental Disorder: Developments in Risk Assessment. Edited by Monaghan J, Steadman HF. Chicago, IL, University of Chicago Press, 1994, pp 101–136

Tinklenberg JR, Roth WT, Kopell BS, et al: Cannabis and alcohol effects on assaultiveness in adolescent delinquents. Ann N Y Acad Sci 282:85–94, 1976

U.S. Department of Justice: Family violence statistics: including statistics on strangers and acquaintances. Washington, DC, U.S. Department of Justice, Office of Justice Programs, Bureau of Justice Statistics, 2001. Available at http://www.ojp.usdoj.gov/bjs/pub/pdf/fvs02.pdf. Accessed October 6, 2005

Vaillant GE: The Natural History of Alcoholism. Cambridge, MA, Harvard University Press, 1983

Vaillant GE: The Natural History of Alcoholism Revisited. Cambridge, MA, Harvard University Press, 1995

Vaillant GE: Alcoholics Anonymous: cult or cure? Aust N Z J Psychiatry 39:431–436, 2005

Virkkunen M, Linnoila M: Serotonin in early onset, male alcoholics with violent behavior. Ann Med 22:327–331, 1990

Volavka J: Neurobiology of Violence, 2nd Edition. Washington, DC, American Psychiatric Publishing, 2002

Volavka J, Dornbush R, Feldstein S, et al: Marijuana, EEG and behavior. Ann NY Acad Sci 191:206–215, 1971

Volavka J, Levine R, Feldstein S, et al: Short-term effects of heroin in man. Arch Gen Psychiatry 30:677–681, 1974

Volpicelli JR, Alterman AI, Hayashida M, et al: Naltrexone in the treatment of alcohol dependence. Arch Gen Psychiatry 49:876–880, 1992

Widom CS, Hiller-Sturmhofel S: Alcohol abuse as a risk factor for and consequence of child abuse. Alcohol Res Health 25:52–57, 2001

Witkiewitz K, Marlatt GA: Therapist's Guide to Evidence-Based Relapse Prevention. Boston, MA, Elsevier Academic, 2007, pp 50–54

World Health Organization: Facts on child maltreatment and alcohol. n.d. Available at http://www.who.int/violence_injury_prevention/violence/world_report/factsheets/ft_child.pdf. Accessed March 2007

Zukin SR, Sloboda Z, Javitt DC: Phencyclidine (PCP), in Substance Abuse: A Comprehensive Textbook, 4th Edition. Edited by Lowinson JH, Ruiz P, Millman RB, et al. Philadelphia, PA, Lippincott Williams & Wilkins, 2005, pp 324–335

CHAPTER 9

Personality Disorders

William H. Reid, M.D., M.P.H.
Stephen A. Thorne, Ph.D.

Personality disorders are enduring, inflexible, and pervasive patterns of inner experience and external behavior that are maladaptive and detrimental to one's overall level of functioning and are in contrast with cultural expectations (American Psychiatric Association 2000). Although personality disorders are associated with a guarded or poor prognosis for change, lumping them into a single, global construct is clinically inappropriate. It is more accurate, and more productive, to view the personality disorders as heterogeneous, having symptoms and behaviors best viewed on a continuum within each diagnosis. There is a great deal of individual variation in the severity and pervasiveness of symptoms. Many individuals with personality disorders live relatively normal lives. Those whose disorders are more severe, those with comorbid mental, physical, or substance abuse disorders, and those whose lives are interrupted by periods of substantial internal or external stress tend to display more severe symptoms and lower levels of functioning.

The association, when there is any, between mental illness and violence has long been a subject of clinical and experimental debate. We do not review in detail the data and arguments on either side of that issue. We examine the assessment and management of violence potential in people with personality disorders whose condition or behavior creates concern. This chapter focuses on understanding and managing some aspects of violence *risk*. It does not address "prediction" or "cure."

Greater awareness of psychological and environmental characteristics associated with violence potential—marked or subtle—in some people with personality disorders should help clinicians and researchers identify patients or evaluees who are more likely than others to engage in violent behavior. We hope that the present chapter will be helpful to mental health professionals involved in forensic work and the criminal justice system and to those who work with personality-disordered patients in inpatient, outpatient, and correctional settings.

Mental Disorders and Violence

Until a few years ago, various authors suggested that people with mental disorders are no more likely to engage in violent behaviors than those in the general population (e.g., Monahan 1981). Rabkin (1979), however, reviewing studies published between 1922 and 1978, found with great consistency that patients released from public psychiatric facilities had higher arrest and conviction rates for violent crimes than did the general population. She concluded that "mental patients are more likely to be arrested for assaultive and sometimes lethal behavior than are other people" (p. 24). Swanson and colleagues' (1990) epidemiological study found that individuals diagnosed with a major mental disorder showed significantly higher rates of violent behavior than individuals with no apparent psychiatric disorder.

Other studies have also supported the notion that, overall and very generically, people with some type of mental disorder are more prone to violent behavior than those in the general population (Krakowski et al. 1986; Mulvey 1994; Nestor 2002; Swanson et al. 1990, 1996; Tardiff et al. 1997). Monahan (1992) himself, in an apparent reversal of some of his previous beliefs, wrote , "I now believe that there may be a relationship between mental disorder and violent behavior, one that cannot be fobbed off as chance or explained away by other factors that may cause them both. The relationship, if it exists, is probably not large, but may be important for both legal theory and…social policy" (p. 511).

Perhaps the most comprehensive search for associations between psychiatric illness and violent behavior came from the MacArthur Foundation study of mental disorders and violence (Monahan et al. 2001), a systematic, prospective, multisite examination of more than 1,100 male and female psychiatric patients. The research team used carefully controlled diagnoses and multiple methods of data collection to assess more than 130 potential risk factors for violence in subjects followed for 20 weeks after discharge from psychiatric facilities. The forms of violence studied included battery resulting in bodily harm, sexual assault, assaultive acts involving weapons, and threats. It came as a surprise to some that after 1 year, "major mental disorder" (such as schizophrenia, major depressive disorder, or history of manic episodes)—*in the absence of a substance abuse diagnosis*—was associated with a *lower* rate of violence (17.9%) than that found in socially and demographically matched control subjects. Dually diagnosed groups with "major mental disorder/substance abuse" and "other mental disorder/substance abuse" (including personality disorders) had higher overall rates of violence (31.1% and 43.0%, respectively) than those with a sole diagnosis of personality disorder.

Personality Disorders and Violence

The simplistic acceptance of a broad, general association between large groups of patients and the many forms of violence must be parsed into specific diagnoses, kinds and levels of symptoms, kinds and levels of violence, and context. The MacArthur Foundation data does this to a laudable extent, but there is a dearth of methodologically sound studies that focus on the relationship between personality disorders per se and violent behavior (Coid 2002; Otto 2000). Otto (2000) commented that the lack of research examining possible relationships between personality disorders and violence risk may, in part, reflect "(1) limitations of the psychiatric nomenclature of personality disorders generally and (2) that assessment of the psychopathy construct (via the PCL-R) is better refined than assessment of any other personality disorder or personality style" (p. 1248).

A review of those studies that do attempt to explore potential relationships between violent behavior and personality disorders suggests a lack of conformity in operational definitions of personality disorder. Some studies include subjects described as having various personality "traits" or merely having endorsed a number of diagnostic criteria. Others incorporate factor or cluster analysis of psychological test data (e.g., defining a personality disorder based on elevated scale scores from the Millon Clinical Multiaxial Inventory, Personality Assessment Inventory, or Minnesota Multiphasic Personality Inventory). Still others refer to personality types or clusters that do not clearly correlate with any DSM-IV-TR (American Psychiatric Association 2000) or ICD-10 diagnosis.

Another factor that can significantly affect research findings, and should call into question the extent to which some findings can be generalized, is the point in time at which the diagnosis was given. Krakowski et al. (1986) pointed out that the "fact that a patient is violent may influence the type of diagnosis which he or she receives. This is particularly true of personality disorder, where the violence itself may serve as a basis for making the diagnosis" (p. 132).

A closer look at study designs suggests that readers must distinguish between *violent* behavior (based on self-report, criminal conviction, and/or review of collateral data) and *hostile/aggressive* behavior. The latter may or may not be the same as violent behavior but is easier to examine in experimental settings.

The MacArthur Foundation project highlights the importance of multiple measures of data collection in violence research. For example, Steadman et al. (1998) observed 1-year violence rates of 4.5% when examining agency records of discharged mental patients, but violence rates for the same subjects were six times greater (27.5%) when three separate sources of information were used (agency records, interviews with patients, and interviews with a collateral source familiar with the subject's behavior in the community).

Other validity and reliability concerns within the violence and risk assessment literature include single-site studies, relatively small sample sizes, limited or nonrepresentative subject populations (including various "extreme" populations), reliance on forensic and psychiatric inpatient populations, and failure to adequately consider common confounding variables such as comorbid psychiatric disorders, substance abuse, and prior history of violence. All of these methodological issues limit the extent to which the results of any study can be viewed with confidence, compared with other research, or accurately generalized to community populations and society.

Lawmakers increasingly appear to be using skewed concepts of diagnosis to support legislation for the management of people whom they consider a threat to society. Sex offenses, in particular, have engendered special, often draconian, commitment statutes and procedures in many states. Most of those procedures, different from ordinary civil commitment of the mentally ill, rest not on a "psychiatric" disorder but on a nonclinical concept of "behavioral abnormality" that often resembles (and sometimes uses) "personality disorder" as evidence of predisposition to sexually violent behavior (*Kansas v. Crane* 2002; *Kansas v. Hendricks* 1997; Leong and Silva 2001).

Variations in Diagnosis-Related Behavior

The presence of a personality disorder diagnosis does not imply that everyone with that diagnosis has the same risk of violence. Although broad similarities can be used for diagnosis and categorization, people with personality disorders are heterogeneous in the variety, consistency, and intensity of their symptoms. Costello (1996) noted that the "use in research of such complex polythetic categories of personality disorder made up of heterogeneous sets of experiences and behaviors makes it very difficult to interpret research findings" (p. 1). In addition, despite the definition and conceptualization of personality disorders as an enduring pattern of inner experience and behavior that is inflexible, pervasive, stable, and of long duration, some have argued against a blanket position that all personality disorders are always stable (Coid 2003; Rogers and Shuman 2005).

Understanding the heterogeneous nature of violence is imperative for clinicians and researchers attempting to develop effective management and treatment approaches and for readers who review their findings. Both ordinary experience and clinical and research findings lead one to view violence itself as a multifaceted construct varying widely in quality, severity, purpose, duration, and frequency. Even very specific forms of violence can have a variety of causes (see Widiger and Trull 1994, p. 212). Swanson et al. (2006) commented on that heterogeneity in their recent study of violence rates among schizophrenics, noting that "[v]iolent behavior occurs within a social-ecological system, involving a whole person with a particular life history and a state of health or disease, interacting with a particular social surround" (pp. 490–491). Each individual's risk level varies with the degree to which his or her personality characteristics and dimensions may or may not be exposed to various environmental variables (Nestor 2002). In general, what accounts for violent behavior in one individual with a given personality disorder does not necessarily portend violent behavior in others with the same diagnosis.

Legal Responsibility and Violence Associated With Personality Disorder

The diagnoses and situations discussed in this chapter are not generally associated with legal exoneration due to mental illness (e.g., being "not guilty by reason of insanity"), but symptoms can mitigate criminal culpability to some extent. Conditions that affect one's *intent* are relevant to legal matters. Perpetrators almost always bear at least some, usually all, responsibility for their behavior, provided they are capable of understanding the harmfulness or illegality of the behavior and that other means of dealing with the situation are more appropriate (such as calling police to handle real or perceived threats, dealing nonviolently with spouses suspected of having affairs, or choosing nonviolent, nondestructive ways to experience personal stimulation or excitement).

Treatment and Management

The treatments discussed in this section are, in most cases, necessarily generic. Psychotherapeutic repair of personality deficit is exceedingly difficult and rarely available to patients even when they are willing to tolerate the emotional, temporal, and financial costs involved. Highly specialized, resource-intensive treatments for some characterological disorders (such as severe borderline traits) may be effective for those who qualify clinically and have access to innovative programs, but such opportunities are a rare exception rather than the rule.

Equally relevant to this chapter, there is no psychiatric treatment or other reasonable clinical answer to violence that is a discrete symptom of a personality disorder (unlike some other forms of violence associated with, for example, certain paraphilias, severe depression, the mood instability of bipolar disorder, frank psychosis, or ictal or other neurological "dyscontrol"). Treatment of problems such as anxiety and depression, unstable mood or affect, psychotic thinking, and inadequate social or relationship skills may decrease the risk of violence as it improves patients' ability to cope with internal and external threat without decompensating.

Setting aside direct treatment for the moment, much of our (mental health professionals') usefulness lies in assisting potential victims, families of real and potential perpetrators and victims, and others who have frequent contact with personality-disordered people (including law enforcement personnel and corrections staffs). Helping members of these groups to better understand potential perpetrators, to modify (or avoid) contact with them, and sometimes to contain and prevent them from harming others is an important part of decreasing the damage done by violence and, in some cases, preventing violence in future generations.

Three Unavoidable Treatment Issues

- *Personality disorders are rarely ego dystonic.* Most people with personality disorders or aberrant character traits do not seek psychiatric help. Those who do are often trying to alleviate symptoms but are unable or unwilling to address characterological issues. They may comply with treatment aimed at anxiety or depression but usually shun serious psychotherapeutic approaches to their maladaptive behaviors and adaptations. Many aspects of personality disorders are simply not amenable to commonly available treatment.
- *Most patients and situations of violence that come to professional attention involve coexisting disorders and conditions.* Treating or managing comorbid

Personality Disorders

or coexisting conditions (many often external to the patient) may alleviate some potential for violence. The presence of a personality disorder usually makes it more difficult to treat accompanying conditions.
- *Violence and risk of violence, with or without a personality disorder, is often associated with intoxication.* Management of simple intoxication and control of damaging behavior associated with it are generally outside the province of the mental health professions. Treatment of substance abuse disorders may reduce violence risk, but personality disorders usually worsen the prognosis. We generally agree with the common principle of first getting the patient clean and sober, then reassessing for personality disorders and other psychiatric conditions. Removing the substance issue often clarifies, and sometimes erases, evidence of other mental disorders.

These bullet points suggest that nonpsychiatric, non–mental health approaches are often more important than mental health professionals in the prevention and management of violence by people with personality disorders and the protection of potential victims from those people.

The discussions in the next section are predicated on personality characteristics, generally without regard to other mental disorders or intoxication. Our examples apply to many situations in the "real world" in which violence related to personality disorders may not come to the attention of mental health professionals or be very amenable to our intervention.

Kinds of Violence Associated With Personality Disorders

We have chosen not to parse violent behaviors by specific personality disorder. The common thread for our purpose is the violence, not the diagnosis. Understanding similarities among kinds of violence is more useful, and better related to common presentations, than separating behavioral and psychological issues by diagnosis (although consideration of DSM-IV-TR "clusters" is sometimes helpful). The categories we have developed and present here are experience-based and practical. They are not mutually exclusive, nor are they intended to create an assessment "decision tree." All examples are taken from actual cases.

Purposeful, Instrumental Violence

Some personality disorders predispose one to violence for obvious personal gain. Disorders that decrease or eliminate a sense of empathy or otherwise diminish the potential perpetrator's thoughtful consideration of other people increase this risk. Antisocial, narcissistic, and borderline disorders are common examples. Such violence is *targeted* rather than random. It includes acts in which violence is a means to a conscious, gainful end (such as a robbery or preventing apprehension after a crime) or designed to manipulate or mislead another into some wanted behavior (such as manipulative behavior by persons with antisocial, narcissistic, or borderline personality). Violence for revenge and violence for hire should be considered here, provided there is a characterological deficit in the perpetrator that allows it to take place.

Case Example 1

A man who met diagnostic criteria for antisocial personality approached an elderly man in an isolated area of a park and demanded money. When the robbery victim resisted giving up his valuables, the perpetrator hit him repeatedly in order to force him to comply. After the victim had been subdued, the perpetrator took his wallet and ran away.

Case Example 2

An injured worker suing his employer for millions of dollars lost his lawsuit because of a somewhat technical judicial decision. His attorney noted that the worker was very upset over the loss, and he referred the client to a psychologist. During a brief course of treatment, the therapist uncovered long-standing signs of paranoia but no frankly delusional material. Believing the sessions to be completely confidential, the patient/plaintiff eventually admitted that since losing the lawsuit, he had rehearsed sabotaging the defense attorney's car, had actually entered the lawyer's property and examined the engine and brake lines, and had a plan to murder the judge.

Case Example 3

A patient with borderline personality was distraught about the possibility of losing custody of her children during a divorce. She told her psychiatrist that her estranged husband had beaten her in front of the children and that she was afraid he would harm them as well. She offered bruises on her neck and arms as evidence. The psychiatrist helped her to contact police and obtain a restraining order prohibiting her husband from visiting her or the children.

As the police and the state child protective agency investigated the matter, attention began to shift to the patient herself. It eventually became clear that she inflicted her own bruises, then invited her husband to her house, started an argument in front of the children, and began hitting him. When he did not hit back and began to leave, she dramatically fell screaming to the floor and loudly proclaimed "Daddy hit me! Daddy's hurting me! Run, or he'll hurt you, too!"

Risk Assessment

An experienced evaluator of antisocial, paranoid, or borderline persons should recognize the presence of some risk, but the level of risk and the probability of violence may be difficult to ascertain, even in patients with substantial aberrant personality traits. Those with histories of violent behavior, paranoid or mildly psychotic thinking in a context of possible gain, and/or marked lack of empathy should raise additional concern.

Treatment/Management of the Violent Behavior

Physical prevention of violence, such as by incarceration, removal of potential victims, or alleviation of risk-laden situations, may be the most practical approach, particularly in the short term. Treatment of symptoms such as psychosis or intolerable anxiety usually decreases risk but should not be considered a lasting solution to personality-based risk. Specialized psychotherapy and psychosocial efforts to address the personality deficit itself, such as helping a characterologically borderline or paranoid patient develop internal alternatives to acting out, are theoretically logical but require expertise, resources, and time that are rarely available. Even in the best cases of psychiatric and psychotherapeutic care, external or pharmacological management, if indicated, should be considered while waiting for insight and change (if insight and change are to be forthcoming at all).

Purposeful, Noninstrumental Violence

Noninstrumental violence may be purposeful, but the injury to others is outwardly *unnecessary*; it is violence for the sake of excitement or stimulation, as contrasted with that aimed toward tangible gain. It may add parenthetically to the pleasure of a stimulating or antisocial activity, but actually injuring others is not integral to the activity's purpose. Bystanders may refer to the violent part of the overall behavior as "senseless" or "random," but it has an emotional purpose, such as stimulation. The targets may be random, but the behavior that places others in danger is intentional.

This concept should not be confused with violence in which the danger to others is unanticipated or not intentional, such as that incidental to impulsively overreacting to an affective state associated with threatened emotional survival (e.g., intolerable anxiety, stifling entrapment, acute abandonment, or marked humiliation; see "Nontargeted, Impulsive Violence Incidental to Emotional Escape" later in this chapter).

Case Example 4

A man who met diagnostic criteria for antisocial personality but not for any Axis I disorder broke into a home and stole several items while the occupants were asleep. He then set fire to the house in order to hide his crime, deflect blame from himself, and destroy evidence that might have incriminated him. The occupants were awakened by a smoke alarm and escaped, but they could easily have been injured or killed.

After his arrest several days later, the robber described setting the fire as necessary to avoid being caught. He denied wanting to harm the occupants, describing the fire as simply a means of avoiding arrest. It was "nothing personal," just "something I had to do whether they [the occupants] were there or not." Warning or awakening them so that they could escape had not crossed his mind.

Case Example 5

A young man with a long history of relatively minor antisocial acts engaged in a drag race on a city street. As he neared the end of the race, he realized he was about to run a red light. Nevertheless, he continued to accelerate, ran the red light, and struck another car. The driver of the other car was killed. When testifying about his reckless behavior, he described it entirely in terms of his taking a thrilling chance with his own life, seeming oblivious to any responsibility for others' safety. He understood the chance of an accident, and the chance that someone might be hurt or killed, but he described the danger of racing purely in terms of a focus on himself, saying "I can live with those odds."

Risk Assessment

This form of violence is overrepresented in those with substantial antisocial and asocial character traits. In addition to lack of empathy or recognition of other's needs and feelings (a common thread in many kinds of violence), the risk of purposeful but noninstrumental violence may be heralded by a potential perpetrator's wish for pleasure or need for stimulation that overshadows his judgment, impulse control, and appreciation of future consequences.

Treatment/Management

When symptoms are recognizable and treatable, the general treatment principles described in the last section apply (e.g., treatment for substance abuse or mood instability).

Purposeful, Targeted, Defensive Violence

Purposeful, targeted, defensive violence is generally a maladaptive attempt to stop some intolerable affect, often associated with humiliation

Personality Disorders | 171

or abandonment. The violent reaction to such a condition, which threatens the integrity of the person's ego, may be rapid (see also the sections "Targeted, Impulsive Violence" and "Nontargeted, Impulsive Violence Incidental to Emotional Escape" in this chapter) or it may be carefully planned. The target may seem illogical to an observer (e.g., it may be related to paranoid ideation or some other idiosyncratic source). The level of violence is often baffling until one realizes its internal meaning. Examples include the sometimes extreme behavior of paranoid stalkers, who may create near-delusional scenarios of competition or abandonment, and paranoid "defenders," who believe they must defend themselves from imagined or exaggerated slights or threats. Dependent, avoidant, and schizoid traits occasionally increase risk. When such thinking becomes more than mildly delusional or other aspects of the person's function are significantly compromised, an Axis I disorder should be considered.

Case Example 6

Frequent arguments between a middle-aged man and his wife, often involving intoxication with alcohol, routinely led to his threatening or assaulting her, her threatening or briefly leaving him, and then his successfully begging her to stay. Eventually, the wife resolved to ignore his entreaties and promises and filed for divorce. He did not believe she would go through with the divorce, but when he came home one night, she had locked him out. He stayed with a friend for a few days, calling her often and thinking she would change her mind.

After several days, he was served with the divorce papers. He drove to her place of work and once again pleaded with her to reconsider. She refused, adding (in front of her coworkers) that he had never been much of a husband and had never satisfied her sexually. He returned to his car, took a shotgun out of the trunk, went back into the building, killed her, and then waited for police to arrive.

Risk Assessment

Characterological paranoia is among the most dangerous personality traits. It is associated with both domestic and general violence. Many people with paranoid personality routinely imagine and rehearse (mentally or literally) violent "solutions" to paranoia-created scenarios. Truly delusional persons with Axis I disorders are much more likely to be seen by a mental health professional than are those with paranoid personality alone. Passive, dependent, or avoidant people do not anticipate violence but may become dangerous when trapped or restrained and unable to escape emotional pressure. However, they usually can adjust their environments to decrease their anxiety (and concomitantly lower their risk of violence). Threatened breach of narcissistic character defenses carries risk as well.

Treatment/Management

Characterologically paranoid people, who go through life with an overdetermined expectation of trouble, are very difficult to manage (and sometimes to recognize) unless or until their public behavior raises concerns. Persons whose personality traits lead them to avoid confrontation and anxiety can usually be relied on to avoid triggering situations *if they have the choice to do so*. Once such a person is in a setting that overwhelms even resilient characterological defenses, such as a perceived inescapable threat or restraint, the best management approaches involve quickly defusing the situation, isolating or containing the potentially violent person, or removing potential victims.

Targeted, Impulsive Violence

Targeted, impulsive violence involves striking out, without planning, at a perceived or psychological threat that others would not consider to warrant the same quality or quantity of violence. The victim is specifically targeted, often in a desperate effort to eliminate (literally or symbolically) the source of an acute psychic threat. Examples of such violence, which erupts in order to escape an intractable situation by eliminating the source, include enraged reactions to acutely perceived humiliation or abandonment. Although severe examples are not common, people who are characterologically paranoid, narcissistic, or exquisitely sensitive to loss (as found in borderline personality) are predisposed, to a greater or lesser extent, to such actions given a triggering setting or environment. Dependent, obsessive-compulsive, and avoidant persons are at less risk but may decompensate into violent behavior under remarkable circumstances (see Coid 2002 and some other studies of prison populations).

Note that we are not referring here to violence whose victims are *incidental* to uncontrolled rage or escape behavior by, for example, "being in the wrong place at the wrong time" (see "Nontargeted, Impulsive Violence Incidental to Emotional Escape" later in the chapter).

Case Example 7

Dr. X, an otherwise competent abdominal surgeon, was known for both his skill and his irritable, narcissistic manner. He led a regimented life, with little warmth for family or friends, the barest superficial acknowledgment of the roles of others in his cases and other achievements, and

Personality Disorders | 173

no tolerance for criticism. The latest of many operating room incidents involved his berating a nurse when she pointed out unacceptable oozing from the omentum as he began to close a laparotomy. Nevertheless, he stopped and dealt with the bleeding before proceeding with the closing. Another nurse commented under her breath, "Saved by a nurse."

The surgeon finished the closing, then calmly asked, "What did you say?"

The nurse who had made the comment said something like "I didn't mean anything disrespectful. I wanted to compliment 'J' [the nurse who noted the bleeding] for making a good catch. She probably saved the patient from reopening."

The surgeon replied hotly, "J works for me. She did her job. Every damned one of you works for me. I'll let you know when you make a good catch and I'll be damned if I'll tolerate anybody in this hospital criticizing my surgery until you've been through medical school and residency yourself."

J came to her colleague's defense. "No problem, Dr. X. We'll just get the patient out of here and awake."

Dr. X then raised his voice and continued to rant in spite of verbal efforts to calm him. Finally, one of the nurses, concerned about the situation and the patient's safety, announced that she was calling for the chief nurse of the surgery suite. Dr. X responded by tossing a tray of bloody sponges in the nurse's direction and storming out of the operating room.

Dr. X was disciplined by the medical staff. He protested their verdict and retained a lawyer to sue for libel and expunge his record. The lawsuit was later dismissed. The medical staff matter was eventually reported to the state medical licensing board, which added its own censure.

Case Example 8

Mr. S was known as a nice, quiet fellow, the adult son of a very aggressive, poorly liked father whose bullying controlled most people close to him. Mr. S behaved in an almost opposite manner, passive and appearing dependent on his father for income and a place to live. In over a decade of adulthood, he had traveled and interacted socially with others but had never held a meaningful job for more than a few weeks, had never married, and had never lived away from his father. Privately, Mr. S dreaded the thought of being like his father, who had abused him during childhood and as an adult.

One night while both were intoxicated, his father began once again to bully and humiliate Mr. S. At some point, the combination of physical and emotional humiliation reached an intolerable level; Mr. S grabbed his father's arms to restrain them. The father laughed derisively, breaking the son's hold, slapped him repeatedly in the face, and called him "my little bitch." Mr. S exploded, pummeled his father to the ground, and finally shot him in the chest with a shotgun kept nearby in case of intruders.

When his father lay obviously dead, Mr. S wrapped him in a bedsheet and bound the body with duct tape, then retreated to his bedroom, locked the door, and went to bed. The next day, he called an attorney and gave himself up to police. Asked later about what he did to the body, Mr. S replied that although he knew his father was dead, he could not feel truly secure until he had wrapped and bound him and locked the bedroom door.

Risk Assessment

Many violent acts of this type occur when an external event threatens poorly defended fears of inadequacy or abandonment. Some people with severely dependent, paranoid, narcissistic, schizotypal, or obsessive-compulsive traits—characteristics that decrease one's ability to marshal and rely upon more efficient internal defenses when trapped in emotionally intractable situations from which one cannot escape—can be very dangerous. Such conditions, particularly inability to escape an intolerable and anxiety-producing situation, increase the likelihood of a violent reaction designed to stop the pain and escape the threat. When conditions are extremely stressful, even schizoid and avoidant persons may revert to primitive, violent actions to defend their egos. Intoxication is a substantial risk factor, as are some kinds of emotional attacks and idiosyncratic emotional triggers (e.g., repeated, inescapable demeaning or "in your face" challenges during arguments with a spouse or competitor).

Treatment/Management

"Treatment" of the characterologic vulnerability, when motivation and resources are present, is described elsewhere. See also the general defusing, separation, and containment principles described above, as well as treatments for coexisting substance abuse, mood instability, and other noncharacterologic factors mentioned earlier in this chapter.

Nontargeted, Impulsive Violence Incidental to Emotional Escape

Impulsive violence incidental to emotional escape is generally nontargeted, although the person who triggers the intractable emotional state may bear the brunt of the violence if he or she is in the path of egress. The purpose of the behavior is rapid escape from a situation that has created an acute, intolerable internal situation for which the personality-disordered person has inadequate emotional defenses and behavioral alternatives. It is different from the type just discussed (targeted,

Personality Disorders | 175

impulsive) in that the anxious or humiliated person does not seek to mitigate or destroy the source of the pain, only to escape from it.

Case Example 9

Ms. T was a 43-year-old woman with borderline personality disorder and very primitive attachment needs. She and her 24-year-old daughter had an extraordinarily hostile-dependent relationship that was often characterized by rather obvious manipulations designed to keep the daughter physically and emotionally bound to the mother. The daughter had tried to move away on several occasions, but each time she had changed her plans to meet her mother's needs and continued to live on her mother's property. At one point, the daughter approached her mother once again—by telephone, to avoid a personal confrontation—to tell her she was moving in with a boyfriend who lived some distance away. She called from her place of work.

The telephone conversation soon deteriorated into a volatile event. Ms. T alternated among superficially rational "suggestions" that the daughter reconsider and have her boyfriend move into the daughter's trailer on the mother's property, pleas that the daughter consider the mother's health conditions (which were not particularly serious), sarcastic comments that the boyfriend would probably leave her, and, eventually, angry threats to rent the daughter's house to someone else so that she could never "come home."

The daughter would not budge. She repeatedly told her mother that she was indeed going to move away and parried each of the manipulative comments and threats with sarcasm and threats of her own (such as "You'll never see your grandchildren" and "You've been sick for years; let me know when it gets really serious"). The daughter finally hung up in the middle of her mother's tirade.

Ms. T got into her car to drive to the daughter's workplace, shaking with anger and anxiety. On the way, she drove very recklessly, failed to yield at an intersection, and hit another car, injuring several people.

Case Example 10

A woman with severe borderline and paranoid traits was being told that she had lost custody of her children. A social worker and a trainee were trying to treat her as gently as possible while making it clear that she would only be allowed to see her children, who had been removed from the home, in a supervised setting. The woman listened for a moment, then began screaming that none of the things they were saying about her was true, that she was a good mother, and that she refused to listen to their lies.

The social work trainee raised her voice and somewhat assertively tried to confront the woman, recounting her past abusive acts in order to make her understand why her parental rights were being terminated. The woman only became more agitated, screamed louder, and bolted from the room, pushing the senior social worker away from the door and into an aquarium, which fell and broke, cutting her arm and neck.

Risk Assessment

This level of fragility and potential for decompensation is not typical of most people with personality disorders and may suggest an Axis I disorder. Those prone to such reactions have marginal egos that are inadequately protected by sometimes superficially resilient, but inwardly brittle, defenses. Their personalities may have substantial, poorly integrated borderline, schizotypal, dependent, obsessive-compulsive, and/or avoidant features. They often seem outwardly stable but have inner worlds kept artificially free of mental controversy that might threaten their emotional lives. They may show stilted or even ritualistic behaviors in order to control the impact of the external environment on those inner lives, or they may simply choose isolation and other defenses as means of avoiding stressors.

Careful examination of such persons' lives may reveal reaction formation, an extraordinary need to defend desperately against discovering in oneself some frighteningly destructive core emotion or self-reviled dependency. For some, that veneer can become dangerously weak under stressful (often idiosyncratic) circumstances such as intoxication, loss, or inescapable humiliation.

Treatment/Management

In case example 10 above, the trainee's confrontational manner increased the pressure on the woman's already assaulted, fragile ego. A less confrontive approach would likely have prevented the accidental injury to her colleague.

Random But Purposeful Violence

People who perform acts of random but purposeful violence derive pleasurable stimulation from violence itself, often to instill a feeling of power. It is neither a means to some profitable end nor merely an adjunct to some other exciting activity (omitting primarily sexual sadism, which we view as an Axis I disorder even though its roots are often characterologic). A particular, repetitive style of violence, such as sniping with a rifle or setting others on fire, is common, but careful review usually reveals other violent or sadistic behavior.

The victim may be stalked or the situation carefully planned in order to set up the violent act (and often to plan escape); however, the victim usually has no direct relationship to the perpetrator, nor is the particular victim associated with revenge or personal gain. He or she is a target of convenience.

Personality Disorders | 177

Randomness of victim choice does not imply random, impulsive, or uncontrolled action. The violence is not a result of neurological dyscontrol, a psychogenic impulse control or explosive disorder, or a thought disorder (better discussed as Axis I or Axis III conditions); rather, it is self-absorbed, antisocial, and uncaring, without empathy or sympathy. A wish to exert or establish power over others, and over the passive portion of one's own psyche, is commonly an important component of the violent purpose.

Case Example 11

Two men decided to play a deadly "urban war game" in which they assumed the roles of assassins. They outfitted a small van in such a way that one of them could drive to an "assassination" location and park the truck while the other sat in the back with a high-powered rifle. The rifle was equipped with a telescopic sight so that shots could be taken from some distance. The driver would spot a faraway victim, chosen at random according to opportunity, and give the shooter a signal. The shooter would then open a side window, fire, and quickly close the window, after which the van would drive away.

The pair were caught after killing several people. Upon evaluation, neither met criteria for any significant psychiatric diagnosis except personality disorder with antisocial and (in one) paranoid traits.

Risk Assessment

As in the case of several other conditions described in this chapter, a history of this kind of violence, in reality or in substantial fantasy (e.g., with "rehearsing" behavior), increases risk of future violence. Those with disorders whose hallmark is a lack of empathy, responsibility, and/or impulse control, such as antisocial, narcissistic, or paranoid personality, are of most concern.

Treatment/Management

Management of persons in this group is generally practical and societal (e.g., judicial, correctional) rather than psychiatric. For those rare cases in which a treatable disorder such as mood instability or substance abuse is relevant, see the treatment comments found earlier in this chapter and elsewhere in the broader treatment literature.

Violence Related to Perceived/Feared Loss or Abandonment

Violence in response to perceived abandonment is a special case of targeted, usually purposeful, and instrumental violence that may be either impulsive or calculated.

Case Example 12

A man and a woman had a 4-month dating relationship that fluctuated between superficial intimacy and loud arguments. The man, who treated the relationship primarily as one of sexual convenience, grew tired of the woman's volatile emotions and demands for proof of his love. The woman clung to the hope that the relationship would lead to a fairy tale marriage. Finally, he stopped calling her and began dating someone else.

The woman was hurt and angry at being abandoned and at losing what she had viewed as a lasting future of love and security. Over time, the loss became less and less tolerable. Her anger grew. She saw no life for herself without (her fantasy of) the ex-boyfriend and convinced herself that their relationship would have a chance if his new girlfriend were gone.

One night, when driving by her ex-boyfriend's house, she noticed the girlfriend's car in the driveway. She stopped and smashed the windshield with a hammer, then drove away. The ex-boyfriend suspected she had broken the windshield and called to confront her. She denied it but took the call as an opportunity to rekindle the relationship and as evidence that she was still in his thoughts. He told her the police had been called and hung up. He continued to date the new girlfriend.

Two weeks later, the woman saw the ex-boyfriend and his new girlfriend in a bar. When they noticed her, they got up to leave. She yelled at them to stop and began to berate the girlfriend. The couple again started to leave, and the woman, who was somewhat intoxicated, attacked the girlfriend. She was restrained and later arrested.

Psychiatric evaluation of the woman revealed these facts as well as a history of significant abuse by a stepfather, very unstable adult relationships, and episodes of depression and self-injury associated with relatively minor losses. No frankly delusional material was evident.

Risk Assessment

People with flagrant manifestations of borderline coping should be viewed with concern. Those with paranoid personality disorder are relatively common perpetrators as well. Severely dependent character traits in the absence of borderline features should raise consideration for violence in some settings and contexts, albeit to a lesser extent. Children with markedly borderline or paranoid parents are especially at risk of either direct abuse or exposure to violent moods and unstable parenting.

Treatment/Management

Treatment of ancillary symptoms of anxiety, mood instability, and occasional psychotic thinking is relatively straightforward and often successful with cooperative patients. Psychotherapy should be designed to teach and reinforce realistic assessment of perceived loss and abandonment, appropriate forms of soothing and coping in lieu of destructive acting out, and use of supportive external resources (including the therapist) rather than reliance on destructive coping mechanisms. Treating professionals who suspect substantial risk of violence should monitor their patients frequently for impending (including symbolic) loss and abandonment, coping difficulties, and deteriorating mood stability.

Violence Related to Chronic Paranoia or Related Misconception

Although we are not addressing chronically delusional or otherwise psychotic states, paranoid and severely narcissistic character features are often associated with episodic violence and enduring levels of tension or threat to others. Some stalkers are paranoid, acting out of a sense of fear or defense against threat rather than erotomania or other signs of an Axis I delusional disorder. Narcissistic individuals may erroneously view others as attempting to undermine their positions (and, more accurately, their highly defensive sense of competence) and react with irritability or outbursts when assailed by reality. Schizotypal persons, usually well defended with self-absorbed isolation when in stable settings, nevertheless often misperceive the nature and purpose of those around them.

Case Example 13

Mr. H was a Vietnam veteran with a stable but childless marriage to a Vietnamese woman whom he had brought to the United States. He was generally domineering, expecting her to be a submissive wife. Once in the United States, she pursued an education, getting a graduate degree and becoming a college teacher, while he remained relatively uneducated and generally unsuccessful in his small business. At home, his wife tried to tolerate his dominating style, dislike for socializing, and noticeable paranoid traits.

One of Mr. H's few hobbies was working with his several dogs, pit bulls who required a large pen and considerable care. He was quite gentle with them, and although he was reclusive and suspicious and had a history of severe childhood beatings from his father, there was no evidence that he had ever physically abused his wife.

As his business failed, Mr. H spent more and more time working on an elaborate backyard structure, the walls of which were created from thick metal plates salvaged from a construction site. He described the structure as a shelter for his dogs. Police would later describe it as a "bunker," but there was no other evidence that he was preparing for some fantasized attack, and he had no known association with antigovernment or "survivalist" groups.

Mr. H legally owned several weapons, some of which he kept at his place of business (which was in an unsavory part of town and vulnerable to robbery). A year before the events that brought him to treatment, he was caught driving with a loaded handgun without a concealed carry permit. The weapon was confiscated and never returned, despite his frequent requests. He told several people that the confiscation was illegal, and although he had excellent relations with the local police through his business, the confiscation remained a sticking point in his interactions with them.

Mr. H's wife finally left him, ostensibly because of the way he treated her and the widening divergence of their interests. He was very upset about her leaving and became noticeably depressed. A family physician prescribed an antidepressant, which he took only sporadically.

Late one night soon thereafter, he was stopped for speeding. The officer noticed a shotgun and a handgun on the passenger seat of the vehicle. He drew his service weapon and retreated to the patrol car. Reports differ at this point, but it appears from patrol car video that soon after he called for a second officer, the first officer fired at the truck, starting an intensive exchange of gunfire. When the second officer arrived, more shots were fired.

No officer was ever wounded, in spite of the police cars' being hit dozens of times by Mr. H's shots. Mr. H was wounded in several places. When he was finally extracted from his truck, several other weapons and a drum of gasoline were found behind the seat.

Mr. H was arrested for attempted murder of a police officer. His defense was that he was trying to commit "suicide by cop" and had been on his way to a police station for that purpose. He had planned, he said, to fire the weapons into the air, then die at the hands of the police whom he respected so much, one of whom would become a "hero" for ending the incident. Criminologic and psychiatric evaluations suggested that the "suicide-by-cop" plan might have been real, but the overall impression was one of paranoid personality with schizotypal features and episodes of depression. It appeared likely that the violent behavior was related more to his paranoia and misperception, triggered by the immediate situation, than to depressive suicidal intent. The first officer's behavior was probably part of the final triggering event, although what might have happened had Mr. H. not been stopped for speeding is unclear.

Risk Assessment

Those with paranoid personality, especially, warrant concern and monitoring, particularly when there is a history of violence or threat. Children in the family are at risk of both direct abuse and exposure to violent moods and cold or unstable parenting. Severe narcissistic and schizotypal traits suggest increased risk as well.

Treatment/Management

There is no specific treatment for patients with histories similar to that of Mr. H. The pain of depression may cause them to seek treatment, but compliance is a difficult issue, and antidepressant approaches do not address the paranoid or other personality traits (although they may alleviate paranoia that stems from a mood disorder). Antidepressant treatment may also contribute to a switch to manic or hypomanic behavior, which, in the context of paranoia or other aberrant personality traits, can be quite dangerous. Adequate monitoring is important. Although one cannot be certain, alleviation of Mr. H's depression might have changed the outcome.

Conclusion

With a few exceptions (e.g., antisocial personality), the potential relationships between personality disorders and violent behavior are poorly studied. We encourage clinicians to view personality disorder as a heterogeneous construct. That heterogeneity raises diagnostic and methodological concerns about the reliability and generalizability of much of the available research. Individual consideration, including understanding setting and context, is vital to improving risk assessment. It follows that recognizing increased risk can allow clinicians to match the problems and needs of individuals to available treatment when appropriate and, perhaps more often, to recommend practical management approaches.

Mental health professionals working with personality-disordered individuals should review critically the better studies of violence risk, particularly those pertaining to personality disorders, then extend that focus beyond diagnosis. The case examples in this chapter highlight characterologic vulnerability but also feature environmental factors related to increased risk. Clinicians who understand the importance of setting and context, and their relationship to the internal vulnerability associated with different personality traits, will have an easier time recognizing and assessing risk than many of their colleagues and will be in a better position to help manage that risk.

Key Points

- Although personality disorders are associated with a guarded or poor prognosis for change, they should not be lumped into a single, global construct. They are heterogeneous, with a variety of symptoms and behaviors within each diagnosis.
- Personality disorders are rarely ego dystonic. Most people with personality disorders or aberrant character traits who seek professional help have coexisting disorders or conditions.
- This chapter focuses on understanding and managing some aspects of violence *risk*. It does not address "prediction" or "cure."
- The presence of a personality disorder diagnosis does not imply that everyone with that diagnosis has the same risk of violence.
- The diagnoses and situations discussed in this chapter do not generally imply lack of responsibility for one's actions. They are rarely associated with exoneration from blame for criminal acts.
- Violence and risk of violence, with or without a personality disorder, is often associated with intoxication of some kind.
- The authors present a new, eight-category typology of characterologic violence, not intended to be mutually exclusive, whose common thread is violence, not diagnosis per se.
    1. Purposeful, instrumental violence
    2. Purposeful, noninstrumental violence
    3. Purposeful, targeted, defensive violence
    4. Targeted, impulsive violence
    5. Nontargeted, impulsive violence incidental to emotional escape
    6. Random but purposeful violence
    7. Violence related to perceived/feared loss or abandonment
    8. Violence related to chronic paranoia or consequent misconception

References

American Psychiatric Association: Diagnostic and Statistical Manual of Mental Disorders, 4th Edition, Text Revision. Washington, DC, American Psychiatric Association, 2000

Coid JW: Personality disorders in prisoners and their motivation for dangerous and disruptive behavior. Crim Behav Ment Health 12:209–226, 2002

Coid JW: Epidemiology, public health, and the problems of personality disorder. Br J Psychiatry 182(suppl):s3–s10, 2003

Costello CG: The advantages of focusing on the personality characteristics of the personality disordered, in Personality Characteristics of the Personality Disordered. Edited by Costello CG. New York, Wiley, 1996, pp 1–23

Kansas v. Crane 534 U.S. 407 (2002)

Kansas v. Hendricks 521 U.S. 346 (1997)

Krakowski M, Volavka J, Brizer D: Psychopathology and violence: a review of literature. Compr Psychiatry 27:131–148, 1986

Leong GB, Silva JA: Sexually violent predator, II. J Am Acad Psychiatry Law 29:340–343, 2001

Monahan J: Predicting Violent Behavior: An Assessment of Clinical Techniques. Beverly Hills, CA, Sage Press, 1981

Monahan J: Mental disorder and violent behavior: perceptions and evidence. Am Psychol 47:511–521, 1992

Monahan J, Steadman H, Silver E, et al: Rethinking Risk Assessment: The MacArthur Study of Mental Disorder and Violence. New York, Oxford University Press, 2001

Mulvey EP: Assessing the evidence of a link between mental illness and violence. Hosp Community Psychiatry 45:663–668, 1994

Nestor PG: Mental disorders and violence: personality dimensions and clinical features. Am J Psychiatry 159:1973–1978, 2002

Otto RK: Assessing and managing violence risk in outpatient settings. J Clin Psychol 56:1239–1262, 2000

Rabkin JG: Criminal behavior of discharged mental patients: a critical appraisal of the research. Psychol Bull 86:1–27, 1979

Rogers R, Shuman DW: Fundamentals of Forensic Practice: Mental Health and Criminal Law. New York, Springer, 2005

Steadman HJ, Mulvey EP, Monahan J, et al: Violence by people discharged from acute psychiatric inpatient facilities and by others in the same neighborhoods. Arch Gen Psychiatry 55:393–401, 1998

Swanson JW, Holzer CE III, Ganju VK, et al: Violence and psychiatric disorder in the community: evidence from the Epidemiologic Catchment Area surveys. Hosp Community Psychiatry 41:761–770, 1990

Swanson JW, Borum R, Swartz M, et al: Psychotic symptoms and disorders and the risk of violent behavior in the community. Crim Behav Ment Health 6:317–338, 1996

Swanson JW, Swartz MS, Van Dorn RA: A national study of violent behavior in persons with schizophrenia. Arch Gen Psychiatry 63:490–499, 2006

Tardiff K, Marzuk PM, Leon AC, et al: Violence by patients admitted to a private psychiatric hospital. Am J Psychiatry 154:88–93, 1997

Widiger TA, Trull TJ: Personality disorders and violence, in Violence and Mental Disorder: Developments in Risk Assessment (The John D. and Catherine T. MacArthur Foundation Series on Mental Health and Development). Edited by Monahan J, Steadman HJ. Chicago, IL, University of Chicago Press, 1994, pp 203–226

CHAPTER 10

Neurological and Medical Disorders

Karen E. Anderson, M.D.
Jonathan M. Silver, M.D.

Violent behavior has long been associated with focal brain lesions as well as with diffuse damage to the central nervous system (CNS). Any condition producing psychosis or mania may have aggression as a concomitant symptom. Medical conditions that do not directly affect the brain can also be a cause of aggressive behavior due to diffuse effects on CNS function. Irritability and aggression are a major source of morbidity for many neurological and medical patients and increase the burden on their families and other caregivers. In this chapter, we discuss common neurological and medical etiologies of aggressive behavior (see Table 10–1). Identification and treatment of the underlying cause is often the first step in treatment of violence related to a neurological or medical disorder.

Dementia

Dementia, a progressive decline in function across multiple cognitive domains, is common, affecting 5%–8% of those over age 65 and nearly 50% of those over 85 (Small et al. 1997). Behavioral disturbances are common in people with many types of dementia. Rabins et al.'s (1982) survey of family and primary caregivers found that the most serious problem reported was aggressive behavior. Families are able to tolerate

TABLE 10–1. Characteristics of aggression associated with neurological or medical disease

Triggered by seemingly inconsequential or previously benign stimuli
Usually not planned
Does not help to fulfill long-term goals or gains
Sudden onset, abrupt offset
Brief outbursts contrasted by long periods of relative calm
After outbursts, patients are upset, concerned, and embarrassed, and may express regret

their relative being forgetful; it is more difficult to manage sudden anger. Aggressive behavior is one of the main factors leading to placement of a demented person in a nursing home (O'Donnell et al. 1992). Hamel (1990) studied predictors of aggression and the reaction of caregivers to aggression in 213 demented outpatients. Aggression was reported in 57.2% of patients; verbal aggression was the most common form, occurring in 51% of cases. Physical aggression, including threatening gestures, was reported in 34% of patients, and sexual aggression, such as inappropriate hugging and kissing, in only 7%. Aggression most often occurred in a situation in which a patient was instructed to do something. A history of aggressive personality traits predicted aggression in patients with dementia. This finding is in agreement with earlier studies by Ryden (1988) and by Morrant and Ablog (1983). A troubled premorbid relationship between patient and caregiver also predicted aggressive behavior. Aggression was endorsed by caregivers as influencing whether they would decide to institutionalize patients, a finding also reported by other groups (Balestreri et al. 2000). Patients with dementia who develop psychosis and subsequent agitation early in the course of the illness should be evaluated for dementia with Lewy bodies, a more rapidly progressive and less common condition than Alzheimer's disease. This is especially true in cases in which parkinsonism or extreme sensitivity to neuroleptics is present.

In a study of agitation and cognitive impairment in nursing home residents, Cohen-Mansfield et al. (1990) studied 408 residents of a large suburban nursing home. Level of impairment in performing activities of daily living (ADLs) and in cognition were associated with increased aggression, with high levels of impairment correlating with problematic behavior. Patel and Hope (1992) found that in 90 inpatients on an extended-stay psychogeriatric unit, levels of aggressive behavior were quite high. Most of the aggressive behavior occurred consistently in relation to morning assistance with ADLs.

Several predictors of aggressive and violent behavior have been found specifically in Alzheimer's disease, the most prevalent form of dementia in the elderly. Devanand et al. (1992) looked at specific behavioral disturbances in 106 outpatients with probable Alzheimer's disease. Aggression and agitation were associated with greater functional impairment but did not correlate with severity of cognitive decline. Deutsch et al. (1991) found that psychotic symptoms were a predictor of aggressive behavior in Alzheimer's patients. The prevalence of delusions and misidentifications was significantly higher in physically aggressive patients.

Imaging studies have revealed correlations among structural and functional deficits and aggression. Burns et al. (1990) studied 178 patients with Alzheimer's disease. Wandering and aggression together were significantly associated with cognitive impairment. Computed tomography scans of subjects' brains were also examined, and a positive correlation was found between temporal lobe atrophy and aggression. A positron emission tomography (PET) study by Sultzer et al. (1995) of 21 Alzheimer's patients found that aggression was correlated with frontal and temporal hypometabolism. Agitation and disinhibition were significantly correlated with global hypometabolism.

Traumatic Brain Injury

Traumatic brain injury (TBI) accounts for substantial morbidity and mortality, especially among those in their mid-teens to mid-twenties. Behavioral symptoms, including aggression, are common both acutely following the injury and as a long-term consequence (Silver et al. 2005). In the acute phase after brain injury, patients often experience a period of agitation and confusion lasting days to months, which is probably best considered a delirium (Sandel and Mysiw 1996). Bipolar disorder secondary to TBI can lead to impulsive aggression. Agitation usually appears within the first 2 weeks of hospitalization and resolves within 2 weeks. Restlessness may appear after 2 months and may persist for 4–6 weeks (Brooke et al. 1992). Subsequently, patients may develop low frustration tolerance and explosive behavior that can be set off by minimal provocation or occur without warning. These episodes range in severity from irritability to outbursts that result in damage to property or assaults on others. In a study of 89 patients assessed during the first 6 months after TBI, Tateno et al. (2003) found aggressive behavior in 33.7% of TBI patients compared with 11.5% of patients with multiple trauma but no TBI. Aggressive behavior was significantly associated with the presence of major depression, frontal lobe lesions, poor premorbid social functioning, and a history of alcohol and substance abuse. In severe cases, affected individuals cannot remain in the community or with their families and often are referred to long-term psychiatric or neurobehavioral facilities.

In the early recovery period, 35%–96% of patients are reported to have agitated behavior (Levin and Grossman 1978; Rao et al. 1985). After the acute recovery phase, irritability or bad temper is common. In a survey of individuals with TBI who were in skilled nursing facilities, Wolf et al. (1996) found that agitation was present in 45% of 140 patients. There has been only one prospective study of the occurrence of agitation and restlessness that has been monitored by an objective rating instrument, the Overt Aggression Scale (Brooke et al. 1992). The authors of this study (Brooke et al. 1992) found that out of 100 patients with severe TBI (Glasgow Coma Scale score less than 8, more than 1 hour of coma, and greater than 1 week of hospitalization), only 11 patients exhibited agitated behavior. Only 3 patients manifested these behaviors for more than 1 week. However, 35 patients were observed to be restless but not agitated.

Studies of mild TBI have evaluated patients for much briefer periods of time; 1-year estimates from these studies range from 5% to 70%. Carlsson et al. (1987) examined the relationship between the number of TBIs associated with loss of consciousness (LOC) and various symptoms and demonstrated that irritability increases with subsequent injuries. Of those men who did not have head injuries with LOC, 21% reported irritability; 31% of men with one injury with LOC and 33% of men with two or more injuries with LOC admitted to this symptom.

An evidence-based review of the TBI literature suggested that TBI patients with frontal lobe injury, a prior history of substance abuse, or impulsive aggression may be at higher risk of post-TBI aggression (Kim et al. 2007). These authors noted that, based on studies to date, it is not possible to define whether there is a relationship between cognitive function and development of aggression after TBI; this may be due to lack of sensitivity to executive dysfunction in neuropsychological testing. They also concluded there was not enough evidence to define the relationship between socioeconomic status and severity of injury to development of post-TBI aggression.

Stroke

Cerebrovascular accidents are an extremely common condition. Despite some decline in cases of stroke due to treatment of hypertension, stroke continues to be a major source of morbidity and mortality, especially in developed countries. Numerous neuropsychiatric symptoms have been described after stroke, including violent behavior. Poststroke mania, a rare behavioral change after stroke, may be associated with right hemisphere lesions; left hemisphere damage is more likely to produce depression (Robinson et al. 1988). In particular, damage to right hemisphere regions with limbic connections may make poststroke mania a more likely phenomenon. Psychosis also occurs with a low prevalence and may be associated with right-sided frontoparietal damage. Patients who have seizures after a cerebrovascular accident may also be at higher risk of developing psychosis. Subcortical atrophy may also play a role in development of psychosis after stroke (Starkstein et al. 1992). Catastrophic reactions are another poststroke behavioral change associated with aggression. The term was coined by Goldstein in 1939 to describe the "inability of the organism to cope when faced with physical or cognitive deficits." Patients with this rare condition seem to lose control of their behavior in a dramatic fashion after stroke. They often have a significant history of prior psychiatric illness and are depressed at the time the behavior occurs. Contrary to earlier work, catastrophic reaction is not necessarily more common in patients with aphasia (Starkstein et al. 1993).

Congenital Brain Disorders and Developmental Disorders

As the life expectancy of persons with mental handicaps increases, management of behavioral problems in this group becomes a pressing issue. Several studies have shown that people with intellectual deficiencies who engage in aggression toward others or self-injurious behavior are more likely to require intensive supervision and management (Hill and Bruininks 1984). Aside from the severity of intellectual impairment, aggression is the most important reason why patients are institutionalized.

Inpatients

Ghaziuddin and Ghaziuddin (1992) studied violent behavior in intellectually impaired persons during 1 year at a 100-bed unit at a university hospital. Of the 106 patients admitted to the unit during the study, 35% were involved in 145 violent incidents. Twelve patients who had associated psychiatric diagnoses were responsible for 86% of the incidents. Sigafoos et al. (1994) studied a population of 2,412 people with intellectual disability in Queensland, Australia. Of the sample, 48% were severely to profoundly mentally retarded, 24% were moderately impaired, and 9.6% were mildly impaired. Most individuals (59%) were male, and 16% of this population lived in institutions. Of the group living in institutions, 35% exhibited aggressive behavior. For those living in group homes, 17% were aggressive. Persons who were identified as aggressive had more profound levels of retardation and lower verbal abilities. Much of the aggressive behavior in this study was directed toward other patients or at other patients and staff.

Outpatients

Variable rates of aggression are reported among mentally handicapped people in outpatient settings. Bouras and Drummond (1992) conducted a study in southeast London, England, of 318 people (190 men, 128 women) with intellectual deficiencies who live in a community setting and were referred to the psychiatry department of a mental handicap service. Most of the patients in the study (54.4%) had a mild mental handicap, 28.6% had moderate mental handicap, and 17% had severe mental handicap. Almost one-third of the patients demonstrated aggression toward others, and 13% engaged in self-injurious behavior. Those people with severe intellectual impairment were more severely and frequently aggressive.

Davidson et al. (1994) studied 199 individuals who were referred to an outpatient crisis intervention program during a 2.5-year period and had an IQ below 70 and concomitant adaptive behavior deficits. All people in the study had at least one severe behavior disorder, and all had behavioral problems that were severe enough to threaten their ability to stay in an outpatient community setting. Half lived with family members, 22% in community residences, and 9% in intermediate community-based facilities for intellectually disabled persons. The remainder of those studied were either in family care or living independently or semi-independently. Intake evaluations, historical data from agency records, and medical records were reviewed as a source of data on aggressive behavior. At the time of the study, 131 individuals were classified as aggressive. This study found that aggressive and nonaggressive patients had similar neurological histories and medical status. CNS disorders, including seizures, were seen with a similar prevalence in both groups. The study concluded that current aggressive behavior was best predicted by past aggressive behavior when found in males with lower cognitive functioning who might have been previously institutionalized.

Epilepsy

Epilepsy has long been felt to be a cause of, or at least a contributor to, acts of violence. However, the literature is far from clear in establishing a strong link between epilepsy and aggression in the vast majority of patients. Many cases of aggressive behavior during or after a seizure are due to the patient's confusion or transient psychosis. In analyzing the occurrence of aggressive behavior in individuals with epilepsy, it is important to note when the behavior occurs. Aggressive acts can be *ictal* (during a seizure), *postictal* (immediately after a seizure), or *interictal* (in the period between seizures).

Ictal Aggression

Ictal aggression occurs most often when persons attempting to assist the patient during a seizure restrain the patient and the patient resists. Treiman (1986) gives several examples of "resistive violence" in response to restraint at the end of a generalized tonic-clonic seizure. Resistive violence has also been observed in animal seizure models. Ictal aggression is rarely directed and does not show elements of planning or premeditation.

Postictal Aggression

Postictal aggression involves violent acts that occur when a patient is still confused following a seizure. Usually, postictal aggression is seen after a general tonic-clonic seizure. It can occur less commonly after a complex partial seizure. Attempts at restraint are the most common cause of aggression during this time. Postictal psychosis is another likely cause of much postictal aggression, especially if the patient experiences frightening hallucinations or feels paranoid during that time (Devinsky and Bear 1984).

Interictal Aggression

Aggressive behavior between seizures is more controversial than ictal or postictal aggression because there is no direct relationship between the aggression and the seizure event. Most epileptologists agree that the majority of patients with epilepsy are psychologically normal between seizures. It is still unclear whether a small subset of persons with epilepsy behave differently between seizures as a result of brain alterations caused by the ictal events. Devinsky et al. (1994) studied 61 adult patients with epilepsy (46 patients with temporal lobe epilepsy, 15 with absence epilepsy) and compared this group with 17 neurologically normal control subjects. This study found no pattern of aggressive or hostile behavior among persons with epilepsy. However, the author did find increased suspiciousness in patients with left temporal lobe epilepsy and increased assaultive behavior in persons with bilateral temporal lobe epilepsy. There was a lack of difference between absence epilepsy and normal groups. These data are in agreement with earlier studies that did not demonstrate an increase in aggressive behavior among persons with epilepsy (Hermann et al. 1984). Mendez et al. (1993) examined 44 patients with epilepsy who were referred for psychiatric evaluation because of violence. They concluded that interictal violence was associated more with underlying psychopathology, such as schizophrenia, or with mental retardation, rather than seizure activity. Stevens and Hermann (1981) critically examined the scientific literature on the association between temporal lobe epilepsy and violent behavior, concluding that damage or dysfunction in the limbic area of the brain was the significant factor in predisposition toward violence.

Central Nervous System Infections

Encephalitis

The influence of viral and other forms of encephalitis on behavior first came to notice during the pandemic of encephalitis lethargica during World War I. Also known as von Economo's encephalitis, the illness was noted to produce a plethora of psychiatric symptoms, including behavioral changes such as aggression, in previously normal persons. Other forms of encephalitis, most notably herpes encephalitis, are now also known to result in aggressive behavior.

Encephalitis Lethargica

Encephalitis lethargica was first described in detail by Constantine von Economo in 1917 (von Economo 1937). Besides producing physical symptoms of an acute CNS infection, encephalitis lethargica could, at times, progress to coma or death. Survivors were sometimes afflicted with parkinsonism or bizarre behavioral disturbances. The agent that causes encephalitis lethargica has not yet been isolated. Some survivors, mostly adolescents, experienced pseudopsychopathic states. Sporadic cases of encephalitis lethargica are still seen infrequently throughout the world.

Herpes Simplex Encephalitis

The herpes simplex virus (HSV-1) can produce a severe form of encephalitis. It is probably the most common cause of nonepidemic encephalitis in temperate zones (Ho and Harter 1982). Mortality rates are as high as 70%. However, with new antiviral treatments, many patients are living longer. These survivors often have severe neurological sequelae, including profound behavioral disturbances. For unclear reasons, the herpes virus tends to produce focal temporal lobe destruction. This can result in a Klüver-Bucy syndrome in which patients are hyperoral and hypersexual and may have an abnormal desire to explore objects (hypermetamorphosis) (Friedman and Allen 1969).

Klüver-Bucy syndrome generally produces passive behavior; however, some patients with temporal lobe damage from the encephalitis are aggressive. The literature on aggressive behavior after herpes encephalitis consists only of case reports. Greer et al. (1989) described a 14-year-old patient with bilateral damage to the temporal lobes (right worse than left on computed tomography scan) due to herpes simplex viral encephalitis. Along with severe intellectual deficits, the patient also had severe, uncontrollable motor activity, including aggressive and self-injurious behavior. He eventually required placement in a residential facility due to his violent behavior. Greenwood et al. (1983) described four patients with herpes simplex encephalitis who exhibited aggressive behavior. The patients all exhibited some bizarre eating and chewing behaviors, mostly related to nonfood items such as bedding or feces. None were hypersexual or sexually inappropriate. All patients looked emotionless and had few facial expressions, but with questioning, three of the four patients flew into unpredictable rages. Greenwood noted that the patient who was the most unpredictably and violently aggressive was also the one with the least memory loss from the encephalitis. When in control, he could sit and play simple board games with staff. Yet when he became angered, he would throw food and feces, shout at staff, and swear. Greenwood suggested that because aggression does not occur in monkeys with bilateral temporal lobectomy, which produces classic Klüver-Bucy syndrome, the aggression in select patients with herpes simplex encephalitis may be due to partial involvement of limbic areas, whereas patients with a classical Klüver-Bucy syndrome have complete destruction of both temporal lobes.

Other Forms of Encephalitis

Because herpes simplex encephalitis is the only encephalitis known to localize to a particular brain area, it is the only encephalitis in which neuropsychiatric symptoms are relatively predictable. Other forms of encephalitis produce more diffuse CNS damage. Subacute encephalitis of various other etiologies causes numerous behavioral syndromes in patients, including marked aggression, sometimes due to psychosis.

These include autoimmune deficiency encephalitis (Beresford et al. 1986; Nurnberg et al. 1984; Snider et al. 1983) and limbic or "paraneoplastic" encephalitis due to remote effects of malignancy (Khan et al. 1994; Newman et al. 1990).

Central Nervous System Tumors

Prior to the widespread availability of neuroimaging, substantial behavioral changes, including aggression, were not infrequently seen with CNS malignancy. With the advent of relatively affordable detailed imaging studies in most developed countries, early diagnosis and treatment are fortunately now the rule. Available data are thus from autopsy studies done early in the last century. When behavioral changes occur due to malignancies, several factors influence what type of behavioral symptoms occur. These include interconnections of structures involved in the pathology, the patient's premorbid level of function, rapidity of tumor growth (which may cause increased intracranial pressure due to rapid expansion) and whether the malignancy produces a single lesion or multiple sites of involvement. Rapidly growing malignancies and those with multiple foci are most likely to cause acute behavioral changes, including psychosis and concomitant aggression (Lishman 1987). Association between tumor histological type and behavioral symptoms has not been shown (Frazier 1935; Keschner et al. 1936). Location of the tumor was found in older, autopsy-based literature to have little correlation with presence or type of psychiatric symptoms observed in patients, due to the factors noted earlier (Keschner et al. 1936). Frontal lobe tumors can produce irritable, labile behavior (McAllister and Price 1987) and psychosis (Strauss and Keschner 1935). Temporal lobe tumors may produce psychotic symptoms, although the literature is conflicting as to whether these symptoms are particularly common in patients with temporal lobe pathology (Davison and Bagley 1969; Mulder and Daly 1952). Parietal and occipital malignancies are relatively less likely to cause psychosis and agitation. Malignancies affecting the diencephalons (thalamus, hypothalamus, and structures surrounding the third ventricle) typically affect the limbic system due to its close proximity and may cause agitation.

Movement Disorders

Movement disorders may result in behavioral changes. Increased irritability and angry outbursts are reported in many movement disorders. Psychotic symptoms, which exacerbate underlying aggression, are also seen. Patients with essential tremor, dystonia, and hereditary ataxias are generally not violent, although exceptions occur.

Parkinson's Disease

Although aggression may not be a common manifestation of Parkinson's disease, per se, it may develop as a result of treatment of motor symptoms with dopaminergic medications, especially if psychosis is a side effect. Patients who develop impulse control disorders—"hedonistic dopaminergic dysregulations" that are at times related to use of dopaminergic medications to treat motor symptoms—may be agitated or impulsive.

Wilson's Disease

Wilson's disease, or hepatolenticular degeneration, is an autosomal recessive disorder involving dysregulation of copper metabolism by the liver. Neurological, renal, and hepatic abnormalities are the usual findings in the disease. In a study of 42 patients with Wilson's disease, Akil et al. (1991) noted that 24 of the patients had psychiatric symptoms as the presenting complaint. Personality changes, including aggression and irritability, were the most common presenting psychiatric complaint. Dening and Berrios (1989) assessed multiple neuropsychiatric symptoms in 195 patients with Wilson's disease. Aggression was definitely present in 17 patients and assessed as possibly present in 11 individuals.

Huntington's Disease

Huntington's disease is an autosomal dominant movement disorder. It typically features choreiform movements and/or psychiatric symptoms. Burns et al. (1990) assessed 26 patients with Huntington's disease and found that 59% of the patients scored significantly on an aggression scale. Aggression and irritability were not correlated with apathy or with each other. Marder et al. (2000) found in a large study of patients at various stages of the disease that aggression was reported by more than half of patients or caregivers.

Gilles de la Tourette Syndrome

Numerous authors have cited behavioral problems as part of the clinical picture in some cases of Tourette's syndrome. Obsessive-compulsive disorder and attention-deficit/hyperactivity disorder are the most commonly described psychiatric symptoms in Tourette's syndrome, but aggressive outbursts have also been described. Robertson et al. (1988) studied the correlation between motor symptoms and behavioral disorders in 90 patients with Tourette's syndrome. They found that 28 patients had been physically aggressive toward people (most typically family members), animals, or objects. Aggressive behavior was significantly associated with symptoms of an urge to touch everything in the immediate surroundings and with copropraxia. There was no significant association between aggression and age at onset, personal or family history of psychiatric illness, electroencephalographic or neurological abnormalities, medication, distribution of tics, hyperactivity, or difficulty in concentration or attention as a child.

White Matter Disorders

White matter, which makes up slightly less than half the volume of the adult human brain, is critical for normal communication between neurons. It is therefore not surprising that pathology of the white matter tracts can lead to aggression. Prediction of whether a particular individual with white matter disease will develop violent behavior is problematic, because most disorders of white matter lead to wide-ranging effects on the brain. Multiple sclerosis, vascular disorders (Binswanger's, cerebrovascular accidents), metabolic conditions (cobalamin deficiency, hypoxia), infections (AIDS),TBI, and neoplasms can all result in white matter damage.

Multiple sclerosis, a demyelinating condition, is the most common adult disorder of white matter. Patients with multiple sclerosis have increased rates of bipolar disorder compared with the general population. Mania is, of course, associated with increased risk of impulsive and aggressive behavior. Temporal lobe demyelination may carry a particular risk of mania in multiple sclerosis, consistent with data discussed earlier regarding temporal lobe pathology and violence (Filley 1996).

Medical Disorders

Numerous medical conditions may result in diffuse brain dysfunction and subsequent aggression. Several authors have discussed the frequency of "minimal brain dysfunction" or poorly characterized "neurological soft signs" in aggressive individuals (e.g., Elliot 1992; Monroe 1978). The most commonly seen disorders are described here; it is well worth pursuing a complete medical workup in any patient who develops aggression suddenly or without a prior history of violent behavior.

Delirium

Delirium, or acute confusional state, is a transient global disorder of cognition; it is a syndrome, not a disease, with multiple causes (see Table 10–2). The condition is a medical emergency associated with increased morbidity and mortality. Decreased attention span and a waxing and waning type of confusion are important features (American Psychiatric Association 2000).

Agitated or violent behavior has been reported in delirium due to many causes, including postoperative confusion (Lepouse et al. 2006). Several conditions associated with delirium are discussed in the following sections.

Toxins

Toxin exposure can produce various neurobehavioral changes, the most common of which are sedation and memory deficits. Toxins that are associated with aggression include alkyltin, arsenic, lead (in adults), manganese, and mercury. Solvents generally cause lethargy and confusion, although toluene exposure may produce excitation and disinhibition. Gas exposure, such as carbon monoxide, causes lethargy and impaired cognition and may cause delirium. Nitrous oxide use is associated with delusions and agitation (Bleecker 1994; Bolla and Roca 1994).

Medication Side Effects

Drug effects and side effects can cause disinhibition or irritability leading to aggression. By far the most common drug associated with aggression is alcohol, during both intoxication and withdrawal. Stimulating

TABLE 10–2. Common causes of delirium

Hypoxia

Metabolic disruption

Hypoglycemia

Hyperthermia

Alcohol or sedative withdrawal

Localized or systemic infections

Structural brain lesions

Postoperative confusion

Medications (may be at therapeutic doses in elderly patients), especially agents with anticholinergic effects drugs such as cocaine and amphetamines, as well as stimulating antidepressants, may produce agitation. Antipsychotic medications may increase agitation through anticholinergic side effects. Agitation and irritability usually accompany severe akathisia. Many other drugs may produce confusional states, especially anticholinergic medications that can cause delirium. Other drugs that may produce aggressive behavior include steroids, which can cause psychosis (prednisone, cortisone, and the anabolic steroids); quinolone antibiotics; analgesics (opiates and other narcotics); and anxiolytics (barbiturates and benzodiazepines). The latter two groups of agents may cause aggression due to disinhibition or medication withdrawal effects.

Rheumatic Diseases

Systemic lupus erythematosus is the autoimmune disorder most closely associated with neuropsychiatric symptoms, including aggression. Behavioral effects of lupus can be due to either direct CNS involvement or effects on other organ systems, such as uremia due to renal impairment, leading to confusion and delirium. Other rheumatological disorders, such as the vasculitides, Sjögren's syndrome, and sarcoidosis, can all produce dementia and psychosis, leading to aggressive behavior (Ovsiew and Utset 1997). As noted earlier, steroids, which are commonly used to treat rheumatological diseases, may cause psychosis and agitation.

Sleep Disorders

There have been a few reports of aggressive behavior during parasomnias, including violent attacks by patients with rapid eye movement behavior disorder (Mahowald et al. 2007). Recognition of this disorder is particularly important due to its association with several other conditions, including Parkinson's disease, Lewy body dementia, and multisystem atrophy. Sleep deprivation can, of course, worsen irritability in many conditions, leading to exacerbation of underlying behavioral problems.

Hypoglycemia

A series of studies conducted by Virkkunen et al. (2007) in Finland has examined biological correlates of aggression in a group of violent prisoners. One consistent finding has been that this group is prone to hypoglycemia and that they have in increase in irritability during these episodes.

Treatment

Assessment and Quantification of Aggressive Episodes

Before therapeutic intervention to treat violent behavior is initiated, clinicians should document the baseline frequency and severity of the occurrences. It is essential to establish a treatment plan that uses objective documentation of aggressive episodes to monitor the efficacy of interventions for both acute and chronic aggression. The Overt Aggression Scale is an instrument of proven reliability and validity that can be used easily and effectively to rate aggressive behavior in patients with a wide range of medical or neurological disorders (Silver and Yudofsky 1991; Yudofsky et al. 1986). The scale comprises items that assess verbal aggression, physical aggression against objects, physical aggression against self, and physical aggression against others. Behavior can be monitored by staff or by family members utilizing this instrument.

Pharmacotherapy

Although no drug is approved by the U.S. Food and Drug Administration specifically for the management of acute or chronic aggression, medications are widely used, and often misused, for this purpose. The use of pharmacological interventions can be considered in two categories: 1) use of the sedating effects of medications, as required in acute situations, so that the patient does not harm him- or herself or others, and 2) use of nonsedating antiaggressive medications to treat for chronic aggression when necessary. Some patients may not respond to just one medication but may require combination treatment. There are few double-blind, placebo-controlled trials conducted in this area to guide the use of medication to treat aggressive behavior (Neurobehavioral Guidelines Working Group et al. 2006). We suggest using the guidelines published by the Expert Consensus Panel for Agitation in Dementia (Alexopolous et al. 1998) as a framework for the assessment and management of agitation and aggression in medical and neurological illness.

Acute Aggression and Agitation

In the treatment of agitation and for treating acute episodes of aggressive behavior, medications that are sedating, such as antipsychotic drugs or benzodiazepines, may be indicated. However, because these drugs are not specific in their ability to inhibit aggressive behaviors, there may be detrimental effects on arousal and cognition. In addition, due to the potential for interference with respiration and thermoregulation, these drugs should be administered only under medical supervision. Therefore, the use of sedation-producing medications must be time limited to avoid the emergence of seriously disabling side effects ranging from oversedation to extrapyramidal side effects.

Chronic Aggression

If a patient continues to exhibit periods of agitation or aggression beyond several weeks, the use of specific antiaggressive medications should be initiated to prevent future episodes. The choice of medication may be guided by the underlying hypothesized mechanism of action (i.e., effects on serotonin system, adrenergic system, kindling) or in consideration of the predominant clinical features. Since no medication has been approved for the treatment of aggression, the clinician must use medications that have been approved for other uses (i.e., for seizure disorders, depression, anxiety, mood stabilization, hypertension).

Table 10–3 summarizes our recommendations for the utilization of various classes of drugs in the treatment of aggressive disorders. In treating aggression, the clinician, when possible, should diagnose and treat underlying disorders and use antiaggressive agents specific for those disorders. When there is a partial response after a therapeutic trial with a specific medication, adjunctive treatment with a medication with a different mechanism of action should be instituted. For example, a patient with a partial response to β-blockers may show further improvement with the addition of an anticonvulsant or a serotonergic antidepressant. Side effects may limit dosing, as in any patient population; patients with disease affecting the brain are often more sensitive to medication side effects. Among the more important side effects, akathisia may occur, with concomitant restlessness and irritability, in patients who are being treated with neuroleptics for suppression of chorea or for psychiatric symptoms. This can potentially worsen aggression if not recognized.

Clinicians should be aware of recent U.S. Food and Drug Administration warnings that the use of atypical antipsychotics was associated with an increased risk of death in a review of data from 5,106 elderly demented patients in randomized, controlled clinical trials (see Kuehn 2005 for an excellent commentary on the "black box" warnings). A mortality rate of 4.5% was seen in those elders receiving atypical agents compared with a rate of 2.6% in those who were given placebo. Deaths were predominantly due to cardiovascular and infectious illnesses. A "black box" warning has been added to labeling of all atypical neuroleptics. As discussed earlier, many of the patients who are most in need of treatment for aggression are elderly and may have memory loss; they may thus be at higher risk of mortality associated with atypical neuroleptic use. Conversely, agitation and violence are associated with significant risk of increased morbidity and mortality. Clinicians should weigh carefully the small possibility of increased mortality associated with atypical antipsychotic use versus the many complications inherent in leaving aggressive symptoms untreated in these patients.

Behavioral Treatment

It is clear that aggression can be caused and influenced by a combination of environmental and biological factors. Because of the unpredictable nature of aggression in neurological and medical disease, caregivers and staff in institutional settings may overreact to aggression when it occurs. Behavioral treatments have been shown to be highly effective in treating patients with organic aggression and may be useful when combined with pharmacotherapy. Behavioral strategies—including a token economy, aggression replacement strategies, and decelerative techniques—may reduce aggression in the inpatient setting and can be combined effectively with pharmacological treatment.

Because irritability is often directed toward individuals known to the patients, education of caregivers in how to identify and avoid situations that trigger irritability and how to minimize its effects if it does occur is crucial. Behavioral interventions may prove helpful in prevention of aggression by removing precipitating factors. This includes adherence to a schedule to avoid surprising the patient and provoking an outburst (Moskowitz and Marder 2001). Caregivers should be advised to stop an activity, such as assistance with ADLs, if aggressive behavior begins to escalate. They should also be counseled not to argue with patients if the behavior begins to escalate. If threats of physical aggression occur, they should quickly remove themselves and other family members from the area where the patient is and contact emergency medical services for assistance. Any ammunition and weapons should be removed from the home. The patient should be prevented from accessing alcohol and illicit drugs because use of these substances, even in small quantities, may contribute greatly to disinhibition in patients with neurological and medical illness. If there is a history of severe aggression against persons or property, law enforcement agencies may need to intervene to prevent injury to the patient or caregivers. Evaluation by a medical professional to rule out medical illness, delirium, medication toxicity, or physical discomfort should be conducted, especially in patients who have not been

TABLE 10–3. Psychopharmacological treatment of chronic aggression

Class of agent	Examples of agents used (dosing range)	Potential side effects	Overall comments
Selective serotonin reuptake inhibitors (SSRIs)	Escitalopram (10–20 mg)	Initially may cause anxiety or agitation	Preferable to start with an SSRI, then add a neuroleptic if needed. However, in cases of acute or extreme aggression, a neuroleptic should be started first. SSRIs may cause or exacerbate apathy in some patients. Higher doses and longer treatment time are needed if anxiety is part of the cause for aggression.
	Sertraline (100–200 mg)	May be more activating than other SSRIs	
Atypical neuroleptics	Olanzapine (2.5–20 mg)	Weight gain, sedation, possible EPS	Standard neuroleptics will provide the most rapid sedation but are more likely to cause EPS and sedation. Recent FDA black box warnings were issued for use of atypical neuroleptics in elderly demented patients.
	Quetiapine (100–400 mg, may go higher in select cases)	Sedation, possible EPS	
Standard (typical) neuroleptics	Haloperidol (0.5–10 mg)	EPS, sedation	Best for acute agitation or delirium; start with small doses. Often used IM in acute situations in conjunction with a benzodiazepine.

TABLE 10–3. Psychopharmacological treatment of chronic aggression *(continued)*

Class of agent	Examples of agents used (dosing range)	Potential side effects	Overall comments
β-Blockers	Propranolol (200–600 mg)	May lower heart rate; contraindicated in bronchospasm, diabetes, thyroid disease, and heart failure	Higher dosages may be needed in select cases. Latency of 4–6 weeks for onset of treatment.
Anticonvulsants/ Mood stabilizers	Valproate (500–1,000 mg)	May cause sedation; need to monitor liver function tests. Blood levels can be monitored.	May be particularly useful in traumatic brain injury and other conditions associated with increased rate of seizures. Abrupt discontinuation of these agents may precipitate seizures in individuals who do not have a prior history of epilepsy.
	Carbamazepine (200–400 mg)	Possible bone marrow suppression	
Benzodiazepines	Lorazepam (0.5–3 mg)	Sedation, disinhibition	Withdrawal from benzodiazepines may precipitate further aggression. Clonazepam is longer acting, causing fewer withdrawal symptoms.
	Clonazepam (0.5–3 mg)	Sedation, disinhibition	

Note. EPS=extrapyramidal symptoms; FDA=U.S. Food and Drug Administration; IM=intramuscular.

violent previously or those with impaired communication abilities. Underlying psychiatric illness should also be considered as a mediating factor, including depression, anxiety, or psychosis. A review of behavioral interventions can be found in Moskowitz and Marder (2001).

Discussion

Aggressive behavior in the presence of medical illness is common and can be highly disabling. Neuroanatomical, neurochemical, and neurophysiological factors may have an etiological or mediating role in the production of violence. The vignettes that follow illustrate some common clinical features of violence in the medical setting.

Case Example 1: Traumatic Brain Injury

Mr. T is a 25-year-old man who sustained a severe TBI in a motor vehicle accident. Damage to his orbitofrontal cortex was visualized on magnetic resonance imaging. When he returned home after a 1-month treatment in a rehabilitation facility, his family noticed a significant change in his temper. Whereas he previously was patient, he now had a "short fuse" and would go into a verbal rage with minimal frustration. Thankfully, he would only occasionally slam a door or throw an object down in anger. The family had been walking around "on eggshells" because they did not know what would provoke the next episode.

The family was educated on the common occurrence of aggression after TBI and told that this is a sequelae of TBI, as is memory problems. They were told to start keeping a diary of the episodes, so that we would know how many occurred during the week. Mr. T was started on propranolol 60 mg/day, with monitoring of his pulse and blood pressure. When the dosage was increased to 240 mg/day, he became much calmer and had a longer "fuse." He described his aggression as like being on a beach and being surprised when a large wave hits you from behind; with the medication, he could see the "wave" approaching and deal with those feelings.

Case Example 2: Huntington's Disease

Mr. H is a 45-year-old married man whose father died of Huntington's disease in his mid-60s after having symptoms of the disease for more than 15 years. Mr. H, who works as a taxicab driver, has been suspended from driving his cab due to several episodes of severe aggression. In one episode he took a baseball bat, which he says he always keeps in his cab for self-defense, and broke the windows on another car after he thought the driver cut him off in traffic. In another episode, he threw a cup of hot coffee at a customer who failed to give him a tip. He began to drink on the job and made inappropriate sexual comments to female passengers. On interview, he admitted he would previously never have reacted in

Neurological and Medical Disorders

this way to fairly minor provocations and expressed regret that he had behaved in such a manner. Mr. H has never been evaluated for Huntington's symptoms clinically and has no wish to know if he has the gene.

This case illustrates the change in behavior of someone who may be developing a neurological disorder. Behavioral changes can be a presenting symptom of Huntington's disease, before onset of motor symptoms. As is typical in aggression in the setting of neurological disease, the patient responds out of proportion to the incident triggering the behavior and is puzzled as to why he reacted in such an extreme manner.

Key Points

- Explosive and violent behavior has long been associated with both focal brain lesions and diffuse damage to the CNS.
- Irritability and/or aggression is a major source of morbidity for individuals with neurological or medical disease and a source of additional stress to their caregivers and families.
- Presence of aggression is often a primary factor when the decision is made to place patients in an institution rather than provide care in a home setting.
- Low frustration tolerance and explosive behavior can be set off by minimal provocation or occur without warning. It is essential that all clinicians be aware of aggression and its assessment and treatment in order to provide effective care to patients with this condition.
- After appropriate evaluation and assessment of possible etiologies, treatment begins with the documentation of the aggressive episodes. Psychopharmacological strategies may be divided into those intended to treat acute aggression and those intended to prevent episodes in the patient with chronic aggression.
- The treatment of acute aggression involves the judicious use of sedation; the treatment of chronic aggression is guided by underlying diagnoses and symptoms.
- Behavioral strategies, including caregiver reassurance and education, remain an important component in the comprehensive treatment of aggression.

References

Akil M, Schwartz JA, Dutchak D, et al: The psychiatric presentations of Wilson's disease. J Neuropsychiatry Clin Neurosci 3:377–382, 1991

Alexopoulos GS, Silver JM, Kahn DA, et al: Treatment of agitation in older persons with dementia. The Expert Consensus Panel for Agitation in Dementia. Postgrad Med (spec no):1–88, 1998

American Psychiatric Association: Diagnostic and Statistical Manual of Mental Disorders, 4th Edition, Text Revision. Washington, DC, American Psychiatric Association, 2000

Balestreri L, Grossberg A, Grossberg GT: Behavioral and psychological symptoms of dementia as a risk factor for nursing home placement. Int Psychogeriatr 12(suppl):59–62, 2000

Beresford TP, Blow FC, Hall RC: AIDS encephalitis mimicking alcohol dementia and depression. Biol Psychiatry 21:394–397, 1986

Bleecker M: Clinical presentation of selected neurotoxic compounds, in Occupational Neurology and Clinical Neurotoxicology. Edited by Bleecker ML, Hansen J. Philadelphia, PA, Williams & Wilkins, 1994, pp 207–233

Bolla KI, Roca R: Neuropsychiatric sequelae of occupational exposure to neurotoxins, in Occupational Neurology and Clinical Neurotoxicology. Edited by Bleecker ML, Hansen JA. Philadelphia, PA, Williams & Wilkins, 1994, pp 133–159

Bouras N, Drummond C: Behaviour and psychiatric disorders of people with mental handicaps living in the community. J Intellect Disabil Res 36 (pt 4):349–357, 1992

Brooke MM, Questad KA, Patterson DR, et al: Agitation and restlessness after closed head injury: a prospective study of 100 consecutive admissions. Arch Phys Med Rehabil 73:320–323, 1992

Burns A, Jacoby R, Levy R: Psychiatric phenomena in Alzheimer's disease, IV: disorders of behaviour. Br J Psychiatry157:86–94, 1990

Carlsson GS, Svardsudd K, Welin L: Long-term effects of head injuries sustained during life in three male populations. J Neurosurg 67:197–205, 1987

Cohen-Mansfield J, Marx MS, Rosenthal AS: Dementia and agitation in nursing home residents: how are they related? Psychol Aging 5:3–8, 1990

Davidson PW, Cain NN, Sloane-Reeves JE, et al: Characteristics of community-based individuals with mental retardation and aggressive behavioral disorders. Am J Ment Retard 98:704–116, 1994

Davison K, Bagley CR: Schizophrenia-like psychoses associated with organic disorders of the central nervous system: a review of the literature, in Current Problems in Neuropsychiatry: Schizophrenia, Epilepsy and the Temporal Lobe (Br J Psychiatry, special publication no 4). Edited by Harrington RN. London, Headley Brothers, 1969, pp 126–130

Dening TR, Berrios GE: Wilson's disease: psychiatric symptoms in 195 cases. Arch Gen Psychiatry 46:1126–1134, 1989

Deutsch LH, Bylsma FW, Rovner BW, et al: Psychosis and physical aggression in probable Alzheimer's disease. Am J Psychiatry 148:1159–1163, 1991

Devanand DP, Brockington CD, Moody BJ, et al: Behavioral syndromes in Alzheimer's disease. Int Psychogeriatr 4 (suppl 2):161–184, 1992

Devinsky O, Bear D: Varieties of aggressive behavior in temporal lobe epilepsy. Am J Psychiatry 141:651–656, 1984

Devinsky O, Ronsaville D, Cox C, et al: Interictal aggression in epilepsy: the Buss-Durkee Hostility Inventory. Epilepsia 35:585–590, 1994

Elliot FA: Violence: the neurologic contribution. An overview. Arch Neurol 49:595–603, 1992

Filley CM: Neurobehavioral aspects of cerebral white matter disorders, in Neuropsychiatry, Edited by Fogel BS, Schiffer RB, Rao SM. Baltimore, MD, Williams & Wilkins, 1996, pp 913–934

Frazier CH: Tumor involving the frontal lobe alone: a symptomatic survey of 105 verified cases. Arch Neurol Psychiatry 35:525–571, 1935

Friedman HM, Allen N: Chronic effects of complete limbic lobe destruction in man. Neurology 19:679–690, 1969

Ghaziuddin M, Ghaziuddin N: Violence against staff by mentally retarded inpatients. Hosp Community Psychiatry 43:503–504, 1992

Greenwood R, Bhalla A, Gordon A, et al: Behaviour disturbances during recovery from herpes simplex encephalitis. J Neurol Neurosurg Psychiatry 46:809–817, 1983

Greer MK, Lyons-Crews M, Mauldin LB, et al: A case study of the cognitive and behavioral deficits of temporal lobe damage in herpes simplex encephalitis. J Autism Dev Disord 19:317–326, 1989

Hamel M, Gold DP, Andres D, et al: Predictors and consequences of aggressive behavior by community-based dementia patients. Gerontologist 30:206–211, 1990

Hermann BP, Whitman S, Gordon AC: Psychopathology in epilepsy: how great is the risk? Biol Psychiatry 19:213–236, 1984

Ho SU, Harter DH: Herpes simplex virus encephalitis. JAMA 247:337, 1982

Hill BK, Bruininks RH: Maladaptive behavior of mentally retarded individuals in residential facilities. Am J Ment Defic 88:380–387, 1984

Keschner M, Bender MB, Strauss I: Mental symptoms in cases of tumor of the temporal lobe. Arch Neurol Psychiatry 35:572–596, 1936

Khan N, Wieser HG: Limbic encephalitis: a case report. Epilepsy Res 17:175–181, 1994

Kim E, Lauterbach E, Reeve A, et al: Neuropsychiatric complications of traumatic brain injury: a critical review of the literature (A report by the ANPA Committee on Research). J Neuropsychiatry Clin Neurosci 19:106–127, 2007

Kuehn BM: FDA warns antipsychotic drugs may be risky for elderly. JAMA 293:2462, 2005

Lepouse C, Lautner CA, Liu L, et al: Emergence delirium in adults in the postanaesthesia care unit. Br J Anaesth 96:747–753, 2006

Levin HS, Grossman RG: Behavioral sequelae of closed head injury: a quantitative study. Arch Neurol 35:720–727, 1978

Lishman WA: Organic Psychiatry: The Psychological Consequences of Cerebral Disorder. New York, Oxford University Press, 1987

Mahowald MW, Schenck CH, Bornemann MA: Pathophysiologic mechanisms in REM sleep behavior disorder. Curr Neurol Neurosci Rep 7:167–172, 2007

Marder K, Zhao H, Myers RH, et al: Rate of functional decline in Huntington's disease. Huntington Study Group. Neurology 54:452–458, 2000 [Erratum in: Neurology 54:1712, 2000]

McAllister TW, Price TR: Aspects of the behavior of psychiatric inpatients with frontal lobe damage: some implications for diagnosis and treatment. Compr Psychiatry 28:14–21, 1987

Mendez MF, Doss RC, Taylor JL: Interictal violence in epilepsy: relationship to behavior and seizure variables. J Nerv Ment Dis 181:566–569, 1993

Monroe RR: Brain Dysfunction in Aggressive Criminals. Lexington, MA, Lexington Books, 1978

Morrant JC, Ablog JR: The angry elderly patient: an approach to understanding. Postgrad Med 74:93–95, 98–100, 102, 1983

Moskowitz CB, Marder K: Palliative care for people with late-stage Huntington's disease. Neurol Clin 19:849–865, 2001

Mulder DW, Daly D: Psychiatric symptoms associated with lesions of the temporal lobe. JAMA 150:173–176, 1952

Neurobehavioral Guidelines Working Group, Warden DL, Gordon B, et al: Guidelines for the pharmacologic treatment of neurobehavioral sequelae of traumatic brain injury. J Neurotrauma 23:1468–1501, 2006

Newman NJ, Bell IR, McKee AC: Paraneoplastic limbic encephalitis: neuropsychiatric presentation. Biol Psychiatry 27:529–542, 1990

Nurnberg HG, Prudic J, Fiori M, et al: Psychopathology complicating acquired immune deficiency syndrome (AIDS). Am J Psychiatry 141:95–96, 1984

O'Donnell BF, Drachman DA, Barnes HJ, et al: Incontinence and troublesome behaviors predict institutionalization in dementia. J Geriatr Psychiatry Neurol 5:45–52, 1992

Ovsiew F, Utset T: Neuropsychiatric aspects of rheumatic diseases, in The American Psychiatric Press Textbook of Neuropsychiatry and Clinical Neurosciences, 4th Edition. Edited by Yudofsky SC, Hales RE. Washington, DC, American Psychiatric Press, 1997, pp 813–850

Patel V, Hope RA: Aggressive behaviour in elderly psychiatric inpatients. Acta Psychiatr Scand 85:131–135, 1992

Rabins PV, Mace NL, Lucas MJ: The impact of dementia on the family. JAMA 248:333–335, 1982

Rao N, Jellinek HM, Woolston DC: Agitation in closed head injury: haloperidol effects on rehabilitation outcome. Arch Phys Med Rehabil 66:30–34, 1985

Robertson MM, Trimble MR, Lees AJ: The psychopathology of the Gilles de la Tourette syndrome: a phenomenological analysis. Br J Psychiatry 152:383–390, 1988

Robinson RG, Boston JD, Starkstein SE, et al: Comparison of mania with depression following traumatic brain injury: causal factors. Am J Psychiatry 145:172–178, 1988

Ryden MB: Aggressive behavior in persons with dementia who live in the community. Alzheimer Dis Assoc Disord 2:342–355, 1988

Sandel ME, Mysiw WJ: The agitated brain injured patient, part 1: definitions, differential diagnosis, and assessment. Arch Phys Med Rehabil 77:617–623, 1996

Sigafoos J, Elkins J, Kerr M, et al: A survey of aggressive behaviour among a population of persons with intellectual disability in Queensland. J Intellect Disabil Res 38 (pt 4):369–381, 1994

Silver JM, Yudofsky SC: The Overt Aggression Scale: overview and guiding principles. J Neuropsychiatry Clin Neurosci 3:22–29, 1991

Silver JM, Yudofsky SC, Anderson KA: Aggressive disorders, in The American Psychiatric Publishing Textbook of Traumatic Brain Injury. Edited by Silver JM, McAllister TW, Yudofsky SC. Washington, DC, American Psychiatric Publishing, 2005, pp 259–278

Small GW, Rabins PV, Barry PP, et al: Diagnosis and treatment of Alzheimer's disease and related disorders: consensus statement of the American Association of Geriatric Psychiatry, the Alzheimer's Association and the American Geriatrics Society. JAMA 278:1363–1371, 1997

Snider WD, Simpson DM, Nielsen S, et al: Neurological complications of acquired immune deficiency syndrome: analysis of 50 patients. Ann Neurol 14:403–418, 1983

Starkstein SE, Fedoroff JP, Price TR, et al: Anosognosia in patients with cerebrovascular lesions: a study of causative factors. Stroke 23:1446–1453, 1992

Starkstein SE, Fedoroff JP, Price TR, et al: Catastrophic reaction after cerebrovascular lesions: frequency, correlates, and validation of a scale. J Neuropsychiatry Clin Neurosci 5:189–194, 1993

Stevens JR, Hermann BP: Temporal lobe epilepsy, psychopathology, and violence: the state of the evidence. Neurology 31:1127–1132, 1981

Strauss I, Keschner M: Mental symptoms in cases of tumor of the frontal lobe. Arch Neurol Psychiatry 33:986–1005, 1935

Sultzer DL, Mahler ME, Mandelkern MA, et al: The relationship between psychiatric symptoms and regional cortical metabolism in Alzheimer's disease. J Neuropsychiatry Clin Neurosci 7:476–484, 1995

Tateno A, Jorge RE, Robinson RG: Clinical correlates of aggressive behavior after traumatic brain injury. J Neuropsychiatry Clin Neurosci 15:155–160, 2003

Treiman DM: Epilepsy and violence: medical and legal issues. Epilepsia 27 (suppl 2):S77–S104, 1986

Virkkunen M, Rissanen A, Naukkarinen H, et al: Energy substrate metabolism among habitually violent alcoholic offenders having antisocial personality disorder. Psychiatry Res 150:287–295, 2007

von Economo C: Encephalitis Lethargica. New York, Oxford University Press, 1931

Wolf AP, Gleckman AD, Cifu DX, et al: The prevalence of agitation and brain injury in skilled nursing facilities: a survey. Brain Inj 10:241–245, 1996

Yudofsky S, Silver JM, Jackson W, et al: The Overt Aggression Scale for the objective rating of verbal and physical aggression. Am J Psychiatry 143:35–39, 1986

CHAPTER 11

Impulsivity and Aggression

Sara T. Wakai, Ph.D.
Robert L. Trestman, Ph.D., M.D.

Aggression is a perplexing phenomenon. It is influenced by many factors (e.g., culture, environment, biology, psychology, neurochemistry) that shape the manner in which it is expressed and perceived. Aggression can have adaptive properties such as self-preservation, protection of one's young, or defense of territory. It is thought to help adolescents develop autonomy, an independent identity, and mastery over their environment (Rome and Itskowitz 1990). In animal models, aggressive behavior has even been demonstrated to serve as a stress management strategy (Williams and Eichelman 1971). Alternatively, aggression can produce destructive behaviors that are directed against others through physical violence or verbal attacks or toward oneself, leading to self-injurious behaviors (SIBs) or suicidality.

Almost every one of us has engaged in an impulsive or aggressive act at some point in our lives, whether it was saying an unkind word we later regretted or making a rash purchase on an extravagant item. Felthous and Barratt (2003) rhetorically posed the question, "Are we not all, mentally disordered or not, capable of acts that are both impulsive and aggressive?" followed by the decisive response "Of course!" (p. 133). They went on to note that the distinguishing feature between pathological and non-pathological behavior is one of severity. Stone (1995) developed a four-zone continuum of aggressive behavior that illustrates this very concept. In Stone's model, severity ranges from culturally sanctioned outbursts of anger and mild aggressive behaviors such as those exhibited on the playing field or at a political rally to severe impulsivity and aggression, which may lead to the commission of felonies.

Theoretical Models of Aggression

Nearly 40 years ago, Moyer (1968) proposed an early and influential classification of seven categories of aggression: 1) fear-induced (aggression associated with fleeing or attacking a perceived threat); 2) maternal (an attack as a means to protect one's young); 3) inter-male (an attack by a male toward another male in the immediate environment as a way to establish dominance or status); 4) irritable (an attack directed toward some source of frustration such as a threat, intimidation, or environmental condition); 5) sex-related (sexual arousal is frequently associated with increased levels of hostility); 6) predatory (an aggressive act aimed at taking down a prey); and 7) territorial (an attack on an intruder who enters into an area claimed by the attacker).

Contemporary definitions refer to *aggression* as "behavior directed by one individual against another individual (or object or self) with the aim of causing harm" (Bond 1992, p. 1). Other researchers have included the notion of intent. For example, Anderson and Bushman (2002) described aggression as behavior that is intended to cause immediate harm to another individual when the intended victim desires to avoid harm. Bjorkvist and Niemela's (1992) definition of aggression not only includes intent to hurt someone or damage something but also adds affective arousal that has the potential to lead to an overtly aggressive act and displays of intimidation.

In the process of developing the Aggression Questionnaire, Buss and Perry (1992) conducted a series of factor analyses resulting in a model with four separate but related categories of aggression. The first category, Overt Physical Aggression, involves a physical attack on another person that results in harm. In Overt Verbal Aggression, an individual uses words to harm another. The third category, Anger, is the emotional element of aggression, described as the "physiological arousal and preparation for aggression" (p. 457). The fourth category, Hostility, is "feelings of ill will and injustice" (p. 457).

The current literature consistently views aggressive behavior as a dichotomous construct. Although the terminology varies greatly, conceptually the two broad classifications result in *premeditated aggression* (also referred to as predatory, instrumental, callous-unemotional, or proactive) and *impulsive aggression* (often called affective, reactive, emotional, hostile, or expressive) (Cornell et al. 1996; Stanford et al. 2003a).

Premeditated aggression is typically purposeful and aimed at obtaining an object such as a reward or advantage for the aggressor (Hartup 1974). These types of behaviors tend to be carried out in a methodical and deliberate fashion, with the aggressor demonstrating limited physiological arousal (Stanford et al. 2003b). Meloy (2000) found that perpetrators often possess a heightened sense of awareness that permits them to effectively stalk their victim, gathering necessary information in preparation for the aggressive act. Studies of incarcerated populations have also demonstrated that premeditated-predatory aggressors are more psychopathic, as measured by the Psychopathy Checklist–Revised (PCL-R), than those classified as impulsive-affective aggressors (Cornell et al. 1996; Woodworth and Porter 2002).

The second prong of the aggression dichotomy is *impulsivity*, which typically is a response to a perceived provocation with immediate and destructive violence. Individuals who display impulsive-affective aggressive behaviors are commonly labeled "unpredictable" and "short fused." Impulsive aggressive behaviors can be carried out involuntarily, in a burst of rage, with no weighing of potential outcomes. Research has found that individuals with impulsivity disorders tend to have lower verbal scores and executive cognitive functioning impairments based on neuropsychological testing (Villemarette-Pittman et al. 2003). It is hypothesized that the limited cognitive resources of impulsive aggressors allow them to become easily overwhelmed by competing stimuli, which leads to feelings of frustration and helplessness. With limited perceived options, the impulsive aggressor frequently acts before thinking about the impact and likely consequences of the behavior (Meloy 2000).

The Etiology of Aggression and Impulsivity

To better understand aggressive and impulsive behaviors, it is helpful to examine the various potential sources and pathways that can contribute to them. These behaviors have multiple causes (e.g., genetics, social learning, environment, mental illness, substance abuse), each with a substantial and valuable body of research. This chapter focuses on prenatal development, early childhood trauma, traumatic brain injury, and neurochemistry as contributors to aggression and impulsivity.

Prenatal Development

Prenatal risk factors such as maternal use of alcohol, tobacco, or cocaine and pregnancy/birth complications have been linked to developmental delays and behavioral problems in children and to antisocial behavior and violent offending in adults (Raine 2002). Exposure to these risk factors may directly or indirectly affect the structure and function of the developing fetal brain, leading to long-term damage to central nervous system neurotransmitter pathways (Ernst et al. 2001). For example, children of mothers who smoked were found to be twice as likely to have a criminal record by age 22 (Räsänen et al. 1999). In addition, 6- or 7-year-old girls who had been exposed to cocaine in utero were significantly more likely to score in the abnormal range on the Aggression subscale of the Child Behavioral Checklist than control subjects (Sood et al. 2005). However, these risk factors are rarely found independent of other psychosocial complications such as poverty, poor parenting skills, and limited access to medical care and educational opportunities.

Childhood Trauma

Childhood trauma has been associated with impulsive and aggressive behaviors, including self-destruction and suicidal behavior in later years (Briere and Runtz 1990). Brodsky et al. (2001) examined 136 adults with major depression and found that participants with a history of physical or sexual abuse were more likely to have made a suicide attempt and had higher levels of impulsivity, aggression, and comorbid borderline personality disorder than participants with no abuse history. The researchers assert that childhood trauma may constitute an environmental risk factor that leads to the development of both suicidality and impulsivity. Similarly, Roy (2005) studied 268 abstinent drug-dependent patients and found a significant positive correlation between impulsivity and risk-taking scores on the Barratt Impulsivity Scale and scores of abuse and neglect on the Childhood Trauma Questionnaire.

Traumatic Brain Injury and Brain Dysfunction

Aggression and impulsivity have been associated with dysfunction in various regions of the brain, most notably the temporal and frontal lobes (Liu and Wuerker 2004). These regions of the brain regulate executive functions, and damage to these regions has been shown to lead to intermittent emotional dyscontrol, an increase in impulsivity, a reduction in self-regulation, and the diminished capacity to consider the outcomes of behaviors (Golden et al. 1996). Violent offenders have been found to have poor functioning in the frontal and temporal regions of the brain as evidenced by neuropsychological tests (Raine 2002), excessive slow-wave electroencephalographic activity (Stoff et al. 1997), and a reduced glucose metabolism in the prefrontal brain region as shown in brain imaging studies (Raine et al. 1997). Grafman et al. (1996) studied Vietnam veterans who had penetrating head injuries and found they had higher verbal aggression scores than control subjects and patients with lesions in other areas of the brain. A study evaluating 89 patients with traumatic brain injury found that those who scored high on the Overt Aggression Scale had a preinjury history of mood disorder, alcohol and drug abuse, and aggressive behaviors (Tateno et al. 2003). These findings indicate that postinjury behavior may be reflective of preexisting impulsive and aggressive tendencies.

Neurochemistry

Neurotransmitters are chemicals that send information between neurons in the brain and help to regulate mood, thinking, and behaviors (Berman and Coccaro 1998). Among the many known neurotransmitters, the most studied in relation to aggression and impulsivity are serotonin, norepinephrine, dopamine, and γ-aminobutyric acid (GABA). The majority of the studies suggest that GABAergic and serotonergic systems inhibit predatory aggression, and the noradrenergic and dopaminergic systems stimulate affective aggression (Eichelman 1988). Low levels of serotonin have been associated with increased rates of aggression, impulsivity, depression, and suicidality. Coccaro (1996) found lower serotonin levels in suicide victims, particularly those who used a violent suicide method, when compared with accident victims. In addition, Coccaro and Kavoussi (1997) examined 40 patients with personality disorders and a history of impulsive aggression and found that fluoxetine, a selective serotonin reuptake inhibitor, reduced scores of aggression and irritability on the Overt Aggression Scale.

The noradrenergic system affects attention to stimuli, arousal levels, and responses to stressors (Berridge and Waterhouse 2003) and is one of the fastest-responding neurochemical systems (Haller et al. 1998). Norepinephrine is involved in the fight-or-flight response and has been linked to aggressive behavior (Haden and Scarpa 2007). In a study measuring aggressive behavior and norepinephrine levels, Gerra et al. (1997) experimentally induced aggression using a free-operant procedure in 15 males with "low normal" and 15 males with "high normal" basal aggressivity (based on scores on the Buss-Durkee Hostility Inventory and other measures). They found no differences between the groups in base rate plasma norepinephrine levels. However, during the task, norepinephrine levels were significantly higher in the high group than the low group. These findings suggest that high-aggressive individuals respond more intensely, and their norepinephrine increases to higher levels when they are presented with frustrating situations, than is the case in low-aggressive individuals.

The remainder of this chapter focuses on formal disorders (i.e., intermittent explosive disorder [IED], pyromania, intellectual disabilities, and autism) and distinct symptoms (i.e., impulsive suicide and SIB) within which aggression or impulsivity are core determinants.

Discussion

Intermittent Explosive Disorder

Case Example 1

> J.W. is a 30-year-old man with a long history of fights and assaultive behavior. He was referred by a judge for anger management classes several years ago. J.W. was walking down the street when he inadvertently bumped into a stranger. The stranger said, "Why don't you watch where you're going!" Infuriated, J.W. turned on the stranger and started pummeling him into unconsciousness. Minutes later, when onlookers pulled him off of his victim, J.W. was upset and remorseful over his behavior.

IED is categorized in DSM-IV-TR (American Psychiatric Association 2000) as an impulse-control disorder not elsewhere classified and is the only diagnosis with recurring acts of aggression as the primary symptom. The inclusion criteria for IED consist of 1) distinct episodes of serious assault against others or destruction of property, 2) behavior that is grossly out of proportion to any precipitating provocation or psychosocial stressor, and 3) explosive episodes that are not better accounted for by another mental disorder, substance use, or a medical condition. As in most of the impulse-control disorders, the individual feels a sense of tension or affective arousal before committing the explosive behavior, may experience pleasure or gratification during the act, and may feel relief or regret after the act.

IED is rare in terms of prevalence, and research has revealed similar rates of lifetime incidence. For example, Coccaro et al. (2004) evaluated 253 participants for the Baltimore Epidemiologic Catchment Area Follow-Up study and found lifetime rates of 4.0%. In a survey of 9,282 U.S. adults, Kessler et al. (2006) found slightly higher rates ranging from 5.4% to 7.3%. IED behaviors typically become apparent in childhood, often in the form of temper tantrums. Explosive outbursts tend to peak during the teen years and to decline after age 30, with only about 7% of new cases occurring after this age (McElroy et al. 1998). Research has found incidents of IED to occur earlier for men (13 years of age) than for women (19 years) (Coccaro et al. 2005).

Impulsivity and Aggression | 217

In a study of 27 individuals who met the criteria for IED, participants described their aggressive impulses as "a need to attack," "an adrenaline rush," "a need to defend oneself," and "an urge to kill" (McElroy et al. 1998). The aggressive episodes were associated with physical or autonomic symptoms such as heart palpitations, chest tightness, head pressure, a loss of awareness, and affective symptoms such as irritability, euphoria, and racing thoughts. The outbursts were often in response to an external stressor (typically a minor disagreement with someone), but many reported that the aggressive episodes were spontaneous. The aggressive episodes occurred approximately nine times per month, and although the duration of a specific episode was relatively brief (22 minutes), the outcomes had devastating repercussions resulting in destruction of property, serious assault on another person, assault with a weapon, attempted homicide, and homicide. Not surprisingly, individuals with IED have difficulties in maintaining employment, financial stability, and meaningful relationships.

The usefulness of classifying IED as a separate diagnosis has come under criticism because aggressive impulses occur in a wide range of psychiatric and medical disorders (Coccaro 2003). McElroy et al. (1998) found a high comorbidity rate among IED patients and mood disorder, anxiety disorders, and other impulse-control disorders. Coccaro et al. (2005) found a substantial amount of lifetime comorbidity among IED patients with mood disorders, anxiety disorders, and alcohol/drug disorders. Nearly a quarter of the patients in a study conducted by Lejoyeux et al. (1999) who met the criteria for alcohol dependence also met the criteria for IED.

Some researchers have raised concerns about the value of the criteria for IED, noting several limitations and ambiguities. For example, Coccaro (2003) pointed out that DSM-IV-TR does not set parameters for the frequency of the aggressive acts, the time span between episodes, or the severity of the outbursts. In addition, it is difficult to determine whether an aggressive outburst is more likely to be caused by another personality disorder, such as antisocial personality disorder. The current definition may be underestimating the number of individuals with IED by excluding individuals with frequent but less severe aggressive actions.

Pyromania

Case Example 2

R.J. is 23 years old and has had a fascination with fires since early childhood. In the past he has set many small, contained fires and enjoyed watching the resultant blazes. Tonight, he is sitting in his room fondling a book of matches. At his ease, he happily remembers the tension and excitement he felt when he set fire to an abandoned garage the previous night.

Pyromania is designated as an impulse-control disorder not elsewhere classified in DSM-IV-TR, along with IED, kleptomania, pathological gambling, trichotillomania, and impulse-control disorder not otherwise specified. The diagnosis itself has an unstable history in DSM: it was included in DSM-I (American Psychiatric Association 1952) as an obsessive-compulsive reaction; omitted from DSM-II (American Psychiatric Association 1968); and reinstated in DSM-III (American Psychiatric Association 1980) as a distinct disorder of impulse control. In DSM-IV-TR it is defined as repeated, deliberate, and purposeful fire setting and is associated with tension before the act; fascination with fire; and gratification when setting, witnessing, or putting out fires. The fire setting is not committed for monetary gain, revenge, as an expression of sociopolitical ideology, to conceal a criminal act, to express anger or vengeance, to improve one's living circumstances, in response to a delusion or hallucination, or as a result of impaired judgment. Finally, the impulse to set fires cannot be better accounted for by another diagnosis.

True pyromania is rare. Rasanen et al. (1995) studied arson defendants in Finland from 1975 to 1993 and found only 4% of their sample to have pyromania. Ritchie and Huff (1999) examined the mental health records and/or prison files of 283 arsonists, and pyromania was diagnosed in only three cases (1.3%). A slightly higher rate was identified in a study conducted by Repo et al. (1997) between 1978 and 1991 in which 14.2% of 304 male Finnish arsonists were diagnosed with pyromania. The low rates of pyromania found in these fairly recent studies calls into question the substantial number of arsonists who were diagnosed with pyromania (39%) in Lewis and Yarnell's (1951) classic work of nearly 1,500 pathological fire setters. The later results almost certainly reflect the changes in diagnostic criteria, which have become more structured and narrowly defined in the intervening decades.

Several risk factors associated with pyromania are consistently found in the literature. Barker (1994) found men to be much more likely than women to have a fascination with fire, and Kafry (1980) found boys to be more interested than girls in fire setting. Large percentages of pathological fire setters are unemployed and live alone (Ritchie and Huff 1999). Lejoyeux et al. (2006) described people with pyromania as individuals with a keen interest in fires who like watching fires and setting off false fire alarms. Their fascination with fires often leads them to seek employment as firefighters. In a study by Lindberg et al. (2005) of

90 arson recidivists, three were diagnosed with pyromania. All three of these arsonists worked as volunteer firefighters.

There is a consistent link reported between fire setting and mental illness. Ritchie and Huff (1999) found that nearly all (90%) of the subjects in their study had a history of mental health issues; 36% of these individuals also had a diagnosis of either schizophrenia or bipolar disorder. Two-thirds of the sample (64%) were abusing alcohol or drugs at the time of the fire setting, and the fire-setting act of half of the sample was judged "very impulsive" by the researchers. In a 5-year study conducted by Leong and Silva (1999) of court-ordered outpatient forensic psychiatric evaluation of individuals charged with arson, nearly half (43.8%) were diagnosed as psychotic, 15.6% as mentally retarded, and 15.6% with alcohol abuse.

Aggressive Behavior in Individuals With Intellectual Disabilities

Case Example 3

W.P. is a 35-year-old woman with moderate intellectual disability deriving from fetal alcohol syndrome. She was recently placed in a group home after the death of her parents several months ago. She has never needed psychiatric care in the past. She does well at her job placement until it is time to leave. At that point, on a fairly consistent basis over the past few weeks, this normally pleasant woman hits anyone who attempts to persuade her to board her minivan for the ride back to her group home.

In contrast to the aforementioned disorders, the following discussion of impulsivity and aggression occurs in the context of other disorders where sudden, unpredictable, and violent behavior may occur. *Intellectual disability* has been defined as "significantly subaverage intellectual functioning resulting in or associated with a concurrent impairment in adaptive behaviour" (Strongman 1985, p. 202). Holland et al. (2002) defined it as significantly impaired intellectual ability and significantly impaired social functioning, with these conditions present from childhood. DSM-IV-TR uses the term *mental retardation* and has three inclusion criteria: a score of 70 or below on an individually administered IQ test, deficits in two adaptive functioning areas (i.e., communication, self-care, home living, social/interpersonal skills, use of community resources, self-direction, functional academic skills, work, leisure, health, and safety), and the onset of the impairment occurring before the age of 18 years.

Aggressive behavior can have a severe negative impact on individuals with intellectual disabilities and their caregivers. Aggression often becomes a barrier to less-restrictive residential options, educational opportunities, competitive employment, and general social acceptability (Bruininks et al. 1994). In addition, aggressive behavior in individuals with intellectual disability is also associated with greater service costs, higher staff turnover rates (Sigafoos et al. 1994), more frequent referrals to mental health professionals (Maguire and Piersel 1992), increased risk for victimization (Rusch et al. 1986), and criminal activity (Crocker and Hodgins 1997). Aggressive behavior may contribute to these individuals being admitted to institutions and being prescribed antipsychotic and behavior control medication (Aman et al. 1987).

The concept of aggressive behavior in individuals with intellectual disability is very broad, and a consistent definition is lacking. McClintock et al. (2003) conducted a meta-analysis of research on aggressive behavior in these individuals, reviewing 86 articles from 1968 to 1997. The researchers found a wide range of terms used to describe aggressive behavior, including physical aggression, threatening others, SIB, destruction of property, and hitting. Deb et al. (2001) considered aggressive behavior to encompass "aggression, destructiveness, self-injurious behavior, temper tantrum, over-activity, screaming/shouting, scattering objects around, wandering, night-time disturbance, objectionable personal habits, antisocial behavior, sexual delinquency, and attention-seeking behaviors" (p. 507). A possible explanation for the variation in describing aggressive behavior is that the descriptions are often based on the perception of caregivers who must manage or endure the behaviors and may be influenced by their coping ability. In addition, the labeling of aggressive behavior may be dependent on the environment. In other words, some behavior may be tolerated in an institutional setting but not in a family setting.

Prevalence rates of aggressive behavior for individuals with intellectual disabilities vary from 2% to 60% based on a variety of factors, such as level of behavioral severity, age, gender, and type of residential environment (Davidson et al. 1994). Males with intellectual disabilities tend to have higher rates of aggressive behavior than females (Harris 1993), and aggressive behavior tends to peak around adolescence (Davidson et al. 1994). Acts of aggression tend to increase with the severity of disability (Davidson et al. 1994); however, higher-functioning individuals tend to act aggressively toward others and lower-functioning individuals tend to engage in SIB (Emerson et al. 1997). Acts of aggression were higher in institutional settings (38%) than in community settings (11%) according to a survey of service providers (Harris 1993).

Notably, deinstitutionalization has not been found to reduce an individual's aggressive behavior (Larson and Lakin 1989).

Individuals with an intellectual disability often have skill deficits in a variety of areas (e.g., attention span, impulse control, memory, neurological functioning, communication skills, and social skills), which may increase the probability of aggression (Allen 2000). For example, in a study measuring the ability of aggressive and nonaggressive individuals with intellectual disabilities to label facial expressions, aggressive individuals were more likely than their nonaggressive peers to mislabel "angry" and "sad" facial expressions, and to label "anger" when they were unsure (Walz and Benson 1996).

Aggressive Behavior in Individuals With Autism

Case Example 4

> M.R. is 28 years old and has been in psychiatric care throughout his life. He is currently on a trial of a new anticonvulsant. He sits quietly rocking back and forth, chewing on his already bleeding left wrist. When Jim, his caregiver, attempts to intervene, this startles him. M.R. then furiously swings his arms, hitting Jim repeatedly.

The term *autism,* derived from the Greek word for "self," was coined by Leo Kanner (1943), a child psychiatrist, to describe the extreme aloneness he viewed as the central trait of the disorder. Autism spectrum disorder (ASD), as it is now called, is currently recognized as a neurodevelopmental disorder (Aicardi 1998). According to DSM-IV-TR, to be diagnosed with autistic disorder an individual must exhibit 6 or more of the 12 identified behaviors, with at least two from the social interaction domain and one each from the communication, repetitive, and stereotyped patterns domains. In addition, delays in social interaction, language, or symbolic or imaginative play must be evident before the age of 3 years.

Prevalence rates of ASD range from 0.7 to 72.6 per 10,000, depending on the diagnostic criteria used in the studies (Williams et al. 2006). Fombonne (1999) reviewed 23 studies on autism and found that prevalence rates significantly increased with publication year, indicating improved diagnostic criteria and methods along with greater availability of services. For example, Croen and Grether (2003) found that 75% of individuals with autism had some level of intellectual disability and proposed that the increase in the prevalence of autism may be attributable to the reclassification of some individuals' diagnoses from intellectual disability to autism. Fombonne (2003) also found a higher rate of boys than girls being affected; intellectual disabilities in about two-thirds of the sample; and a relatively high rate of epilepsy.

Aggression is a common behavioral characteristic of autism and may include impulsivity, aggression toward others, SIB, destruction of property, disruption to the environment, stereotypy, and other socially unacceptable behaviors (McDougle et al. 2003). Although the inappropriate or aggressive behavior may be objectionable, the intention of the behavior is not necessarily malicious (Dewey 1991). The impairments in brain functioning and neurological activity commonly found in autism may reduce one's capacity for social interaction, verbal and nonverbal communication, and the ability to alter behavior and emotional states in response to another's action or perceived feelings. For example, Williams et al. (2005) compared the memories of non–intellectually disabled adults with autism and a control group. The participants with autism did not demonstrate any deficits in word pairs, stores, or verbal working memory. However, on tests measuring immediate and delayed recall of faces and family scenes, there was significant impairment. The research suggests that a lack of social connectiveness and empathy may predispose individuals with autism toward acts of aggression (Rogers et al. 2006).

Impulsive Suicide

Case Example 5

After 65 years of life, K.T. has coped with several serious illnesses and repeated bouts of depression. He has been treated by a psychiatrist for the past few years, with only modest symptomatic improvement. The past 3 months have been filled with unremitting depression. K.T. feels hopeless and has intermittently considered ending his life. The three drinks he just had seem to make the decision easier. He hits the car's accelerator and aims head on for the gap in the guard rail, with the river 100 feet below.

Suicide ranks among the top 10 causes of death for individuals in all age groups in several Western countries (World Health Organization 2006). *Suicide attempts* have been defined as "potentially self-injurious behavior with a nonfatal outcome, for which there is evidence (either implicit or explicit) that the person intended at some (nonzero) level to kill himself/herself" (O'Carroll et al. 1996, p. 247). Terms such as *parasuicide, deliberate self-harm,* and *suicidal gestures* are considered SIBs that may have the appearance of a suicide attempt but may not have the associated intention of ending one's life. Using data from the National Comorbidity Survey of 5,877 respondents, Nock and Kessler (2006) found

Impulsivity and Aggression | 223

4.6% of the sample had made a suicide attempt, 2.7% reported doing so with the intent to die, and 1.9% committed the act as a way to communicate distress to others with no intent to die.

To date, a prior suicide attempt is among the best predictors of eventual death by suicide (Goldstein et al. 1991). In a 5-year follow-up of 1,573 suicide attempters, Nordstrom et al. (1995) found the risk of recurrent suicidal behavior to be 11% for attempted suicide and 6% for ultimately completed suicide. Rates were highest among young men. Johnsson-Fridell et al. (1996) reported a 13% suicide completion rate among inpatients within 5 years of attempted suicide. In a study examining lifetime history of suicide attempts and methods of 1,397 suicides in Finland, Isometsä and Lonnqvist (1998) found that 56% of fatal suicides occurred on the first attempt (62% of males and 38% of females), and the risk of suicide completion was highest during the first year after a suicide attempt. With such high fatality figures, particularly for men, using previous suicide attempt as a predictor of suicide completion has limited preventive value.

Risk factors associated with suicidal behavior include male gender, fewer years of education, being young, and residence in the southern or western regions of the United States (Nock and Kessler 2006). Based on psychological autopsies, a 6-month prevalence rate of an Axis I diagnosis has been found in 88% of suicide completers (Lesage et al. 1994). Specifically, depressive (major depressive episode and mania), impulsive (drug abuse and dependence), and aggressive (conduct disorder and antisocial personality disorder) behaviors and psychiatric comorbidity increase the risk of suicide attempts (Nock and Kessler 2006), with major depression being the most common psychiatric disorder associated with suicide and attempted suicide (Henriksson et al. 1993). Childhood trauma has been associated with self-destruction and suicidal behavior in later years (Briere and Runtz 1990) and contributes to a younger age of onset of suicidal behaviors, often beginning in childhood or adolescence (Brodsky et al. 2001).

Impulsivity has been conceptualized as action without planning or reflection; it differs from premeditated behavior by having a short response time, lack of reflection, and a dissociation between action and consequence (Barratt et al. 1999). Impulsivity, along with other disinhibiting moderators such as substance use or significant current distress, is strongly associated with self-destructive behaviors, including suicidal behavior (Dumais et al. 2005). *Impulsive suicidal behavior* has been defined as a suicide attempt with less than 5 minutes of premeditation (Simon et al. 2001). Using this definition of impulsive suicidality, prevalence rates range from 24% for nearly lethal suicide attempts by individuals 13–34 years old (Simon et al. 2001) to 40% for hospital patients treated for self-injury (Williams et al. 1980).

Individuals who engage in impulsive suicidal behavior tend to use more violent methods, such as firearms, hanging, cutting, and jumping (Simon et al. 2001), than their nonimpulsive counterparts. At the same time, impulsive suicide attempters have lower expectations of dying from their actions (Swann et al. 2005). Despite the impulsive attempters' lower expectations of dying than nonimpulsive attempters, the destructive outcomes are comparable in terms of severity of injuries, reversibility of condition, and admission into intensive care (Simon et al. 2001). The incongruous thought process involved in these attempts is consistent with a defining construct of impulsivity: the disconnect between action and intention (Swann et al. 2005).

Impulsivity does not appear to increase the risk of suicide independently. Simon et al. (2001) suggested that suicidal behavior may be associated with the inability to control aggression-related impulsive behavior rather than with impulsivity in general. For example, the researchers examined indicators of impulsive behavior such as prior arrests, quitting a job without a source of income, having multiple sex partners, and alcohol use within 3 hours of the suicide attempt and found no relationship to impulsive suicidal behavior. However, being in a physical fight in the past year was associated with impulsive suicide attempts. Zouk et al. (2006) examined the psychiatric records of 164 suicide cases using the Barratt Impulsivity Scale. Individuals who scored 75 or higher (which was the 70th percentile for the group) were labeled impulsive and scored significantly higher on the Buss-Durkee Hostility Inventory than their nonimpulsive peers (defined by a score equal to or below the 30th percentile on the Barratt scale), suggesting that aggression is a serious risk factor for impulsive suicidal behavior. Dumais et al. (2005) found impulsive and aggressive behaviors to be associated with suicidality in 104 males diagnosed with major depression. However, they asserted that the relation of aggressive and impulsive behaviors and suicide may be better explained by Cluster B personality disorder and alcohol/drug abuse.

Self-Injurious Behaviors

Case Example 6

B.D. has been in psychiatric care for a decade. Her problems have included an eating disorder, emotional instability, intense unstable relationships, and SIBs. Finding a space on her inner thigh not already scarred, the 25-year-old cuts herself. As she watches the blood flow, the intense roiling emotions she had felt moments before give way to a sense of relaxation and peace.

SIB involves deliberate and often repetitive harm to one's own body without suicidal intent (Favazza 1998). A typical pattern for SIB begins with an overwhelming psychological distress such as anger, anxiety, tension, fear, or a sense of loss. An individual often responds to the overwhelming emotion by isolating and dissociating. In carrying out SIB, there is an absence of suicidal intent and often a lack of pain. The precipitating tension is relieved by the SIB, and individuals report feeling a sense of calm, often followed by disgust and/or guilt (Suyemoto 1998).

SIBs can be very diverse in terms of specific behaviors, severity, and frequency. Simeon and Favazza (2001) proposed four classifications of SIBs—major, stereotypic, compulsive, and impulsive—as a way to help understand and treat the disorder. *Major* SIBs tend to be severe, potentially lethal, and irreversible, such as castration, eye enucleation, and amputation of extremities. This category of SIB is relatively rare and is associated with schizophrenia, intoxication, neurological conditions, bipolar disorder, and severe personality disorders. The impetus for major SIB is often associated with sin, religious delusions, sexual temptation, punishment, and salvation (DeMuth et al. 1983). *Stereotypic* SIBs tend to be repetitive and lack symbolism or affect. The behaviors can be occasional or chronic, such as head banging, eyeball pressing, and finger biting (Favazza and Simeon 1995). These types of SIBs are common in individuals with mental retardation (Griffin et al. 1986), autism (Christie et al. 1982), and Tourette's syndrome (Robertson et al. 1989). *Compulsive* SIBs are ritualistic and repetitive behaviors such as trichotillomania, nail biting, skin picking, and skin scratching (Simeon 2006). Individuals with this type of behavior often report that the behaviors occur unintentionally. The behaviors are typically associated with mounting anxiety followed by relief. *Impulsive* SIBs include skin cutting, skin burning, poisoning, and self-hitting. These behaviors tend to provide short-term relief from unbearable psychological states (Simeon 2006).

The prevalence of any SIB in the general public has been estimated to be 4% (Briere and Gil 1998). However, prevalence rates vary greatly based on selected populations. For example, in a study of 15- and 16-year-old students in England, researchers (Hawton et al. 2002) found that 6.9% of their sample had engaged in at least one act of deliberate self-harm in the previous year. The primary method of harm was cutting (two-thirds) and poisoning (less than one-third). Multiple acts of

SIB were reported by about half of those acknowledging SIB. Matsumoto et al. (2005) studied 201 adolescents in a juvenile detention center in Japan and found 16.4% had cut their wrists or forearms at least once, and 28.4% had burned themselves at least once. This was found to be significantly higher than the incidence among Japanese university students, where the overall rate was 3.3% (males 3.1% and females 3.5%; Yamaguchi et al. 2004). Prevalence rates for U.S. college students have ranged from 12% (Favazza et al. 1989) to 17% (Whitlock et al. 2006). In a study of male prisoners, Shea (1993) found prevalence rates of 6.5%–25%. SIB in adult psychiatric populations can range from 4% (Darche 1990) to 20% (Langbehn and Pfohl 1993). In adolescent inpatients the prevalence rate can range from 40% (Darche 1990) to 61% (DiClemente et al. 1991). SIB may occur in up to 60% of individuals with Tourette's syndrome (Eisenhauer and Woody 1987). The differences in prevalence rates may be attributed to the various definitions of SIB, different study populations, and the reporting mechanisms for SIB.

SIB can serve multiple functions simultaneously. Paris (2005) identified five psychological functions of SIB: 1) relief from negative mood states; 2) distraction, encouraging the individual to refocus attention from psychological pain to physical pain; 3) communication of distress, as the behaviors come to the attention of significant others or therapists; 4) expression of emotions such as guilt or anger; and 5) dissociation from the current state while engaging in SIB.

SIB has been associated with psychological disorders such as borderline personality disorder (Paris 2005), antisocial behavior (Suyemoto 1998), and eating disorders (Paul et al. 2002). Other indicators of SIB include depression, anxiety, impulsivity, and low self-esteem (Herpertz et al. 1997). In a study of adolescent students in England, researchers (Hawton et al. 2002) found that SIB was more common in females than in males, and the presence of SIB increased with greater consumption of cigarettes, alcohol, and drugs. SIB has been associated with childhood adversities such as physical abuse, sexual abuse, and parental neglect. It is also related to environmental factors such as being bullied, having a family member who had attempted suicide, and knowing a peer who had engaged in SIB. Individuals who engage in SIB have also been found to have impulsive behavioral traits (Simeon et al. 1992). For example, individuals who carried out SIB had fewer future-oriented problem-solving abilities and were more likely to be involved with other impulsive behaviors such as suicide attempts, substance abuse, bingeing, and promiscuity (Herpertz et al. 1997).

Key Points

- Impulsivity and aggression may be useful or destructive behaviors, depending on the context. They are characteristic of a range of disorders and of symptoms of mental illness that may result in significant functional impairment, morbidity, and mortality.
- Intermittent explosive disorder (IED), an impulse-control disorder, is the only DSM-IV-TR diagnosis with recurrent aggressive acts as the primary symptom. People with IED describe "a need to attack," "an adrenaline rush," "a need to defend oneself," and "an urge to kill." Episodes may be infrequent and brief but can have devastating results such as destruction of property, serious assault, or even homicide. People with IED have difficulties maintaining employment, financial stability, and meaningful relationships.
- Pyromania is the repeated failure to resist the impulse to set motiveless fires. Risk factors associated with pyromania are male gender, unemployment, living alone, and a keen interest in fires.
- For people with intellectual disabilities, aggressive behavior can have a severe negative impact on residential, education, and employment opportunities. Acts of aggression tend to increase with severity of disability, but higher-functioning individuals tend to act aggressively toward others and lower-functioning individuals to engage in self-injurious behavior (SIB). Skill deficits in attention span, impulse control, memory, neurological functioning, communication skills, and social skills may be present and may increase the probability of aggression.
- In individuals with autism, aggression is common and may include impulsivity, aggression toward others, SIB, destruction of property, disruptiveness, stereotypy, and other socially unacceptable behaviors, not necessarily with malicious intent. Impairments commonly found in autism may reduce the capacity for social interaction, communication, and ability to alter behavior and emotional states in response to another's action or perceived feelings.
- Suicide is a major public health concern and is a leading cause of death in several Western countries. A prior suicide attempt is one of the best predictors for eventual death by suicide; however, the preventive value of this is limited because more than half of fatal suicides occur on the first attempt. Those who engage in impulsive suicide (with less than 5 minutes of premeditation) use more violent methods, have lower expectations of dying from their actions, and have comparable destructive outcomes to their non-impulsive counterparts.

- Self-injurious behavior is deliberate, repetitive harm (e.g., cutting, burning, poisoning) to one's own body without suicidal intent. A typical pattern for SIB is an initial overwhelming distress with subsequent emotional dissociation; a lack of pain while carrying out the SIB; and relief of tension, possibly followed by a sense of guilt. SIB can serve psychological functions, such as relief from negative mood states, distraction, communication of distress, expression of emotions, and dissociation from one's current psychological state.

References

Aicardi J: Diseases of the Nervous System in Children, 2nd Edition. Cambridge, England, Cambridge University Press, 1998

Allen D: Recent research on physical aggression in persons with intellectual disability: an overview. J Intellect Dev Disabil 25:41–57, 2000

Aman MG, Richmond G, Stewart AW, et al: The Aberrant Behavior Checklist: factor structure and the effect of subject variables in American and New Zealand facilities. Am J Ment Defic 91:570–578, 1987

American Psychiatric Association: Diagnostic and Statistical Manual: Mental Disorders. Washington, DC, American Psychiatric Association, 1952

American Psychiatric Association: Diagnostic and Statistical Manual of Mental Disorders, 2nd Edition. Washington, DC, American Psychiatric Association, 1968

American Psychiatric Association: Diagnostic and Statistical Manual of Mental Disorders, 3rd Edition. Washington, DC, American Psychiatric Association, 1980

American Psychiatric Association: Diagnostic and Statistical Manual of Mental Disorders, 4th Edition, Text Revision. Washington, DC, American Psychiatric Association, 2000

Anderson CA, Bushman BJ: Human aggression. Annu Rev Psychol 53:27–51, 2002

Barker AF: Arson: A Review of the Psychiatric Literature. Oxford, UK, Oxford University Press, 1994

Barratt ES, Stanford MS, Dowdy L, et al: Impulsive and premeditated aggression: a factor analysis of self-reported acts. Psychiatry Res 86:163–173, 1999

Berman ME, Coccaro EF: Neurobiologic correlates of violence: relevance to criminal responsibility. Behav Sci Law 16:303–318, 1998

Berridge CW, Waterhouse BD: The locus coeruleus-noradrenergic system: modulation of behavioral state and state-dependent cognitive processes. Brain Res Rev 42:33–84, 2003

Bjorkvist K, Niemela P: Of Mice and Women: Aspects of Female Aggression. New York, Academic Press, 1992

Bond AJ: Pharmacological manipulation of aggressiveness and impulsiveness in healthy volunteers. Prog Neuropsychopharmacol Biol Psychiatry 16:1–7, 1992

Briere J, Gil E: Self-mutilation in clinical and general population samples: prevalence, correlates, and functions. Am J Orthopsychiatry 68:609–620, 1998

Briere J, Runtz M: Differential adult symptomatology associated with three types of child abuse histories. Child Abuse Negl 14:357–364, 1990

Brodsky BS, Oquendo M, Ellis SP, et al: The relationship of childhood abuse to impulsivity and suicide behavior in adults with major depression. Am J Psychiatry 158:1871–1877, 2001

Bruininks RH, Olson KM, Larson SA, et al: Challenging behaviors among persons with mental retardation in residential settings, in Destructive Behavior in Developmental Disabilities: Diagnosis and Treatment. Edited by Thompson TE, Gray DBE. Thousand Oaks, CA, Sage, 1994, pp 24–48

Buss A, Perry M: The Aggression Questionnaire. J Pers Soc Psychol 63:452–459, 1992

Christie R, Bay C, Kaufman IA, et al: Lesch-Nyan disease: clinical experience with nineteen patients. Dev Med Child Neurol 24:293–306, 1982

Coccaro EF: Neurotransmitter correlates of impulsive aggression in humans. Ann NY Acad Sci 794:82–89, 1996

Coccaro EF: Intermittent explosive disorder, in Aggression: Psychiatric Assessment and Treatment. Edited by Coccaro EF. New York, Marcel Dekker, 2003, pp 149–199

Coccaro EF, Kavoussi RJ: Fluoxetine and impulsive aggressive behavior in personality disorder subjects. Arch Gen Psychiatry 54:1081–1088, 1997

Coccaro EF, Schmidt CA, Samuels JF, et al: Lifetime and 1-month prevalence rates of intermittent explosive disorder in a community sample. J Clin Psychiatry 65:820–824, 2004

Coccaro EF, Posternak MA, Zimmerman M: Prevalence and features of intermittent explosive disorder in a clinical setting. J Clin Psychiatry 66:1221–1227, 2005

Cornell DG, Warren J, Hawk G, et al: Psychopathy in instrumental and reactive violent offenders. J Consult Clin Psychol 64:783–790, 1996

Crocker AG, Hodgins S: The criminality of noninstitutionalized mentally retarded persons: evidence from a birth cohort followed to age 30. Crim Justice Behav 24:432–454, 1997

Croen LA, Grether JK: Response: a response to Blaxill, Baskin, and Spitzer on Croen et al. (2002). The changing prevalence of autism in California. J Autism Dev Disord 33:227–229, 2003

Darche MA: Psychological factors differentiating self-mutilating and non-self-mutilating adolescent inpatient females. Psychiatr Hosp 21:31–35, 1990

Davidson PW, Cain NN, Sloane-Reeves JE, et al: Characteristics of community-based individuals with intellectual disability and aggressive behavioral disorders. Am J Ment Retard 98:704–716, 1994

Deb S, Thomas M, Bright C: Mental disorder in adults with intellectual disability, 2: the rate of behaviour disorders among a community-based population aged between 16 and 64 years. J Intellect Disabil Res 45:506–514, 2001

DeMuth GW, Strain J, Lombardo-Maher A: Self-amputation and restitution. Gen Hosp Psychiatry 5:25–30, 1983

Dewey M: Living with Asperger's syndrome, in Autism and Asperger Syndrome. Edited by Frith U. Cambridge, UK, Cambridge University Press, 1991, pp 184–206

DiClemente RJ, Ponton LE, Hartley D: Prevalence and correlates of cutting behavior: risk for HIV transmission. J Am Acad Child Adolesc Psychiatry 30:735–739, 1991

Dumais A, Lesage AD, Alda M, et al: Risk factors for suicide completion in major depression: a case-control study of impulsive and aggressive behaviors in men. Am J Psychiatry 162:2116–2124, 2005

Eichelman B: Toward a rational pharmacotherapy for aggressive and violent behavior. Hosp Community Psychiatry 39:31–39, 1988

Eisenhauer GL, Woody RC: Self-mutilation and Tourette's disorder. J Child Neurol 2:265–267, 1987

Emerson E, Alborz A, Reeves D, et al: The HARC Challenging Behaviour Project, Report 2: The Prevalence of Challenging Behaviour. Manchester, England, Hester Adrian Research Centre, University of Manchester, 1997

Ernst M, Moolchan ET, Robinson ML: Behavioral and neural consequences of prenatal exposure to nicotine. J Am Acad Child Adolesc Psychiatry 40:630–641, 2001

Favazza AR: The coming of age of self-mutilation. J Nerv Ment Dis 186:259–268, 1998

Favazza A, Simeon D: Self-mutilation, in Impulsivity and Aggression. Edited by Hollander E, Simeon D. New York, Wiley, 1995, pp 185–200

Favazza AR, DeRosear L, Conterio K: Self-mutilation and eating disorders. Suicide Life Threat Behav 19:352–361, 1989

Felthous AR, Barratt ES: Impulsive aggression, in Aggression: Psychiatric Assessment and Treatment. Edited by Coccaro EF. New York, Marcel Dekker, 2003, pp 123–148

Fombonne E: The epidemiology of autism: a review. Psychol Med 29:769–786, 1999

Fombonne E: The prevalence of autism. JAMA 289:87–89, 2003

Gerra G, Zaimovic A, Avanzini P, et al: Neurotransmitter-neuroendocrine responses to experimentally induced aggression in humans: influence of personality variable. Psychiatry Res 66:33–43, 1997

Golden CJ, Jackson ML, Peterson-Rohne A, et al: Neuropsychological correlates of violence and aggression: a review of the clinical literature. Aggression and Violent Behavior 1:3–25, 1996

Goldstein RB, Black DW, Nasrallah A, et al: The prediction of suicide: sensitivity, specificity, and predictive value of a multivariate model applied to suicide among 1906 patients with affective disorders. Arch Gen Psychiatry 48:418–422, 1991

Grafman J, Schwab K, Warden D, et al: Frontal lobe injuries, violence, and aggression: a report of the Vietnam Head Injury Study. Neurology 46:1231–1238, 1996

Griffin JC, Williams DE, Stark MT, et al: Self-injurious behavior: a state-wide prevalence survey of the extent and circumstances. Appl Res Ment Retard 7:105–116, 1986

Haden SC, Scarpa A: The noradrenergic system and its involvement in aggressive behaviors. Aggression and Violent Behavior 12:1–15, 2007

Haller J, Makara GB, Kruk MR: Catecholaminergic involvement in the control of aggression: hormones, the peripheral sympathetic and central noradrenergic systems. Neurosci Biobehav Rev 22:85–97, 1998

Harris P: The nature and extent of aggressive behaviour amongst people with learning difficulties (mental handicap) in a single health district. J Intellect Disabil Res 37 (pt 3):221–242, 1993

Hartup WW: Aggression in childhood: developmental perspectives. Am Psychol 29:336–341, 1974
Hawton K, Rodham K, Evans E, et al: Deliberate self harm in adolescents: self report survey in schools in England. BMJ 325:1207–1211, 2002
Henriksson MM, Aro HM, Marttunen MJ, et al: Mental disorders and comorbidity in suicide. Am J Psychiatry 150:935–940, 1993
Herpertz S, Sass H, Favazza A: Impulsivity in self-mutilation behavior: psychometric and biological findings. J Psychiatry Res 31:451–465, 1997
Holland T, Clare IC, Mukhopadhyay T: Prevalence of criminal offending by men and women with intellectual disability and the characteristics of offenders: implications for research and service development. J Intellect Disabil Res 46 (suppl 1):6–20, 2002
Isometsä ET, Lonnqvist JK: Suicide attempts preceding completed suicide. Br J Psychiatry 173:531–535, 1998
Johnsson Fridell E, Ojehagen A, Träskman-Bendz L: A 5-year follow-up study of suicide attempts. Acta Psychiatr Scand 93:151–157, 1996
Kafry D: Playing with matches: children and fires, in Fires and Human Behavior. Edited by Canter D. Chichester, UK, Wiley, 1980, pp 47–62
Kanner L: Autistic disturbances of affective contact. Nerv Child 2:217–250, 1943
Kessler RC, Coccaro EF, Fava M, et al: The prevalence and correlates of DSM-IV intermittent explosive disorder in the National Comorbidity Survey replication. Arch Gen Psychiatry 63:669–678, 2006
Langbehn DR, Pfohl B: Clinical correlates of self-mutilation among psychiatric inpatients. Ann Clin Psychiatry 5:45–51, 1993
Larson SA, Lakin KC: Deinstitutionalization of persons with mental retardation: behavioral outcomes. J Assoc Pers Sev Handicaps 14:324–332, 1989
Lejoyeux M, Feuché N, Loi S, et al: Study of impulse-control disorders among alcohol-dependent patients. J Clin Psychiatry 60:302–305, 1999
Lejoyeux M, McLoughlin M, Ades J: Pyromania, in Clinical Manual of Impulse-Control Disorders. Edited by Hollander E, Stein DJ. Washington, DC, American Psychiatric Publishing, 2006, pp 229–250
Leong GB, Silva JA: Revisiting arson from an outpatient forensic perspective. J Forensic Sci 44:558–563, 1999
Lesage AD, Boyer R, Grunberg F, et al: Suicide and mental disorders: a case-control study of young men. Am J Psychiatry 151:1063–1068, 1994
Lewis ND, Yarnell H: Pathological firesetting (pyromania). Nervous and Mental Disease Monographs no 82, 1951
Lindberg N, Holi MM, Tani P, et al: Looking for pyromania: characteristics of a consecutive sample of Finnish male criminals with histories of recidivist fire-setting between 1973 and 1993. BMC Psychiatry 5:47, 2005
Liu J, Wuerker A: Biosocial bases of aggressive and violent behavior: implications for nursing studies. Int J Nurs Stud 42:229–241, 2004
Maguire KB, Piersel WC: Specialized treatment for behavior problems of institutionalized persons with mental retardation. Ment Retard 30:227–232, 1992
Matsumoto T, Yamaguchi A, Chiba Y, et al: Self-burning versus self-cutting: patterns and implications of self-mutilation. A preliminary study of differences between self-cutting and self-burning in a Japanese juvenile detention center. Psychiatry Clin Neurosci 59:62–69, 2005

McClintock K, Hall S, Oliver C: Risk markers associated with challenging behaviours in people with intellectual disabilities: a meta-analytic study. J Intellect Disabil Res 47:405–416, 2003

McDougle CJ, Stigler KA, Posey DJ: Treatment of aggression in children and adolescents with autism and conduct disorder. J Clin Psychiatry 64(suppl):16–25, 2003

McElroy SL, Soutullo CA, Beckman DA, et al: DSM-IV intermittent explosive disorder: a report of 27 cases. J Clin Psychiatry 59:203–212, 1998

Meloy JR: Violence Risk and Threat Assessment: A Practical Guide for Mental Health and Criminal Justice Professionals. San Diego, CA, Specialized Training Services, 2000

Moyer KE: Kinds of aggression and their physiological basis. Commun Behav Biol 2:65–87, 1968

Nock MK, Kessler RC: Prevalence of and risk factors for suicide attempts versus suicide gestures: analysis of the National Comorbidity Survey. J Abnorm Psychol 115:616–623, 2006

Nordström P, Samuelsson M, Asberg M: Survival analysis of suicide risk after attempted suicide. Acta Psychiatr Scand 91:336–340, 1995

O'Carroll PW, Berman AL, Maris RW, et al: Beyond the Tower of Babel: a nomenclature for suicidology. Suicide Life Threat Behav 26:237–252, 1996

Paris J: Understanding self-mutilation in borderline personality disorder. Harv Rev Psychiatry 13:179–185, 2005

Paul T, Schroeter K, Dahme B, et al: Self-injurious behavior in women with eating disorders. Am J Psychiatry 159:408–411, 2002

Raine A: Annotation: the role of prefrontal deficits, low autonomic arousal, and early health factors in the development of antisocial and aggressive behavior in children. J Child Psychol Psychiatry 43:417–434, 2002

Raine A, Buchsbaum M, LaCasse L: Brain abnormalities in murderers indicated by positron emission tomography. Biol Psychiatry 42:495–508, 1997

Räsänen P, Hakko H, Väisänen E: Arson trend increasing: a real challenge to psychiatry. J Forensic Sci 40:976–979, 1995

Räsänen P, Hakko H, Isohanni M, et al: Maternal smoking during pregnancy and risk of criminal behavior among adult male offspring in the Northern Finland 1996 Birth Cohort. Am J Psychiatry 156:857–862, 1999

Repo E, Virkkunen M, Rawlings R, et al: Criminal and psychiatric histories of Finnish arsonists. Acta Psychiatr Scand 95:318–323, 1997

Ritchie EC, Huff TG: Psychiatric aspects of arsonists. J Forensic Sci 44:733–740, 1999

Robertson MM, Trimble MR, Lees AJ: Self-injurious behavior and the Gilles de la Tourette syndrome: a clinical study and review of the literature. Psychol Med 19:611–625, 1989

Rogers J, Viding E, Blair RJ, et al: Autism spectrum disorder and psychopathy: shared cognitive underpinnings or double hit? Psychol Med 36:1789–1798, 2006

Rome S, Itskowitz R: The relationship between locus of control and type of aggression in middle-class and culturally deprived children. Pers Individ Dif 11:327–333, 1990

Roy A: Childhood trauma and impulsivity: possible relevance to suicidal behavior. Arch Suicide Res 9:147–151, 2005

Rusch RG, Hall JC, Griffin HC: Abuse-provoking characteristics of institutionalized mentally retarded individuals. Am J Ment Defic 90:618–624, 1986

Shea S: Personality characteristics of self-mutilating male prisoners. J Clin Psychol 49:576–585, 1993

Sigafoos J, Elkins J, Kerr M, et al: A survey of aggressive behaviour among a population of persons with intellectual disability in Queensland. J Intellect Disabil Res 38:369–381, 1994

Simeon D: Self-injurious behavior, in Clinical Manual of Impulse-Control Disorders. Edited by Hollander E, Stein D. Washington, DC, American Psychiatric Publishing, 2006, pp 63–86

Simeon D, Favazza AR: Self-injurious behaviors: phenomenology and assessment, in Self-Injurious Behaviors: Assessment and Treatment. Edited by Simeon D, Hollander E. Washington, DC, American Psychiatric Publishing, 2001, pp 1–28

Simeon D, Stanley B, Frances A, et al: Self-mutilation in personality disorders: psychological and biological correlates. Am J Psychiatry 149:221–226, 1992

Simon OR, Swann AC, Powell KE, et al: Characteristics of impulsive suicide attempts and attempters. Suicide Life Threat Behav 32 (1, suppl):49–59, 2001

Sood BG, Nordstrom Bailey B, Covington C, et al: Gender and alcohol moderate caregiver reported child behavior after prenatal cocaine. Neurotoxicol Teratol 27:191–201, 2005

Stanford MS, Houston RJ, Mathias CW, et al: Characterizing aggressive behavior. Assessment 10:183–190, 2003a

Stanford MS, Houston RJ, Villemarette-Pittman NR, et al: Premeditated aggression: clinical assessment and cognitive psychophysiology. Pers Individ Dif 34:773–781, 2003b

Stoff D, Breiling J, Maser J: Handbook of Antisocial Behavior. New York, Wiley, 1997

Stone MH: Psychotherapy in patients with impulsive aggression, in Impulsivity and Aggression. Edited by Hollander E, Stein D. New York, Wiley, 1995, pp 313–331

Strongman KT: Emotion in mentally retarded people. Aust NZ J Dev Disabil 10:201–213, 1985

Suyemoto KL: The functions of self-mutilation. Clin Psychol Rev 18:531–554, 1998

Swann AC, Dougherty DM, Pazzaglia PJ, et al: Increased impulsivity associated with severity of suicide attempt history in patients with bipolar disorder. Am J Psychiatry 162:1680–1687, 2005

Tateno A, Jorge RE, Robinson RG: Clinical correlates of aggressive behavior after traumatic brain injury. J Neuropsychiatry Clin Neurosci 15:155–160, 2003

Villemarette-Pittman NR, Stanford MS, Greve KW: Language and executive function in self-reported impulsive aggression. Pers Individ Dif 34:1533–1544, 2003

Walz NC, Benson BA: Labeling and discrimination of facial expressions by aggressive and nonaggressive men with mental retardation. Am J Ment Retard 101:282–291, 1996

Whitlock J, Eckenrode J, Silverman D: self-injurious behaviors in a college population. Pediatrics 117:1939–1948, 2006

Williams CL, Davidson JA, Montgomery I: Impulsive suicidal behavior. J Clin Psychol 35:90–94, 1980

Williams DL, Goldstein G, Minshew NJ: Impaired memory for faces and social scenes in autism: clinical implications of memory dysfunction. Arch Clin Neuropsychol 20:1–15, 2005

Williams JG, Higgins JP, Brayne CE: Systematic review of prevalence studies of autism spectrum disorders. Arch Dis Child 91:8–15, 2006

Williams RB, Eichelman B: Social setting: influence on the physiological response to electric shock in the rat. Science 174:613–614, 1971

Woodworth M, Porter S: In cold blood: characteristics of criminal homicides as a function of psychopathy. J Abnorm Psychol 111:436–445, 2002

World Health Organization: Suicide prevention, 2006. Available at http://www.who.int/mental_health/prevention/suicide/suicideprevent/en/index.html. Accessed February 5, 2007

Yamaguchi A, Matsumoto T, Odawara T, et al: Prevalence of self-mutilation in Japanese university students: a study using self-reporting questionnaire. Seishin Igaku 46:473–479, 2004

Zouk H, Tousignant M, Seguin M, et al: Characterization of impulsivity in suicide completers: clinical, behavioral and psychosocial dimensions. J Affect Disord 92:195–204, 2006

PART III

Treatment Settings

CHAPTER 12

Outpatient Settings

James C. Beck, M.D., Ph.D.

For the vast majority of psychiatric patients potential violence is not an issue, but when it is, the clinician is obliged to deal with it. This chapter focuses on voluntary outpatient treatment, with brief comments, when relevant, on involuntary or otherwise coerced outpatient treatment.

Violence in this chapter is defined according to the MacArthur group criteria—purposeful physical assault against a person. *Serious violence* refers to assault with a weapon, assault that causes significant injury, or sexual assault (Monahan and Steadman 1994).

Potential violence is a topic that concerns every clinician, and it frightens some clinicians more than others. In discussions of this issue, people often look for clear answers to the question of whether there is a risk of violence, and if there is a risk, whether there is a clear basis for deciding what to do about it. Many clinicians would like to believe that there are clear rules for making decisions or that "This risk assessment tool will provide me with the guidance I need to proceed." In this vein, a clinician once said, "In our clinic it is policy that whenever a patient makes a threat, we warn the threatened person." The *wish* for certainty is understandable, and probably harmless, but the *rigid warning policy* of that clinic is pernicious. It carries the risk of serious harm to patients, and responsible clinicians and agencies should avoid policies like these.

General Principles

There is no substitute for clinical judgment in assessing the risk of violence and in making the many decisions involved in treatment.

Actuarial methods are helpful as background, but only as background. For example, it helps to know that young people are more often violent than older people, that men are more often violent than women, that people brought up in violent circumstances are more likely to be violent than those brought up in safety, and so on. However, knowing all the actuarial data will not in the end serve to reduce the necessity for making a clinical assessment of risk. The person in the clinical encounter is unique; the circumstances of his or her life are unique and may be changing, rapidly or slowly, in ways that affect risk. It is the clinician's responsibility, difficult as this may be, to learn about this person and the circumstances of his or her life, and on this basis to make the best estimate of risk. This is true in all clinical settings.

This chapter does not review the literature on risk assessment instruments or recommend one particular risk assessment method. Instead, it presents a conceptual framework that should help guide the clinician's assessment.

Whether the clinician is concerned about violence or not, two useful screening questions are "Are you angry at anyone?" and "Have you hurt anyone?" If the answer is "No" to both questions, the risk of violence is almost always low—unless the interview or other data suggest contrary facts. This is an example of a general principle of clinical assessment: to find out the answer to a question about a patient, ask the patient the question. If concerned about potential violence, ask "Are you thinking about hurting someone?" This does not imply that the clinician should always believe the answer—here, as elsewhere, clinical judgment is required. Yet this approach yields quite a lot of useful information, and it can be far more efficient than sniffing around the problem by asking a number of supposedly related questions.

A corollary of this principle is that the more the clinician knows about the person, the more confidence the clinician can have in his or her assessment of the answers to these questions. An interview after 1 year of weekly psychotherapy is a different situation from an initial interview in an emergency service.

If the interview develops evidence that the person is having violent fantasies, or is thinking about hurting someone, it is useful to ask something like, "Do you think this is something you might actually do, or are you just thinking about it?" (This question is useful in assessing risk of suicide or other self-harmful behavior when a patient has expressed suicidal ideation.) Patients are often able to answer this question in ways that provide useful guidance to the clinician in assessing risk. Second, assess the affect associated with the answer. Is the patient frightened that he might actually hurt his separated wife? Or excited about possibly getting revenge on her and her new boyfriend? Or is this a fantasy with little or no affective charge of any kind? It is essential to attend to the affect associated with the answers to these questions and not only to the content of the answer.

Conceptual Framework and Case Example

Kurt Lewin, often recognized as the father of social psychology, first wrote the following simple equation, quoted in Hall and Gardner (1978):

$$B = f(P,E)$$

Expanded, it means that *behavior* (B) is a function of the *person* (P) and the *environment* (E). Too often, clinical training focuses on the individual person, P, ignoring or giving too little attention to the facts of the person's situation or environment, E. The description of a patient as a "violent person" is common but not terribly helpful. It is true that some people are more likely to be violent than others, but the likelihood of violence depends to a substantial extent on the person's environment or situation, and the clinician should not neglect gathering the relevant facts about the person's situation. This conceptual framework is useful not only for assessment, but also for treatment, as in this case example.

Case Example

Mr. A, a 37-year-old single white male, was first diagnosed with paranoid schizophrenia at age 19. He receives disability payments and lives with his mother, whom he believes is poisoning his food. He gives as his reason that his food tastes funny. He adds that when he complains, his mother tells him there is nothing wrong with the food—there must be something wrong with him.

He tells his clinician that he is frightened and that he has begun to think about killing his mother. He denies that he has any concrete idea of how to kill her or any plan for what he might do, but he acknowledges that this thought does not cause him any anxiety. He denies being angry at anyone else, and he has no known history of violence. He denies any substance abuse. He says that he is taking his medication and attending outpatient treatment and a drop-in center regularly. His health is good.

His past history shows that he was a quiet child with few friends. His chart contains no mention of fighting, truancy, or oppositional behavior. He had one brief romantic relationship at age 19, and he has a long history of unemployment—he last worked 15 years ago, part time, bagging groceries. In the past he has taken his medication inconsistently, and when he has stopped his medicine he has also stopped coming to outpatient appointments.

What is to be done for this patient? As a first step in assessing risk, the clinician might review one of the published methods of risk assessment. The HCR-20, a 20-item instrument, is a good choice (Webster 1997). It serves as a reminder-checklist for things we need to know in weighing risk. The authors of the HCR-20 suggest that each item be rated absent (0), possibly present (1), or definitely present (2). The authors wrote, "Put simply, it is reasonable for assessors to conclude that the more factors present in a given case, the higher the risk for violence" (Webster 1997, p. 22). But, they added, "Even here, though, assessors must be cautious" (p. 22), implying that they recognized that a simple quantitative approach is not an adequate basis on which to assess risk. Published studies show correlations of about 0.30 between scores on the HCR-20 and future violence (Webster 1997). This means that the HCR-20 predicts less than 10% of the variance in future violence. It is useful for helping us gather the data we need, but it is not a substitute for clinical judgment.

There are three scales in the HCR-20: 10 historical items *(H)*, 5 clinical items *(C)*, and 5 risk items *(R)*. Rating the H items for the patient in the case example, we have the following:

- Major mental illness: Yes
- Early maladjustment: Possible
- Employment problems: Possible
- Five negatives: A history of violence, substance abuse, intimate relationship instability (this patient's history is considered to show paucity rather than instability), psychopathy, and personality disorder
- Two not applicable: Age at first violence and failed supervision ("supervision" refers to probation or other involuntary supervision)

Rating the clinical items for this patient, we have

- Three positives: Lack of insight, negative attitude (toward mother), active symptoms of mental illness
- Two negatives: No evidence for impulsivity, and patient is responsive to treatment currently. However, if past history of inconsistent medication compliance is factored in, this might better be scored "possible."[1]

---

[1] This illustrates that so-called objective rating scales often require clinical judgments in making the ratings. However, since the inconsistent response is rated "possible" as a risk-management factor as well, rating it as possible here may be double counting. Thus "negative" is more accurate.

Outpatient Settings

Rating the five risk-management items for Mr. A, we find that he has

- No positive indicators
- One negative: No feasible plan
- One possible: Variable past compliance with treatment
- Three items we have *not* evaluated: Exposure to destabilizers, lack of personal support, and current stress

This exercise reveals that evaluation to this point has focused almost exclusively on *P* (person) items in attempting to assess *B*—that is, future violent behavior—and has almost totally ignored *E* (environment). In the HCR-20, three of the five risk-management items refer to environmental variables: exposure to destabilizers, lack of personal support, and stress. At this point, these have not been adequately assessed.

This analysis points in the appropriate direction. The clinician can either re-interview Mr. A or, if she will agree, interview his mother. Note here I did not say to interview the mother if *Mr. A* agrees. Interview the mother regardless of whether he agrees. Why? Because, as a general rule, safety issues override confidentiality issues. When the clinician is seriously concerned about the potential for harm to either the patient or anyone else, he or she should attempt to gather whatever data is relevant to the assessment of risk. Here, the mother is likely to provide useful information, and the concern is about a potential killing, so the clinician must interview her.

Too often, when a senior clinician consults about a patient's potential for suicide or for violence toward others and asks what the family says, the answer is, "Oh, we haven't talked with the family. The patient wouldn't give us permission." This occurs most often on inpatient units. This is wrong. Safety is more basic than confidentiality. This does not mean that the clinician has *carte blanche* to violate confidentiality. It *does* mean that when the clinician has done a thorough assessment with the patient and safety remains an important issue, the clinician must look further to whatever other sources of information may be accessible.

To add one clinical note to this aside, the clinician should *almost* always, except in the most unusual circumstances (e.g., a delirious patient), explain to the patient what he or she is going to do and why. There are data showing that therapy is disrupted not when the clinician breaches confidentiality to seek additional sources of information but rather when the clinician fails to inform the patient of what he or she is doing (Beck 1981). When the clinician goes behind the patient's back to breach confidentiality, the patient feels betrayed. The result is that the patient distrusts the clinician, will end the contact if possible, and is likely to avoid the mental health system in the future (Beck 1981; *Tarasoff v. Regents of the University of California* 1976).

Returning to Mr. A, and recalling the missing information, here are two alternative scenarios.

> In the first scenario, Mr. A and his mother live alone with no immediate family nearby. Mr. A is not sure whether his mother is angry with him or not. When the clinician interviews the mother, she says that she is quite annoyed with her son—she cannot understand why he is complaining about her cooking, and she is quite unsympathetic. She says, "With all I do for him, he is really ungrateful. I tell him if he doesn't like the food here he should 'go to another hotel.'" Mr. A is worried about his situation at home. He wonders if his mother means he should leave. Asked about outside social supports, Mr. A says his only regular contact is the drop-in center and that he has recently had an argument with one of the other patients and has not been back for several weeks.

In terms of the missing data, each of the three risk-management variables converts to positive. Mother's suggestion that he can "go to another hotel" destabilizes the living situation because the patient is actively worried about it. We have no evidence for other social supports, and his argument at the drop-in center is evidence of additional current stress.

> In the alternate scenario, the clinician learns Mr. A's divorced sister lives downstairs with her 10-year-old son and Mr. A has a good relationship with them. He often eats there, especially if there has been an argument at home. Mother (or sister) says that Mr. A has been talking for years about his fear of being poisoned but that his sister is able to reassure him, and the family takes all this in stride as part of Mr. A's illness. Mr. A has no close friends, but he does have coffee almost every day at the local Dunkin' Donuts, and he is doing fine in his drop-in center.

The assessment of risk in these two scenarios is quite different. In the first scenario, the patient's mother is a destabilizing influence with her angry implied threat that he should leave. There are no other balancing family members who can be a source of support, and he has an unstable social situation at the drop-in center that is an additional source of stress. In this case, hospitalization seems clearly to be indicated. In the second scenario, however, a number of positive features are present: a relationship with other family members that provides both support and respite; a family that is apparently able to deal with this member without becoming alarmed; and a stable social situation at the drop-in center. In this case some clinicians might still be inclined to hospitalize, but others might conclude that there is no risk of imminent harm and that a longer-term plan might be contemplated while the patient continued in the community. Here the issue of prior knowledge is important. If the assessing clinician has been seeing this person for medication management for several years and knows the family, outpatient management is more likely. If the mother has brought the patient to an emergency department where he is unknown, and the outpatient psychiatrist is unavailable, hospitalization is more likely.

It may be necessary to hospitalize this man acutely and perhaps adjust his medication. Medication may reduce the strength of the delusion or it may not. He may take his medication as prescribed, or he may not. For the long term, the critical intervention that will reduce risk, under the first, more dangerous set of facts, is to separate Mr. A and his mother. If the patient is agreeable to moving to a group home or other setting, and if this can be accomplished, the risk of violence can be reduced to tolerable levels. This man has never threatened anyone except his mother as far as we know, and he has one very specific paranoid delusion—thus, removing him from the source of perceived threat may be adequate to control risk.

This example illustrates a fundamental point. If $B=f(P,E)$, and the B (behavior) in question is serious violence, we can reduce the risk of violence by changing either P (the individual) or E (the environment). Changing P may involve depot medication or new psychosocial treatment such as day treatment, a group, or a rehabilitation program. Changing E may involve changing the patient's physical environment or interpersonal situation or, as in Mr. A's example, changing both.

Assessing Risk in Patients With a Past History of Violence

When called on to assess potential future violence in the case of a patient who has been violent, a simple but often helpful rule is, "The best predictor of what will happen in the future is what happened in the past, *unless something is different.*" This rule is not absolute, but it focuses attention where it should be placed—on what has happened and what has or has not changed. If someone has been violent in this or a similar environment, then the immediate question is whether the person or the situation has changed sufficiently that the risk is acceptably low. The critical question to ask is, "What has changed?"

The situation often arises in outpatient practice that the clinician is asked to accept an about-to-be discharged inpatient into some kind of outpatient follow-up treatment. If the patient had been hospitalized in part because of violent behavior, the clinician should be satisfied, before accepting the patient, that the risk of violence has been reduced to an acceptable level. At the present time, when managed care dictates brief hospitalizations, very little if anything is likely to have changed between pre-admission and discharge except that a week has passed since the patient was removed from his or her environment to the hospital. Now the hospital is proposing to discharge the patient to outpatient care. If the outpatient clinician is part of an organizational network caring for such patients, she or he may have something to say about whether enough has changed that this patient is safe for outpatient treatment. The value of $B=f(P,E)$ in this situation is that it helps the clinician ask a broad range of questions and consider a range of potentially useful interventions or changes that may reduce the risk.[2]

Assessing Imminence of Risk

Assume that the clinician has assessed risk and decided that the patient in this situation is at risk for violence. In this context, assessing *imminence of risk* is critical. If risk is imminent, the clinician must make a definitive intervention **now**. If risk is not imminent, there is the luxury of time in which to try to engage the patient in treatment or to otherwise intervene.

As with everything else, assessment of imminence requires assessment of both P and E. For example, a patient who insists that he plans to blow up the post office but who appears to have no access to, or experience with, explosives and no knowledge of how to build them is probably not at imminent risk. The clinician may decide to hospitalize this patient, but unless there is reason to believe the patient may be contemplating some other imminent violent act, the choice is not forced.

When the clinician is convinced that there is a risk of imminent violence, and the patient is mentally ill, then action is necessary, and usually the best choice is hospitalization. If the patient agrees to be hospitalized, the decision is easy. If the patient refuses voluntary hospitalization and the clinician judges that failure to hospitalize would create a likelihood of serious harm by reason of mental illness, then the clinician has the legal power to hospitalize the patient involuntarily.

---

[2] Although the focus of this analysis is on danger to others, it is equally useful in assessing risk of self-harmful behavior. For example, a man who worked in the same office with his girlfriend became suicidally depressed after she dumped him. This patient improved significantly after he changed his job situation. Not seeing the ex-girlfriend every day gave the patient and the clinician time to provide treatment addressing the person's vulnerability to loss and related depression. Changing E-related risk reduced the risk of self-harmful B and gave the psychiatrist the freedom to work on enduring P variables with her patient.

Outpatient Settings

This implies the responsibility to use one's best judgment in deciding how to use that power.

Involuntary hospitalization involves not only treatment but also a deprivation of liberty. This deprivation is a very serious matter. In the United States, imminent risk of serious harm by reason of mental illness is the only condition under which a person may be deprived of liberty without having been charged with a crime. Clinicians are likely to focus on the good they can do by providing treatment, whether voluntary or not; they are much less likely to weigh the seriousness of depriving the patient of his or her liberty. Good clinical practice is to hospitalize involuntarily only if the risk of serious harm is imminent. Yet a question arises for which scales or algorithms provide no guidance: how to define imminent risk?

According to the *Oxford English Dictionary* (1991), *imminent* means "impending, threateningly, overhanging (almost always of evil intent)...close at hand...coming on shortly." A useful operational definition of *imminent* is "within 24 hours." In other words, if in best clinical judgment this patient is likely to act violently *within the next 24 hours*, then there is a basis to hospitalize involuntarily. If the estimated time frame is longer or more vague—there is a risk of violence, but not tomorrow, maybe the day after tomorrow or next week—then it is wrong to hospitalize involuntarily because there are treatment choices that do not involve depriving this person of his or her liberty.

When violence is a concern but judged not to be imminent, then it is possible, for example, to start the patient on medicine and have him or her come back tomorrow or start day treatment. Where this gets tricky is when the patient refuses to come back tomorrow. Then, if the clinician is worried about potential violence *the day after* tomorrow but thinks the patient will not come back to be reevaluated *tomorrow*, this gets into a gray area in which the clinician will not be able to evaluate imminence going forward. If violence is judged not imminent today, but the clinician's best estimate is that she or he will not be able to reevaluate imminence tomorrow, then involuntary hospitalization *today* may be called for.

Preventive Action to Reduce Risk

When the clinician knows that the patient has threatened someone else, and the clinical assessment is that these threats are not just talk or fantasy but behavior for which the patient is at risk, then the clinician has a responsibility to do whatever is possible to prevent the future violence. The clinician's first responsibility is to make sure the patient understands the limits on confidentiality—that the clinician is obligated to do whatever is judged to be necessary to prevent threatened violence.

Preventive action can include breaching the patient's confidentiality to warn the victim or the authorities, and the patient needs to understand this as a condition of his or her further discussions with the clinician. This does not mean that breach of confidentiality is always called for; often it is not, but the patient needs to know the ground rules.

If the clinician judges the threatened violence not to be imminent, there are several options. As always, the basic principle is to treat the threatened violence **primarily as a clinical problem,** and only secondarily as a legal issue. Just as the clinician would not stand by when judging a patient to be a risk to self, so, equally, the clinician must try to prevent violence when a patient is judged to be a risk to others. The first effort should be to involve the patient in a discussion of these impulses and of possible ways to avoid violence. It is critical to assess the emotional charge associated with the thoughts, beliefs, fantasies, or threatened behavior that has raised concern about future violence. If risk assessment were only a matter of asking, "Are you thinking of hurting anyone?" then interviewers with minimal training could be hired to screen for this.

When patients perceive that the clinician is interested in their welfare and not just in protecting the potential victim, it is often possible to use the alliance to reduce risk. If a man is threatening his significant other, he may agree that the clinician should let the threatened partner know how angry he is and what he is thinking about doing. If the potential victim and the patient will agree, perhaps both can meet with the clinician. In the context of threatened violence, this sounds like an extreme intervention. In more usual circumstances, it is called "couples therapy."

This brief discussion illustrates that there are no bright-line rules for deciding what to do when potential violence is an issue. Potentially violent patients present difficult clinical problems. In the end, it is the clinician's best judgment based on careful clinical assessment that the profession must rely on. It is tempting for clinicians, when in doubt about imminence, to hospitalize the patient, even when they are in serious doubt, because this is the "conservative" thing to do. It is a safer choice for the clinician in regard to the threat of being sued. However, the cost of this conservative approach is the deprivation of another's liberty. If successful, this chapter will help clinicians assess these risks more comfortably so that they are less often in the kind of doubt that leads to unnecessary hospitalization.

Legal Aspects of Potential Violence

Since the *Tarasoff* decision, clinicians have been concerned about the risks of being sued for future harm done by a patient who is currently in treatment. There is an extensive literature on this topic that is not reviewed here, but see, for example, Herbert (2002) and Walcott et al. (2001). Here, it is enough to comment that when the clinician focuses on the clinical issues and does a careful risk assessment, the likelihood of being found negligent for a patient's future violent acts is very small. There is a standard for risk assessment. There is no standard for risk prediction. Therefore, if the clinician has done a careful risk assessment along the lines suggested in this chapter, then there is no basis to find the clinician negligent. If violence occurs, it is an unfortunate outcome for which the clinician cannot be held legally responsible.

Currently, there are laws on the books in 29 states that sharply limit the basis on which a clinician can be sued for harm done by a patient. These laws are all broadly similar. They state that the clinician's duty to protect is limited to cases in which the patient has made a threat to the therapist (or, in California, to a credible third party who informs the therapist) or in which there is other reason, based on the patient's history of serious violence, to believe the patient constitutes a threat. The clinician then discharges the duty either by hospitalizing the patient or warning the victim or appropriate authorities. An equally important provision is that if the clinician's communication to third parties has been made in good faith, then the clinician is immune from suit for breach of confidentiality. In the past 10 years, almost no clinician has been found liable for a breach of the duty to protect.

This is not to say that there are no legal risks. In America, anyone can sue anyone else for almost anything, and there are underemployed lawyers who will take bad cases. Being a defendant is always a difficult experience, and there is no guarantee that good clinical work will protect you from all eventualities. Good clinical work will, however, keep you safe from all reasonable risks associated with the assessment of potentially violent patients. It is true that that there are risks, however small, associated with potential violence that are not present in other clinical work. These come with the territory, and a clinician who is not at least tolerably comfortable with them should think about working in situations where patients who present such risks are rare.

Threats to Patients

The focus of this chapter is on assessing risk of possible violence that the patient may commit in the future, and how to assess that. Much of the relevant data is elicited from the patient in the clinical interview. This section addresses risk assessment when the patient is worried about being a victim of violence, for example if she is being stalked. For an excellent discussion of threats as risk factors for violence related to stalking, see McEwan et al. (2007) and Mullen et al. (2006).

In a recent lecture, Paul Mullen, a distinguished Australian professor of forensic psychiatry, commented on a relevant finding. His group asked persons who had been threatened with violence whether the threats had seriously frightened them. Only 3% of respondents said that they had been seriously frightened. Clinicians should take this seriously in assessing risk. It is true that some people have a much lower threshold for being frightened than others; but, just as assessing the affect of the potentially violent person is important, this result points to the importance of assessing the affect of the *threatened* victim. One should try to make allowances for potential victims who appear to be somewhat dramatic or hysterical, but in general it is prudent to take more seriously a threat that the *potential victim* takes more seriously. As with assessing patients as possible actors, so in assessing patients as possible victims it is critical to assess the emotional charge associated with the thoughts, beliefs, fantasies, or threatened behavior that has raised the patient's concern.

Risk of Violence to the Clinician

Very occasionally the therapist may be concerned about being assaulted by the patient. In that context, physical safety for the therapist is an essential consideration. Location and time of day are the critical issues to consider related to the therapist's potential isolation.

Outpatient locations vary widely in the extent to which they provide physical safety. At one potentially dangerous extreme, the therapist in individual practice may have a private office in an isolated building— for example, a home office or an office in a small building with few or absent tenants. Not much better, from a safety standpoint, are single offices in large buildings where there are no organizational connections between the many offices and their occupants. Safer are therapist offices within an institutional structure—outpatient clinics or offices physically related to inpatient services.

An office is only as safe as the nearest available help. Any office is unsafe at times of day when no one else is around. Similarly, any situation is unsafe if the clinician fails to use good sense. Not to belabor the obvious, but where the clinician and the patient sit can be important. A young resident once was working in an emergency department interviewing a rather agitated patient. The resident was sitting on a low stool in front of the patient, who was in a chair. It suddenly occurred to this resident that the patient could easily kick him in the face. At that moment he moved to a more prudently placed chair.

Outpatient Settings

With a paranoid patient the question of who sits nearer the door may be important. If the clinician is not worried about violence toward him- or herself, it may be best to let the patient have a clear path to the door, so that the patient can leave without going through the clinician if he or she becomes frightened. On the other hand, if the clinician is concerned about violence, there may be greater risk to placing the patient between the door and the clinician.

When in doubt about your own physical safety, *ask the patient.* That is, raise a concern about the patient's current volatility and your own safety in the patient's presence and try to negotiate an agreement on how to further conduct the interview. This could mean leaving the door open. In extreme cases it could mean arranging to meet in an emergency department or other hospital setting. The point is that the clinician should never meet with a patient in a situation in which the clinician feels unsafe.

This last point leads to another critical assessment—namely, the clinician's assessment of his or her own comfort in dealing with potential violence. Clinicians vary widely in how tolerant they are of dealing with patients with histories of serious violence and in how comfortable they are working in settings such as emergency services or prisons in which potentially violent patients are a significant part of the caseload. It is important to know one's own level of comfort or discomfort with the issue of violence and to try to arrange a professional life in which the expected level of assessment of potential violence is within a zone of comfort.

Again, no physical location is safe if no one else is present. It is essential when seeing patients identified as potentially violent that other people are within earshot and that they are aware of the issue. If the clinician is worried, he or she can arrange to keep the office door partly open if this is the best that can be done in a particular setting. Clinics can install "panic buttons" that the clinician can use to alert staff to difficulties. A clinician once interviewed a patient in a prison setting in which the guards placed a small tower-shaped buzzer on the desk. "If this gets knocked down," they said, "40 people will come running in." In emergency services, weapons checks or metal detectors may be appropriate.

The recent tragic death of a senior psychiatrist—killed by a patient whom he saw in a physically isolated office on a Sunday morning—illustrates the potential dangers of seeing patients in isolation. It is not good for patients to be violent, and it is certainly not good for therapists to be victims. Commitment to patients is good, but professional services should be provided only in a context that keeps the clinician safe.

Axis I Diagnosis and Violence

Clinicians need to know the evidence relating violence to particular mental disorders as part of their own knowledge base when conducting risk assessments. However, they must also be able to discuss this issue knowledgably with members of the public. Here it is important to know the evidence, but it is also important to know what the public believes. Several studies have documented that the general public believes mental disorder and violence are associated (Wahl 2003). This belief is supported by portrayals of mentally ill people on television (Diefenbach 2007) and also by the media attention to random killings perpetrated by mentally ill persons. Our understanding of the relationship between mental disorders and violence has evolved significantly over the past 15 years, and for that reason it is summarized here.

Swanson et al.'s 1990 paper providing self-report data on violence in relation to mental disorder marks the beginning of the current understanding of the relationship between violence and mental disorder. Relying on interview data in a community sample of more than 10,000 people, they found that 2% of respondents without evidence of mental disorder reported having been violent in the past year. In comparison, violence was reported by 10%–12% of people with schizophrenia or bipolar disorder; 25% of people who abused alcohol; and 33% of people with substance abuse. The data also showed a steady increase in self-reported violence for people with multiple diagnoses (Swanson et al. 1990).

That paper has been followed by epidemiological studies on four continents (Arseneault et al. 2000; Brennan et al. 2000; Corrigan and Watson 2005; Stueve and Link 1998; Wessely et al. 1994) and by case register (Wessely et al. 1994) and other studies of clinical samples, almost all of which have produced consistent findings: people with schizophrenia are more likely to be violent or seriously violent than comparison samples. Comorbidity of substance abuse with schizophrenia increases these risks. Similar risks of violence apply for persons with bipolar disorder (Buchanan et al. 1993; Commander et al. 2005).

More recent work suggests that much of the risk of violence associated with schizophrenia is actually related to the presence of comorbid antisocial personality or conduct disorder, both of which are more common in association with schizophrenia than in the general population (Bland et al. 1987; Swanson et al. 1990). For example, Mueser et al. (2006) studied patients with schizophrenia or bipolar disorder and comorbid substance abuse. Of those who also met criteria for comorbid antisocial personality disorder, more than two-thirds had a criminal history of one or more violent offenses. Similar but less dramatic results held for patients who had a comorbid conduct disorder.

Hodgins et al. (1999) also reported that antisocial personality was associated with violence among patients with schizophrenia, but in contrast to Mueser et al. (2006), Hodgins's group did not find that antisocial personality was associated with violence among patients with bipolar disorder. For the bipolar patients, substance abuse was associated with violence, and compliance with treatment decreased the risk of violence.

Recent data establish quite clearly that the violence associated with schizophrenia is strongly related to the presence of comorbid conduct disorder or antisocial personality disorder (Hodgins et al. 2005). In a sample of 248 men with schizophrenia or schizoaffective disorder, approximately 20% had comorbid conduct disorder, and almost all men with conduct disorder also met criteria for antisocial personality disorder. "In childhood and adolescence, conduct disorder was associated with poor academic performance, physical abuse, substance misuse, institutionalization, and being raised in a family characterized by criminality and substance misuse" (Hodgins et al. 2005, p. 323). Conduct disorder was associated with an increased risk of violent crime such that for each additional symptom of conduct disorder, the risk of violent crime increased by 1.2. This was true after controlling for diagnoses of drug or alcohol misuse. Notably, there was no association between violence and positive or negative symptom level in this sample, and current substance abuse was equally common in conduct disorder patients and others. The clinical implication of these findings is clear: the clinician should routinely assess for a history of symptoms of conduct disorder or antisocial personality.

A body of work exists showing that delusions of threat (paranoia) or control-override (delusions of thought insertion, or that one's behavior is controlled by outside forces) are associated with violence (Hodgins et al. 2003; Link et al. 1992, 1998). These symptoms are associated with violence after controlling for gender, age, ethnicity, antisocial personality disorder, and years of education. This association is another example of the general principle that violence is associated with anger. It seems likely that most people would be angry if they thought someone was trying to harm them or was inserting thoughts into their mind.

Inquiring about the emotional charge associated with delusions is critical (Buchanan et al. 1993). Buchanan et al. (1993) studied delusional patients with the aim of better understanding why patients acted on delusions. They found that patients were more likely to act on delusions when feeling sad, anxious, or frightened as a result of the delusion. The authors noted that Bleuler, in 1924, had already found affect to be an important determinant of delusionally driven action.

In a multisite/multinational study of 128 men with schizophrenia discharged from the hospital and followed up for 2 years, Hodgins et al. (2003, 2005) found that aggressive behavior was associated with severe positive symptoms and in particular with threat or control-override symptoms. This relationship held true when psychopathy and substance abuse were held constant. Depot medication did not reduce the risk of violence for these patients. Again, the clinical implication is clear: inquire about threat or control-override symptoms with care in patients who show evidence of a psychotic disorder.

Fava and Rosenbaum (1999; Fava et al. 1993) studied anger attacks as a symptom of depressive disorders. More than one-third of depressed outpatients reported anger attacks, and 30% of those said that they threw things or destroyed property. Personality disorders were more common in patients with anger attacks than in those without. A small study of women with psychosis in the community (Dean et al. 2006) found more Cluster B personality disorders (impulsive, dissocial, histrionic, and borderline) in violent compared with nonviolent patients. These data show that clinicians should not imagine that patients are too depressed to be violent. They reinforce also the importance of assessing personality characteristics as risk factors for violence.

What to conclude from all this? First, that the risk of violence associated with schizophrenia in the absence of antisocial personality or conduct disorder or substance abuse is probably not much higher than the risk for persons without mental disorder—an informed guess is that the risk is perhaps doubled. Risk for future violence is greater when, in addition to schizophrenia, there is evidence for antisocial personality disorder, conduct disorder, substance abuse, symptoms of threat or control override, past history of victimization, or exposure to violence in the current environment. These are variables that are critical to evaluate when assessing any patient for risk of future violence.

Personality Traits and Risk of Violence

Some personality traits may increase the risk of violence, regardless of whether the person meets criteria for a personality disorder. *Narcissism* and *impulsivity* are both of concern, because narcissistic people can feel entitled to do whatever they want in order to get their way, and impulsive people may not have the usual controls on violent behavior when they are angry. Conversely, traits that militate against violence include capacity for empathy, and strongly held religious beliefs.

Gender and Risk of Violence

In the community at large, men are more violent than women, but this relationship is significantly attenuated in patient samples. Women patients are more likely to be violent than women in general. This is clinically important. The clinician cannot assume that just because a patient is a woman she is unlikely to have been violent. Many people come to evaluation or treatment in part because they have been violent. Thus it is important for the clinician not to assume that risk assessment has to do mostly with men. For example, Stueve and Link (1998) examined the relationship between gender and violence in an Israeli sample of 2,700 persons with mental disorder. In the sample as a whole, men were four times as likely as women to report fighting in the past 5 years (10% vs. 2.5%), but for people who had recently been psychiatric patients, men were only twice as likely as women to report violence.

Environmental Variables

Swanson et al. (2002) reported on the relationship between environmental variables and violence in a study of 802 inpatients and outpatients with psychotic or major mood disorders. They found that 1-year rates of serious violence were related to three variables: 1) substance abuse, 2) past history of victimization, and 3) exposure to violence in the current environment. When all three were present, 30% of patients reported serious violence; when none were present, almost no patients reported serious violence. When one of these factors was present, 2% reported violence, and when two were present, 8%–10%.

Treatment Variables

As a general principle, there is no specific treatment for aggression. One exception to this may be the treatment of impulsive aggression. Barratt et al. (1997) showed that in a prison sample, phenytoin decreased impulsive aggression but not planned aggression. Medications that reduce affect dysregulation may reduce the likelihood of aggression. Examples of these medications include oxcarbazepine, gabapentin, lamotrigine, and other medications initially developed to treat seizure disorders.

Although there is no treatment for violence per se, there is treatment for mental disorders, and to the extent that aggression is associated with active symptoms of mental disorder, successful treatment of the mental disorder may reduce the risk of violence. Clozapine has been shown to reduce the risk of violent behavior among inpatients, when compared with olanzapine and haloperidol (Krakowski et al. 2006). However, in an earlier study of atypical versus typical antipsychotic medications, Swanson et al. (2004) found that clozapine, olanzapine, and risperidone all reduced the rate of violent behavior in 229 outpatients with schizophrenia spectrum disorders, when compared with treatment with typical antipsychotics. However, the study was not sufficiently powered to determine whether one atypical agent was more effective than another.

Violence in the community among psychotic patients was strongly related to perceived need for treatment in a study of 1,011 outpatients with major mental disorder in treatment in public sites in five states (Elbogen et al. 2006). Patients were asked if they needed treatment, whether treatment helped, and whether they had been compliant. Of those who answered yes to all three, only 8% reported having behaved violently; of those who answered no to all three, 40% reported violence. Interestingly, 7.5% of men and 5% of women reported serious violence, but more women (17%) than men (11%) reported non-serious violence.

In a sample of recidivist inpatients, those randomly assigned to involuntary outpatient treatment who received at least 6 months of involuntary treatment were less likely to be violent in the year after discharge than patients in treatment as usual (Swanson et al. 2000). Violence was much less likely for patients who were compliant with regular outpatient treatment and who did not abuse substances.

In the study of anger attacks in depressed outpatients, these attacks diminished or disappeared in more than half of patients treated with selective serotonin reuptake inhibitors (Fava and Rosenbaum 1999; Fava et al. 1993).

Key Points

- Risk assessment is first and foremost a process of clinical assessment. Applying an algorithm or using a rating scale may be a useful part of the process, but in the end it is the clinician's assessment of the unique facts that characterize *this* person in *this* situation that will determine the recommended course of action.
- The clinician should *always, always, always* attend to his or her own safety. Never work in isolation with patients about whom there are any safety concerns.
- Assessing the person is important, but it is not the whole story— behavior (*B*) is a function of the person (*P*) and the environment (*E*).

Outpatient Settings | 255

- A past history of violence is a strong predictor of future violence, especially if there has been no change in either *P* or *E* since the violent *B*.
- Current mental status—anger, impulsiveness, delusions held with strong affect—is a more important determinant of near-term behavior than enduring characteristics of the person such as age, gender, or diagnosis.
- Antisocial personality disorder and conduct disorder, whether alone or as comorbid conditions, are associated with violence.
- Treat violence as a clinical issue primarily. Clinical assessment, not legal concerns, should drive the decisional process.

References

Arseneault L, Moffitt TE, Caspi A, et al: Mental disorders and violence in a total birth cohort: results from the Dunedin Study. Arch Gen Psychiatry 57:979–986, 2000

Barratt ES, Stanford MS, Felthous AR, et al: The effects of phenytoin on impulsive and premeditated aggression: a controlled study. J Clin Psychopharmacol 17:341–349, 1997

Beck JC: When the patient threatens violence: an empirical study of clinical practice after *Tarasoff*. Bull Am Acad Psychiatry Law 10:199–201, 1981

Bland RC, Newman SC, Orn H: Schizophrenia: lifetime co-morbidity in a community sample. Acta Psychiatr Scand 75:383–391, 1987

Brennan PA, Mednick SA, Hodgins S: Major mental disorders and criminal violence in a Danish birth cohort. Arch Gen Psychiatry 57:494–500, 2000

Buchanan A, Reed A, Wessely S, et al: Acting on delusions, II: the phenomenological correlates of acting on delusions. Br J Psychiatry 16:377–381, 1993

Commander M, Sashidharan S, Rana T, et al: North Birmingham assertive outreach evaluation: patient characteristics and clinical outcomes. Soc Psychiatry Psychiatr Epidemiol 40:988–993, 2005

Corrigan PW, Watson AC: Findings from the National Comorbidity Survey on the frequency of violent behavior in individuals with psychiatric disorders. Psychiatry Res 136:153–162, 2005

Dean K, Walsh E, Moran P, et al: Violence in women with psychosis in the community: prospective study. Br J Psychiatry 188:264–270, 2006

Diefenbach DL: The portrayal of mental illness on prime time television. J Community Psychol 25:289–302, 2007

Elbogen EB, Van Dorn RA, Swanson JW, et al: Treatment engagement and violence risk in mental disorders. Br J Psychiatry 189:354–360, 2006

Fava M, Rosenbaum JF: Anger attacks in patients with depression. J Clin Psychiatry 60(suppl)15:21–24, 1999

Fava M, Rosenbaum JF, Pava JA, et al: Anger attacks in unipolar depression, part 1: clinical correlates and response to fluoxetine treatment. Am J Psychiatry 150:1158–1163, 1993

Hall G, Gardner L: Theories of Personality. New York, John Wiley, 1978

Herbert PB: The duty to warn: a reconsideration and critique. J Am Acad Psychiatry Law 30:417–424, 2002
Hodgins S, Hiscoke UL, Freese R: The antecedents of aggressive behavior among men with schizophrenia: a prospective investigation of patients in community treatment. Behav Sci Law 21:523–546, 2003
Hodgins S, Lapalme M, Toupin J: Criminal activities and substance use of patients with major affective disorders and schizophrenia: a 2-year follow-up. J Affect Disord 55:187–202, 1999
Hodgins S, Tiihonen J, Ross D: The consequences of conduct disorder for males who develop schizophrenia: associations with criminality, aggressive behavior, substance use, and psychiatric services. Schizophr Res 78:323–335, 2005
Krakowski MI, Czobor P, Citrome L, et al: Atypical antipsychotic agents in the treatment of violent patients with schizophrenia and schizoaffective disorder. Arch Gen Psychiatry 63:622–629, 2006
Link BG, Andrews H, Cullen FT: The violent and illegal behavior of mental patients reconsidered. Am Sociol Rev 57:275–292, 1992
Link BG, Stueve A, Phelan J: Psychotic symptoms and violent behaviors: probing the components of "threat/control-override" symptoms. Soc Psychiatry Psychiatr Epidemiol 33(suppl):S55–S60, 1998
McEwan T, Mullen PE, Purcell R: Identifying risk factors in stalking: a review of current research. Int J Law Psychiatry 30:1–9, 2007
Monahan J, Steadman HJ: Violence and Mental Disorder: Developments in Risk Assessment. Chicago, IL, University of Chicago, 1994
Mueser KT, Crocker AG, Frisman LB, et al: Conduct disorder and antisocial personality disorder in persons with severe psychiatric and substance abuse disorders. Schizophr Bull 12:626–636, 2006
Mullen PE, Mackenzie R, Ogloff JR, et al: Assessing and managing the risks in the stalking situation. J Am Acad Psychiatry Law 34:439–450, 2006
Oxford English Dictionary. Oxford, UK, Oxford University Press, 1991
Stueve A, Link BG: Gender differences in the relationship between mental illness and violence: evidence from a community-based epidemiological study in Israel. Soc Psychiatry Psychiatr Epidemiol 33(suppl):S61–S67, 1998
Swanson JW, Holzer CE III, Ganju VK, et al: Violence and psychiatric disorder in the community: evidence from the Epidemiologic Catchment Area surveys. Hosp Community Psychiatry 41:761–770, 1990
Swanson JW, Swartz MS, Borum R, et al: Involuntary out-patient commitment and reduction of violent behaviour in persons with severe mental illness. Br J Psychiatry 176:324–331, 2000
Swanson JW, Swartz MS, Essock SM, et al: The social-environmental context of violent behavior in persons treated for severe mental illness. Am J Public Health 92:1523–1531, 2002
Swanson JW, Swartz MS, Elbogen EB: Effectiveness of atypical antipsychotic medications in reducing violent behavior among persons with schizophrenia in community-based treatment. Schizophr Bull 30:3–20, 2004
Tarasoff v. Regents of the University of California. 17 Cal 3d. 425, 551 P 2d. 334 (1976)
Wahl OF: News media portrayal of mental illness. Am Behav Sci 46:1594–1600, 2003

Walcott DM, Cerundolo P, Beck JC: Current analysis of the *Tarasoff* duty: an evolution towards the limitation of the duty to protect. Behav Sci Law 19:325–343, 2001
Webster CD: HCR-20: Assessing Risk for Violence. Vancouver, BC, Canada, Simon Fraser University, 1997
Wessely SC, Castle D, Douglas AJ, et al: The criminal careers of incident cases of schizophrenia. Psychol Med 24:483–502, 1994

CHAPTER 13

Inpatient Settings

Cameron D. Quanbeck, M.D.
Barbara E. McDermott, Ph.D.

Inpatient violence is widely recognized as a serious problem in need of evidence-based solutions. Among mental health professionals working in outpatient settings, psychiatrists are the most likely to be assaulted. In inpatient settings, however, the vast majority of assaults target the nursing staff working most closely with psychiatric patients (Tardiff 1995). Public psychiatric nursing is a hazardous occupation; each year, one in four nurses suffers a disabling injury from a patient assault (Love and Hunter 1996). Assaulted staff experience emotional distress, as evidenced by high rates of substance misuse, anxiety disorders, poor morale, and job burnout (Quintal 2002). Aggressive psychiatric inpatients are adversely affected as well. Seclusion and restraints are frequently used to manage violent behavior, even though their use poses physical risks to patients and can be psychologically damaging (Frueh et al. 2005; Kaltiala-Heino et al. 2003). Past research in a variety of inpatient settings has consistently shown that a small percentage of patients are responsible for the majority of assaults (Kraus and Sheitman 2004); this subset of repetitively assaultive patients is 10 times more likely than other patients to inflict serious injuries (Convit et al. 1990).

Characteristics of Assaultive Inpatients

Past behavior is the best predictor of future behavior. A history of assaultive behavior or violent crime is the most robust long-term predictor of inpatient violence (Steinert 2002). Research has shown that men are more violent than women in the community (Swanson et al. 1990); however, this gender difference is not observed in a psychiatric inpatient setting. Women are just as likely as men to assault, and their risk of violence should not be discounted (Lam et al. 2000). Other diagnostic, historical, developmental, and neurological factors associated with inpatient violence are shown in Table 13–1.

Short-Term Risk Factors for Inpatient Assault

The characteristics of assaultive inpatients just described help the clinician identify which inpatients are at highest risk for assault. Once such patients are identified, it becomes critically important to be cognizant of the symptoms and behaviors that indicate an inpatient is at increased risk for assault so that preventative measures can be taken. Although psychiatric clinicians have been criticized for the inability to predict long-term violent recidivism, the ability of these clinicians to correctly identify which inpatients will be aggressive in the short term (i.e., hours, days) is somewhat accurate (Nijman et al. 2002). Clinical, rather than sociodemographic, risk factors have been shown to best predict aggression in the short term (McNiel et al. 2003).

A number of studies have shown the following symptoms and behaviors to be short-term risk factors for inpatient aggression: 1) recent physical violence and threats of violence (McNiel and Binder 1989; McNiel et al. 1988); 2) poor therapeutic alliance (Beauford et al. 1997), for instance, failure to cooperate with an initial assessment (Swett and Mills 1997); 3) a hostile attitude and irritable mood (Linaker and Busch-Iversen 1995; McNiel and Binder 1994); 4) psychomotor agitation (Lanza et al. 1996; Whittington and Patterson 1996); and 5) attacks on objects or property damage. In patients with a psychotic disorder, severe positive symptoms and thought disorder are short-term violence risk factors (Hoptman et al. 1999; Krakowski et al. 1999; Nolan et al. 2005).

Environmental Risk Factors

Certain situational or environmental factors have been associated with inpatient assaults. Assaults are more likely to occur during the week, when activity demands are higher (Smith et al. 2005). They occur more frequently during times of transition and increased staff–patient interaction, such as meal times, changes of shift, and medication administration (Carmel and Hunter 1989). The early afternoon is a peak time for assault (Manfredini et al. 2001). Assaults occur most often in crowded,

TABLE 13–1. Long-term risk factors for inpatient aggression

Axis I diagnosis (Binder and McNiel 1988; Hoptman et al. 1999; Lehmann et al. 1999; Miller et al. 1993; Tardiff and Sweillam 1982)

    Schizophrenia

    Mania

    Substance misuse disorder

    Dementia and other organic mental disorders

Axis II diagnosis (Hill et al. 1996; Miller et al. 1993; Soliman and Reza 2001; Tardiff and Sweillam 1982)

    Antisocial personality disorder and psychopathy

    Borderline personality disorder

    Mental retardation

Past suicide attempts (using violent methods) (Convit et al. 1988; Soliman and Reza 2001)

Developmental factors (Convit et al. 1988; Hoptman et al. 1999)

    Parental substance misuse or psychiatric illness

    Childhood physical abuse

    Placement into foster care

    School truancy

Neurological abnormalities (Barratt et al. 1997; Krakowski and Czobor 1997; Krakowski et al. 1989)

    Abnormal P300 wave amplitude

    Impairment in integrative sensory and motor functions (in those with schizophrenia)

    Frontal lobe deficits

---

high-traffic areas such as hallways, dayrooms, bedrooms, and in front of the nursing station (Chou et al. 2002).

Staffing ratios and ward atmosphere are also linked to rates of assault. There is an inverse relationship between the number of nursing staff and patient assaults (Lanza et al. 1994). Different wards or units have different rates of violence. Higher rates of violence have been observed on units where staff functions are not clearly defined and the schedule of activities is unpredictable; conversely, units with strong psychiatric leadership, clearly defined roles, and a predictable, repetitive routine have lower rates of violence (Katz and Kirkland 1990).

Motivations for Assault

Until recently, aggressive inpatients have been viewed as a homogeneous group. Recent research, however, indicates that it is important to differentiate between acts of aggression and to categorize assaults based on their various motivating factors. Two primary subtypes of aggression have been identified in both animals and humans (Weinshenker and Siegel 2002): 1) an uncontrolled outburst of aggressive behavior driven by intense emotion (varyingly termed impulsive, affective, reactive, or overt) or 2) a controlled, purposeful, and planned act of aggression (organized, predatory, premeditated, psychopathic, or covert). *Impulsive aggression* refers to spontaneous, unplanned aggressive acts that are externally provoked; feelings of remorse and confusion often follow the violent act. Persons who are impulsively aggressive often are described as "hot-blooded" or are said to have "anger control problems." In contrast, premeditated aggressive acts are not usually considered to have a large emotional component but are more "cold-blooded" in nature; the aggression is goal directed and requires a degree of forethought or planning. This type of aggression has been linked with individuals described as more antisocial and/or psychopathic (Woodworth and Porter 2002).

A study conducted in a New York psychiatric state hospital examined inpatient assaults to determine whether these two types of aggression were adequate in describing inpatient violence (Nolan et al. 2003). Assaults occurring in a common area of the inpatient unit were videotaped so that motivations and triggers for the aggression could be examined. After the assault, the assailant and victim were interviewed separately in an attempt to identify the underlying reason for the aggressive act. Three primary factors motivating assaults were identified: 1) disordered impulse control, 2) psychopathy, and 3) symptoms of psychosis. Psychotic assaults were generally committed by an individual acting under the influence of delusions, hallucinations, or disordered thinking.

A recent study attempted to determine the types of aggression occurring at a large psychiatric state hospital (Quanbeck et al. 2007). Nearly a thousand assaults committed by a large sample of randomly selected chronically aggressive inpatients were categorized as impulsive, organized, or psychotic in motivation. Impulsive assaults were the most common (54%) and the most likely to target staff. Assaults on staff were precipitated by the following interpersonal interactions: 1) attempting to change a patient's behavior, such as by enforcing unit rules, and 2) refusing a patient's request. Organized or planned assaults (29%) and psychotic assaults (17%) were less common but were more likely to target other patients in the facility. Acts of organized aggression were frequently motivated by the patient's desire to retaliate against or "get even with" another patient or staff member. Psychotic aggression was

Inpatient Settings

usually committed by patients acting under the paranoid ideation that the victim intended to harm (e.g., by poisoning), was stealing from, or was talking about/laughing at the assailant. This research suggests that the affective/reactive and predatory/planned subtyping of aggressive behavior is also valid when examining institutional violence. However, for a more accurate characterization, a third type should be included: psychotically motivated aggression. It is critical to characterize aggression exhibited on inpatient units so that appropriate and effective interventions can be developed. The different characteristics of the three types of aggression are summarized in Table 13–2.

The following three case examples illustrate these various forms of aggression. Each case is followed by a discussion of appropriate clinical interventions.

Case Example 1

Ms. Smith is a 23-year-old woman with borderline personality disorder. She was brought by police into an acute psychiatric hospital after cutting her wrists in an apparent suicide attempt. Ms. Smith had become distraught after discovering her boyfriend was involved with another woman. On the unit, she exhibits agitated behavior. She is seen pacing rapidly though the hallways of the unit, her emotions ranging from intense anger to hysterical crying. She exclaims repeatedly, "How could he do this to me?!" Suddenly, she approaches the nursing station and demands to use the phone so she can call her boyfriend. The nurse on duty sternly responds, "No! Calling him right now is not a good idea, you just need to go to your room right now and calm down!" Ms. Smith, not pleased with the nurse's response, becomes more hostile and yells, "Give me your phone! I need to call him right now! I'm gonna kill you, bitch!" The nurse, attempting to control the situation, stands up and barks out an order: "Go to your room immediately!" Ms. Smith then jumps over the desk and begins to strike the nurse repeatedly in the head and face.

This is an example of an impulsive assault, the most common type of aggression in an inpatient setting and the most likely to target staff (Quanbeck et al. 2007). This assault occurred immediately after the nurse refused a patient request; the vast majority of assaults on staff are preceded by an aversive interpersonal stimulus to the patient (Whittington and Wykes 1996). Put simply, patients lash out in frustration after being told to do something they do not want to do or being told they cannot have something they want. Because the assault is precipitated by an interpersonal situation, the staff–patient interaction that preceded the assault warrants close examination. Nurses with an authoritarian attitude, a tendency to externalize blame, high levels of anxiety, less

TABLE 13–2. Characteristics of impulsive, organized, and psychotic assaults

	Assault type		
	Impulsive	**Organized**	**Psychotic**
Precipitant	Spontaneous reaction to interpersonal provocation	Opportunity arises to use violence to advantage	Paranoia peaks in intensity and assailant feels compelled to act
Behaviors preceding assault	Psychomotor agitation, hostile and irritable mood, verbal abuse and threats	Distinct lack of emotional display; controlled; assault occurs with little warning	Paranoid delusions accompanied by anger and fear; command auditory hallucinations
Motivation for assault	Threat reduction	A desire to assert social advantage or obtain items of value	A desire to protect oneself against a perceived persecutor
Insight regarding assaultive behavior	Remorse may follow act; recognizes that control was lost	Remorse lacking; little concern for victim; may deny or justify violence	Insight is typically poor, but fluctuates with level of psychotic symptoms

Inpatient Settings

experience, and less formal training are the most likely to be assaulted (Flannery et al. 2001; Ray and Subich 1998). Furthermore, when asked about the underlying reasons for staff assaults, patients cite as precipitants poor communication with staff or the perception that staff are too controlling (Duxbury 2002).

Research has shown that if psychiatric clinicians learn the clinical skills needed to "de-escalate" emotion in patients who are agitated, staff assaults can be reduced (Forster et al. 1999). A key component of this technique is the ability to recognize early signs that indicate a patient is "escalating" in a process that may ultimately result in physical violence (Maier 1996). The escalating process has been characterized as follows: 1) tension in minor muscles; 2) verbal abuse, verbal threats, and hostility; 3) tension in major muscles; 4) physical violence; and, finally, 5) relaxation and exhaustion. Experienced nurses viewed as experts in de-escalation techniques cite the importance of intervening in the first two stages of the process in order to avert an attack (Johnson and Hauser 2001). Effective de-escalation techniques are summarized in Table 13–3. Interventions clinicians can use to help gain control of a patient's dangerous behavior are outlined in Table 13–4. (For a more detailed discussion of seclusion and restraints, see Chapter 17.) If de-escalation fails and a staff assault occurs, it is important to engage the clinicians involved in a debriefing session (Secker et al. 2004). The goals of this debriefing session should be to 1) determine what triggered the assault; 2) review the interventions taken and why they failed; and 3) examine what was learned and what can be done differently next time. Finally, the physical and psychological impact on the involved staff should be evaluated; a significant decline in rates of assault has been noted after psychiatric facilities implement a program that provides psychological support for staff who have been assaulted (Flannery et al. 1998).

Case Example 2

Mr. Jones is a 34-year-old man with schizophrenia, paranoid type. He was transferred from an acute facility to a psychiatric state hospital for long-term treatment. The first several months of his stay were uneventful. Nursing staff then began to note deterioration in his clinical condition. Mr. Jones began to complain that other patients were saying negative things about him behind his back. He began to isolate himself in his room throughout the day and was often observed talking to himself. He accused nursing staff of putting poison in his medications and occasionally refused to take his scheduled antipsychotic. While waiting in line for medications a few weeks later, he became very angry and agitated and exclaimed, "Stop giving out drugs and syringes to kids; it's illegal!"

TABLE 13–3. De-escalation techniques to prevent an impulsive assault: approaching an agitated patient

Notice early signs of agitation and read the situation.
  Identify what is upsetting the patient.
Verbally connect with the patient using a calm voice.
  Listen to the patient and attempt to understand and empathize with the patient's perspective.
    "I notice you are upset; what is bothering you?"
    "What might help you calm down?"
  Agree with the patient if possible.
    "Yes, your medication does cause some annoying side effects."
  Avoid taking an authoritarian stance with the patient; getting into an argument will only fuel the escalating process.
Interventions designed to give the patient a sense of control can be helpful.
  Show respect by asking permission to speak with the patient.
  Divide energy by giving the patient choices:
    "Would you like to move to a different area and talk?"
    "Would you like to take some medication [as needed]?"
    "Would you like to listen to some music?"
Increase the personal space between yourself and the patient; do not make an escalating patient feel cornered.
  Locate an escape route and summon help if necessary.
Accompany the patient to a calmer space and observe patient for signs of relaxation.

> He then threw his medications at nursing staff. A few days later, he frantically dialed 911 and demanded an ambulance be sent to get him because his life was in jeopardy. Early the next day, he approached the unit psychiatrist from behind and struck him in the head while yelling, "You poured kerosene on me last night!"

This long-term psychiatric inpatient committed an assault while acting under the influence of a paranoid delusion. Persons with schizophrenia are the most likely to act on persecutory delusions (Swanson et al. 2006). There are multiple other factors associated with violent behavior and delusions. Inpatients are more likely to act on delusions if they feel frightened, anxious, unhappy, or angry as a consequence of the delusional belief (Appelbaum et al. 1999). A history of acting violently in response to a delusion increases the future likelihood of acting on delusions (Monahan et al. 2001). Inpatients who are both psychotic and violent have poorer insight into their psychotic symptoms than those who

TABLE 13–4. Measures of control in inpatient settings

Medications (oral or intramuscular)
One-to-one staff observation
Seclusion (open or closed)
Restraints

---

are not violent (Arango et al. 1999). Inpatients with treatment-resistant schizophrenia exhibit a significant increase in the positive symptoms of psychosis 3 days prior to the occurrence of an aggressive incident (Nolan et al. 2005).

A patient experiencing an auditory hallucination that issues a command to harm others is at increased violence risk. Command hallucinations double the risk a patient will be assaultive (McNiel et al. 2000). An inpatient is more likely to act on command hallucinations if the voice is familiar to the patient, if there is a delusion associated with the hallucination, and if coping strategies to diminish the hallucination are not successful (Cheung et al. 1997). Indicators that a patient with psychosis is at increased risk for assault are summarized in Table 13–5.

Management strategies for preventing psychosis-related aggression can include separating the inpatient from the perceived persecutor and the use of cognitive therapies that may reduce the patient's conviction that the delusional belief is true (Turkington et al. 2006). The most effective approach to reducing violence in individuals with a psychotic disorder is pharmacological; clozapine is superior to other antipsychotic agents in reducing aggressive behavior (Volavka et al. 2004).

TABLE 13–5. Psychotic violence: indicators of impending assault

Persecutory or paranoid delusions are closely linked to violence

Delusions causing fear, unhappiness, or anger are more likely to be acted on

Past aggression based on delusions is predictive of future similar acts

An increase in positive symptoms has been observed in the days before an assault

Command hallucinations increase the risk of violent behavior

  Patients are more likely to behave aggressively if
    —The voice is familiar
    —A delusion is associated with the hallucination
    —Coping strategies are not successful

Case Example 3

Mr. Green is a 28-year-old man who was admitted to a Veterans Affairs psychiatric hospital after going to the emergency department and reporting that voices were telling him to kill himself and others. His urine toxicology screening was positive for cocaine. His preliminary diagnosis was psychotic disorder not otherwise specified. On the unit, Mr. Green frequently came to the nursing station complaining of anxiety and received several doses of lorazepam (Ativan) as needed. Several days later, Mr. Jackson (another patient on the unit) approached the charge nurse and reported that Mr. Green was threatening to harm patients unless they "cheek" their benzodiazepines and give them to him. The nurse notified the unit psychiatrist, and Mr. Green's order for lorazepam was discontinued based on the suspicion that he was abusing it.

Later in the day, Mr. Green approached the nursing station complaining of agitation and requested lorazepam. The nurse on duty informed Mr. Green that his lorazepam had been discontinued by the psychiatrist. When Mr. Green asked why it was stopped, the nurse replied, "I don't know, you'll have to ask the doctor tomorrow during rounds." Visibly irritated, Mr. Green walked away and entered his room. He returned to the nursing station 1 hour later and calmly told the nurse, "You have a really pretty face, I'd hate to see it get all cut up, but you never know what could happen around here. Now, I want you to work on getting my Ativan reordered." Later, on the night shift, nurses rushed to Mr. Jackson's room after hearing a lot of commotion and yelling. They found Mr. Jackson (the patient who had reported Mr. Green's extortion scheme to nursing staff) with a bloodied and broken nose. Mr. Jackson immediately exclaimed, "He hit me when I was sleeping!" and pointed to Mr. Green standing in the hallway. Mr. Green smiled at the nursing staff and said, "The voices made me do it."

Predatory violence is dangerous because it usually occurs without warning and is difficult to predict and prevent (Meloy 1987). Persons who engage in organized aggression may have a limited capacity to empathize with others. Thus, they are comfortable using violence as a tool to gain control over others, assert dominance, and obtain desired goals. In this case, the patient made a "cold threat" against the unit nurse (Quanbeck et al. 2007). A *cold threat* is defined as a threat of future violence delivered in an unemotional, controlled manner and intended to frighten another into doing what the threatener wants. This type of threat is seen with increasing frequency in psychiatric facilities and can distress and demoralize clinicians (Flannery et al. 1995). Cold threats should be managed differently than the "hot threats" that foreshadow an impulsive assault (Maier 1996). Because of the personal nature and gravity of the threat, psychiatric clinicians have a tendency to hide the threat from colleagues and may isolate themselves from peers. This response, however, is exactly what the threatener desires, because it only

Inpatient Settings

serves to increase the level of control the patient holds over the clinician. To deal with these threats, psychiatric units can maintain a "threat book" in which staff can document threats received that day. At the end of the shift, staff meet as a group to assess the clinical meaning of the threat in the context of the patient's clinical condition. Two staff members then later confront the patient who made the threat, attempt to get him or her to accept responsibility for making the threat, and suggest more effective ways of getting what the patient wants. Clinicians working in long-term and forensic settings must develop approaches to this type of aggression because, unlike in short-term community settings, immediate discharge is not an option.

A controversial approach to inpatient assaults is criminal prosecution (Appelbaum and Appelbaum 1991). Filing criminal charges against violent inpatients is a recent phenomenon, with the first case report appearing in the literature in 1978 (Schwarz and Greenfield 1978). In the past, prosecution has not been considered a viable option because of the prevailing belief that hospitalized psychiatric patients are, by virtue of their situation, not responsible for their actions (Norko et al. 1991). Furthermore, taking an action that moves a patient out of a therapeutic milieu and into the punitive atmosphere of a jail or prison creates an ethical dilemma. Mental health professionals are expected to act in patients' best interests and respect their autonomy, and physicians have a duty to "do no harm" (Appelbaum and Appelbaum 1991).

Over recent years, however, the number of inpatients prosecuted for assaults has increased on the basis of several countervailing ethical viewpoints (Dinwiddie and Briska 2004):

- The Supreme Court has determined that psychiatric inpatients are entitled to safe conditions, and statutes based on the *Tarasoff* case obligate mental health professionals to protect endangered third parties (Appelbaum and Appelbaum 1991). Organized or predatory inpatients preferentially target other patients in the facility (Quanbeck et al. 2007). An involuntarily confined patient who is being victimized by another patient is unable to escape the situation. Thus, removing the dangerous patient from the hospital is ethically justified because it creates a safer environment for all patients.
- Psychiatric institutions also have an interest in providing for the safety of hospital personnel. Ignoring assaults can lead to poor staff morale and performance, which interferes with the therapeutic aims of the hospital (Coyne 2002).
- If patients who engage in acts of aggression that are planned and designed to meet their own needs go unpunished, the antisocial

behavior may be positively reinforced (Dinwiddie and Briska 2004). Many argue that a psychiatric patient, even though he or she is living in a hospital environment, should be held responsible for his or her conduct and live by societal rules. Criminal prosecution can set firm limits on antisocial behaviors and result in positive change (Coyne 2002; Miller and Maier 1987). Allowing such behavior to continue unchecked may ultimately harm these patients when they reenter society with the belief that acts of violence do not result in serious consequences (Dinwiddie and Briska 2004).

Psychiatric facilities should develop clear, consistent guidelines for prosecuting inpatients (Norko et al. 1991). Before a policy is implemented, gaining the cooperation of local law enforcement is essential. The district attorney may be reluctant to view inpatient assaults as a criminal matter because the community is not endangered; hospital administrators can meet with local law officials to educate them about the issue and determine the type of information needed to pursue prosecution. A prosecution policy should give inpatients an opportunity to change their behavior though treatment before resorting to the filing of criminal charges. At admission, when patients are provided written material explaining their rights and responsibilities, a statement should be included that notifies the patient that respect for others and the law is expected in the hospital and that a failure to conform could result in criminal charges. Other elements of a model prosecution policy are summarized in Table 13–6. Note that these policy recommendations are intended for repetitively assaultive patients who have not yet disrupted the milieu to a substantial degree. There may be instances when a single act of violence is so egregious that prosecution is a viable option even without a history of assaults, such as an assault causing severe physical trauma or sexual assaults on patients and staff (Dinwiddie and Briska 2004).

TABLE 13–6. Key elements and clinical considerations in determining whether prosecution is appropriate

After an inpatient assault, perform a thorough assessment of the assailant's state of mind and motivation for the violence.

Determine whether the assault was motivated by impulsivity, psychopathy, or psychosis, and document your findings in detail (see Table 13–2).

—Assaultive behavior stemming from a patient's illness (severe mood dysregulation or psychosis) may respond to clinical intervention.

—Because violence motivated by a patient's antisocial characteristics is less likely to respond to treatment, prosecution (or the threat to prosecute) may be the best strategy (Reid and Gacono 2000).

On the basis of the assessment, implement appropriate clinical interventions in the patient's individualized treatment plan.

If the interventions fail and the assaultive behavior continues, contact a hospital administrator to determine whether further acts of violence should be prosecuted.

—The administrator could have an independent clinician or forensic specialist review the case.

—If a decision is made to pursue prosecution, the assaultive patient should be placed on notice; the creation of "probationary status" itself may be effective (Hoge and Gutheil 1987).

A decision to prosecute a particular assault should be based on careful consideration of the following factors:

—Nature and severity of the violence

—Adequacy of prior treatment attempts and results

—Likelihood of response to further treatment

—Clinical impact of incarceration on the patient

—Chances of conviction

—Potential negative effects and risks to staff and other patients if assailant remains in the hospital

Key Points

- Inpatient aggression is an important problem because it has damaging psychological and physical effects on both psychiatric patients and staff.
- A small minority of psychiatric inpatients are responsible for the majority of inpatient assaults, including the most serious assaults; this subset of repetitively assaultive patients warrants greater attention in the form of systematic study.
- The most robust long-term risk factor for inpatient violence is a history of inpatient assaults or violent crime.
- Certain psychiatric symptoms and behaviors indicate an inpatient is at increased risk for assault in the short term; recognizing these clinical risk factors and making appropriate interventions can help prevent aggression.
- The clinical management of an aggressive inpatient should be guided by the type of violence in which a patient engages. It is important to characterize the primary factor motivating aggressive behavior.
- Impulsively aggressive inpatients should be observed for signs of escalation so that measures can be taken to de-escalate patients early in the process. Because most impulsive assaults are precipitated by an aversive interpersonal interaction, clinicians should critically examine how they approach patients.
- In inpatients with a history of assaults motivated by psychosis, increased assault risk is indicated by paranoid or persecutory delusions (with or without commanding auditory hallucinations) and accompanying anger, fear, or sadness.
- Among inpatients whose aggression is motivated by antisocial or self-serving interests, it is important to confront the behavior and to attempt to get the patient to assume responsibility for his or her actions. Criminal prosecution may be ethically justified in managing this type of patient.
- When a clinician is assuming care of an inpatient with a history of violence, time spent investigating past motivations for aggressive behavior through record review and clinical interview can be valuable. Knowing the precipitants, situations, and symptoms that have led to violence in the past can be useful in preventing future assaults. After an inpatient assault, a debriefing session can yield critical information that can be used to develop different approaches effective in preventing subsequent violence.

References

Appelbaum KL, Appelbaum PS: A model hospital policy on prosecuting patients for presumptively criminal acts. Hosp Community Psychiatry 42:1233–1237, 1991

Appelbaum PS, Robbins PC, Roth LH: Dimensional approach to delusions: comparison across types and diagnoses. Am J Psychiatry 156:1938–1943, 1999

Arango C, Calcedo Barba A, Gonzalez, et al: Violence in inpatients with schizophrenia: a prospective study. Schizophr Bull 25:493–503, 1999

Barratt ES, Stanford MS, Felthous AR, et al: The effects of phenytoin on impulsive and premeditated aggression: a controlled study. J Clin Psychopharmacol 17:341–349, 1997

Beauford JE, McNiel DE, Binder RL: Utility of the initial therapeutic alliance in evaluating psychiatric patients' risk of violence. Am J Psychiatry 154:1272–1276, 1997

Binder RL, McNiel DE: Effects of diagnosis and context on dangerousness. Am J Psychiatry 145:728–732, 1988

Carmel H, Hunter M: Staff injuries from inpatient violence. Hosp Community Psychiatry 40:41–46, 1989

Cheung P, Schweitzer I, Crowley K, et al: Violence in schizophrenia: role of hallucinations and delusions. Schizophr Res 26:181–190, 1997

Chou KR, Lu RB, Mao WC: Factors relevant to patient assaultive behavior and assault in acute inpatient psychiatric units in Taiwan. Arch Psychiatr Nurs 16:187–195, 2002

Convit A, Jaeger J, Lin SP, et al: Predicting assaultiveness in psychiatric inpatients: a pilot study. Hosp Community Psychiatry 39:429–434, 1988

Convit A, Isay D, Otis D, et al: Characteristics of repeatedly assaultive psychiatric inpatients. Hosp Community Psychiatry 41:1112–1115, 1990

Coyne A: Should patients who assault staff be prosecuted? J Psychiatr Ment Health Nurs 9:139–145, 2002

Dinwiddie SH, Briska W: Prosecution of violent psychiatric inpatients: theoretical and practical issues. Int J Law Psychiatry 27:17–29, 2004

Duxbury J: An evaluation of staff and patient views of and strategies employed to manage inpatient aggression and violence on one mental health unit: a pluralistic design. J Psychiatr Ment Health Nurs 9:325–337, 2002

Flannery RB Jr, Hanson MA, Penk W: Patients' threats: expanded definition of assault. Gen Hosp Psychiatry 17:451–453, 1995

Flannery RB Jr, Hanson MA, Penk WE, et al: Replicated declines in assault rates after implementation of the Assaulted Staff Action Program. Psychiatr Serv 49:241–243, 1998

Flannery RB Jr, Stone P, Rego S, et al: Characteristics of staff victims of patient assault: ten year analysis of the Assaulted Staff Action Program (ASAP). Psychiatr Q 72:237–248, 2001

Forster PL, Cavness C, Phelps MA: Staff training decreases use of seclusion and restraint in an acute psychiatric hospital. Arch Psychiatr Nurs 13:269–271, 1999

Frueh BC, Knapp RG, Cusack KJ, et al: Patients' reports of traumatic or harmful experiences within the psychiatric setting. Psychiatr Serv 56:1123–1133, 2005

Hill CD, Rogers R, Bickford ME: Predicting aggressive and socially disruptive behavior in a maximum security forensic psychiatric hospital. J Forensic Sci 41:56–59, 1996

Hoge SK, Gutheil TG: The prosecution of psychiatric patients for assaults on staff: a preliminary empirical study. Hosp Community Psychiatry 38:44–49, 1987

Hoptman MJ, Yates KF, Patalinjug MB, et al: Clinical prediction of assaultive behavior among male psychiatric patients at a maximum-security forensic facility. Psychiatr Serv 50:1461–1466, 1999

Johnson ME, Hauser PM: The practices of expert psychiatric nurses: accompanying the patient to a calmer personal space. Issues Ment Health Nurs 22:651–668, 2001

Kaltiala-Heino R, Tuohimaki C, Korkeila J, et al: Reasons for using seclusion and restraint in psychiatric inpatient care. Int J Law Psychiatry 26:139–149, 2003

Katz P, Kirkland FR: Violence and social structure on mental hospital wards. Psychiatry 53:262–277, 1990

Krakowski M, Czobor P: Violence in psychiatric patients: the role of psychosis, frontal lobe impairment, and ward turmoil. Compr Psychiatry 38:230–236, 1997

Krakowski M, Convit A, Jaeger J, et al: Neurological impairment in violent schizophrenic inpatients. Am J Psychiatry 146:849–853, 1989

Krakowski M, Czobor P, Chou JC: Course of violence in patients with schizophrenia: relationship to clinical symptoms. Schizophr Bull 25:505–517, 1999

Kraus JE, Sheitman BB: Characteristics of violent behavior in a large state psychiatric hospital. Psychiatr Serv 55:183–185, 2004

Lam JN, McNiel DE, Binder RL: The relationship between patients' gender and violence leading to staff injuries. Psychiatr Serv 51:1167–1170, 2000

Lanza ML, Kayne HL, Hicks C, et al: Environmental characteristics related to patient assault. Issues Ment Health Nurs 15:319–335, 1994

Lanza ML, Kayne HL, Pattison I, et al: The relationship of behavioral cues to assaultive behavior. Clin Nurs Res 5:6–27, 1996

Lehmann LS, McCormick RA, Kizer KW: A survey of assaultive behavior in Veterans Health Administration facilities. Psychiatr Serv 50:384–389, 1999

Linaker OM, Busch-Iversen H: Predictors of imminent violence in psychiatric inpatients. Acta Psychiatr Scand 92:250–254, 1995

Love CC, Hunter ME: Violence in public sector psychiatric hospitals: benchmarking nursing staff injury rates. J Psychosoc Nurs Ment Health Serv 34:30–34, 1996

Maier GJ: Managing threatening behavior: the role of talk down and talk up. J Psychosoc Nurs Ment Health Serv 34:25–30, 1996

Manfredini R, Vanni A, Peron L, et al: Day-night variation in aggressive behavior among psychiatric inpatients. Chronobiol Int 18:503–511, 2001

McNiel DE, Binder RL: Relationship between preadmission threats and later violent behavior by acute psychiatric inpatients. Hosp Community Psychiatry 40:605–608, 1989

McNiel DE, Binder RL: The relationship between acute psychiatric symptoms, diagnosis, and short-term risk of violence. Hosp Community Psychiatry 45:133–137, 1994

McNiel DE, Binder RL, Greenfield TK: Predictors of violence in civilly committed acute psychiatric patients. Am J Psychiatry 145:965–970, 1988

McNiel DE, Eisner JP, Binder RL: The relationship between command hallucinations and violence. Psychiatr Serv 51:1288–1292, 2000

McNiel DE, Gregory AL, Lam JN, et al: Utility of decision support tools for assessing acute risk of violence. J Consult Clin Psychol 71:945–953, 2003

Meloy JR: The prediction of violence in outpatient psychotherapy. Am J Psychother 41:38–45, 1987

Miller RD, Maier GJ: Factors affecting the decision to prosecute mental patients for criminal behavior. Hosp Community Psychiatry 38:50–55, 1987

Miller RJ, Zadolinnyj K, Hafner RJ: Profiles and predictors of assaultiveness for different psychiatric ward populations. Am J Psychiatry 150:1368–1373, 1993

Monahan J, Steadman HJ, Silver E, et al: Violence and the clinician: assessing and managing risk, in Rethinking Risk Assessment: The MacArthur Study of Mental Disorder and Violence. New York, Oxford University Press, 2001, pp 129–143

Nijman H, Merckelbach H, Evers C, et al: Prediction of aggression on a locked psychiatric admissions ward. Acta Psychiatr Scand 105:390–395, 2002

Nolan KA, Czobor P, Roy BB, et al: Characteristics of assaultive behavior among psychiatric inpatients. Psychiatr Serv 54:1012–1016, 2003

Nolan KA, Volavka J, Czobor P, et al: Aggression and psychopathology in treatment-resistant inpatients with schizophrenia and schizoaffective disorder. J Psychiatr Res 39:109–115, 2005

Norko MA, Zonana HV, Phillips RT: Prosecuting assaultive psychiatric inpatients. Hosp Community Psychiatry 42:193–194, 1991

Quanbeck CD, McDermott BE, Lam J, et al: Categorization of aggressive acts committed by chronically assaultive state hospital patients. Psychiatr Serv 58:521–528, 2007

Quintal SA: Violence against psychiatric nurses: an untreated epidemic? J Psychosoc Nurs Ment Health Serv 40:46–53, 2002

Ray CL, Subich LM: Staff assaults and injuries in a psychiatric hospital as a function of three attitudinal variables. Issues Ment Health Nurs 19:277–289, 1998

Reid WH, Gacono C: Treatment of antisocial personality, psychopathy, and other characterologic antisocial syndromes. Behav Sci Law 18:647–662, 2000

Schwarz CJ, Greenfield GP: Charging a patient with assault of a nurse on a psychiatric unit. Can Psychiatr Assoc J 23:197–200, 1978

Secker J, Benson A, Balfe E, et al: Understanding the social context of violent and aggressive incidents on an inpatient unit. J Psychiatr Ment Health Nurs 11:172–178, 2004

Smith GM, Davis RH, Bixler EO, et al: Pennsylvania State Hospital system's seclusion and restraint reduction program. Psychiatr Serv 56:1115–1122, 2005

Soliman AE, Reza H: Risk factors and correlates of violence among acutely ill adult psychiatric inpatients. Psychiatr Serv 52:75–80, 2001

Steinert T: Prediction of inpatient violence. Acta Psychiatr Scand Suppl 412:133–141, 2002

Swanson JW, Holzer CE III, Ganju VK, et al: Violence and psychiatric disorder in the community: evidence from the Epidemiologic Catchment Area surveys. Hosp Community Psychiatry 41:761–770, 1990

Swanson JW, Swartz MS, Van Dorn RA, et al: A national study of violent behavior in persons with schizophrenia. Arch Gen Psychiatry 63:490–499, 2006

Swett C, Mills T: Use of the NOSIE to predict assaults among acute psychiatric patients: Nurses' Observational Scale for Inpatient Evaluation. Psychiatr Serv 48:1177–1180, 1997

Tardiff K: The risk of being attacked by patients: who, how often, and where? in Patient Violence and the Clinician. Edited by Eichelman BS, Hartwig AC. Washington, DC, American Psychiatric Press, 1995, pp 13–32

Tardiff K, Sweillam A: Assaultive behavior among chronic inpatients. Am J Psychiatry 139:212–215, 1982

Turkington D, Kingdon D, Weiden PJ: Cognitive behavior therapy for schizophrenia. Am J Psychiatry 163:365–373, 2006

Volavka J, Czobor P, Nolan K, et al: Overt aggression and psychotic symptoms in patients with schizophrenia treated with clozapine, olanzapine, risperidone, or haloperidol. J Clin Psychopharmacol 24:225–228, 2004

Weinshenker N, Siegel A: Bimodal classification of aggression: affective defense and predatory attack. Aggression and Violent Behavior 7:237–250, 2002

Whittington R, Patterson P: Verbal and non-verbal behavior immediately prior to aggression by mentally disordered people: enhancing the assessment of risk. J Psychiatr Ment Health Nurs 3:47–54, 1996

Whittington R, Wykes T: Aversive stimulation by staff and violence by psychiatric patients. Br J Clin Psychol 35:11–20, 1996

Woodworth M, Porter S: In cold blood: characteristics of criminal homicides as a function of psychopathy. J Abnorm Psychol 111:436–445, 2002

CHAPTER 14

Emergency Services

Jean-Pierre Lindenmayer, M.D.
Anzalee Khan, M.S.

Psychiatric emergency services (PESs) usually provide a systematic care process in which patients who present psychiatric emergencies are optimally evaluated and managed. A *psychiatric emergency* is defined as a disturbance in thoughts, feelings, or behaviors for which immediate assessment and treatment are necessary. An emergency can not only be declared by the care delivery system but also by the patient, family, community, or a friend who may present the patient as having an emergency. Staff in the emergency setting will then assess and attend to the patient and decide on a course of action to further ascertain the problem and its origins. The systematic care process includes sequential steps such as assessment, problem identification, treatment planning, interventions, ongoing monitoring, and discharge. However, resolution of the emergency usually does not occur in the emergency setting itself; most often it is post-emergency care that leads to resolution.

PESs usually consist of acute hospital-based psychiatric service delivery models that are available for mental health emergencies. They are generally open 24 hours a day in the United States and in some form or other in most developed countries. In the United States the 1963 Community Mental Health Act mandated emergency psychiatric care as one of "five essential services" in all federally funded community mental health service systems (Gerson and Bassuk 1980). Such a service was believed to be critical "to prevent unnecessary [re]hospitalizations that might, in turn, foster chronicity and dependence on institutional care" (Solomon and Gordon 1986–1987, pp. 119–120).

Bassuk and Gerson (1979) suggested that the PES's role was to "reconcile the complex needs of the local population with the traditional organizational structure of [local treatment options]" (p. 35), suggesting that definitions of appropriate use of such services should include a broad array of treatments. A competing and classically medical-surgical viewpoint is that these costly services ought to be reserved for those who legitimately cannot wait for psychiatric intake appointments. This perspective would suggest that a narrow definition of "emergency" conditions is more appropriate to justify help-seeking in the PES, perhaps including only illness episodes "characterized by surprise, time constraints, high stakes, and pressure for action" (Murdach 1987, pp. 268–269). That definition is supported, in part, by a 1988 review of psychiatric decision making in the emergency department (Marson et al. 1988), which concluded that acuteness of symptoms and inherent dangerousness, such as acute aggressive or agitated states, were the variables that most strongly predicted the decision to hospitalize.

The service delivery model for providing hospital-based PES appears to vary widely by site and state. Some hospital emergency departments in large urban areas have designated separate areas for handling psychiatric patients; such areas often are linked to a 24- or 72-hour holding facility for patients requiring extended observation. As an example of such expanded services, New York State has introduced the Comprehensive Psychiatric Emergency Program (CPEPs), which provides a range of psychiatric emergency services including brief overnight observation stays. These programs coordinate the delivery of a full range of psychiatric crisis and emergency care within a distinct geographic area. Such programs are required to provide four components of service: hospital-based crisis intervention, extended-observation beds, mobile crisis outreach services, and crisis residences. These integrated programs attempt to alleviate the overcrowding in emergency rooms, provide alternatives to inpatient admissions, and maintain a community-based focus. The objectives are to provide crisis intervention in the community—consisting of timely triage, assessment, intervention, and links to other community-based mental health services—and to control inpatient admissions.

Smaller facilities utilize referral to an on-call mental health specialist as needed but maintain the patient in the general emergency department population. Regardless of the service delivery model used, research indicates that hospital-based PES facilities receive a broad array of service requests, many of which at times appear to be nonemergent

Emergency Services

(Kooiman et al. 1989; Oyewumi et al. 1992; Vaslamatzis et al. 1987; Vigiser et al. 1984), such as requests for social services, requests for treatment of substance abuse, or referral requests for psychological treatments.

The following types of services are included in PES:

- Psychiatric treatment to stabilize and/or ameliorate acute symptoms of mental illness/emotional crisis
- Evaluation and referral for inpatient psychiatric hospitalization
- Medical screening and referral to acute medical services
- Continued observation and assessment in the Extended Observation Unit
- Transfer to other facilities for further assessment and/or care
- Referral to an outpatient facility and/or treatment program
- Referral to assistance in resolving a situational crisis
- Evaluations for patients of private practitioners, psychiatrists, social workers, counselors (second opinion) in crisis situations. The patient is referred back to the primary therapist.

Case Example 1:
An Agitated Patient and the Delivery of Emergency Psychiatric Care

Initial evaluation. A 24-year-old male is brought by the local police and ambulance to an emergency psychiatric facility within a medical emergency setting for bizarre and uncontrolled behavior at home. His mother had contacted the police because she was afraid for her life and that of her son. She reported that he had not slept for the past 3 nights, was not eating, and was pacing the apartment "damning people to hell" and stating "God is here." He had begun to throw plates, glasses, and furniture around the apartment. The patient also admitted to visual hallucinations of seeing God in the shape of a white male. Both mother and patient denied any drug use. The patient had no prior medical history, was not on any medications, and had no allergies. He was initially evaluated by the emergency psychiatric nurse, who also interviewed the mother. The nurse reported that the patient did not have any significant past psychotic episodes or hospitalizations, and she referred him to be seen by the medical doctor and the psychiatrist.

Medical evaluation. The patient's physical examination results were within normal limits, as was his laboratory workup.

Psychiatric evaluation. The patient was examined by the psychiatrist and psychiatric resident. The psychiatric assessment resulted in the diagnosis of acute schizophrenic episode. Following the diagnosis, the patient was referred to a social worker and case manager on staff for further evaluation of available support structures and past history, which he refused, saying, "The people here are going to kill me." One staff member with whom he had bonded convinced the patient that no harm would come to him. However, the patient refused to be further examined and instead paced up and down the hallway outside yelling, "God is here, come and get me." The emergency department psychiatrist recommended that the patient be admitted to the inpatient psychiatric facility for observation because he was thought to present a risk of harm to himself or others. A short-acting intramuscular antipsychotic for his agitated behavior was prescribed. The patient eventually agreed to take the medication and to go to the inpatient psychiatric unit.

Psychiatric Emergency Services Delivery Models

Psychiatric Emergency Room

The psychiatric emergency room is a key component of a PES. Its primary function is the care of "true emergency" psychiatric patients who are acutely distressed and disturbed, with rapidly changing mental status situations. Brief intake evaluation, crisis intervention, and appropriate subsequent referral are the primary tasks of this service.

The emergency room is usually housed in easily accessible, fairly spacious quarters. An appropriately structured psychiatric emergency room will usually provide a quiet environment and procedures to manage patients who may want to escape; who would require restraint or seclusion because of dangerous, assaultive behavior; and who may want to harm themselves (Allen 2002). A typical emergency room has several different areas, each specialized for patients with particular severities of psychiatric illness, as described in the following paragraphs.

In the *triage area*, patients receive a preliminary evaluation by psychiatry-trained nurses and/or psychiatric social workers. After triage, patients are usually taken directly to one of four functional treatment areas based on the nature of the emergency: nonthreatening psychiatric emergencies, life-threatening psychiatric emergencies, extremely agitated behavior requiring physical restraint, or extremely agitated behavior requiring seclusion. Suicidal patients may bypass triage and are seen directly by the emergency room psychiatrist.

The *seclusion area* is an important area of an emergency room. There may be separate rooms for voluntary and unlocked seclusion, often termed a "quiet room," as well as locked seclusion rooms and available restraint. The seclusion rooms should have no furniture or accessories and have visual observational capacity for the staff.

The *general medical area* is for stable patients who still need to be followed-up but may not pose a serious physical threat. This area usually contains several interviewing rooms that offer privacy but are in close proximity to ancillary staff as well as a physical examination room with life safety equipment. The surrounding area is often very busy, filled with patients with a wide range of psychiatric problems. Many will require further investigation and possible admission. Patients who are not in need of immediate treatment are sent to a different area to await disposition or discharge.

Generally, a PES within a hospital should be designed to increase overall efficiency while providing a calming, open setting that minimizes the crowded environment and resulting anxiety that often characterize emergency visits. Emergency rooms should be focused on maximum patient privacy and optimum comfort because these features are essential for an emergency psychiatric patient. This can be enhanced by aesthetically pleasing design features throughout the emergency room, such as an interior glass wall between waiting and patient registration areas to provide a sense of security to the staff and a monitoring capability of the entire emergency area.

An efficient emergency room layout is important to the rapid administration of services. The following design features should be available: 1) separate entrances for life-threatening emergencies, such as threats of suicide and self-harm; 2) entry/registration/waiting/triage functions located in close proximity to one another to decrease distance; and 3) entrances to patient interview rooms that allow maximum access by psychiatric and medical staff for patients to be taken directly to the treatment areas. It is very important to note that all doors should have locks but that doors are usually kept open to avoid creating a sense of crowding for paranoid patients. All sharp objects should be out of the reach of patients and their families. Articles of furniture should be installed so as to prevent them from being used as a weapon. Additional comfort is provided by appropriate reading materials, televisions, and availability of telephones. Televisions and telephones should be secured to their respective structures, and the television should be out of the reach of patients.

There also needs to be an area where safety personnel, usually local police officers, can wait while the paperwork for patients whom they have brought to the emergency room is being processed. A cardinal rule is that no loaded weapons can be brought in by law enforcement officers. Most emergency departments also have their own safety officer supervising the waiting and examination areas.

Goals of the Psychiatric Emergency Room

The psychiatric emergency room acts as a central assessment and acute treatment agency with the possibility of referrals to various mental, medical, and social services. The emergency services branch out to the inpatient admissions service, all outpatient clinics, day programs, and, if possible, to case management systems, transitional housing, and substance abuse treatment programs. The mere presence of a receptive and helpful PES is often a tremendous relief to these other services and their patients. Thus the psychiatric emergency room is able to facilitate patients' connecting or reconnecting with various services without the complexity of an inpatient admission. However, in many circumstances inpatient admission is still indicated. An admission to inpatient services should not be construed as a failure of the emergency team.

Staff

Most large emergency rooms include a number of psychiatrists (M.D.s) and at times psychiatric residents, registered nurses (R.N.s), psychologists (Ph.D.s), social workers (M.S.W.s), psychiatric technicians (e.g., hospital orderlies), clerical staff, and security officers. PES staff should be trained in making thorough assessments of patients' problems and in identifying appropriate dispositions and referrals. To conduct these assessments, Summers and Happell (2002) argued that the psychiatric nurses may be a core service provider in the emergency room. Similarly, Osborne (2003) and McDonough et al. (2004) reported that the use of a mental health triage nurse reduced lengthy waiting times and crowding in waiting rooms. In addition, studies found that the use of psychiatric triage scales contributed to reduced wait times, more efficient and effective treatment of mental health patients, and improved referral to appropriate resources (Broadbent et al. 2004; Happell et al. 2002).

A key focus of PES staff is the safe management of the psychiatric and behavioral emergencies. Staff should be trained in emergency procedures, including seclusion and physical restraint. Trained safety officers should also be present and should be under the supervision of the psychiatrist and medical and nursing personnel.

The psychiatric emergency team is led by the psychiatrist. This leadership position is built on the specific medical-psychiatric diagnostic background and the psychopharmacological expertise of the psychiatrist. However, many psychiatric emergency rooms, particularly those that do not offer comprehensive services, cannot provide continuous coverage by a psychiatrist (Allen 1999). Consequently, psychiatric nurses, social workers, and at times trained psychologists will provide crisis intervention and emergency psychotherapy, if necessary.

Most psychiatric emergency rooms also have a physician available to evaluate psychiatric emergencies with a medical component. This is particularly important in medical emergencies that may have been misidentified as a psychiatric emergency by the patient, friend, or family member. A general medical evaluation should be assured for all registered patients. When specific medical conditions are identified, it is important to have rapid access to appropriate medical care. Thus it is advantageous to have the psychiatric emergency room contiguous to the medical emergency department and to have policies in place concerning the movement of patients and consultants between these two services. Good communication between the medical staff and the psychiatric staff is also important (McClelland 1983).

Flow of Assessments in the Emergency Room

The process for determining patient needs in psychiatric emergency rooms optimally includes six steps (Coristine et al. 2007):

1. A person arriving in the PES undergoes triage for mental health complaints by an emergency room nurse using standardized risk assessment criteria (e.g., Mental Health Triage Scale or the National Triage Scale [Dreyfus 1987]) or another standardized triage procedure.
2. If the person threatens to hurt him- or herself or others, or if the person is at risk for escape or for violence to others, he or she should be seen immediately by the emergency room psychiatrist.
3. If none of the risks in item 2 is present, a triage assessment is conducted, including recording a complete set of vital signs, history of significant mental illness, medical history, recent history of alcohol or substance abuse, disorientation, clouding of consciousness, appearance of intoxication with alcohol or drugs, malnourishment, unkempt appearance, or any other concerns of a medical nature.
4. If the assessment confirms the presence of any of these signs, the person is triaged to be medically assessed by the emergency department physician. Once the person is medically cleared, the emergency medical doctor will refer him or her for more intensive mental health assessment by the psychiatrist in conjunction with the PES team. This team then provides a full mental assessment and the most appropriate disposition, such as discharge, referral to an outpatient program, admission to an inpatient unit, or transfer to another facility.
5. If all observations are negative, the patient is fast-tracked to the case worker or social worker, who screens the patient about problems with housing, finances, legal issues, or social supports. The case worker or social worker conducts an assessment and reports to the

emergency room psychiatrist regarding referral to appropriate community resources.
6. Case worker or social worker referrals may be made to any of several community mental health agencies that provide case management, housing, social supports, and crisis management services.

Extended Services

Research on PES delivery systems has documented persistent growth in demand, with concomitant increased pressure on psychiatric emergency room operations and personnel. Factors contributing to this demand are the shift to the community mental health service delivery model and the reduction of available long-term inpatient beds in state psychiatric facilities; insufficient community mental health supports; and recidivism among people with persistent mental illness identified as socially disadvantaged (Ellison and Blum 1986; Smart et al. 1999; Solomon and Davis 1985). The delineation of these factors provides the arena in which to test new PES delivery strategies, such as the introduction of Assertive Community Treatment teams and Intensive Case Management models, liaison with community agencies (Sundheim and Ryan 1999), and utilization of psychiatric nurses to create an integrated care pathway (Wynaden et al. 2003).

Case Example 2:
Psychiatric Evaluation in an Emergency Setting

Initial symptoms. A day after his prison release, Mr. A became agitated at home and began staring at others and not communicating. Upon registration at the PES, and after initial review by the nurse, he was seen by the psychiatric resident. He reported that other people could read his mind and broadcast his thoughts. He also reported that he heard voices outside his window at home telling him that he was "not a good man" and would "not succeed." Mr. A also reported that he heard his neighbors talking about him. He had threatened and confronted some individuals, which resulted in an altercation.

Past history. Mr. A had no history of psychiatric symptoms or legal problems until his early 40s, when he was incarcerated for a nonviolent offense for 6 months. During the incarceration, his mental status deteriorated. He began exhibiting depression, ideas of hopelessness, and paranoid delusions. He was hospitalized in the prison infirmary and treated with venlafaxine and haloperidol, with subsequent stabilization. He was released after serving his full sentence.

Initial examination. Mr. A was noted to be staring blankly without looking at the interviewer. His speech was monosyllabic. He showed marked psychomotor retardation, and he made negativistic statements about his life. He denied experiencing auditory hallucinations. He was oriented to time, place, and person but had poor insight and judgment.

Treatment and course of illness. Mr. A was given an evaluation including the Mini-Mental State Examination and the Structured Guide for the Assessment of Violence. His cognitive status was reported as "fair." Mr. A was seen by the emergency psychiatrist, who conferred with the nurse. A diagnosis of psychotic depression was made. Mr. A was hospitalized in the 72-hour bed service program at the emergency psychiatric facility and began antidepressant and antipsychotic pharmacotherapy. Mr. A's mental status improved progressively after the first day, and he became cooperative and well groomed. His condition began to deteriorate at day 3, when he again reported that he was "not a good person" and that people were threatening him. He also reported auditory hallucinations, primarily in the evening. Mr. A was admitted to the inpatient unit. After 3 weeks of treatment, his condition stabilized and he was discharged to a residential facility.

Extended Psychiatric Observation Services

Extended psychiatric observation services typically use a designated short length of stay to stabilize and observe patients with unclear and unstable psychiatric presentations. These units are most often integrated in the PES, are small in size, and may offer a length of stay between 24 hours and 3 days. Several studies have suggested that most patients admitted to these programs show improvement in the severity of their psychiatric symptoms, are able to be discharged in the designated time frame, express high satisfaction with the program (Schneider and Ross 1996), and have a low rehospitalization rate (Allen 2002; Rhine and Mayerson 1971; Weisman et al. 1969). These observation beds are often used as an adjunct to the initial psychiatric emergency room evaluation; patients needing definitive psychiatric hospitalization will be transferred to a separate inpatient facility for hospitalization of several days or weeks.

The option of offering brief admission to short-stay beds within a PES provides a model that meets a variety of patient and system needs. Brief admission within a PES 1) allows emergency staff more time to develop alternatives to hospitalization or gain diagnostic clarity; 2) enables difficult patients to remain in the community by offering respite for both the patient and community providers; 3) provides selected patients with a setting that does not gratify dependency needs in the same manner as a hospital stay might; and 4) makes available a targeted treatment modality for patients whose presenting symptomatology can be ameliorated within a brief period of time (e.g., those who become disorganized following an acute stressor). However, a key admission criterion for such short-term PES units is that the patient be cooperative and voluntary. Involuntary admission can only be done to an acute inpatient admissions unit. The main emphasis of such units is on maintaining patients' functioning in and ties to the community. Herz et al. (1979), in a series of papers, developed the idea that the results of brief hospitalization can be comparable with standard hospitalization, with the advantage of fostering less regression and better maintenance of community survival skills.

Observations

Several different models exist for short-term observation assessment and stabilization units, including the 23-hour observation bed, the crisis stabilization unit, and the 72-hour observation bed. Such units are usually in close proximity to PESs.

23-Hour Observation Bed, Psychiatric

A 23-hour observation bed is a facility-based crisis stabilization unit that provides a medically safe environment for a limited period of up to 23 hours for individuals experiencing a crisis or acute psychiatric emergency condition. Individuals are monitored, assessed, and evaluated to ensure appropriate care and disposition within the given time period. The observation facility is located in the emergency department and is configured to provide primary emergency care during periods of peak demand. It provides rapid resolution of many crises (e.g., filtering of substance use emergencies [Breslow et al. 1996]).

Crisis Stabilization Unit

The crisis stabilization unit is generally a small unit located adjacent to the emergency department. The service provides extended 24-hour observation, treatment, and support up to a total of 72 hours for patients seen in the emergency department. The purpose of a crisis stabilization unit is to stabilize and redirect a client to the most appropriate and least restrictive community setting available, consistent with the client's needs. Crisis stabilization units may screen, assess, and admit for stabilization those persons who present themselves to the unit on a voluntary basis or who are brought to the unit. Patients are referred to the crisis stabilization unit by a physician or psychiatrist at the emergency department. A multidisciplinary treatment team including physicians, registered nurses, licensed clinicians, and mental health technicians provide the patient with the following:

Emergency Services

- Crisis intervention/stabilization
- Psychiatric nursing assessment
- Physical assessments
- Medication/somatic services
- 24-hour observation
- Individual and group counseling
- Linkage and referrals to longer-term services
- Education for safe return to the community

A client's discharge from the crisis stabilization unit is based on his or her self-assessment and a clinically appropriate disposition reached by the treatment team.

Case Example 3: Extended Observation

Initial assessment. Mr. B is a 38-year-old man with three prior psychiatric hospitalizations with the diagnosis of major depression, the last having been 2 months prior to his admission to the extended observation unit. A conflict with his mother more than a year ago led to a suicidal episode in which Mr. B took various prescription drugs and was subsequently hospitalized. After discharge, and prior to the emergency department presentation, Mr. B had frequent episodes of anxiety and suicidal ideation during which he reported wanting to die. He would buy "all the drugs he could find." In addition to his psychiatric follow-up, Mr. B was followed up by a social worker who immediately took the patient to the psychiatric emergency room, where he was again evaluated. His physical and neurological evaluation, magnetic resonance imaging scans, and electroencephalogram were all negative.

Psychiatric evaluation. The emergency room psychiatrist concluded that Mr. B would be a danger to himself and decided to keep him in the 72-hour extended observation unit. During his time in the unit, Mr. B received antidepressant pharmacotherapy. He responded well to both the antidepressant and psychotherapy. After discharge he was followed up at the outpatient psychiatric clinic. Two months after discharge Mr. B developed an acute paranoid episode with suicidal and homicidal ideation during which he believed that his mother was coming to find him and hurt him for not calling her while he was in the hospital. Mr. B's psychiatrist again recommended admission to the extended observation unit that had previously worked so well for him. Mr. B was admitted to the unit, and antipsychotic medication was added to his regimen. He was greatly relieved by the availability of this additional support (psychotherapy, psychiatric follow-up, and observation) to help him control himself. During his stay in the unit, his paranoid symptoms markedly improved and the suicidal and homicidal ideas resolved. Mr. B agreed to remain on his antipsychotic medication and was discharged to return to his psychiatric follow-up.

72-Hour Observation Bed, Psychiatric

Only designated personnel in a psychiatric emergency setting can place a person in a 72-hour mental health hold. Such personnel include police officers, members of a "mobile crisis team," or other mental health professionals authorized by their county. One of three conditions must be present for an individual to be placed on a 72-hour hold. The designated personnel must believe there is probable cause that, due to a psychiatric disorder, the individual is 1) a danger to him- or herself; 2) a danger to others; or 3) gravely disabled (unable to provide for his or her basic personal needs for food, clothing, or shelter).

The person placed in a 72-hour hold must be advised of his or her rights. Most facilities require an application stating the circumstances under which the person's condition was called to the attention of the professional; what probable cause there is to believe the person is a danger to self or others or is gravely disabled (due to a mental disorder); and the facts upon which this probable cause is based. Mere conclusions without supporting facts are not sufficient. When a person is detained for up to 72 hours, the hospital is required to do an evaluation, taking into account the patient's medical, psychological, educational, social, financial, and legal situation. The hospital does not have to hold the patient for the full 72 hours if it is thought that the patient no longer requires evaluation or treatment. By the end of the 72 hours, one of the following must happen:

- The person is released;
- The person signs in as a voluntary patient to the hospital; or
- The person is put on a 14-day involuntary hold (a "certification for intensive treatment"), the structure of which will depend on the local mental hygiene state laws.

A mental health patient being held involuntarily must be informed of his or her rights in a language or manner that he or she can understand, in accordance with the local laws.

In addition, the patient has the right to be informed fully of the risks and benefits of the proposed treatment and to give his or her informed consent to the treatment. A patient has the right to refuse medication unless there is an emergency condition or the patient is found to lack capacity to make an informed decision after a judicial hearing. If a patient is found in a hearing to lack capacity to consent to medication, the judge may then order medication over the patient's objection (Oldham and DeMasi 1995; Weisman et al. 1969). In recent years, in New York State,

13%–15% of all patients in an emergency psychiatric service have been admitted to extended observation units (Allen 2002).

Psychiatric Emergency Services in the Community

Community services providers may offer short-term case management services to psychiatric patients who have been seen in the psychiatric emergency department. These services (usually funded by municipal, county, private, or hospital-affiliated providers) include

- Availability of crisis residences and mobile response teams
- Outreach
- Help with basic needs (food, clothing, emergency housing, identification)
- Assistance in connecting or reconnecting with healthcare and mental healthcare providers and programs
- Counseling and support

Crisis Residence

A crisis residence offers a supervised residential setting for persons requiring extended stabilization during a mental health crisis. The expected length of stay could be up to 21 days. Crisis beds are usually linked to local psychiatric emergency rooms and acute inpatient programs. Follow-up care is provided after discharge by community resources and supports. The major goal of crisis residences is to stabilize the situation and return the patient to his or her home quickly, rather than to provide long-term care. Emphasis is on maintaining the relationships the patient has in the community, with family, the referral agency, and with those resources that have provided services previously. Services that can be provided in the community will not be duplicated in the residence. Each program provides a highly structured, individually designed intervention for each resident in accordance with the needs of patients.

Crisis Response Services

Persons with serious and long-term psychiatric illness may experience recurrent crises even when comprehensive and continuous community support services are available. As a result, the capacity to provide crisis assistance is a critical aspect of a community support system. Crisis response services have 24 hours a day, 7 days a week telephone services to provide counseling and support to relieve a crisis situation. If a face-to-face contact is indicated, these services refer a trained professional to visit the patient/client in the community.

Crisis response services assist individuals to alleviate and resolve emotional distress or situational disturbances that affect their ability to cope. The goals of a crisis response service are to use the least intrusive, most effective intervention to provide immediate support, information, and referrals; to facilitate problem solving to assist in the alleviation of a mental health crisis; and to develop an intervention plan with individuals in crisis that meets their needs, mobilizes their strengths and resources, and averts hospitalization and contact with police.

Crisis Respite

Crisis respite is the lowest level of treatment intensity in the crisis residence program. The crisis respite programs serve patients with housing problems. Sledge et al. (1996) described an arrangement linking respite with day hospitalization programs designed for the severely and persistently mentally ill. The respite component provides housing for up to four clients, using mental health workers and Master's-level program directors.

Mobile Crisis Intervention Team

A mobile crisis intervention team (MCIT) program partners a mental health professional and a police officer who respond to 911 emergency and police dispatch calls involving emotionally disturbed persons. The goal of the MCIT is to enable individuals experiencing a psychiatric crisis or distress to access a range of crisis intervention services in a timely and effective manner in their own environment or the environment of their choice. An additional goal is to provide a consistent integrated response to a psychiatric crisis in the community, regardless of which service identifies the individual in crisis. MCIT also serves to improve overall capacity of the community to address the concerns of individuals experiencing a mental health crisis at their living site, through provision of support, information, and education to caregivers. MCIT usually coordinates response to an emergency call with the PES to support and triage over the phone and through mobile visits. The services offered include

- Assessment of the presenting crisis, current supports, and resources
- Supportive, collaborative planning for solution-focused options
- Referral to appropriate follow-up services
- Consultation/advocacy with existing supports and services
- Short-term crisis management as necessary

Although mobile crisis models overlap to some extent, they also differ in terms of readiness, tactical training, equipment, and cross-training of police in psychiatric techniques and vice versa. Stroul (1993) found that 80% of mobile crisis models were accessible on a 24-hour basis. These services can cover wide areas and may be particularly useful in rural communities where mental health services are distant (Allen 2002).

Assessment Issues in the Emergency Setting

Safety Considerations

One of the main goals of PESs is safety; the evaluating clinician and patients must be safe. At a minimum, patients must have been searched and disarmed before meeting with the evaluating clinician in the psychiatric emergency room. A clear route of rapid egress from the examination room must be ensured, and security personnel must be available, ideally through a panic button or other communication means. Safety considerations may require that the patient be in restraints or that a physical barrier be present between patient and clinician. In addition to the patient's history and presentation, the clinician's own experience and anxiety level ought to be among the determining factors in deciding the extent of safety precautions in place during a particular evaluation.

The importance of a full assessment of the patient to ensure safety cannot be overstated. In the case of a suicidal patient, a determination of what will keep the patient safe must be made as soon as possible. In the patient with acute psychosis, medical comorbidities and substance abuse should be considered early in the differential diagnosis and treated (Buckley 1994).

Seclusion and Restraints

Seclusion

Seclusion can be useful for agitated patients and external stimulation; it also allows the patient a period of "time-out" to regain behavioral control. A seclusion room must be safe and free of objects that could be used to injure self or others. Medical conditions that are unstable and require close physical interactions or monitoring preclude the use of seclusion. Only staff who have been trained in using seclusion techniques are authorized to implement the procedure. At first the door can remain open, but if the patient continues to be agitated, the door is locked for safety. The patient must always be aware of the consequences of his or her behavior and be given periodic opportunities to comply with defined behavioral parameters in order to be released from seclusion. Medications can be offered to avoid further restrictive measures. Patients in seclusion should be monitored by closed-circuit television if possible. Seclusion is always time limited, depending on the local mental health policies; usually the duration does not exceed 4 hours, after which the patient has to be reevaluated by the physician and a new order has to be written. For patients under age 18 this duration is reduced to 2 hours. During seclusion or restraints, staff is required to conduct 15-minute checks to assess vital signs, any signs of injury, and the patient's psychological state and readiness to discontinue seclusion or restraints. Staff must clearly document in the medical record the need for seclusion, intervening steps, and medications given (Hill and Petit 2002).

Restraints

The implementation of restraints is a difficult procedure, but an important option, generally reserved for those situations in which there is the potential for imminent harm to patient or staff through patients' behavior and where other interventions of a lesser degree of intensity and restrictiveness have been unsuccessful. The specific definition by the Joint Commission for the Accreditation of Healthcare Organizations (JCAHO; 2002, p. 123) for use of restraint is "a direct application of force without permission to restrict freedom of movement."

Once the decision to use restraint is made, the overriding principle is that it be done swiftly and humanely and that the patient be reassured that it is done in his or her best interest. As is the case for seclusion, only staff members trained in applying restraints are allowed to use them. The implementation of physical restraints is a dangerous procedure, both for staff and patient. It should never be attempted unless there is sufficient staff present to ensure that it can be done with a minimum of struggle. Using at least five staff members is recommended, one for each limb and an extra person as team leader. The presence of a critical group of staff may also assist in calming the patient, thus aborting the need for restraints. Once the decision is made to proceed, implementation must be completed and negotiations temporarily suspended. The team leader, just as in team resuscitation, oversees the staff and ensures safety. It is usually best that the physician avoid physical participation in subduing a combative patient because this may interfere with the therapeutic relationship. The same time limitations are placed on restraints as they are on seclusion. During restraints, staff is required to conduct 15-minute checks to assess vital signs, any signs of injury, and the patient's psychological state and readiness to discontinue seclusion or restraints.

If possible, the patient or family should be provided with an ongoing explanation of the reasons for the procedure and what to expect.

After a seclusion or restraint episode is resolved, a debriefing note needs to be added to the medical record that documents precipitants to the incident and alternative treatments, modifications of the treatment plan, and the patient's psychological and physical well-being after the intervention. Debriefing is also important to ascertain any trauma to staff as a result of the intervention and the offering of support to staff after a serious violent incident (Lindenmayer et al. 2002).

JCAHO's (2002, p. 123) recommendations describe procedures of seclusion and restraints as "aversive experience with potential for serious physical and emotional consequences including death." Organizations are "required to continually explore ways to decrease and eliminate use through training, leadership commitment and performance improvement." (See also Chapter 17, "Seclusion and Restraint.")

Case Example 4: Seclusion in Emergency Psychiatric Services

Initial assessment. A 31-year-old male university graduate was escorted by police officers involuntarily because of delusional thinking and aggressive behavior during the previous 24 hours. The patient violated a restraining order from his ex-wife, whom he had harassed and threatened to physically assault. He had bizarre and rigid thinking that was sexually inappropriate; he was noted to walk 10–25 miles daily exposing himself to others. The initial screening evaluation completed by the emergency room triage nurse indicated that he was disheveled and showed grandiose delusions.

Medical evaluation. The patient did not have any significant medical history, and he had not been in psychiatric treatment. The neurological examination was normal. There was no history of alcohol or illicit drug use. Blood and urine tests were normal.

Psychiatric assessment. Mental status examination showed the patient to be disheveled and to have marked flight of ideas and belligerence. The most striking features were grandiose delusional thinking and significant paranoia centering on the police in his community. His affect was inappropriate during the interview; at times he would laugh when asked a serious question and at times he would cry. He was fully oriented but would not cooperate with formal mental status testing. The initial diagnosis was acute mania with psychosis.

Patient behavior. Upon admission to the emergency room, the patient was extremely uncooperative, verbally threatening staff members and other patients and making sexually explicit remarks to a female nurse, with occasional verbal outbursts. During the time of his outbursts, less restrictive methods of modifying the patient's behavior, such as "talking him down," had failed. The doctrine of "the least restrictive method of restraint" was employed. The patient was provided with options for modifying his behavior. Four emergency room nursing aides were in clear view of the patient but remained 10 feet distant. The emergency room psychiatrist spoke to the patient in a firm but nonthreatening voice, stating that the continuation of the patient's uncontrolled and disruptive behavior would not be allowed and that the patient would be restrained by staff unless he cooperated with the medical and psychiatric staff. He was told that he could choose whether he wanted to be restrained or secluded as a result of his behavior. He agreed to seclusion over physical restraints. He also received emergency intramuscular haloperidol. He was calmed by the medication to some extent, as well as by a brief seclusion episode of 15 minutes. He then allowed further diagnostic evaluation.

Suicidal Risk

Suicide and suicide attempts are among the most serious outcomes of psychiatric illness, and the most extreme intervention (e.g., involuntary hospitalization) may have to be used if these events are at high risk. The national rate of suicide has remained fairly consistent at 1.1%–1.4%. Suicidal ideation and behavior are the most common presenting complaints of patients seeking treatment at psychiatric emergency facilities, and these patients are at a considerable risk of subsequent suicide (Dhossche 2000). Substance use disorders have been consistently recognized as chronic risk factors for suicide (Pages et al. 1997). Patients presenting to the emergency room with complaints of suicidal ideation or suicidal command hallucinations, or presenting after a suicide attempt, have to be carefully evaluated. Both state-related risk factors, such as ideas of hopelessness or worthlessness, and trait-related risk factors, such as age or a previous serious suicide attempt, need to be fully assessed. The intensity of current suicidal ideation should be explored, and the presence of protective factors against suicidal acting out should also be assessed. The result of this in-depth evaluation will dictate the final treatment decision.

Case Example 5: Use of Restraints for Suicidal Ideation in Emergency Service Settings

Initial assessment. Mr. R is a 50-year-old man with a long history of recurrent depressions and multiple hospitalizations dating back to age 19. The patient had been discharged from an inpatient psychiatric facility 3 months earlier and voluntarily presented himself to the hospital emergency room indicating that his medication was not helping him and that he was having frequent thoughts of wanting to hurt himself. The patient had a history of three suicide attempts in the past: at age 29 he took an overdose of hypnotics, at age 38 he attempted to overdose on a combination of medications, and he made a final attempt at age 49, when he lacerated his arm with a pin. The patient was followed at the local outpatient department by a psychiatrist and a social worker on a monthly basis and was receiving antidepressant medication. However, he had not visited the clinic since his hospital discharge.

Psychiatric evaluation. Mr. R was assessed by the psychiatrist and diagnosed with acute depression with suicidal ideation. Mr. R indicated that he was feeling tense and depressed and was considering hurting himself by hitting his head on the bathroom wall. The patient was evaluated on the InterSept Scale for Suicidal Thinking (Lindenmayer et al. 2003) and showed a score of 18 (out of a total of 24). During this time the patient was monitored one to one. Mr. R later also reported that he was hearing command voices telling him to hurt himself. During the psychiatric evaluation, Mr. R began hitting his head on the desk and saying he no longer wanted to live. He became extremely agitated. Hospital emergency staff immediately tried to restrain him; however, he broke loose and proceeded to hit his head against the wall. The staff utilized wrist-to-belt restraints, and Mr. R was given intramuscular ziprasidone 20 mg and lorazepam 4 mg for severe agitation secondary to his psychotic depressive disorder. He was then maintained on one-to-one monitoring for suicidal behavior and ideation. After approximately 24 hours he was able to calm down. He was admitted to the inpatient unit and continued on one-to-one observation.

Key Points

- Psychiatric emergency services (PESs) comprise a large spectrum of acute psychiatric service delivery systems that are available for the assessment, acute stabilization, and initial treatment of mental health emergencies.
- PESs usually function on a 24-hour-a-day basis and provide extremely important clinical services.
- The psychiatric emergency room is traditionally the main venue for the delivery of emergency services; however, PESs cover extensive and comprehensive mental health delivery systems and do not function in isolation.
- Such delivery systems are critical to prevent unnecessary hospitalizations that might, in turn, foster chronicity and dependence on institutional care.
- The crisis situation leading up to an emergency presentation by a patient is rarely completely resolved after evaluation and treatment in the PES.

- Often, the services provided by PESs represent patients' entry portal or referral place for longer-term care in an appropriate inpatient or outpatient setting where various psychiatric and social supportive services can be delivered and contribute to the resolution of the crisis.

References

Allen MH: Level 1 psychiatric emergency services: the tools of the crisis sector. Psychiatr Clin North Am 22:713–734, 1999

Allen MH (ed): Emergency Psychiatry. Washington, DC, American Psychiatric Publishing, 2002

Bassuk EL, Gerson S: Into the breach: emergency psychiatry in the general hospital. Gen Hosp Psychiatry 1:31–45, 1979

Breslow RE, Klinger BI, Erickson BJ: Characteristics of managed care patients in a psychiatric emergency service. Psychiatr Serv 47:1259–1261, 1996

Broadbent M, Jarman H, Berk M: Emergency department mental health triage scales improve outcomes. J Eval Clin Pract 10:57–62, 2004

Buckley PF: Dualism in psychiatry. Lancet 343:1102, 1994

Coristine RW, Hartford K, Vingilis E, et al: Mental health triage in the ER: a qualitative study. J Eval Clin Pract 13:303–309, 2007

Dhossche DM: Suicidal behavior in psychiatric emergency room patients. South Med J 93:310–314, 2000

Dreyfus JK: Nursing assessment of the ED patient with psychiatric symptoms: a quick reference. J Emerg Nurs 13:278–282, 1987

Ellison J, Blum NR: Repeat visitors in the psychiatric emergency service: a critical review of the data. Hosp Community Psychiatry 37:37–41, 1986

Gerson S, Bassuk EL: Psychiatric emergencies: an overview. Am J Psychiatry 137:1–11, 1980

Happell B, Summers M, Pinikahana J: The triage of psychiatric patients in the hospital emergency department: a comparison between emergency department nurses and psychiatric nurse consultants. Accid Emerg Nurs 10:65–71, 2002

Herz MI, Endicott J, Spitzer RL: Brief hospitalization: a two-year follow-up. Arch Gen Psychiatry 134:502–507, 1979

Hill SL, Petit J: The violent patient. Emerg Med Clin North Am 18:301–315, 2002

Joint Commission on the Accreditation of Healthcare Organizations: Hospital Accreditation Standards. Oakbrook Terrace, IL, Joint Commission Resources, 2002

Kooiman CG, Van de Wetering BJ, Van der Mast RC: Clinical and demographic characteristics of emergency department patients in The Netherlands: a review of the literature and a preliminary study. Am J Emerg Med 7:632–638, 1989

Lindenmayer JP, Crowner M, Cosgrove V: Emergency treatment of agitation and aggression, in Emergency Psychiatry. Edited by Allen MH. Washington, DC, American Psychiatric Publishing, 2002, pp 115–149

Lindenmayer JP, Czobor P, Alphs L, et al: The InterSePT scale for suicidal thinking reliability and validity. Schizophr Res 63:161–170, 2003

Marson DC, McGovern MP, Pomp HC: Psychiatric decision making in the emergency room: a research overview. Am J Psychiatry 145:918–925, 1988

McClelland PA: The emergency psychiatric system. Psychiatr Clin North Am 6:225–232, 1983

McDonough S, Wynaden D, Finn M, et al: Emergency department mental health triage consultancy service: an evaluation of the first year of the service. Accid Emerg Nurs 12:31–38, 2004

Murdach AD: Decision making in psychiatric emergencies. Health Soc Work 12:267–274, 1987

Oldham JM, DeMasi ME: An integrated approach to emergency psychiatric care. New Dir Ment Health Serv 67:33–42, 1995

Osborne J: Mental health triage. Emerg Nurs 11:14, 2003

Oyewumi LK, Odejide O, Kazarian SS: Psychiatric emergency services in a Canadian city, I: prevalence and patterns of use. Can J Psychiatry 37:91–95, 1992

Pages KP, Russo JE, Roy-Byrne PP, et al: Determinants of suicidal ideation: the role of substance use disorders. J Clin Psychiatry 58:510–517, 1997

Rhine MW, Mayerson P: Crisis hospitalization within a psychiatric emergency service. Am J Psychiatry 127:1386–1391, 1971

Schneider SE, Ross IM: Ultra-short hospitalization for severely mentally ill patients. Psychiatr Serv 47:137–138, 1996

Sledge WH, Tebes J, Rakfeldt J, et al: Day hospital/crisis respite care versus inpatient care, part I: clinical outcomes. Am J Psychiatry 153:1065–1073, 1996

Smart D, Pollard C, Walpole B: Mental health triage in emergency medicine. Aust N Z J Psychiatry 33:57–69, 1999

Solomon P, Davis J: Meeting community service needs of discharged psychiatric patients. Psychiatr Q 57:11–17, 1985

Solomon P, Gordon B: The psychiatric emergency room and follow-up services in the community. Psychiatr Q 58:119–127, 1986–1987

Stroul BA: Psychiatric Crisis Response Systems: A Descriptive Study. Rockville, MD, Center for Mental Health Services, National Institutes of Mental Health, 1993

Summers M, Happell B: The quality of psychiatric services provided by an Australian tertiary hospital emergency department: a client perspective. Accid Emerg Nurs 10:205–213, 2002

Sundheim ST, Ryan RM: Amnestic syndrome presenting as malingering in a man with developmental disability. Psychiatr Serv 50:966–968, 1999

Vaslamatzis G, Kontaxakis V, Markidis M, et al: Social and resource factors related to the utilization of emergency psychiatric services in the Athens area. Acta Psychiatr Scand 75:95–98, 1987

Vigiser D, Apter A, Aviram U, et al: Overutilization of the general hospital emergency room for psychiatric referrals in an Israeli hospital. Am J Public Health 74:73–75, 1984

Weisman G, Feirstein A, Thomas C: Three-day hospitalization: a model for intensive intervention. Arch Gen Psychiatry 21:620–629, 1969

Wynaden D, Chapman R, McGowan S, et al: Emergency department mental health triage consultancy service: a qualitative evaluation. Accid Emerg Nurs 11:158–165, 2003

PART IV

Treatment and Management

CHAPTER 15

Psychopharmacology and Electroconvulsive Therapy

Leslie Citrome, M.D., M.P.H.

The use of medications and other somatic treatments in the care of patients who exhibit violent behavior is complex. Prior chapters have outlined the different diagnostic entities that may be associated with violent behavior. In addition, comorbidity is common: patients with schizophrenia or bipolar disorder can also have a substance use disorder or a personality disorder. There may be an additional superimposed nonpsychiatric medical disorder that has been overlooked. Careful attention to the differential diagnosis will lead to the formation of a list of the medication approaches most likely to be effective in treating the underlying core disorder—and also in ameliorating the violent behavior, if it is a consequence of the disorder. If this approach fails, consideration should be given to the possibility of a missed diagnosis or of having underestimated the importance of a secondary diagnosis as a cause of the noxious behavior. Problems can also arise when the indicated treatment for the underlying disorder has adverse behavioral consequences. An example of this would be akathisia secondary to the use of first-generation antipsychotics. Akathisia can be mistaken for anxiety and agitation, resulting in an increase in the dosage of the antipsychotic, thus leading to more severe akathisia, which can ultimately result in violent behavior.

In acute emergencies, where the goal is the rapid resolution of agitated behavior, there are many different effective pharmacological interventions. A careful differential diagnosis is still important—for example, a patient whose violent behavior is secondary to alcohol withdrawal would be better served by a drug treatment that has cross-tolerance with alcohol. This chapter discusses the options currently available for the short-term management of agitation, including the newly available intramuscular formulations of second-generation antipsychotics. Emphasis is placed on these agents particularly because they are relatively new and have received regulatory approval in many countries for the specific indication of agitation associated with schizophrenia and/or bipolar mania and thus are being marketed extensively by their manufacturers for this purpose.

Once the acute episode is safely managed, longer-term treatment is necessary to decrease the likelihood of future episodes and to diminish the intensity of future outbursts should they still occur. Here, attention to the underlying disorder (or disorders) is crucial in achieving this goal. Addressing all comorbid conditions and environmental stressors is essential.

This chapter emphasizes data from randomized studies, preferably double blind. Where such information is not available, references to naturalistic studies or case series are judiciously made.

Case Example

John is a 40-year-old white male, diagnosed at different times as having schizophrenia, bipolar disorder, or schizoaffective disorder. His first psychiatric hospitalization was at age 18 when he was brought to the hospital emergency department in an acute psychotic state with paranoid delusions. He has had several known hospitalizations since then, the most recent after he was arrested for assault. In the emergency department he was acutely agitated and required intramuscular medication to control his behavior. He was given an intramuscular injection of haloperidol 5 mg combined with lorazepam 2 mg in the same syringe. After 45 minutes he appeared calmer, but he complained of stiffness in his neck and tongue and was drooling. He received diphenhydramine 50 mg intramuscularly for this dystonic reaction, followed by oral benztropine 2 mg. Toxicology screen in the emergency department came back positive for cocaine and cannabis.

John was admitted to the psychiatric inpatient unit and refused all oral medications, saying he was "allergic to Haldol" and that "nothing really works." On the second day of hospitalization he asked to smoke a cigarette, and when told the unit was now "smoke free," he began shouting at the staff, threatened to sue them, and made a fist. Because he was not taking any oral medications, a decision was made to give him a "stat" dose of ziprasidone 20 mg intramuscular. After the injection, John was substantially calmer. He was able to articulate that he felt less anxious, and he acknowledged he did not feel any restlessness or stiffness that he usually felt after receiving intramuscular haloperidol. He agreed to continue taking the "new" medication.

Despite the initial success with ziprasidone, John continued to feel paranoid and uncomfortable. He was unable to sleep. He was subsequently prescribed a number of different other antipsychotics, including quetiapine and olanzapine. Although he was free of any extrapyramidal side effects, symptom relief was incomplete and he continued to be intermittently agitated, often with little provocation. John was ultimately placed on clozapine, which did decrease the frequency of his outbursts. John's aggression became exclusively verbal, never physical, and he was more easily reassured. Adjunctive valproate and adjunctive lamotrigine treatment were also attempted but did not make a substantial difference in his impulsivity.

John's diagnostic history is confusing: it is unclear whether he has schizophrenia or bipolar disorder. The diagnostic uncertainty is accentuated by his comorbid substance use and nonadherence to medication treatments. John presents the clinician with two distinct problems: 1) how to best manage his acute behavioral dyscontrol and 2) how to prevent these behavioral problems from happening again. John is an experienced patient; he knows what has not worked in the past and is keenly aware of the discomforts he has had with different medications. This plays into his paranoid outlook on life and makes establishing a therapeutic alliance a significant challenge for the clinician treating him. Fortunately for John, there are new pharmacological tools to use that were not available when he first became ill. For acute emergencies there are medications that are better tolerated than haloperidol, and for longer-term use there are medications that have greater efficacy.

Medications for Psychiatric Emergencies

Psychiatric emergencies such as acute states of agitation and overt aggressive behavior are commonly treated with the use of sedating agents. These treatments have evolved over the years from the use of agents such as sodium amytal to the administration of benzodiazepines and antipsychotics (often simultaneously). Intramuscular administration of medications yields higher maximum plasma concentrations than that achieved with oral formulations. Moreover, these maximum concentrations are reached much more quickly with intramuscular formulations. Table 15–1 outlines several intramuscular options for the pharmacological treatment of acute agitation.

TABLE 15–1. Selected intramuscular medications for the treatment of acute agitation

Agent	Dose, mg	Half-life in nonelderly adults, h	Comments
Lorazepam	0.5–2.0	10–20	The only benzodiazepine that is reliably absorbed intramuscularly. Useful for symptoms of alcohol withdrawal.
Haloperidol	5–10	12–36	The most commonly used anti-agitation intramuscular antipsychotic, but associated with substantial risk for acute dystonia, akathisia, and tremor. Other first-generation antipsychotics are also available in intramuscular preparations but are associated with hypotension (chlorpromazine) and a decrease in seizure threshold (all).
Droperidol	2.5–5	2	Association with QT prolongation has led to its removal from the U.K. market and a "black box" warning in U.S. labeling.
Ziprasidone	10–20*	2.2–3.4	Lower risk of extrapyramidal adverse events than first-generation agents.
Olanzapine	10*	34–38	Lower risk of extrapyramidal adverse events than first-generation agents.
Aripiprazole	9.75*	75	Lower risk of extrapyramidal adverse events than first-generation agents.

*Recommended dose in U.S. product labeling

Head-to-head double-blind comparisons of these intramuscular agents for the treatment of agitation are not generally available, with the exception of recent registration studies (see Table 15–2) comparing olanzapine or aripiprazole with either haloperidol (in patients with schizophrenia) or lorazepam (in patients with bipolar mania). A quantitative review of these registration studies can be found elsewhere (Citrome 2007). In terms of combinations, the extant controlled evidence is one three-arm study that compared haloperidol intramuscular 5 mg, lorazepam intramuscular 2 mg, or both haloperidol and lorazepam in combination, in 98 psychotic and agitated patients (Battaglia et al. 1997).

Sodium amytal entails the risk of respiratory depression, and essentially this agent has been supplanted by lorazepam. Although lorazepam also can result in a decrease in respiratory drive, particularly in patients with a history of lung disease or sleep apnea, it is otherwise relatively well tolerated. Advantages include its relatively short half-life, lack of active metabolites, and cross-tolerance to alcohol, making it the dominant choice in patients whose agitation is secondary to acute alcohol withdrawal. Disadvantages include the potential for behavioral disinhibition that may paradoxically increase agitation (Dietch and Jennings 1988). Another disadvantage to using intramuscular lorazepam is its lack of substantial antipsychotic effect; thus lorazepam is inadequate in treating any underlying core psychotic disorder. Long-term use of a benzodiazepine will also result in physiological tolerance, leading to potential rebound anxiety or agitation in between doses or when doses are missed. Abrupt withdrawal of benzodiazepines is associated with a risk for epileptic seizures.

Given the limitations of intramuscular lorazepam for patients with schizophrenia or bipolar disorder, intramuscular antipsychotics may be preferred for treating acute agitation. The combination of intramuscular haloperidol and lorazepam is commonly used, with the rationale that combining these agents will improve the sedative effect as well as decrease the likelihood of extrapyramidal adverse events such as acute dystonia, akathisia, or tremor. Our patient in the above case example received the combination of haloperidol and lorazepam and had marked reduction in agitation but developed an acute dystonic reaction that required additional interventions, including an additional injection. This complicated course in the emergency department set him up to be overtly noncompliant with medications once admitted to the psychiatric inpatient unit. There are now three second-generation antipsychotics available in rapidly acting intramuscular formulations that can be considered. All have a lower propensity for extrapyramidal adverse

TABLE 15–2. Registration studies for intramuscular formulations of second-generation antipsychotics

Reference	Agent and indication	N	Study arms (N)	Results vs. placebo or placebo equivalent
Lesem et al. 2001	Ziprasidone; schizophrenia	117	Ziprasidone 2 mg (54), 10 mg (63)	10 mg superior on Behavioral Activity Rating Scale at 0–2 hours, but not by Clinical Global Impression–Severity
Daniel et al. 2001	Ziprasidone; schizophrenia	79	Ziprasidone 2 mg (38), 20 mg (41)	20 mg superior on Behavioral Activity Rating Scale at 0–4 hours and by Clinical Global Impression–Severity at 4 hours
Breier et al. 2002	Olanzapine; schizophrenia	270	Olanzapine 2.5 mg (48), 5 mg (45), 7.5 mg (46), 10 mg (46); haloperidol 7.5 mg (40); placebo (45)	All doses of olanzapine superior to placebo on PANSS-EC; effect larger and more consistent for 5, 7.5, and 10 mg
Wright et al. 2001	Olanzapine; schizophrenia	311	Olanzapine 10 mg (131); haloperidol 7.5 mg (126); placebo (54)	Olanzapine superior to placebo on PANSS-EC
Meehan et al. 2001	Olanzapine; bipolar manic or mixed	201	Olanzapine 10 mg (99); lorazepam 2 mg (51); placebo (51)	Olanzapine superior to placebo on PANSS-EC
Meehan et al. 2002	Olanzapine; dementia*	272	Olanzapine 2.5 mg (71), 5 mg (66); lorazepam 1 mg (68); placebo (67)	Both olanzapine doses superior to placebo on the PANSS-EC

TABLE 15–2. Registration studies for intramuscular formulations of second-generation antipsychotics *(continued)*

Reference	Agent and indication	N	Study arms (N)	Results vs. placebo or placebo equivalent
Andrezina et al. 2006a	Aripiprazole; schizophrenia	448	Aripiprazole 9.75 mg (175); haloperidol 6.5 mg (185); placebo (88)	Aripiprazole superior to placebo on PANSS-EC
Tran-Johnson et al. 2007	Aripiprazole; schizophrenia	357	Aripiprazole 1 mg (57), 5.25 mg (63), 9.75 mg (57), 15 mg (58); haloperidol 7.5 mg (60); placebo (62)	All but the 1-mg dose of aripiprazole were superior to placebo on PANSS-EC
Zimbroff et al. 2007	Aripiprazole; bipolar, manic or mixed	301	Aripiprazole 9.75 mg (78), 15 mg (78); lorazepam 2 mg (70); placebo (75)	Both doses of aripiprazole superior to placebo on PANSS-EC

Note. PANSS-EC=Positive and Negative Syndrome Scale, Excited Component.
*Not FDA approved for this indication.

effects compared with the older antipsychotics and are discussed in the following paragraphs.

Ziprasidone

Ziprasidone mesylate was approved in 2002 by the U.S. Food and Drug Administration (FDA) for the indication of acute agitation in patients with schizophrenia, on the basis of two 1-day, double-blind trials (Daniel et al. 2001; Lesem et al. 2001) of agitated hospitalized subjects with a primary diagnosis of schizophrenia, schizoaffective disorder, bipolar disorder with psychotic features, delusional disorder, or psychotic disorder not otherwise specified (DSM-IV-TR; American Psychiatric Association 2000). Approximately 80% of the subjects had schizophrenia or schizoaffective disorder. Doses tested were ziprasidone 10 mg versus 2 mg (Lesem et al. 2001) and 20 mg versus 2 mg (Daniel et al. 2001). There was no placebo arm, per se, nor were active comparators such as haloperidol or lorazepam used. The 2-mg dose of ziprasidone can be considered as a placebo-equivalent. The 20-mg dose yields a higher percentage of responders and a greater degree of response in terms of reduction of agitation than the 10-mg dose; however, product labeling recommends the range of 10–20 mg per injection.

Safety concerns specific to intramuscular ziprasidone, as noted in product labeling, include caution in patients with impaired renal function because the cyclodextrin excipient is cleared by renal filtration. Because of ziprasidone's dose-related prolongation of the QT interval and the known association of fatal arrhythmias with QT prolongation by some other drugs, ziprasidone is contraindicated in patients with a known history of QT prolongation (including congenital long QT syndrome), recent acute myocardial infarction, or uncompensated heart failure. However, more than 5 years of clinical availability has not resulted in evidence that ziprasidone by itself poses a substantial clinical problem in this regard (Zimbroff et al. 2005). Comparative intramuscular antipsychotic data on QT_c are available; the product information (Pfizer 2005) includes details of a study evaluating the QT_c-prolonging effect of intramuscular ziprasidone, with intramuscular haloperidol as a control, and reveals a mean increase in QT_c from baseline for ziprasidone of 4.6 msec following the first injection and 12.8 msec following the second injection, compared with 6.0 msec and 14.7 msec for haloperidol, and with no patients having had a QT_c interval exceeding 500 msec.

The patient in the case example did not have any history of cardiac conduction problems. When the need developed for an intramuscular injection of an anti-agitation medication, ziprasidone was selected over the combination of haloperidol and lorazepam because of his past adverse experience with an acute dystonic reaction. John did not develop akathisia or any other extrapyramidal symptoms after the injection. Because of the improved immediate tolerability over haloperidol, he agreed to continue an oral preparation of this "new" medication.

Olanzapine

Olanzapine was approved in 2004 by the FDA for the indication of agitation associated with schizophrenia and bipolar I mania, on the basis of three 1-day, placebo-controlled inpatient trials with active comparators (Breier et al. 2002; Meehan et al. 2001; Wright et al. 2001). A fourth pivotal trial was done in patients age 55 or older with agitation associated with dementia, though regulatory approval was not pursued (Meehan et al. 2002). Superior onset of efficacy for intramuscular olanzapine 10 mg was demonstrated compared with intramuscular haloperidol 7.5 mg in patients with schizophrenia (Wright et al. 2001) and intramuscular lorazepam 2 mg in patients with bipolar mania (Meehan et al. 2001). In the bipolar trial, olanzapine was superior to lorazepam at all time points up to and including 2 hours postinjection. In the schizophrenia trial examining olanzapine 10 mg (Wright et al. 2001), olanzapine was superior to haloperidol at 15, 30, and 45 minutes postinjection. In the study comparing multiple fixed doses of intramuscular olanzapine with intramuscular haloperidol 7.5 mg (Breier et al. 2002), patients treated with 5.0, 7.5, or 10.0 mg of olanzapine had greater mean improvement in agitation than those given placebo at all time points, but the groups given 2.5 mg of olanzapine or haloperidol did not show greater mean improvement compared with those given placebo until 60 minutes after the first injection. In the pivotal trials, no adverse event was significantly more frequent for intramuscular olanzapine compared with intramuscular haloperidol or intramuscular lorazepam. The recommended dose in product labeling is 10 mg (with lower doses of 2.5–5.0 mg for vulnerable patients such as the elderly or medically infirm) (Eli Lilly 2006).

Safety concerns specific to intramuscular olanzapine, as noted in product labeling, include hypotension, bradycardia with or without hypotension, tachycardia, and syncope as reported during the clinical trials. As per the product label, patients should remain recumbent if drowsy or dizzy after injection until examination has indicated that they are not experiencing postural hypotension, bradycardia, and/or hypoventilation. Simultaneous injection of olanzapine intramuscular and parenteral benzodiazepines is not recommended. Data from the first 21 months of post-marketing safety experience with olanzapine intramuscular were presented in a poster (Sorsaburu et al. 2006) in which 29 fatalities were reported among an estimated worldwide patient exposure of 539,000. The fatalities were complicated by multiple concomitant medications, including benzodiazepines or other antipsychotics, and medically significant risk factors.

Aripiprazole

Aripiprazole intramuscular was approved by the FDA in late 2006 for the indication of agitation associated with schizophrenia or bipolar mania, on the basis of three 1-day, placebo-controlled inpatient trials with active comparators (Andrezina et al. 2006a; Tran-Johnson et al. 2007; Zimbroff et al. 2007). The schizophrenia studies utilized haloperidol intramuscular as an active comparator, with mixed results in terms of relative efficacy. In the study comparing intramuscular aripiprazole 9.75 mg with intramuscular haloperidol 6.5 mg (Andrezina et al. 2006a), analysis according to the non-inferiority hypothesis indicated that aripiprazole was non-inferior to haloperidol. However, for the aripiprazole group, decrease in agitation differed significantly from placebo at 1 hour after the first injection, whereas a significant difference was achieved at 45 minutes in the haloperidol group. There was no significant difference in the improvement in the agitation scores between the aripiprazole and haloperidol groups at these time points, nor at 30 minutes or 2 hours; however, the difference at 90 minutes was significant in favor of haloperidol ($P=0.022$). Aripiprazole performed somewhat better in the study that compared multiple fixed doses of intramuscular aripiprazole with intramuscular haloperidol 7.5 mg (Tran-Johnson et al. 2007). In that study, changes in agitation scores were statistically significant as early as 45 minutes for the aripiprazole 9.75-mg group, whereas a significant difference between haloperidol and placebo was first seen at 105 minutes. In the study comparing aripiprazole versus lorazepam and placebo in agitated patients with bipolar disorder, lorazepam evidenced superiority over placebo as early as 45 minutes after injection and aripiprazole at 60 minutes (Zimbroff et al. 2007). In product labeling, the usual recommended dose is 9.75 mg (Bristol-Myers Squibb 2006).

Safety concerns specific to intramuscular aripiprazole, as noted in product labeling, include greater sedation and orthostatic hypotension with the combination of lorazepam and aripiprazole as compared with that observed with aripiprazole alone.

The pivotal registration trials of the intramuscular formulations of the second-generation antipsychotics suffer from the limitation that the subjects were generally not as severely ill as some patients commonly seen in clinical practice. Moreover, patients with comorbid medical conditions and prescribed multiple psychotropic medications are generally excluded from registration trials. In addition, the studies did not enroll children or adolescents. Thus, generalizability of these studies may be limited. Some information is now available in terms of naturalistic studies for ziprasidone (Preval et al. 2005) and olanzapine (San et al. 2006) that enrolled more severely agitated patients than the registration studies. In the ziprasidone mesylate naturalistic study, 119 patients who presented to a psychiatric emergency department received either intramuscular ziprasidone 20 mg ($n=110$) or conventional intramuscular antipsychotics ($n=9$). Ziprasidone was effective in reducing agitation among patients with and without alcohol and substance abuse. In the olanzapine naturalistic study, 92 patients attending psychiatric emergency settings were enrolled, all receiving intramuscular olanzapine 10 mg; however, patients with active drug and alcohol use were screened out. Olanzapine was effective in reducing agitation, with 96% receiving a single injection and 4% receiving two. In a retrospective chart review of 100 hospitalized patients younger than 18 years of age treated with intramuscular ziprasidone or intramuscular olanzapine, both agents resulted in similar reductions of agitation or aggression (Khan and Mican 2006).

For the second-generation antipsychotics that are available in intramuscular form, several studies have been published that describe the transition from intramuscular to oral administration for ziprasidone (Brook et al. 2000, 2005; Daniel et al. 2004), olanzapine (Wright et al. 2003), and aripiprazole (Andrezina et al. 2006b).

For patients whose level of agitation does not mandate the use of intramuscular medication, oral administration can be considered first line. For patients who are actively refusing oral medication, such as our case patient, this is not an option. Controlled clinical trials have been reported on the use of risperidone liquid (Currier et al. 2004) and olanzapine tablets (Baker et al. 2003) for patients with agitation. The risperidone trial enrolled patients with schizophrenia, schizoaffective disorder, mania with psychotic features, acute paranoid reaction, or delusional disorder. The olanzapine trial enrolled patients with schizophrenia, schizoaffective disorder, schizophreniform disorder, or bipolar I disorder, manic or mixed episode (not necessarily with psychotic features). Regarding olanzapine, dosages that exceeded the product label recommended maximum of 20 mg/day were found to be useful in the short-term management of agitation (Baker et al. 2003).

Medications for Long-Term Treatment

Long-term treatment of violent behavior is geared toward the prevention of future episodes of agitation and aggression. For this goal to be attained, future episodes must be reduced in both frequency and intensity. If the aggressive behavior is secondary to uncontrolled psychosis, treating these symptoms with an antipsychotic will have the desired effect in reducing aggressive behavior. However, violent behavior is often multifactorial in origin, with contributing factors such as the influence of street drugs, an underlying problem with poor impulse control, and environmental triggers. Another level of complexity exists when the violent behavior is *instrumental*—that is, premeditated—and a means for the aggressor to obtain an advantage of some sort. John, the patient in our case example, exhibited aggression related to both an uncontrolled psychotic disorder refractory to first-generation antipsychotics and poor impulse control that persisted even during times he was free of hallucinations and delusions. These characteristics make treatment planning difficult. In an effort to address the psychosis, antipsychotics have been prescribed with varying success based on efficacy and tolerability issues. To address the impulsivity, and possibly the substance abuse, John received a trial of an anticonvulsant, valproate, with little success. He ultimately was placed on clozapine, a second-generation antipsychotic commonly reserved for patients with treatment-refractory schizophrenia but also approved for the indication of recurrent suicidal behavior in patients with schizophrenia. The available controlled evidence is reviewed for these long-term treatment options.

Antipsychotics

In the United States several second-generation antipsychotics are available: clozapine, risperidone, olanzapine, quetiapine, ziprasidone, aripiprazole, and paliperidone. All seven are approved by the FDA for the treatment of schizophrenia, and all, except for clozapine and paliperidone, are also approved for the treatment of bipolar mania. Second-generation antipsychotics have also been used off-label for a variety of conditions (Tremeau and Citrome 2006). Of special interest is the possibility that these agents have specific anti-hostility effects, with clozapine having the strongest evidence supporting this.

Clozapine's usefulness for patients with aggressive behavior was initially suggested by case series and retrospective studies in which a reduction in the number of violent incidents and/or a decrease in the use of seclusion or restraint was observed among inpatients once they began clozapine treatment (Citrome et al. 2004b). The reductions in hostility (Volavka et al. 1993) and aggression (Buckley et al. 1995) after clozapine treatment were *selective* in the sense that they were (statistically) independent of the general antipsychotic effects of clozapine. This was confirmed in two double-blind, randomized clinical trials. The first was a 14-week study that compared the specific anti-hostility effects of clozapine with those of olanzapine, risperidone, or haloperidol in 157 inpatients with schizophrenia or schizoaffective disorder (Citrome et al. 2001) and found that clozapine had significantly greater anti-hostility effect than haloperidol or risperidone. This effect on hostility was specific: it was independent of antipsychotic effect on delusional thinking, formal thought disorder, or hallucinations, and independent of sedation. Further analyses of these data, including measures of overt aggression (Volavka et al. 2004), showed that patients exhibiting overt aggression had less overall improvement of psychopathology but that antipsychotic efficacy of clozapine was greatest in aggressive patients, whereas the opposite was true for risperidone and olanzapine. A key finding was that a therapeutic dosage of clozapine was necessary to achieve superior effects on the frequency and the severity of overt aggression. Because it can take many days to titrate clozapine to a therapeutic dosage, it is important not to terminate a clozapine trial prematurely. However, this study enrolled patients who were not necessarily aggressive, which limits its generalizability. A second study was undertaken that enrolled 110 patients who had been physically aggressive and subsequently randomly assigned to receive double-blind clozapine, olanzapine, or haloperidol for up to 12 weeks (Krakowski et al. 2006). Patients assigned to clozapine had statistically significant lower endpoint aggression scores than patients assigned to either olanzapine or haloperidol. Patients in the olanzapine group had statistically significant lower endpoint aggression scores than patients in the haloperidol group. However, no differences were seen among the three groups in terms of reduction of psychopathology as measured by the total Positive and Negative Syndrome Scale (PANSS) score, suggesting that clozapine's advantage was related to a specific anti-aggressive effect.

No other double-blind, randomized clinical trials are available that report on the efficacy of other second-generation antipsychotics in reducing aggressive behavior among patients specifically selected because of such behavior. In the absence of these studies, post hoc analyses have been done using data gathered during other studies for risperidone (Czobor et al. 1995), olanzapine (Kinon et al. 2001), quetiapine (Arango and Bernardo 2005; Chengappa et al. 2003), ziprasidone (Citrome et al. 2006), and aripiprazole (Volavka et al. 2005). Results varied from superiority to haloperidol (for risperidone, olanzapine, quetiapine, and ziprasidone) to equivalency to haloperidol (for aripiprazole) in terms of anti-hostility or anti-aggressive effect. Compared with haloperidol, the second-generation antipsychotics were associated with fewer extrapyramidal effects and thus were considered more tolerable and overall more effective. Methodologies varied, however, and specific anti-hostility or anti-aggressive effect was not always determined (for olanzapine [Kinon et al. 2001]) or was inconsistently demonstrated (for quetiapine [Arango and Bernardo 2005; Chengappa et al. 2003]).

Anticonvulsants

Mood stabilizers such as lithium and anticonvulsants are extensively used, including off-label use among patients with a diagnosis of schizophrenia (Citrome et al. 2002). There is an expectation that adjunctive mood stabilizers can reduce aggressive and impulsive behavior (Citrome 1995). There are expert consensus guidelines suggesting the use of adjunctive mood stabilizers in those with schizophrenia with agitation, excitement, aggression, or violence (McEvoy et al. 1999), but the supporting evidence for this indication is based almost entirely on uncontrolled studies and case reports. The most commonly used mood stabilizer is valproate (Citrome et al. 2000, 2002). Our case patient had a trial of adjunctive valproate, but it did not have a substantial impact on his psychopathology or degree of impulsivity. A review of the use of valproate in violence and aggressive behaviors in a variety of diagnoses (Lindenmayer and Kotsaftis 2000) did reveal a 77.1% response rate (defined by a 50% reduction in target behavior) based on 17 reports (164 patients, approximately one-half with dementia). Double-blind controlled studies that tested and support this are few in number but do include a varied array of diagnoses, including borderline personality disorder (Hollander et al. 2001, 2005), Cluster B personality disorders as a group (Hollander et al. 2003), and children and adolescents with explosive temper and mood lability (Donovan et al. 2000).

Positive symptoms were reduced with adjunctive valproate in a 28-day double-blind, randomized study with olanzapine and risperidone among 249 patients with an acute episode of schizophrenia (Casey et al. 2003). A post hoc secondary analysis from this study found that combination therapy with divalproex had significantly greater anti-hostility effect at 3 days and at 7 days than antipsychotic monotherapy ($P<0.05$), as measured by the PANSS hostility item (Citrome et al. 2004a). The effect on hostility was statistically independent of antipsychotic effect on other PANSS items that reflect delusional thinking, a formal thought disorder, or hallucinations. Adequate dosing may be important and may explain why valproate 480 mg/day did not differentiate from placebo on measures of aggressive-behavior patients with dementia (Sival et al. 2002). Other negative data come from an 84-day study that failed to replicate the 28-day double-blind, randomized study with olanzapine and risperidone (Abbott Laboratories 2007) and from a randomized, open-label label study of risperidone with and without valproate that did not demonstrate an advantage for combination therapy on psychopathology rating scales or measures of aggression (Citrome et al. 2007).

The strategy of adding lamotrigine to antipsychotics was supported by promising results from a double-blind trial of adjunctive lamotrigine in patients with treatment-refractory schizophrenia unresponsive to clozapine monotherapy (Tiihonen et al. 2003). Although specific effect on hostility was not reported, improvement in positive symptoms was seen. Subsequent studies have not been encouraging; the usefulness of adjunctive lamotrigine in patients with schizophrenia was not supported by two large trials undertaken by its manufacturer (GlaxoSmithKline 2005, 2006; Goff et al. 2007).

Evidence supporting the use of carbamazepine for persistent aggressive behavior is limited (Volavka 2002), with the largest randomized clinical trial of carbamazepine failing to detect a significant improvement on the total Brief Psychiatric Rating Scale but showing differences in suspiciousness, uncooperativeness, and excitement (Okuma et al. 1989). Studies have also been done in nursing home patients with agitation and dementia (Tariot et al. 1998), with significant short-term efficacy of carbamazepine for agitation and aggression and with generally good safety and tolerability.

In the absence of mania, lithium may not be efficacious in reducing aggressive behavior, as evidenced in a study in which lithium was added to antipsychotics for the treatment of patients with resistant schizophrenia who were classified as "dangerous, violent or criminal" (Collins et al. 1991). However, there are case reports of lithium being helpful in cases of akathisia among patients with schizophrenia (Shalev et al. 1987). There are also case reports of patients with paranoid schizophrenia with aggressive or disorderly behaviors who responded to the addition of lithium to their antipsychotic treatment, deteriorated after the lithium was discontinued, and subsequently improved when it was reinstituted (Prakash 1985). In another population, lithium treatment reduced the number of violent infractions in 66 nonpsychotic, impulsively aggressive prisoners in a double-blind, placebo-controlled study (Sheard et al. 1976).

Other Medication Approaches

The use of β-adrenergic blockers has been reported in randomized clinical trials in several different disease states to reduce violent behavior (Volavka 2002). Although propranolol has been the agent most studied, others such as nadolol may be simpler to titrate (starting at 40 mg at bedtime and then up to 80 mg and 120 mg at bedtime over the span of several days, depending on parameters such as heart rate and blood pressure). Other possible medication choices include serotonin-specific reuptake inhibitors, for which one double-blind, randomized clinical trial in patients with schizophrenia and aggressive behavior revealed an advantage with the adjunctive use of citalopram (Vartiainen et al. 1995). This is consistent with an open-label study of citalopram in patients with DSM-IV-TR Cluster B personality disorder or intermittent explosive disorder (Reist et al. 2003) and a double-blind trial of fluoxetine in the treatment of impulsive aggressive behavior in non–major depressed, non-bipolar or schizophrenic, personality-disordered individuals (Coccaro and Kavoussi 1997).

The prolonged use of benzodiazepines for aggression and schizophrenia is discouraged because of the problems with physiological tolerance and dependence. For example, missing scheduled doses of lorazepam may result in withdrawal symptoms that can lead to agitation or excitement as well as irritability and a greater risk for aggressive behavior. Moreover, a controlled study of adjunctive clonazepam in patients with schizophrenia demonstrated no additional therapeutic benefit, and several patients demonstrated violent behavior during the course of clonazepam treatment (Karson et al. 1982).

The Role of Electroconvulsive Therapy

Adjunctive electroconvulsive therapy (ECT) may help individuals who have inadequately responsive psychotic symptoms (Fink and Sackeim 1996), in particular, patients with persistent aggressive behavior. Controlled studies have not been reported, but an open trial of ECT in combination with risperidone in male patients with schizophrenia and aggression resulted in a reduction in aggressive behavior for 9 of the 10 patients (Hirose et al. 2001).

Nonpsychotic Patients Who Exhibit Violent Behavior

A nonpsychotic outpatient may present with episodic violent behavior. A differential diagnosis and workup are required to rule out a somatic cause of the aberrant behavior. Psychological testing may also be helpful in discerning the impact of a personality disorder. Intermittent explosive disorder (IED) is also a possibility, and its lifetime prevalence was noted to be 7.3% in a recent report of a nationally representative sample in the United States (Kessler et al. 2006). Despite this high prevalence, there are no positive published double-blind, randomized clinical trials of medication treatments for DSM-IV-TR–defined IED. Even so, the use of the agents described earlier can be considered; for example, the off-label use of clozapine has been described in nine adolescents with IED (Kant et al. 2004). Another option is the use of serotonin-specific reuptake inhibitors, for which case reports for IED can be found (Feder 1999) as well as a double-blind clinical trial that enrolled patients with a personality disorder and impulsive aggressive behavior (Coccaro and Kavoussi 1997).

Outpatients with personality disorders and impulsive aggressive behavior may benefit from treatment with mood stabilizers such as valproate at mean modal dosages of about 1,500 mg/day (Hollander et al. 2003, 2005). Notably, the study that found improvement with valproate versus placebo in Cluster B personality disorders did not find the same advantage in the entire enrolled sample, which also included patients with IED and posttraumatic stress disorder (Hollander et al. 2003).

Although long-acting benzodiazepines are sometimes used in an attempt to manage aggressive behavior, there are no supporting controlled clinical trials and many cautionary reports regarding behavioral disinhibition.

Behavioral and psychotherapeutic interventions, including cognitive-behavioral modification (Meichenbaum and Goodman 1971) and dialectical behavior therapy (Linehan 1987), remain important components in the treatment of aggressivity, particularly among nonpsychotic individuals (Citrome et al. 2004b).

Key Points

- Attempts to manage violent behavior by using medication geared to the primary diagnosis may fail if the violent behavior is due to an unidentified comorbid psychiatric or medical disorder.
- Medication options for management of an acute episode of agitation have expanded to include several different rapid-acting formulations of second-generation antipsychotics. These agents are less likely than first-generation antipsychotics to cause extrapyramidal side effects. Extrapyramidal symptoms especially relevant in the emergency setting are akathisia (introduces an iatrogenic cause for worsening of agitation) and acute dystonia (complicates treatment course and impairs the therapeutic alliance).
- Long-term treatment requires addressing all comorbidities. For patients with schizophrenia, use of clozapine appears to be the best option to decrease aggressivity. The evidence base for the other second-generation antipsychotics is not as compelling as that for clozapine. Adjunctive use of anticonvulsants, β-adrenergic blockers, and serotonin-specific reuptake inhibitors can be considered, as can electroconvulsive therapy. The long-term use of benzodiazepines is discouraged.
- Psychotherapeutic approaches remain an important part of managing patients with impulsive aggressive behavior, particularly for outpatients with personality disorders, although the use of certain agents such as valproate and serotonin-specific reuptake inhibitors shows promise in controlled clinical trials.

References

Abbott Laboratories: ABT-711 M02–547 clinical study report. Available at http://www.clinicalstudyresults.org/documents/company-study_782_0.pdf. Accessed March 19, 2007

American Psychiatric Association: Diagnostic and Statistical Manual of Mental Disorders, 4th Edition, Text Revision. Washington, DC, American Psychiatric Association, 2000

Andrezina R, Josiassen RC, Marcus RN, et al: Intramuscular aripiprazole for the treatment of acute agitation in patients with schizophrenia or schizoaffective disorder: a double-blind, placebo-controlled comparison with intramuscular haloperidol. Psychopharmacology (Berl) 188:281–292, 2006a

Andrezina R, Marcus RN, Oren DA, et al: Intramuscular aripiprazole or haloperidol and transition to oral therapy in patients with agitation associated with schizophrenia: sub-analysis of a double-blind study. Curr Med Res Opin 22:2209–2219, 2006b

Psychopharmacology and Electroconvulsive Therapy | 319

Arango C, Bernardo M: The effect of quetiapine on aggression and hostility in patients with schizophrenia. Hum Psychopharmacol 20:237–241, 2005

Baker RW, Kinon BJ, Maguire GA, et al: Effectiveness of rapid initial dose escalation of up to forty milligrams per day of oral olanzapine in acute agitation. J Clin Psychopharmacol 23:342–348, 2003

Battaglia J, Moss S, Rush J, et al: Haloperidol, lorazepam, or both for psychotic agitation? A multicenter, prospective, double-blind, emergency department study. Am J Emerg Med 15:335–340, 1997

Breier A, Meehan K, Birkett M, et al: A double-blind, placebo-controlled dose–response comparison of intramuscular olanzapine and haloperidol in the treatment of acute agitation in schizophrenia. Arch Gen Psychiatry 59:441–448, 2002

Bristol-Myers Squibb: Abilify product information (revised October 2006). Available at http://www.abilify.com. Accessed December 13, 2006

Brook S, Lucey JV, Gunn KP: Intramuscular ziprasidone compared with intramuscular haloperidol in the treatment of acute psychosis. J Clin Psychiatry 61:933–941, 2000

Brook S, Walden J, Benattia I, et al: Ziprasidone and haloperidol in the treatment of acute exacerbation of schizophrenia and schizoaffective disorder: comparison of intramuscular and oral formulations in a 6-week, randomized, blinded-assessment study. Psychopharmacology (Berl) 178:514–523, 2005

Buckley P, Bartell J, Donenwirth K, et al: Violence and schizophrenia: clozapine as a specific antiaggressive agent. Bull Am Acad Psychiatry Law 23:607–611, 1995

Casey DE, Daniel DG, Wassef AA, et al: Effect of divalproex combined with olanzapine or risperidone in patients with an acute exacerbation of schizophrenia. Neuropsychopharmacology 28:182–192, 2003

Chengappa KN, Goldstein JM, Greenwood M, et al: A post hoc analysis of the impact on hostility and agitation of quetiapine and haloperidol among patients with schizophrenia. Clin Ther 25:530–541, 2003

Citrome L: Use of lithium, carbamazepine, and valproic acid in a state-operated psychiatric hospital. J Pharm Technol 11:55–59, 1995

Citrome L: Comparison of intramuscular ziprasidone, olanzapine, or aripiprazole for agitation: a quantitative review of efficacy and safety. J Clin Psychiatry 68:1876–1885, 2007

Citrome L, Levine J, Allingham B: Changes in use of valproate and other mood stabilizers for patients with schizophrenia from 1994 to 1998. Psychiatr Serv 51:634–638, 2000

Citrome L, Volavka J, Czobor P, et al: Effects of clozapine, olanzapine, risperidone, and haloperidol on hostility among patients with schizophrenia. Psychiatr Serv 52:1510–1514, 2001

Citrome L, Jaffe A, Levine J, et al: Use of mood stabilizers among patients with schizophrenia, 1994–2001. Psychiatr Serv 53:1212, 2002

Citrome L, Casey DE, Daniel DG, et al: Effects of adjunctive valproate on hostility in patients with schizophrenia receiving olanzapine or risperidone: a double-blind multi-center study. Psychiatr Serv 55:290–294, 2004a

Citrome L, Nolan KA, Volavka J: Science-based treatment of aggression and agitation, in The Science, Treatment, and Prevention of Antisocial Behaviors, Vol 2. Edited by Fishbein D. Kingston, NJ, Civic Research Institute, 2004b

Citrome L, Volavka J, Czobor P, et al: Efficacy of ziprasidone against hostility in schizophrenia: post hoc analysis of randomized, open-label study data. J Clin Psychiatry 67:638–642, 2006

Citrome L, Shope CB, Nolan KA, et al: Risperidone alone versus risperidone plus valproate in the treatment of patients with schizophrenia and hostility. Int Clin Psychopharmacol 22:356–362, 2007

Coccaro EF, Kavoussi RJ: Fluoxetine and impulsive aggressive behavior in personality-disordered subjects. Arch Gen Psychiatry 54:1081–1088, 1997

Collins PJ, Larkin EP, Shubsachs AP: Lithium carbonate in chronic schizophrenia: a brief trial of lithium carbonate added to neuroleptics for treatment of resistant schizophrenic patients. Acta Psychiatr Scand 84:150–154, 1991

Currier GW, Chou JCY, Feifel D, et al: Acute treatment of psychotic agitation: a randomized comparison of oral treatment with risperidone and lorazepam versus intramuscular treatment with haloperidol and lorazepam. J Clin Psychiatry 65:386–394, 2004

Czobor P, Volavka J, Meibach RC: Effect of risperidone on hostility in schizophrenia. J Clin Psychopharmacol 15:243–249, 1995

Daniel DG, Potkin SG, Reeves KR, et al: Intramuscular (IM) ziprasidone 20 mg is effective in reducing acute agitation associated with psychosis: a double-blind, randomized trial. Psychopharmacology (Berl) 155:128–134, 2001

Daniel DG, Zimbroff DL, Swift RH, et al: The tolerability of intramuscular ziprasidone and haloperidol treatment and the transition to oral therapy. Int Clin Psychopharmacol 19:9–15, 2004

Dietch JT, Jennings RK: Aggressive dyscontrol in patients treated with benzodiazepines. J Clin Psychiatry 49:184–188, 1988

Donovan SJ, Stewart JW, Nunes EV, et al: Divalproex treatment for youth with explosive temper and mood lability: a double-blind, placebo-controlled crossover design. Am J Psychiatry 157:818–820, 2000

Eli Lilly: Zyprexa product information (revised November 13, 2006). Available at http://pi.lilly.com/us/zyprexa-pi.pdf. Accessed December 13, 2006

Feder R: Treatment of intermittent explosive disorder with sertraline in 2 patients. J Clin Psychiatry 60:195–196, 1999

Fink M, Sackeim HA: Convulsive therapy in schizophrenia. Schizophr Bull 22:27–39, 1996

GlaxoSmithKline: A multicenter, double-blind, placebo-controlled, randomized, parallel group evaluation of the efficacy of a flexible dose of lamotrigine versus placebo as add-on therapy in schizophrenia. Available at http://ctr.gsk.co.uk/Summary/lamotrigine/III_SCA30926.pdf. Accessed November 5, 2005

GlaxoSmithKline: A multicenter, randomized, double-blind, parallel group study to evaluate the efficacy and safety of a flexible dose of lamotrigine compared to placebo as an adjunctive therapy to an atypical antipsychotic agent(s) in subjects with schizophrenia. Available at http://ctr.gsk.co.uk/Summary/lamotrigine/III_SCA101464.pdf. Accessed May 27, 2006

Goff DC, Keefe R, Citrome L, et al: Lamotrigine as add-on therapy in schizophrenia: results of 2 placebo-controlled trials. J Clin Psychopharmacol 27:582–589, 2007

Hirose S, Ashby CR, Mills MJ: Effectiveness of ECT combined with risperidone against aggression in schizophrenia. J ECT 17:22–26, 2001

Hollander E, Allen A, Lopez RP, et al: A preliminary double-blind, placebo-controlled trial of divalproex sodium in borderline personality disorder. J Clin Psychiatry 62:199–203, 2001

Hollander E, Tracy KA, Swann AC, et al: Divalproex in the treatment of impulsive aggression: efficacy in Cluster B personality disorders. Neuropsychopharmacology 28:1186–1197, 2003

Hollander E, Swann AC, Coccaro EF, et al: Impact of trait impulsivity and state aggression on divalproex versus placebo response in borderline personality disorder. Am J Psychiatry 162:621–624, 2005

Kant R, Chalanani R, Chengappa KN, et al: The off-label use of clozapine in adolescents with bipolar disorder, intermittent explosive disorder, or posttraumatic stress disorder. J Child Adolesc Psychopharmacol 14:57–63, 2004

Karson CN, Weinberger DR, Bigelow L, et al: Clonazepam treatment of chronic schizophrenia: negative results in a double-blind, placebo-controlled trial. Am J Psychiatry 139:1627–1628, 1982

Kessler RC, Coccaro EF, Fava M, et al: The prevalence and correlates of DSM-IV intermittent explosive disorder in the National Comorbidity Survey Replication. Arch Gen Psychiatry 63:669–678, 2006

Khan SS, Mican LM: A naturalistic evaluation of intramuscular ziprasidone versus intramuscular olanzapine for the management of acute agitation and aggression in children and adolescents. J Child Adolesc Psychopharmacol 16:671–677, 2006

Kinon BJ, Roychowdhury SM, Milton DR, et al: Effective resolution with olanzapine of acute presentation of behavioral agitation and positive psychotic symptoms in schizophrenia. J Clin Psychiatry 62:17–21, 2001

Krakowski M, Czobor P, Citrome L, et al: Atypical antipsychotic agents in the treatment of violent patients with schizophrenia and schizoaffective disorder. Arch Gen Psychiatry 63:622–629, 2006

Lesem MD, Zajecka JM, Swift RH, et al: Intramuscular ziprasidone, 2 mg versus 10 mg, in the short-term management of agitated psychotic patients. J Clin Psychiatry 62:12–18, 2001

Lindenmayer JP, Kotsaftis A: Use of sodium valproate in violent and aggressive behaviors: a critical review. J Clin Psychiatry 61:123–128, 2000

Linehan MM: Dialectical behavior therapy for borderline personality disorder: theory and method. Bull Menninger Clin 51:261–276, 1987

McEvoy JP, Scheifler PL, Frances A: The expert consensus guideline series, treatment of schizophrenia 1999. J Clin Psychiatry 60:43, 1999

Meichenbaum DH, Goodman J: Training impulsive children to talk to themselves: a means of developing self-control. J Abnorm Psychol 77:115–126, 1971

Meehan K, Zhang F, David S, et al: A double-blind, randomized comparison of the efficacy and safety of intramuscular injections of olanzapine, lorazepam, or placebo in treating acutely agitated patients diagnosed with bipolar mania. J Clin Psychopharmacol 21:389–397, 2001

Meehan KM, Wang H, David SR, et al: Comparison of rapidly acting intramuscular olanzapine, lorazepam, and placebo: a double-blind, randomized study in acutely agitated patients with dementia. Neuropsychopharmacology 26:494–504, 2002

Okuma T, Yamashita I, Takahashi R, et al: A double-blind study of adjunctive carbamazepine versus placebo on excited states of schizophrenic and schizoaffective disorders. Acta Psychiatr Scand 80:250–259, 1989

Pfizer: Geodon product information (revised May 2005). Available at http://www.pfizer.com/pfizer/download/uspi_geodon.pdf. Accessed December 13, 2006

Prakash R: Lithium-responsive schizophrenia: case reports. J Clin Psychiatry 46:141–142, 1985

Preval H, Klotz SG, Southard R, et al: Rapid-acting IM ziprasidone in a psychiatric emergency service: a naturalistic study. Gen Hosp Psychiatry 27:140–144, 2005

Reist C, Nakamura K, Sagart E, et al: Impulsive aggressive behavior: open-label treatment with citalopram. J Clin Psychiatry 64:81–85, 2003

San L, Arranz B, Querejeta I, et al: A naturalistic multicenter study of intramuscular olanzapine in the treatment of acutely agitated manic or schizophrenic patients. Eur Psychiatry 21:539–543, 2006

Shalev A, Hermesh H, Munitz H: Severe akathisia causing neuroleptic failure: an indication for lithium therapy in schizophrenia? Acta Psychiatr Scand 76:715–718, 1987

Sheard MH, Marini JL, Bridges CI, et al: The effect of lithium on impulsive aggressive behavior in man. Am J Psychiatry 133:1409–1413, 1976

Sival RC, Haffmans PM, Jansen PA, et al: Sodium valproate in the treatment of aggressive behavior in patients with dementia: a randomized placebo controlled clinical trial. Int J Geriatr Psychiatry 17:579–585, 2002

Sorsaburu S, Hornbuckle K, Blake DS, et al: The first 21 months of safety experience with post-marketing use of olanzapine's intramuscular formulation. Poster NR432 presented at the 159th Annual Meeting of the American Psychiatric Association, Toronto, ON, Canada, May 2006

Tariot PN, Erb R, Podgorski CA, et al: Efficacy and tolerability of carbamazepine for agitation and aggression in dementia. Am J Psychiatry 155:54–61, 1998

Tiihonen J, Hallikainen T, Ryynanen OP, et al: Lamotrigine in treatment-resistant schizophrenia: a randomized placebo-controlled trial. Biol Psychiatry 54:1241–1248, 2003

Tran-Johnson TK, Sack DA, Marcus RN, et al: Efficacy and safety of intramuscular aripiprazole in patients with acute agitation: a randomized, double-blind, placebo-controlled trial. J Clin Psychiatry 68:111–119, 2007

Tremeau F, Citrome L: Antipsychotics for patients without psychosis? What clinical trials support. Current Psychiatry 5:33–44, 2006. Available at http://www.currentpsychiatry.com/pdf/0512/0512CP_Article2.pdf. Accessed March 19, 2007

Vartiainen H, Tiihonen J, Putkonen A, et al: Citalopram, a selective serotonin reuptake inhibitor, in the treatment of aggression in schizophrenia. Acta Psychiatr Scand 91:348–351, 1995

Volavka J: Neurobiology of Violence, 2nd Edition. Washington, DC, American Psychiatric Publishing, 2002

Volavka J, Zito JM, Vitrai J, et al: Clozapine effects on hostility and aggression in schizophrenia. J Clin Psychopharmacol 13:287–289, 1993

Volavka J, Czobor P, Nolan KA, et al: Overt aggression and psychotic symptoms in patients with schizophrenia treated with clozapine, olanzapine, risperidone, or haloperidol. J Clin Psychopharmacol 24:225–228, 2004

Volavka J, Czobor P, Citrome L, et al: Efficacy of aripiprazole against hostility in schizophrenia and schizoaffective disorder: data from 5 double-blind studies. J Clin Psychiatry 66:1362–1366, 2005

Wright P, Birkett M, David SR, et al: Double-blind, placebo-controlled comparison of intramuscular olanzapine and intramuscular haloperidol in the treatment of acute agitation in schizophrenia. Am J Psychiatry 158:1149–1151, 2001

Wright P, Meehan K, Birkett M, et al: A comparison of the efficacy and safety of olanzapine versus haloperidol during transition from intramuscular to oral therapy. Clin Ther 25:1420–1428, 2003

Zimbroff DL, Allen MH, Battaglia J, et al: Best clinical practice with ziprasidone IM: update after 2 years of experience. CNS Spectr 10(suppl):1–15, 2005

Zimbroff DL, Marcus RN, Manos G, et al: Management of acute agitation in patients with bipolar disorder: efficacy and safety of intramuscular aripiprazole. J Clin Psychopharmacol 27:171–176, 2007

CHAPTER 16

Psychotherapeutic Interventions

John R. Lion, M.D.

This chapter describes general psychodynamic principles applicable to the inpatient or outpatient therapy of patients who are physically violent. This quite heterogeneous group includes spousal abusers, those who hurt animals, temper-prone individuals, persons convicted of criminal acts of violence such as murder, aggressive paraphiliacs, and arsonists. The common denominator among these patients is that they all translate the affect of anger into dangerous behavior, be it assaultive or destructive. Diagnostically, aggression can be seen within a wide variety of mood, thought, and personality disorders (Stone 1995). What is described here focuses more on patients who are characterologically disordered than those who are psychotic and may, for example, have command hallucinations urging them to hurt someone. Although psychotic patients may well benefit from psychotherapy, the main effort with such patients is pharmacological suppression of pathology rather than insight-driven treatment. The following comments refer to traditional, individual therapy. For a description of group therapy for violent patients—the mainstay of institutional care and offender-based clinics—the reader is referred to descriptions of prison-based programs such as those at Patuxent Institution in Jessup, Maryland (Coldren 2004), or Herstedvester in Denmark (Sturup 1968).

Clinical Inexperience

A word should be said about aggression as a "stepchild" entity in clinical psychiatry. Despite its commonplace occurrence in society and its frequent occurrence in hospital inpatient settings, violence largely remains a behavior of the criminal realm and a subject of interest to sociologists or students of law enforcement. Indeed, few clinicians enter the field of psychiatry anticipating that the patients they treat will be violent or dangerous; the discipline is, after all, a "talking" specialty with verbal interventions. A resident's early exposure to the emergency department may correct some of this distortion, but denial is still possible, particularly because most aggressive patients are managed by nursing staff and technicians. Restraint and seclusion, although medical interventions, are not routinely taught to physicians. Indeed, in residency training programs little formal education is provided about the management of violent patients when compared with teachings about the psychotherapy of anxiety or depression or the pharmacological treatment of the schizophrenias (Dubin and Lion 1992). The elective of forensic psychiatry delves into the subject of violence, but few psychiatric residencies have formal links with jails or prisons.

A therapist thus can easily emerge from training with limited awareness of the world of antisocial conduct. Many psychiatrists have never examined a rapist or a murderer, let alone treated one. This inexperience often leads the beginning therapist to avoid confrontation with the patient's aggressiveness. The therapist may not properly delve into past behaviors or may avoid probing subjects or feelings that evoke anger; a false delicacy may descend on the therapy. It is recommended that clinicians who undertake work with violent patients peruse the journals of the forensic sciences and criminology. Psychiatrists rarely see these periodicals and should be acquainted with the vocabularies and concepts of this entirely different clinical world.

The phenomenology of violence leads to further complexity. Unless the patient is still in the throes of a manic illness or has otherwise demonstrated frequent outbursts on a hospital unit, he or she generally is not violent when seen by the clinician. For example, jails and prisons house men and women who have been very violent. However, that violence is over; when seen by the clinician, they are typically nonviolent. This is not the case with a depressed patient who enters treatment in the midst of an observable melancholic state. Not viewing the pathological or deviant behavior makes it difficult for a clinician to appreciate the gravity of a patient's case or his or her dangerousness. Because violent patients easily disclaim their violent propensities even when confronted with overwhelming data and documentation, therapists can find themselves colluding with the patient's denial. This is particularly true with paraphiliac males who minimize their aggressive predatoriness.

Case Example 1

A therapist was sent to a local prison to review the case of a child molester. The patient presented as a mild-mannered man who rejected any idea that he was guilty of multiple assaults on children and who insisted that he had been falsely incarcerated. The therapist easily believed him until such time as he began to read a very thick chart filled with accounts of violent paraphiliac behavior.

Spouse abusers also often insist that they are no longer violent and that they love those whom they have hurt and would never harm them again. One-time murderers may describe a rich circumstantiality that absolves them of their actions. A therapist, faced with such disavowal of violent tendencies, may dismiss the act as a "one-time" event and excuse future propensities. Thus it is vital to review the violent act. If a police report exists, an attempt should be made to procure it and read it. If the patient committed murder, the autopsy report of the victim should be studied. These efforts bring home the seriousness of the behavior. Another common reaction on the part of unseasoned therapists is to boast about the patient's violent deeds, as if they were treating individuals of distinction (e.g., "He's the one who brutally murdered all those children..."). Such a statement converts fear into awe, diminishes repugnance, and rationalizes the clinician's involvement in a case that other colleagues might view as belonging in the sphere of antisocial behavior and more fittingly dealt with by a prison psychologist than by someone in a suburban practice.

Fears and Liabilities

An issue that arises early in treatment is the problem of agency. Many violent patients are court mandated to attend therapy. This immediately poses problems of agency for the patient, creating a negative view of the therapist that is a powerful deterrent to trust and to the revelation of intimate thoughts. This skew must be periodically acknowledged, for only after some time has passed will the patient come to believe in the therapist's sincerity. In the meantime, the clinician has to deal with his or her own anxieties about treating someone who can harm others. This transcends the usual worries felt in the therapy of suicidal patients, where it is more or less accepted that failure might occur. In effect, the risk of death by suicide parallels the risk involved in treating any inherently fatal disease. However, in the case of outwardly directed aggression, the patient can hurt or kill others; the violence thus moves beyond the boundaries of therapy and can affect more or less innocent bystanders. Liability, always on the mind of today's clinician, has the potential to escalate dramatically. The average psychotherapy patient talks about becoming violent or dreams of violence but does not act on those urges. The violent patient, in contrast, has "crossed the line" from contemplation to response. Therapists must worry about things going very wrong. They must concern themselves with the safety of potential victims, with weaponry, with *Tarasoff* issues, with liability, and with the patient's use of alcohol or other disinhibitory or stimulant substances.

Vectors of Violence

A common misconception is that the violent patient is exempt from suicide and vice versa. However, violent patients can hurt others and themselves as well; they can commit both homicide and suicide. The disorder of unregulated aggression, then, is a disease unto itself, and there is some evidence that it reflects central nervous system serotonin deficits (Markowitz and Coccaro 1995). It is the vector, then, that often becomes a focus of treatment. The psychological burden of treating violent patients, whether they be suicidal or homicidal, is significant, and the therapist must worry about patients' inwardly and outwardly directed aggression. No homicidal patient is ever immune from committing suicide, just as no suicidal patient with violent tendencies is exempt from channeling anger outwardly. Vectors of aggression can shift abruptly, depending on the availability of the victim or of a weapon such as a handgun.

Case Example 2

A man who was being treated for an ear infection became delusional and thought that his doctor was poisoning him. He decided to kill himself in front of the doctor in order to illustrate his plight. He brought a loaded pistol to his appointment, took it out, and pointed it at his head, but at the last moment he turned the muzzle toward the doctor and shot and killed him.

In one sense, the development of depression is a goal of treating violent patients. Therapy aims at helping patients tolerate painful affects associated with loss and with injuries to self-esteem. Improperly modulated, however, the despair may become overwhelming.

Case Example 3

A young adolescent girl stabbed and killed her abusive mother during an argument. The court mandated inpatient psychiatric treatment, and the girl remained on a university teaching unit for more than a year. Because her case was an unusual one, she became the subject of intensive psychotherapy. Upon her release, she continued outpatient treatment but became increasingly depressed and ultimately committed suicide by hanging.

Postpsychotic depression has been described as emerging in the therapy of schizophrenia at a point when the patient comes to relinquish his or her psychosis and realizes how ill and dysfunctional he or she has been (McGlashan and Carpenter 1976). Violent patients can go through the same phase. Therapists should predict this to the patient and should outline the goals of fostering introspection. Patients given to behaviorally "acting out" may find the passivity of therapy alien and difficult, because they may not understand how talking and feeling can possibly help them in their lives.

Goals and Strategies of Therapy

The goals of psychotherapy of violent patients are relatively straightforward: they are to help patients understand the origins of their need to destroy or hurt and wound and to appreciate their inner affective state before it erupts. This urge springs from severe injury in childhood, neglect to the point of rage, a long-standing pathological detachment, or an aberration in the choice of object, as seen in paraphiliac disturbances. Some origins are easier to identify than others. Spouse abuse, for example, often reflects intolerable ambivalence toward a lover and can often be traced back to earlier abuse or neglect by a parental figure. Aggressive pedophilia, on the other hand, has as yet undetermined biological origins; although some components such as love-seeking can be identified, a clear resolution of dynamics usually remains elusive. However, the therapist can still help the patient identify emotional trigger points and inner yearnings that fuel a need to act. Treatment of fire setting, which often is not identified as violence, requires that patients understand when they are feeling angry or empty. Temper proneness, as seen in intermittent explosive disorder, requires identification of recurring precipitants that lead to the rage.

Case Example 4

An investment broker entered treatment after erupting in rage at a country club wedding and loudly calling his girlfriend a whore. In the past, he had once begun to choke her. It became apparent that a recurring stressor was abandonment; at the country club, she had left his side to interact with other family members, and he recalled feeling isolated and becoming furious.

The therapy of these conditions is a mixture of insight-oriented and cognitive therapy. The task of eliciting affect can be a very pedestrian one. It requires that the clinician continually probe what the patient is feeling and has the quality of learning a new language of expression. Affective recognition is the most crucial task of treatment. To the extent that the therapist begins to probe deeper issues, exploring the various degrees of sadism is a central effort as well. Patients who break glass, draw the blood of others, or create pain all receive some satisfaction from the intimidation they create. Beginning therapists can easily view the violent acts as "mistakes" by the patient, rather than as the products of an intrinsic derangement of empathy. That is, it may be that a patient not only has the capacity to harm or destroy but also is gratified by the act and will seek to do it again unless a repair takes effect. It is necessary to explore with a patient all the various manifestations of sadism, even to the tiniest detail. The results are often surprising.

Case Example 5

A schoolteacher stabbed her husband during an argument. He later died, and she adamantly maintained that she had not intended to kill him. Indeed, when the police arrived, she was administering cardiopulmonary resuscitation to him. She presented as a demure woman and was much prone to intellectualize. It was only after the therapist explored her history of violence for some 9 hours that she admitted, sheepishly, that she disliked ants in her house and would pour flammable fluids on them and light them on fire. In time, she also related that she had burned herself on the ankle with cigarettes, something she hid with ankle bracelets.

Even the most hardened criminal may be ashamed of admitting to behaviors that reflect sadism, brutality to children or animals, or sexual excitement in connection with the infliction of pain. In the elicitation of such pathology, the therapist must bridge a gap between expressing revulsion and exhibiting detachment. Some dismay can be shown, together with a therapeutic desire to help the patient overcome such malignant behaviors. The origins of sadism must be explored if they are ever to be changed; such exploration once again involves a review of childhood events that unleashed the need to be cruel.

This issue of sadism raises a larger question of whether it is ever unrealistic to treat someone whose crimes or behaviors are extremely heinous. The therapist obviously must decide whether therapeutic intervention is feasible, but this is not a simple task. As with gravely injured patients in a wartime battle situation, some patients cannot be salvaged. This is particularly the case with intractably aggressive persons who lack a conscience or use projection and denial to the point of therapeutic impenetrability. Sometimes, a trial of therapy is needed to confirm whether or not the patient is introspective or responsive to insight. Remorse, guilt, sorrow, and the capacity for empathy may not emerge for a long time.

Deranged Transferences

Assuming that the violent person becomes a willing patient and meaningfully partakes in treatment, the transference must be carefully monitored. Physical rage usually reflects the most desperate helplessness, and it can easily be rekindled, particularly within the nurturing process of psychotherapy. Patients with primitive character structures can begin to relate to a therapist in the same way they responded to parents or authority figures. Small prohibitions on the part of the therapist may become magnified; for example, the clinician who will not renew a benzodiazepine drug may be perceived as very cruel and withholding. Perhaps the greatest danger stems from the vicissitudes of intimacy. As the violent patient comes to feel closer to the therapist, an intolerable yearning may arise that is frustrated by the constraints of treatment. Loss of the therapist may arise as a risk. The simple dependency of the patient on the therapist can become overwhelming. These dynamics must be regularly explored, as must the specific fantasies that the patient has about the therapist.

Case Example 6

A social worker treated a woman with a borderline personality disorder in a public clinic setting. The patient was demanding and often paranoid but came regularly to sessions and developed a clear dependency on the therapist. In time, this dependency changed into wishes to be with the therapist outside of the hour. These urges were not fully explored. One evening, the patient appeared outside the therapist's home wielding a loaded handgun. She fired a shot that missed the therapist, at which time the therapist tackled her and subdued her until the police arrived.

Deranged transferences are frightening events, seemingly appearing out of thin air; however, there are usually warning signs, such as a patient's view of the therapist as cold and uncaring, a perception that mirrors childhood neglect or violence. This perception can lead to anger and an emerging desire to harm the therapist. Conversely, the intimacy of treatment may spawn a desire in the patient to be closer to the therapist, manifested as driving by the therapist's home or engaging in stalking behavior (Lion and Herschler 1998). Even a patient's spending excess time in the therapist's waiting room can signal some form of attachment that warrants exploration and intervention. The issue here is pathological attachment, but such an attachment is often a silent one. The patient will not talk about it because he or she senses it is not proper and fears alienating the clinician. As the patient's needfulness spirals out of control, the unattainability of the sought closeness liberates anger. This is the point at which violence can erupt. The only way to guard against the development of a deranged transference is to *periodically ask the patient about it;* the question takes the form of asking the patient how he or she is feeling about therapy in general and about the clinician in particular.

Where therapy is conducted bears mention. Many therapists see patients in the evening or on weekends when office buildings are empty. This may create too intimate a setting for seeing some patients, and the clinician generally would be safer working in a more public space where there is traffic and other signs of external controls. At the very least, the first intake session should occur when other staff are nearby. Very little attention is given to the safety of the settings in which the clinician practices (Lion et al. 1996). Most clinics, for example, have no buzzer alarm system in place, nor are staff trained in how to summon help in an emergency. Interview rooms may be poorly configured, placing the clinician behind a desk against a wall rather than near the door so that, in a crisis, he could exit. Weapons screening practices, although more in keeping with emergency departments, still warrant consideration when the population being treated is very ill or the clinician serves an offender population.

Countertransference Issues

It can happen that a therapist becomes irrationally fearful of a violent patient, as the following case illustrates.

Case Example 7

A psychiatrist sought consultation because he found himself frightened of a violent patient without good cause. No threat had been made, nor was the patient menacing or otherwise intimidating. As he discussed the case and the consultant asked him about his own experiences with violence, the clinician stated that he once had gone on vacation and parked at an overlook atop a mountain. Another car drove up and a man got out of the car, walked toward the psychiatrist, took out a revolver, and aimed it at him. He managed to push the man over the ledge in self-defense and called for the police. The man was found and returned to a prison from which he had escaped. The psychiatrist had actually not remembered this upsetting event, and talking about it resolved his uneasiness with the patient who had obviously kindled the recollection.

Such an event is rare in the lives of most clinicians, but less dramatic instances of violence may be evoked during treatment, leading to skews in the perception of the patient (Lion 1998). For certain therapists, sexual deviance such as that shown by a child molester is so repulsive that no meaningful treatment can be undertaken. Clinicians must make an inner appraisal of their own experiences with aggression as they labor with the patient before them.

Victims

Treating a violent patient without consideration of an existing victim is an error. In spouse abusers, for example, the therapist must monitor how the patient is behaving at home, and this can only be done by asking the wife about the patient. A useful strategy with identified victims is to invite them into an evaluative session with the patient present. This minimizes any breach of confidentiality while allowing the therapist to observe how the two parties interact. It is sometimes the case that the would-be victim's behaviors are so provocative that treatment is indicated. In cases where the patient has been violent toward children or animals, a corroborating source of information should be sought, such as a case worker or relative. Again, the therapy of the violent patient is conducted with less privacy than that operative in more traditional individual treatment. In some sense, it is like the treatment of an actively suicidal patient, in which the therapist comes to rely on the family for feedback and participation.

Warning victims about incipient violence is now a standard of care under most *Tarasoff*-based state statutes. Although imminence of a threat prevails as the qualifier for warning, there should be some concept of reasonableness in the mind of the treating clinician. Certainly, a patient who wishes to harm a non–family member presents a dire situation in which warning may be indicated. More frequently, however, the patient is already enmeshed in a troubled relationship with a clearly identified other such as a lover or spouse. If a threat is made, the clinician should seek, whenever possible, to invite the spouse or lover into a treatment session. This is far superior to issuing a sudden formal warning by phone or letter. Such a warning is a clearly alienating event and leads to little or no possibility of therapeutic resolution. In general, it makes little clinical sense to wait until a major interpersonal crisis occurs before intervening; the therapist must engage in prophylactic work and introduce the potential victim into the treatment setting early on. Otherwise, that person is distanced from the treatment and cannot easily enter into it to inform the therapist about the patient's behavior.

Controversy about warning has recently arisen in the case of college students whose suicidal or homicidal thoughts come to the attention of administrators. However, institutions can come to see their role as a private one, and misguided notions of confidentiality can prevail, leading the college to withhold notification of a patient's violent urges at possible risk to the public or to the patient him- or herself. Very few patients are "imminently" homicidal (or even suicidal) to the point of equipping themselves with a loaded weapon. Rather, they talk first about emerging thoughts, much as any patient describes angry feelings about someone else. Unchallenged, the thoughts escalate. The point here is that the clinician should adopt a lower threshold for "warning" a victim or notifying family so that preventive action can be taken.

The Uses of Medication

The pharmacological treatment of violence is discussed in Chapter 15 of this book. Some principles, however, bear mention. No specific antiaggressive drug exists. Rather, it may be helpful to use a drug that affects a target symptom conducive to violence. If the patient, for example, begins to ruminate about a perceived insult made by his spouse and becomes agitated in the process, he may benefit from a benzodiazepine taken upon recognition of his escalating anxiety. This may short circuit the buildup of anger. Anxiety, in fact, is a key factor in the production of rage. Just as the condition of anxiety increases the risk of suicide in a despondent patient, so panic states can fuel rage in someone so predisposed. In general, "fuse lengthening" is a goal of treatment, but it can only be effective if the patient comes to identify the affect that swirls within. Similar rationales support the use of anticonvulsant drugs that attenuate "ictal" expressions of explosive violence such as those seen in intermittent explosive disorder. Some violent patients appear to have behavioral lability that mirrors mood changes; in such instances, an antidepressant or mood stabilizer may be of benefit. In other instances, a quenching agent can be useful, such as a short-acting benzodiazepine

Psychotherapeutic Interventions

that the patient keeps in his or her wallet and uses when the anger starts building up. Perhaps the only exception to the nonspecificity of treatment is the use of antiandrogens or hormonal agents to treat the heightened drive state seen among pedophiles or rapists.

Assessing the efficacy of a drug is often difficult. A patient may claim that he or she is no longer violent when the spouse reports otherwise, and a dosage adjustment may be necessary. This is another reason why it is useful to periodically (once a month, for example) solicit information from a victim. One matter to be cognizant of is a reduction in alertness resulting from too high a dosage of medication. Because violent patients are often hypervigilant, they may be noncompliant with any drug that makes them feel vulnerable to the world around them. Small dosages, titrated upward, is the rule of thumb. Patients can be told that the initial amount of medication given may be ineffective and that the clinician will slowly increase it.

Supervision

Psychiatry tends to be practiced in isolation. With violent patients, it is useful to talk things over with another clinician, provided that the latter has some experience in the management of aggression.

Case Example 8

A resident treated a paranoid patient who became threatening to her, threw a pillow at her during a session, and ultimately made a homicidal threat. The resident had been reporting this to her supervisor, a psychoanalyst. The latter was dismissive of the danger involved and suggested that the resident was both unconsciously eliciting the threats and magnifying the risk of them. The resident sought consultation with a forensic psychiatrist, who became appropriately alarmed. He recommended that the resident notify the police of the threat and helped the resident hospitalize the woman and halt therapy with her.

Unstable Treatment Situations

There may come a time, as the previous example illustrates, when the clinician should consider disengagement from the patient. This is obviously not a simple matter.

Case Example 9

A young man prone to temper smoked marijuana frequently. He lived by himself but was pressured by his family to find a stable job and get married. Arguments often erupted between the patient and his father, an attorney. However, when the parents went on vacation, the patient typically became anxious and used more drugs. During one such holiday, the patient complained bitterly to his therapist about the parents. The therapist acknowledged his dependence and anger, at which point the patient took out a large pocket knife, opened the blade, and held it to his own abdomen. The therapist immediately stated that he was frightened by the patient's actions and asked that he put away the knife. The patient complied, ran out of the office, went home, and began to destroy his apartment. Police were called and the patient was hospitalized. The therapist decided that the patient posed a danger and could no longer be safely managed in a private outpatient setting but should be treated in a more public setting. He arranged for the patient to be transferred to a hospital-based clinic.

It is clear that there may come a time when limits with a patient are reached and it becomes prudent to relinquish treatment. Assuming that the situation does not reflect a countertransference element as described earlier, the clinician should shift care to another setting. This is not simple to accomplish, because a truthful revelation of what occurred will deter many prospective therapists from taking on the case. It is useful in these instances to hospitalize the patient and meet on several occasions with the treatment team and the future therapist. It is important to explain to the patient why transfer is taking place—that is, to admit to the patient directly that he or she has become too frightening. Patients are often surprised to hear this, but the comment has clear therapeutic value, particularly in a critical situation when physical confrontation by the patient occurs. If a patient becomes threatening, not revealing the impact of the threat can lead the patient to become more menacing because he or she senses no response. This advice seems counterintuitive to security and law enforcement personnel who would never admit to others that they are fearful. However, in the clinical realm, the message can halt dangerous behavior.

Key Points

- Many therapists lack experience with aggressive patients. It is recommended that clinicians who undertake work with violent patients peruse the journals of the forensic sciences and criminology.

- Violent behavior typically is not on display during therapy, and this can make it difficult for a clinician to appreciate a patient's dangerousness. Thus it is important to review the patient's past violent acts.

- Therapists treating violent patients must concern themselves with the safety of potential victims, with weaponry, with *Tarasoff* issues, with liability, and with the patient's use of alcohol or other drugs that may contribute to violence.
- No homicidal patient is immune from committing suicide. Likewise, suicidal patients may turn aggression outward.
- The goals of psychotherapy of violent patients are to help patients understand the origins of their need to destroy or hurt and to appreciate their inner affective state before it erupts.
- To guard against the development of a deranged transference, the therapist must periodically ask the patient how he or she is feeling about therapy in general and about the clinician in particular.
- The therapist must be aware of duty to warn potential victims of a violent patient. Warning victims about incipient violence is now a standard of care under most *Tarasoff*-based state statutes.
- Supervision is useful to therapists who are treating violent patients, and the possibility that the best course will be disengaging from the patient should be recognized.
- Psychotic patients may benefit from psychotherapy, but the main effort with such patients is pharmacological suppression of pathology.

References

Coldren JR: Patuxent Institutions: An American Experiment in Corrections. New York, Peter Lang Publishing Group, 2004

Dubin WR, Lion JR (eds): Clinician Safety. Task Force Report No 33. Washington, DC, American Psychiatric Press, 1992

Gellerman DM, Suddath R: Violent fantasy, dangerousness, and the duty to warn and protect. J Am Acad Psychiatry Law 33:484–495, 2007

Lion JR: Countertransference in the treatment of the antisocial patient, in Countertransference Issues in Psychiatric Treatment. Edited by Gabbard GO (Review of Psychiatry Series, Vol 18; Oldham JM and Riba MB, series eds). Washington, DC, American Psychiatric Press, 1998, pp 73–84

Lion JR, Herschler JA: The stalking of clinicians by their patients, in The Psychology of Stalking: Clinical and Forensic Perspectives. Edited by Meloy JR. San Diego, CA, Academic Press, 1998, pp 165–172

Lion JR, Dubin WR, Futrell DE (eds): Creating a Secure Workplace. Chicago, IL, American Hospital Publishing, 1996

Markowitz PH, Coccaro PI: Biological studies of impulsivity, aggression, and suicidal behavior, in Impulsivity and Aggression. Edited by Hollander E, Stein DJ. Chichester, UK, Wiley, 1995, pp 71–90

McGlashan TH, Carpenter WT: Postpsychotic depression in schizophrenia. Arch Gen Psychiatry 33:231–239, 1976

Stone MH: Psychotherapy in patients with impulsive aggression, in Impulsivity and Aggression. Edited by Hollander E, Stein DJ. Chichester, UK, Wiley, 1995, pp 313–332

Sturup GK: Treating the "Untreatable": Chronic Criminals at Herstedvester. Baltimore, MD, Johns Hopkins University Press, 1968

CHAPTER 17

Seclusion and Restraint

Kenneth Tardiff, M.D., M.P.H.
John R. Lion, M.D.

Seclusion and restraint are "hands-on" techniques that can be used to manage violent patients within psychiatric inpatient units and emergency rooms. Being often the sole means of initially controlling very combative and assaultive individuals before medications become effective, and even when used in conjunction with drugs, restraint and seclusion are destined to remain controversial. This is because the techniques so dramatically infringe on the physical freedom of patients and because they are historically associated with the inhumane practices of older times. Seclusion and restraint have thus received intense scrutiny by the lay public as well as by psychiatrists themselves. The first effort by the psychiatric profession to address the utility of restraint and seclusion was undertaken by a task force of the American Psychiatric Association during the years 1981–1985. The findings of this group were published in 1985 and still remain a standard of care (Tardiff 1984), although a second task force met during the years 2003–2005 and issued a revised report that has not yet been fully approved by the American Psychiatric Association at the time of this writing (American Psychiatric Association 2006). Portions of the report, however, will appear as a correctional mental health commentary in the *Journal of the Academy of Psychiatry and the Law* (J.L. Metzner, personal communication, October 14, 2007). The most recent task force (herein called "the APA task force") was convened to address new directives issued by Medicaid and Medicare agencies and the Joint Commission for the Accreditation of Healthcare Organizations (JCAHO). These directives are commented upon in the following discussion.

Studies of Seclusion and Restraint

The 1984 task force studied the extent of the use of restraint and seclusion in various states and found great variability in terms of how structured and specific the guidelines were. Some states had very detailed formal policies; others had virtually no guidelines. In some published studies in which restraint and seclusion were used primarily to halt physical violence toward other persons, rates of usage ranged from 2% to 10% (Mattson and Sacks 1978; Soloff and Turner 1981; Tardiff 1981; Wells 1972). In other studies done within acute psychiatric inpatient units, there was a greater frequency of restraint and seclusion, ranging from 18% to 37% (Binder 1979; Convertino et al. 1980; Oldham et al. 1983; Plutchik et al. 1978; Schwab and Lahmeyer 1979). The latter settings were found to be more likely to use physical intervention for other reasons in addition to halting physical violence, such as to manage agitation and anger, poor impulse control, threats, or property damage.

In 1986, Way conducted a survey of all state hospitals in New York. He found that 59% of such facilities used restraints and 46% used seclusion. Most of the hospitals used only one or the other technique for the control of disruptive behaviors. Emergency medication was used with seclusion or restraint in 56% of the hospitals, but there was great variability in the use of such drugs. Restraint or seclusion was used more frequently in response to physical attacks toward staff (30%) or other patients (21%) than for threatening behavior (16%) or agitated behavior (16%). Later, in 1992, Ray and Rappaport (1995) surveyed 125 state hospitals and psychiatric units in general hospitals within New York. Some 33% of general hospitals and 14% of state hospitals used seclusion or restraints, but they used these for fewer than 1% of their patients. Swett (1994) studied all admissions to the only state hospital in New Hampshire during a 1-year period in 1991–1992. A total of 114 (31%) of admissions had at least one episode of seclusion or restraint, usually because the patients were harmful to themselves or others. Crenshaw and Francis (1995; Crenshaw et al. 1997) conducted a survey of state hospitals in 44 states and the District of Columbia in 1991 and repeated the survey in 1994. They found that smaller hospitals had greater use of seclusion and restraint than larger hospitals. These authors attributed their findings to the fact that smaller hospitals treated more acutely ill patients for shorter time periods, whereas larger hospitals had more chronic patients. Lavoie (1992) studied the use of seclusion and restraint in the emergency department of an urban university hospital in Kentucky and found that 9% of patients were secluded, whereas 26% were restrained. Studying the overall use of restraint and seclusion, Busch and Shore (2000) reviewed the literature from 1994 through 1999 and found a variation in the frequency of restraint and seclusion that appeared independent of the socioeconomic and clinical characteristics of patients. Staff decision making was inconsistent, but other nonpharmacological interventions (such as behavior modification) lowered the use of seclusion and restraint. Sailas and Fenton (2000), in reviewing the literature, found no controlled studies of the use of seclusion or restraint as an intervention in the treatment of psychiatric emergencies and no studies regarding the effects of seclusion or restraint upon patients with schizophrenia or other serious psychiatric disorders.

Other countries have looked at the use of restraint and seclusion. Ahmed and Lepnurm (2001) studied the use of seclusion in a Canadian forensic hospital and found that patients with acute psychosis represented 11.8% of seclusions, whereas those with agitation or disruptive behavior represented 12.7% of episodes of seclusion. Suicide threats or self-harm gestures were the reasons for secluding a patient in 27.4% of episodes. Diagnostically, substance-related disorders accounted for 41% of seclusion episodes, whereas patients with schizophrenia accounted for 28% of seclusion episodes. Kaltiala-Heino et al. (2003) studied the reasons for the use of seclusion and restraint in the psychiatric inpatient units within Finland and found results similar to those of the Canadian study by Ahmed and Lepnurm.

New Governmental Guidelines

In 1999, the Health Care Financing Authority, now known as the Centers for Medicare and Medicaid Services (CMS), defined rules for the use of seclusion and restraint in facilities that participated in Medicare and Medicaid (U.S. Department of Health and Human Services 1999, 2001). CMS maintains a narrow indication for restraint and seclusion, stating that these interventions can be used only to manage severely aggressive or destructive behavior that places the patient or others in imminent danger. CMS has published directives on who can order restraint and seclusion, who can review the process, and when such a review should take place. However, JCAHO has also entered the field and defined its own parameters (Joint Commission on Accreditation of Healthcare Organizations 2002). Table 17–1, from the unpublished report of the most recent American Psychiatric Association Task Force on Restraint and Seclusion [2006], provides a synthesis of these parameters

TABLE 17–1. Time parameters for restraint or seclusion interventions

	Length of time or frequency
Time from initial order to face-to-face evaluation by **physician** (preferable) or **LIP**	1 hour
Subsequent face-to-face evaluations by **LIP**	Every 12 hours
Maximum length of time before new order is required	
Adult	4 hours
Age 9–18 years	2 hours
Child	1 hour
Maximum length of time before chief physician must review	24 hours
Visual observations by **trained staff**	**Every 15 minutes**; continuous if in four-point restraints or restraint plus seclusion
Face-to-face evaluations by **clinical staff**	Every 2 hours

Note. This table synthesizes JCAHO and CMS recommendations. These two agencies have differing definitions of *staff*.
  A **licensed individual practitioner (LIP)** is a clinician state licensed to write orders for restraint and seclusion and trained in emergency care techniques.
  A **clinical staff member** is a degreed nurse or nursing assistant.
  A **trained staff member** has some degree of mental health training, such as a mental health assistant.
Source. Adapted from American Psychiatric Association Task Force on Seclusion and Restraint 2006.

and definitions. Unfortunately, the fact that these two institutions have differing standards has made the subject of restraint and seclusion more confusing. Added to this complexity is the fact that states vary in which regulations they follow. Thus the clinician must know the written guidelines applicable to the state in which he or she practices.

Indications for Seclusion and Restraint

Described here are the principles on the use of seclusion and restraint as detailed in the revised APA task force report. The main changes made since 1985 pertain to the matter of who authorizes the restraint and seclusion, who reviews its use or continuation, and when such reviews occur. Also addressed in the revised report is how long a patient can be kept in restraints and seclusion (see Table 17–1). Although CMS guidelines state that seclusion or restraint can be used only in emergency situations, the recent task force expands on this, emphasizing the maintenance of the milieu and specifically adding that seclusion and restraint can be used to prevent imminent harm to other persons as well as the patient and to prevent serious disruption of the treatment environment. For example, a patient may be a danger to him- or herself in two ways: first, in terms of deliberate suicidal acts or self-mutilation, or second, by a degree of excitement or behavioral dyscontrol that, if it continues, will result in exhaustion or injury. The patient can be a danger to another by deliberately trying to assault that person or by unintentional violence as a result of marked disorganization of behavior, such as that seen in an agitated paranoid delusional state. Under certain circumstances, seclusion of a patient may be indicated both for the patient's benefit and that of the environment. The delicate balance of competing interests between the patient, other patients, and the milieu is often difficult to achieve. Patients who are seriously disruptive to the environment or who are seriously interfering with the rights of other patients generally do so because of the underlying disease process. Certain events, such as uncontrollable screaming or abuse, public masturbation, nude behavior, uncontrolled intrusiveness on others, or fecal smearing may indeed constitute indications for seclusion or restraint.

Before using seclusion or restraint, the staff should have considered or tried other means of control, particularly verbal and environmental interventions. Appropriate use of antipsychotic, mood-stabilizing, or anxiolytic drugs should be considered as well. With appropriate documentation, staff may rely on the patient's known history of violent episodes and their known predecessors, such as escalating, excited motor behavior, increase in muscle tone or generalized tension, pacing, or loud or profane speech. The key to the medically appropriate use of restraint and seclusion is documentation and review. Why such interventions were used should always be stated in the record, together with what other interventions failed. Any institution using restraint and seclusion must keep records of usage and review those records on an annual basis. Although there exists no "average" use of these modalities, changes in usage can signify a changing population, staffing problems, or a change in treatment philosophy.

Initiation of Seclusion and Restraint

Portions of the following sections are taken from the current Task Force Report on Seclusion and Restraint (American Psychiatric Association 2006) submitted to the American Psychiatric Association.

Initiation of a restraint procedure or placement of a patient in seclusion is usually an emergency procedure carried out by nursing and other professional staff in accordance with established hospital policy for seclusion and restraint. CMS guidelines now specify the need for a "licensed independent practitioner" (LIP) to initiate and monitor restraint and seclusion. Such clinicians are described as being trained in emergency care techniques and licensed by their state to write orders for restraint and seclusion. JCAHO guidelines make no such comments about manpower and qualifications. According to CMS, a patient should be seen face-to-face by the LIP within 1 hour after initiation of restraint and seclusion and at least every 4 hours thereafter. If a patient is released from seclusion before the initial assessment, the LIP must still render an evaluation within that first hour's time. JCAHO is more lenient in its requirements, stating that an initial face-to-face evaluation must be done within 4 hours in the case of an adult and within specified shorter periods for younger patients. The task force has adopted the CMS 1-hour interval as a maximum permissible time period between the initiation of restraint or seclusion and an in-person evaluation. In the first edition of the APA task force report, the physician was identified as the person needed to make such an assessment. Neither CMS nor JCAHO makes this requirement, and the task force acknowledges the LIP as qualified to assess the patient. However, the task force continues to view restraint and seclusion as medical procedures and identifies the physician as the preferred person responsible for evaluating the patient within the first hour as well as countersigning the initiation and subsequent orders. Furthermore, the task force states that the physician should maintain a leadership role in formulating all policies and practices of restraint and seclusion. If a clinician other than one on the patient's treatment team orders restraint or seclusion, the patient's treating doctor should be notified.

CMS and JCAHO requirements vary considerably. The initial order for restraint or seclusion, according to CMS, cannot exceed a duration of 4 hours for adults, 2 hours for adolescents between the ages of 9 and 18, and 1 hour for children under 9 years of age. After the first specified time period, a new order for another term of restraint or seclusion is required. On the basis of clinical information that can be conveyed by telephone, CMS allows additional restraint or seclusion orders without face-to-face evaluations for up to 24 hours. JCAHO mandates a face-to-face evaluation every 8 hours for patients 18 and older and every 4 hours for younger patients, but it does not comment on total time limits. In its first edition, the APA task force described the initial order for restraint or seclusion as valid for 12 hours and orders of longer than

Seclusion and Restraint | 345

72 hours as requiring higher administrative approval. The task force adheres to its original recommendation of 12 hours for the period between initiation of restraint or seclusion and subsequent in-person evaluations after the first 1-hour check and now recommends 24 hours as the time limit after which higher administrative approval is required by a chief physician (see Table 17–1).

The task force recognizes that there may be individuals so disturbed that more time in seclusion or restraint will be needed beyond 24 hours. In such instances, the chief physician of the institution or his or her designee must review the treatment plan and concur with additional restraint or seclusion. Some patients will require more frequent face-to-face visits than every 4 hours. Examples are patients with concurrent medical problems, those with organic brain syndrome such as related to drugs or alcohol, and situations in which hyperthermia may occur. CMS has commented that in cases of unusual self-mutilation, such as Lesch-Nyhan syndrome, a patient can be kept in long-term restraints as part of medical management, not behavioral management. The task force further recommends that orders be time and behavior specific, with a stated goal (e.g., "Four-point restraints for 1 hour or until patient is no longer agitated and combative"). Standing orders for restraint or seclusion are not allowed. The clinician must document in the patient's record the failure of less restrictive alternatives and the justification for continued seclusion or restraint. This decision takes into account the mental and physical status of the patient, his or her degree of agitation, and the adverse effects of seclusion (both physical and emotional). Debriefing at the end of each restraint or seclusion episode is mandatory. The patient should be asked about the experience and appropriate comments documented.

Techniques for Seclusion and Restraint Maneuvers

The APA task force makes the following recommendations concerning the maneuvers for restraint and seclusion, based on the realization that uniform techniques and standards are lacking nationwide.

First, the technique of restraint practiced within a particular facility should be rehearsed and approved by the hospital staff, including the chief of service of the institution. If the particular technique and modality, such as four-point leather restraints, is viewed as normal practice, that should be specifically noted in the policy manual of the hospital. Details of the specific technique should be disseminated to all members of the clinical staff as part of the service training. Written instructions, photographs, and videotapes are desirable. A certification process should be in place, with documentation that each clinical staff member has been taught restraint and seclusion and been recertified on an annual basis. Hands-on training is requisite. Identified instructors should be designated within a hospital facility to teach these skills to both new and existing clinical staff and as part of in-service training. Physicians should also take part in training procedures. This matter, along with the general subject of staff protection, is extensively covered in an American Psychiatric Association monograph on the subject of clinician safety (Dubin and Lion 1993).

A variety of restraint devices are marketed, including Velcro and leather limb restraints, body vests, and full body jackets (Lion and Danto 1996). Presently, no data exist concerning the relative efficacy of any devices. JCAHO regulations recommend the gathering of such data in keeping with "evidence-based" medical practices, but the task force realizes that such an effort is exceedingly difficult. The choice of which apparatus to use is left up to the individual institution. Legal representatives for the institution should be consulted regarding the use of the particular restraint methods and their acceptability within the prevailing regulations and law of the hospital and state. JCAHO, but not CMS, recommends that families be informed of the institution's practices and policies regarding restraint and seclusion. Both agencies concur, however, on the need for restraint and seclusion practices to be a part of the patient's treatment plan. The APA task force concurs with some of these recommendations. For instance, family knowledge about an institution's policy on restraint and seclusion appears reasonable. However, on the matter of the treatment plan, it should be recognized that restraint and seclusion are emergency procedures. Thus, their employment cannot be anticipated in most treatment plans unless the patient's history of previous restraint needs is known to staff. On the other hand, new patients should be informed about existing restraint and seclusion techniques and policies on the unit to which they are assigned.

Specific Techniques of Seclusion and Restraint

Once the decision has been made to proceed with seclusion or restraint of an agitated or disruptive patient, a seclusion or restraint "leader" is chosen among available clinical staff. Sufficient personnel consists of at least one person per limb. Staff should gather in a "show of force." Rather than appear "combat ready," the supporting staff should convey an air of confidence and calm, a measured control, reflecting a detached and professional approach to a routine and familiar procedure. A seclusion monitor is designated to clear the area of other patients and phys-

Seclusion and Restraint | 347

ical obstructions to entering the seclusion room. In addition, the monitor stands clear of the physical action, noting any and all injuries or difficulties with physical technique, thus allowing for an accurate critique of the seclusion procedure after the event.

Any confrontation with the patient begins with a clear statement of purpose and rationale for the seclusion or restraint. The patient is given few and clear behavioral options without undue verbal threat or provocation. For example, the patient is told that his or her behavior is out of control and that a period of seclusion is required to assist the patient to regain control. The patient is then asked to walk quietly to the seclusion room accompanied by staff. Because the decision for seclusion has already been made, negotiation or psychodynamic interpretation at this juncture is superfluous and leads only to an escalation of disruptive behavior, potentially aggravating the violence of the event. At this point the team should position itself around the patient in such a manner as to allow rapid access to the patient's extremities. At a predetermined signal from the leader, physical force commences, with each staff member seizing and controlling the movement and each limb restrained at the joint by a member of the team. The patient's head must be controlled to prevent him or her from biting. With the patient completely restrained on the ground, additional staff may be called to secure the limbs and to prepare to move the patient to the seclusion room or to apply mechanical restraints. In the most violent of cases, staff may need to carry the patient into the seclusion room. This involves physically lifting the patient in the recumbent position with arms pinned to sides, legs held tightly at the knees, head controlled, and force applied uniformly to the back, hips, and legs.

If the patient is taken to seclusion, he or she should be positioned on his or her back with the head toward the seclusion door and feet in the opposite direction. An assessment should be made regarding transfer to a hospital gown, and special attention should be paid to rings, belts, shoelaces, and other potentially destructive objects. Medication may be injected at this time while the patient is physically restrained. For the most violent patients, the cross-arm-vise maneuver is again established, allowing attendants to control the head and both arms in preparation for leaving the seclusion room. The staff exit in a coordinated fashion, one at a time, releasing legs first and arms last.

Mention should be made as to whether the patient is restrained face up or face down. The face-down posture is safer because the patient is less apt to bite or aspirate. However, the task force is aware of instances in which patients have suffocated from being so restrained. This is a particular risk in obese patients or in instances where there is a medical illness such as a goiter or another medical condition that can obstruct breathing. Such patients should be restrained face up. In any event, caution should be exercised in the placing of knees on any patient's back so as to avoid compromising breathing. The monitoring of breathing adequacy is critical to any restraint process.

A debriefing follows each seclusion or restraint maneuver to review the technique and progress of the event and allow an emotional release of tension for the staff members. The restraint or seclusion should be discussed openly among the patient population to allay or uncover fears associated with the eruption of violence and staff use of force. The patient should also be asked about the experience and whether it contributed to or worsened his or her sense of control. Documentation of the restraint episode is undertaken and written in the chart or on an incident form.

Observation

During the period of time the patient is in restraints or seclusion, observations regarding behavior should be made every 15 minutes by appropriately trained nursing staff. For those patients in four-point restraints or in lesser degrees of restraint in combination with seclusion, observations must be continuous. In the first edition of its report, the APA task force considered 15-minute observations as satisfied by visual checks and recommended in-person evaluation every 2 hours minimally. JCAHO mandates 15-minute checks and allows seclusion monitoring to be done by video camera, whereas CMS makes no comment on technique or frequency of observations, deferring to parameters spelled out in hospital policy. The APA task force adheres to the 15-minute observation rule, although it recommends more frequent monitoring if clinically indicated, for example, in instances of self-destructiveness that may involve headbanging. The task force recognizes that continuous television monitoring of patients in seclusion is common, and it approves such methods of observation provided that appropriate use is made of the monitor. The screen itself should be placed in an area of the nursing station conducive to privacy. Visual observation checks (as opposed to in-person assessments) should comment on the patient's behavior while ascertaining that the patient is not injuring him- or herself. Observations should also determine that the patient is not at risk for physical exhaustion or hyperpyrexia due to exertion while taking psychotropic drugs.

Patients should be seen in person every 2 hours—more often if clinically indicated, such as if the patient is banging his or her head. If agitated patients are to be approached in the seclusion room, the same

Seclusion and Restraint | 349

number of staff should enter the room as were required in the first instance to subdue the patient (e.g., one for each extremity). Once a patient is quiet, direct observation with the seclusion room door open should be made so that the state of the patient and a description of verbal interchange can be documented on the patient's chart. If the patient is in restraints, the pulse, blood pressure, and range of motion of extremities should be assessed. Table 17–1 summarizes times regarding orders and observations.

Care of the Patient in Seclusion or Restraints

Toileting of the patient should be allowed at least every 4 hours. The design of some seclusion room facilities is such that the patient may have to physically exit to accomplish this, or the patient may have to be removed from restraint devices. In situations in which this cannot be carried out for reasons of danger, toileting can be done through use of the urinal or bedpan. Privacy should be considered. Meals should be brought to the patient at regular intervals when the remainder of the ward is served. All articles should be blunt; plastic knives and forks can be used as weapons. Mealtime can be dangerous for belligerent patients, who can use food as a weapon. In certain rare instances with severely regressed patients, the food tray may be placed within the room and the patient allowed access to it without staff persons being present. However, the rationale for this solitary meal should be strictly documented in nursing notes. Whenever possible, feeding should be a time of interaction between patient and staff.

The proper administration of fluids is vital for patients in restraint or seclusion, particularly for those who perspire profusely and are prone to dehydration. Documentation of fluid intake, although often difficult with regressed patients, is still requisite.

Patients in restraint and seclusion may exhaust themselves from the physical activity of pushing or pulling against restraint devices or walking or running around the seclusion room itself. Some severely regressed patients may be menstruating or prone to fecal soiling. Although not dangerous, such behaviors are often sufficiently repugnant to others to cause avoidance. Hence, the patient is ignored and approached with trepidation. Negligence is thus a potential hazard in the seclusion of such patients.

There is the possibility of a worsening of a psychosis due to decreased sensory stimulation inherent in seclusion room use. The patient may become more delusional as a function of being isolated. It has been suggested that the emotional impact of seclusion is severe and that some debriefing is necessary following removal from seclusion to mitigate painful memories (Wadeson and Carpenter 1976).

Seclusion Room Design

A full awareness should exist regarding the hazards of the seclusion room. Presently, no standard seclusion-room architecture exists. Theoretically, the seclusion room is an empty cubical with a high ceiling and recessed lamp fixtures. All walls and ceilings should be made of material that cannot be gouged out by a patient intent upon self-harm. For example, plasterboard walls are not acceptable. Padded walls can be used, provided that the integrity of the material used is high and the surfaces are clean; however, there are insufficient data available to make this a formal recommendation of the APA task force. Although fire laws sometimes dictate otherwise, the door to the room should open out so that a patient cannot barricade him- or herself inside. Protuberances within the room, such as oxygen jets, are dangerous. Windows must be constructed of safety Plexiglas or otherwise shielded from breakage. The mattress should be the only furnishing in the room; a full bed, even when bolted to the floor, poses a danger because the patient can jump from it and injure him- or herself. The mattress should be constructed of durable foam and not fiber or another substance that the patient could conceivably use for hanging or self-suffocation. The mattress should not be flammable. Patients should always be searched before being placed alone in seclusion. The issue here is that a violent patient may become self-destructive when placed in isolation. Self-mutilative acts can occur, headbanging can occur, or a patient can throw him- or herself against a wall if unrestrained.

Removal From Seclusion and Restraint

Patients may be released from seclusion when the goals of the treatment have been achieved—that is, when a patient's behavior is under control and no longer poses a threat to self or others or a further disruption to the therapeutic milieu. The relative ability of a patient to control his or her behavior is observable many times during the course of seclusion. At each exit from and reentry into the seclusion room for the purpose of feeding, bathing, or examining the patient, responsiveness to verbal direction can be judged. The patient can be asked about his or her control of feelings. Cooperation with physical examinations are also important. All these parameters form a data base for deciding to wean the patient from restraints and seclusion. However, removal from restraint and se-

Seclusion and Restraint | 351

clusion does not have to be abrupt. Indeed, graduated steps toward freedom are often safer. Patients can also have their restraints partially removed first and then be observed for a period of time, or the door of the seclusion room can be opened. Reactions to these events then form the basis for further release procedures.

Emergency Medication

Confusing definitions and recommendations regarding medication have been put forth by CMS and JCAHO. CMS allows medications to be used "as part of an approved treatment plan for the patient's diagnosis." If, however, a medication is not so used, the intervention becomes a "chemical restraint" and is thus viewed the same as a physical restraint and subject to CMS regulations. JCAHO considers the use of medication to restrict a patient's freedom of movement to be improper. The APA task force believes that psychotropic medication may or may not restrict movement but that it can be a powerful aid to patients who are struggling to control behavior. The task force does not endorse the term *chemical restraint* because it is both a misnomer and pejorative. The use of medication obviously depends on the nature of the patient's condition, the degree of agitation, and the qualitative nature of the aggressiveness. If the patient is flagrantly psychotic or in an extremely agitated manic state, medication may be indicated. Medication, if rationally used, may shorten the length of stay in seclusion by helping the patient to gain mastery over aggressive urges. One hazard, however, of medicating assaultive patients is that the patient may be rendered so lethargic that he or she becomes disorganized and combative as a function of organic impairment. Thus clinicians need to navigate between under- and over-medication and document specific target symptoms that respond to psychotropic agents.

Some patients in restraint and seclusion can be offered medication orally, a tactic more conducive to dignity than other routes. On the other hand, it is well known that there are some patients so flagrantly ill that a parenteral injection is needed. Parenteral medication is rarely curative of an underlying psychosis but is used basically to induce symptomatic improvement. Further and more vigorous treatment must ensue before the core symptoms such as delusions and hallucinations abate.

"As-needed" dosing of drugs should be avoided. If drugs are used during the restraint and seclusion process, the goals of administration should be spelled out in specific orders, for example, "Haldol 5 mg po q4h until belligerence and aggressiveness abates." Clinicians who are involved in the care of violent patients should be familiar with a variety of parenteral drugs, including benzodiazepines, for use in the management of aggression (Tardiff 1996).

Unique Restraints

It is possible to use various restraint devices in a creative fashion that allows the patient to mingle with others on a ward or within the room. The use of garments that restrain extremities or that bind older patients to a wheelchair may allow the individual to participate in group meetings and receive milieu enrichment that would not occur in a seclusion room. The use of PADS (Protective Aggression Devices) allows a belt-like device to be applied to the waist and wrists or to the ankles but in a manner that permits some range of motion, including ambulation (Van Rybroek et al. 1987). An advantage of these devices is that they enable the patient to take part in ward activities while still restricting potentially dangerous arm or leg movements. There is flexibility in the use of PADS, so that the nondominant hand can even be released from the belt line as a function of improved behavior.

Contraindications to Seclusion and Restraint

Restraint and seclusion may be contraindicated on the basis of the patient's clinical condition. For example, unstable medical status resulting from infection, cardiac illness, disorders of thermoregulation, or metabolic illness may make restraint a preferable intervention to the isolation of seclusion. In some conditions of delirium or dementia, the patient's vulnerability to sensory deprivation as a pathogenic force may lead to worsening of the total clinical state. Patients prone to serious and uncontrollable self-abuse and self-mutilations are also at risk in seclusion. With physical restraints, circulatory obstruction is always a hazard, but this can be minimized by temporarily releasing one of the four-point restraints every 15 minutes. When a patient is lying on his or her back while restrained, aspiration is always a risk.

Seclusion of a patient as a purely punitive response is contraindicated, nor should a patient ever be secluded for the convenience of the staff or because of staffing difficulties or shortages.

Danger and Injury

The implementation of seclusion and restraint procedures places staff and patients at high risk for injury. One-half of all assaults on staff occur during the process of secluding or restraining disruptive patients or in the initiation of seclusion (Mattson and Sacks 1978; Tardiff 1981). Well-rehearsed restraint and seclusion techniques are the best safeguards against this. Patient injuries can occur from improperly worn restraint devices that can potentially restrict breathing. Thus, high chest vests should be avoided. Even when placed in restraints that restrict arm movement, some very thin patients can wriggle their hands and arms with sufficient mobility to engage in self-mutilation such as scratching of their eyes.

Forensic Aspects of Seclusion and Restraint

Seclusion and restraint are high-profile techniques, and both the public and some clinicians have high hopes of abolishing these hands-on treatments in the future. Indeed, some psychiatric facilities pride themselves on using virtually no restraint and seclusion. Although in these instances diligent use of behavior modification plans may be effective, a question is always raised concerning admission criteria, transfer to other facilities in the case of violence, or overzealous use of medication. It seems reasonable to the APA task force that if a hospital elects to treat violent and/or self-destructive mental patients, it will need to have available to it restraint appliances and seclusion rooms. Generally speaking, of the two modalities, restraint is the more hazardous intervention because it involves subjugation of the patient during which injury or death can occur. Cases of litigation have arisen from suffocation induced by holding an obese patient to the ground, face down, without proper observation. Occasionally, a restrained patient may be hurt by another patient who takes advantage of the former's immobility. However, failure to restrain can also arise as a cause of litigation, as when a patient who is not properly controlled becomes violent toward others or injures him- or herself. The patient who is unrestrained in seclusion may be capable of self-injury as well.

Restraint and Seclusion Committee

A new recommendation made by the APA task force is the formation of a local monitoring agency for restraint and seclusion use. In a specific local area, such a group of administrators or clinicians could oversee the extent of practices, review complicated protocols such as those needed for long-term restraint, and review any injuries that might occur. The documentation of injuries is already part of JCAHO policy.

Key Points

- Seclusion and physical restraint are techniques to manage violent patients in hospitals that are regulated by governmental agencies and the psychiatric profession.
- Seclusion and restraint are used in emergencies to prevent imminent harm to other persons, as well as to the patient, and to prevent serious disruption of the treatment environment.
- Seclusion or restraint may be contraindicated on the basis of the patient's clinical condition and should not be used as a punitive response or for the convenience of the staff.
- Seclusion and restraint must be ordered by a physician or, in some situations, by another licensed independent practitioner who must see the patient face to face within one hour after initiation of seclusion or restraint.
- The duration of seclusion or restraint is limited on the basis of the patient's age.
- Clinicians must know and adhere to the policies of the hospital in which they practice in regard to other parameters such as techniques of using and renewing seclusion and restraint.
- The patient in seclusion or restraint must be observed properly and receive adequate nursing care and medical care, including the use of medication.
- Patients may be released from seclusion or restraint when the patient's behavior is under control and no longer poses a threat to self or others or a further disruption of the treatment environment.

References

Ahmed MB, Lepnurm M: Seclusion practice in a Canadian forensic psychiatric hospital. J Am Acad Psychiatry Law 29:303–309, 2001

American Psychiatric Association: Seclusion and Restraint: Report No 22 of the American Psychiatric Association Task Force on Seclusion and Restraint. Washington, DC, American Psychiatric Association, 1985

American Psychiatric Association Task Force on Seclusion and Restraint: Seclusion and Restraint: Report of the American Psychiatric Association Task Force on Seclusion and Restraint (unpublished). Submitted to the American Psychiatric Association, 2006

Binder RL: The use of seclusion on an inpatient crisis intervention unit. Hosp Community Psychiatry 30:266–269, 1979

Busch A, Shore MF: Seclusion and restraint: a review of the recent literature. Harv Rev Psychiatry 8:261–270, 2000

Convertino K, Pinto RP, Fiester AR: Use of inpatient seclusion at a community mental health center. Hosp Community Psychiatry 31:848–850, 1980

Crenshaw WB, Francis PS: A national survey on seclusion and restraint in state psychiatric hospitals. Psychiatr Serv 46:1026–1031, 1995

Crenshaw WB, Cain KA, Francis PS: An updated national survey on seclusion and restraint. Psychiatr Serv 48:395–397, 1997

Dubin W, Lion JR (eds): Clinician Safety: American Psychiatric Association Task Force Report No. 33. Washington, DC, American Psychiatric Press, 1993

Joint Commission on Accreditation of Healthcare Organizations: The Official Handbook. Oakbrook Terrace, IL, Joint Commission on the Accreditation of Healthcare Organizations, 2002

Kaltiala-Heino R, Tuohimaki C, Korkeila J, et al: Reasons for using seclusion and restraint in psychiatric inpatient care. Int J Law Psychiatry 26:139–149, 2003

Lavoie FW: Consent, involuntary treatment, and the use of force in an urban emergency department. Ann Emerg Med 21:25–40, 1992

Lion JR, Danto BL: The hardware of violence containment, in Creating a Secure Workplace. Edited by Lion JR, Dubin WR, Futrell DE. Chicago, IL, American Hospital Publishing, 1996, pp 195–208

Mattson MR, Sacks MH: Seclusion: uses and complications. Am J Psychiatry 135:1210–1213, 1978

Oldham JM, Russakoff LM, Prusnofsky L: Seclusion: patterns and milieu. J Nerv Ment Dis 171:645–650, 1983

Plutchik R, Karasu TB, Conte HR, et al: Toward a rationale for the seclusion. J Nerv Ment Dis 166:571–579, 1978

Ray KN, Rappoport ME: Use of restraint and seclusion in psychiatric settings in New York State. Psychiatr Serv 46:1032–1037, 1995

Sailas E, Fenton M: Seclusion and restraint for people with serious mental illnesses. Cochrane Database Syst Rev(2):CD001163, 2000

Schwab PJ, Lahmeyer RN: Uses of seclusion on a general hospital psychiatric unit. J Clin Psychiatry 40:228–231, 1979

Soloff PH, Turner SM: Patterns of seclusion: a prospective study. J Nerv Ment Dis 169:37–44, 1981

Swett C: Inpatient seclusion: description and causes. Bull Am Acad Psychiatry Law 22:421–430, 1994

Tardiff K: Emergency measures for psychiatric inpatients. J Nerv Ment Dis 169:614–618, 1981

Tardiff K (ed): The Psychiatric Uses of Seclusion and Restraint. Washington, DC, American Psychiatric Press, 1984

Tardiff K: Assessment and Management of Violent Patients. Washington, DC, American Psychiatric Press, 1996

U.S. Department of Health and Human Services: 42 CFR Part 482. Medicare and Medicaid programs; hospital conditions of participation; final rule. Fed Regist 64:36069–36089, 1999

U.S. Department of Health and Human Services: 42 CFR Part 483.358. Orders for the use of restraint or seclusion. Fed Regist 66:71477164, 2001

Van Rybroek GJ, Kuhlman TL, Maier GJ, et al: Preventive aggression devices (PADS): ambulatory restraints as an alternative to seclusion. J Clin Psychiatry 48:401–405, 1987

Wadeson H, Carpenter WT: Impact of the seclusion room experience. J Nerv Ment Dis 163:318–328, 1976

Way BB: The use of restraint and seclusion in New York State psychiatric centers. Int J Law Psychiatry 8:383–393, 1986

Wells DA: The use of seclusion on a university hospital psychiatric floor. Arch Gen Psychiatry 26:410–413, 1972

PART V

Special Populations

CHAPTER 18

Children and Adolescents

Peter Ash, M.D.

Violence is surprisingly common among children and adolescents: four longitudinal studies in the United States using youth self-reports have shown that by age 17, 30%–40% of boys and 16%–32% of girls have committed a serious violent offense, defined as an aggravated assault, robbery, gang fight, or rape (U.S. Department of Health and Human Services 2001). Only a small fraction of these offenses resulted in arrest. Despite the dramatic drop in youth homicide rates since 1993, homicide remains the second leading cause of death in 15- to 19-year-olds, after accidents and ahead of suicide, accounting for approximately 1,900 deaths in the United States per year between 1999 and 2004—a rate of 9.3 per 100,000 (Centers for Disease Control and Prevention 2007). Violence in youth appears in many forms, ranging from the benign, relatively friendly wrestling on the schoolyard playground through such varieties as bullying and dating violence to the more extreme gang-related killings and school shootings with multiple victims. Developmentally, the onset of violence is a phenomenon of childhood and adolescence: if a person has not committed a serious violent offense by his or her early 20s, the likelihood that he or she will ever do so is quite low.

Although mental health clinicians tend to look at violence as a mental health problem or symptom, it is not at all clear that youth violence is best thought of as caused by mental health problems or that the most efficacious interventions are traditional mental health interventions. Youth violence is a major public health concern and a focus of the juvenile justice system in addition to being a problem facing mental health clinicians. It is therefore important for clinicians dealing with violent youth to keep other perspectives—and other types of intervention—in mind. Few now look at adult criminals and expect the mental health system to prevent their recidivism, whereas delinquent youth are seen as more amenable to mental health intervention, and a central mission of the juvenile court is to rehabilitate them. Those whose violence is a product of a psychotic illness make up only a small minority of youth whose violence is a focus of attention. Therefore, although many of the general principles pertinent to the assessment and management of adults detailed elsewhere in this volume are relevant to the assessment and treatment of violent youth, because of youths' developmental differences, different living circumstances, different precipitants, and different legal status, approaches to younger patients are often different from those utilized with adults. Key differences are shown in Table 18–1.

Epidemiology

Aggression is a common behavior in a child's development. A high percentage of an 18-month-old's peer interactions involve aggression, often in reaction to frustration or wanting something another child has. By age 2½, after the child has developed more social skills and language, the frequency of physical peer aggression drops significantly, and it continues to decrease until age 6 as most children shift to verbal types of aggression. Most of the preschool child's aggression is directed at peers. Much of how a child learns to handle aggression is mediated by parenting, so children who deviate from normal development and are identified early can often be helped by parental interventions.

Aggression remains common in elementary school children. Data from a large-scale longitudinal survey of Canadian children indicated that parents rated as "sometimes" or "often true" that more than one-third of boys and about 30% of girls ages 4–11 get into many fights and about 20% of boys and 10% of girls physically attack people (Offord et al. 2001). Of the 15 DSM-IV-TR criteria for conduct disorder, seven code for physical aggression (American Psychiatric Association 2000), so rates of conduct disorder give some indication of the frequency of rates of maladaptive aggression in elementary school–aged children. Epidemiological studies report rates of conduct disorder in elementary school–aged boys as approximately 3%–7% (Loeber et al. 2000), with considerably lower rates in girls.

Violence is common throughout adolescence: in the United States, about 30% of 12-year-old boys and 25% of 17-year-old boys surveyed in a large-scale study in 2005 reported having gotten into a serious fight in the past year (U.S. Department of Health and Human Services 2006). For girls, the rates were only about one-third lower. In the same study, about

TABLE 18–1. Key differences between violent behavior in adults and adolescents

Category	Compared with adults, for adolescents:
Epidemiology	Violence is much more common.
	Homicide accounts for a higher proportion of all deaths.
	Violent careers are shorter.
	The first episode of serious violence most commonly occurs in adolescence, sometimes in childhood, and rarely in adulthood.
Diagnostic differences	Conduct disorder is specific to children and adolescents and is diagnosed on Axis I.
	Antisocial personality disorder cannot be diagnosed in those younger than age 18 and is diagnosed on Axis II.
	Psychotic disorder is much less common.
Behavior patterns	Violent behavior occurs more in groups.
Treatment	Peer group considerations are key.
	Family involvement in treatment is more important.
Legal status	Confidentiality and consent issues are more complex because minors typically cannot consent, control record release, or waive rights against self-incrimination.
	Legal consent for treatment needs to be provided by someone other than patient.
	Hospitalization over the patient's objection can often be accomplished without resorting to civil commitment.
	Patient's responsibility for treatment compliance is reduced.
	Much criminal behavior is adjudicated in juvenile court.

10% of adolescent boys and 3%–4% of girls reported that in the past year they attacked someone with intent to seriously hurt the victim. Bullying is a common middle school variant of violent behavior, practiced by about 13% of sixth to tenth graders (Nansel et al. 2001). Adolescent dating violence also occurs with high frequency. In a nationally representative sample of high school students, about 9% of both girls and boys reported being physically hit by a boyfriend or girlfriend in the previous year (Centers for Disease Control and Prevention 2006). Interestingly, the rates of dating violence were not significantly different for boys and girls, unlike most other forms of violent behavior. Dating violence was most strongly associated with the risk factors of being sexually active and having attempted suicide. The cumulative prevalence of committing a serious violent offense by age 17 is estimated at 30%–40% for boys and 16%–32% for girls. Although African American youth are arrested at much higher rates than white youth, the self-report data cited above show much smaller racial differences. The peak age for the onset of violent behavior occurs in adolescence, around age 16 for boys (Elliott 1994).

These rates of violence appear to have been fairly stable over the past several decades (U.S. Department Health and Human Services 2001). However, adolescent homicide rates have been quite variable: rates for white males tripled from 1964 to 1991 and then over the ensuing 10 years fell back to the rates of the 1970s (National Center for Health Statistics 2004). Thus, although the frequency of violence has remained fairly constant, the *lethality* of that violence has varied considerably. Both the increase and decrease of adolescent homicide rates were linked to changing rates of using firearms by adolescents (Snyder and Sickmund 2006). The involvement of youth in the crack trade and increased gang activity led to an increase in youth homicide. Despite the fact that possession of a handgun by an adolescent is illegal, fear on the street led more youth to carry handguns for protection, which led to more homicides and a spiraling cycle of yet more fear (Blumstein 2002). In the mid-1990s, one study showed almost all incarcerated male delinquents owned a handgun (Ash et al. 1996). Possession of a handgun markedly raises the potential lethality of a violent confrontation. After the mid-1990s youth (and, to a lesser extent, adult) violent crime rates dropped markedly. The reasons for the crime drop remain controversial but appear related to increases in the prison population, increases in the number of police, the decline of crack, and legalized abortion (Levitt 2004). The cycle of fear went into reverse, and firearm carrying by youth decreased. The central role of guns in the lethality of youth violence obviously has major implications for intervention.

Developmental Trajectories

Much of what we know about the development of violence has been learned from longitudinal studies of youth. The majority of researchers recognize at least two main patterns: an early-onset trajectory in which the youth engages in serious violence before puberty, and a late-onset group who do not engage in serious violence until adolescence (Moffitt 1993; National Institutes of Health 2004; U.S. Department of Health and

Human Services 2001). Significant differences between these two trajectories are shown in Table 18–2. Those with early onset have more severe and longer courses and are more difficult to treat. With research currently available, the late-onset group cannot be identified prospectively from preadolescent symptoms, although in retrospect they experienced many childhood risk factors.

Children first learn to manage their aggression from their parents in toddlerhood, and poor parenting in this period sets the stage for later problems (Tremblay et al. 2004). Poor parenting may involve abusive parental behavior, neglect, coercive parenting, parenting by antisocial parents, poor limit setting, or general family dysfunction. Oppositional defiant disorder (ODD) is a frequent precursor of more serious aggressive behavior, and about 30% of those with early-onset ODD progress to conduct disorder (Connor 2002; Loeber et al. 2000). Of those with conduct disorder, about 40% will progress to antisocial personality disorder (Zoccolillo et al. 1992). The most potent risk factors for preadolescent violence are general, nonviolent criminal offenses and preadolescent substance abuse (Hawkins et al. 2000), whereas peer effects become the most potent risk factor in adolescent-onset violence. For both early-onset and adolescent-onset types, there appears to be a developmental progression of offenses, beginning with minor crime such as vandalism and shoplifting, then progressing to aggravated assault, then robbery, and then rape (Elliott 1994). That robbery precedes rape in more than 70% of cases is some of the strongest evidence that rape is a crime of violence, not a crime of sex. Longitudinal studies suggest that most serious violent crime—in fact, most youth crime of all types—is committed

TABLE 18–2. Comparison of developmental trajectories toward violence

Characteristic	Early onset	Late onset
Onset of offending	Before puberty	After puberty
Serious violent offenders, %	30±15	70±15
Violent career longer than 2 years, %	13	2
Strongest risk factors (effect size $r > 0.30$)	General offenses Substance use	Weak social ties Antisocial delinquent peers Gang membership

Source. Data excerpted from *Youth Violence: A Report of the Surgeon General* (U.S. Department of Health and Human Services 2001).

by a relatively small minority of offenders. Whereas more than one-third of adolescents have committed a serious violent offense, about 5%–10% of youth are committing more than 75% of the violent crimes (U.S. Department of Health and Human Services 2001).

Substance abuse, especially alcohol and marijuana, and mental disorder are common among incarcerated delinquents. Excluding conduct disorder, about two-thirds of incarcerated delinquents meet diagnostic criteria for an Axis I mental disorder (Marsteller et al. 1997; Teplin et al. 2002) and exhibit rates of disorder about triple that of the normal population. Axis II personality disorders are also more common among adolescent offenders (Johnson et al. 2000). However, whether there is a causal link between mental disorder and violence in adolescence remains unclear.

The good news is that for most youth, violence is limited to adolescence: even in the early-onset type, fewer than one in seven continue as serious violent offenders into adulthood. The fact that so much violence is limited to adolescence has important implications for social policy. Zimring (2005) suggested that we consider adolescents as having a "learner's permit" to experiment, recognizing that experimentation will bring with it mistakes. Juvenile justice policy, in his view, should aim to minimize the harm of those mistakes and help those who have trouble learning from them, rather than focusing on punishment.

Risk Factors

The high rates of violence in adolescents, compared with the general population, indicate that adolescence itself is a risk factor. The considerable literature on risk factors for youth violence demonstrates numerous risk factors at the levels of individual, family, and community (Connor 2002; Hann 2002; Hawkins et al. 2000). The risk factor literature is complex for several reasons. First, violence is a heterogeneous group of behaviors, and risk factors differ for different types of violence. Second, not only are there numerous risk factors in different domains, but given the dynamic nature of development, different risk factors become salient at different ages. For example, having a delinquent peer group is a potent risk factor for adolescents but not for preadolescents. Third, risk factors may interact: for example, there is considerable evidence from twin and adoption studies that some genetic risk factors, such as having an antisocial biological parent or having the low–monoamine oxidase A allele, are much more likely to be expressed in violent behavior when an adopted child is raised in an adverse home environment (Caspi et al. 2002; Foley et al. 2004). Finally, as with suicidality, no combination of risk factors can predict with much

Children and Adolescents

confidence whether a particular individual will become violent. From a public health perspective, knowledge of risk factors guides prevention efforts; from a clinical perspective, risk factors provide a structure for obtaining information and may point toward areas needing intervention.

Some of the many risk factors for violence noted in the literature are listed in Table 18–3.

Case Examples

Case 1: Early-Onset Course

Bruce, age 13, was referred for treatment as a condition of probation for carrying a handgun while "on duty" as a lookout for a drug seller. He presented as an irritable teenager who initially resented having to come, but he was quite talkative in the initial evaluation session. He had been in foster care for 3 years beginning at age 4 when his mother was sent to prison on a drug charge, but he was returned to her care when he was 7. His father was unknown. His mother reported oppositional behavior at home after age 7 and theft from other youths at school. Despite this history, he had obtained a C average in school. When he was 9, he got mad and killed a dog with a baseball bat, and a year later, he got angry during a baseball game and hit another player with a bat. The school reported he was a bully and hung out with a peer group that harassed other students. He had recently joined a gang and proudly showed the evaluator the gang tattoo on his shoulder.

Case 2: Possible School Shooter

Jeremy, age 13, was suspended from school pending "psychiatric clearance" when a teacher found him doodling pictures of guns on a piece of paper that was entitled "Hit List" and listed six students in his class. Jeremy had no known history of violence, but he did have a long history of not fitting in with peers. A previous therapist had diagnosed him with pervasive developmental disorder not otherwise specified. Academically he had obtained average grades. He had complained to his parents that "lots of kids make fun of me" and that he had been bullied at school on numerous occasions. At the request of the evaluator, his parents checked his computer for recent sites visited and found that he had visited a number of sites dedicated to the Columbine and Virginia Tech school shootings. His father liked to hunt and had four rifles in the home.

Assessment

Violence, both prospective and completed, encompasses a wide range of behaviors that call for differing approaches to assessment and intervention. Violent youth are involved in multiple systems, and depending on the referral, a clinician may take one of a variety of roles, such as

TABLE 18–3. Risk factors for violence

History of prior criminal acts, including nonviolent offenses
Individual factors
  Biological factors
    Physiological under-arousal, including lowered heart rate
    Impairments in frontal lobe functioning
    Abnormal serotonin levels
    Temperament
    Antisocial biological parent
  Psychopathology
    Psychopathy
    Oppositional defiant disorder, conduct disorder
    Attention-deficit/hyperactivity disorder, substance abuse, mood disorder
  Poor social skills
  Poor school performance
    Learning disabilities
    Low IQ
Family factors
  Poor parenting, including abuse and neglect
  Antisocial parent
  High family dysfunction
Negative peer relations
  Delinquent peers
  Gang membership
Community factors
  Neighborhood crime
  School tolerance of bullying and antisocial behavior
  Disadvantaged neighborhoods
  Availability of drugs

primary therapist, medication manager, or forensic evaluator, each of which will call for a different type of assessment. Table 18–4 highlights some of the dimensions in assessment that provide important information for assessing risk and developing a treatment plan. In a full assessment, it is important to obtain information from collateral sources, including parents, schools, and often peers.

The assessment should take place in an environment where both the clinician and patient can feel safe. For high-risk youth, this requires a setting where the youth can be screened for weapons, where no objects

Children and Adolescents | 367

TABLE 18–4. Dimensions to consider in assessing youth violence

Clinical component	Example issues
History of past violence	Developmental trajectory, age at onset, recent behaviors
Social setting	Individual versus group offending
	Nature of relationship to victim (intrafamilial–stranger)
	Gang involvement
Psychiatric diagnosis	Comorbid conditions such as attention-deficit/hyperactivity disorder, posttraumatic stress disorder, mood disorders, pervasive developmental disorder, or psychopathic personality traits
Risk factors	See Table 18–3
Protective factors	Intolerant attitude toward delinquent behaviors, high IQ, commitment to school
Intent	Impulsive versus predatory
Potential lethality	Carrying weapons
Imminence of risk	Near future, long-range risk

are present that can be used as weapons, and where others are rapidly available in the case of an impending assault from the patient.

Consent and Confidentiality

In discussing past violence with a youth, the interviewer may be hearing about criminal acts, and because such information could potentially be used to further criminal prosecution, issues regarding informed consent and confidentiality need to be thought through carefully. Consent issues are more complex with minors for a number of reasons. First, minors typically are not deemed competent to provide legal consent and do not control access to their medical records. Second, minors are less able to understand the implications of material that could constitute a confession and are more likely than adults to defer to the wishes of authority to provide incriminating information. Third, because of the rehabilitative mission of juvenile courts, juvenile courts have looser standards for admissibility, and juvenile judges have considerable discretion in how they utilize mental health information in apportioning rehabilitative services and punishment. Finally, even when information is obtained in a relatively confidential treatment context, if the youth later enters the custody of the juvenile justice system, such information may be released. The evaluator therefore balances the need to obtain relevant information, the ability of the youth to understand the confidentiality and self-incrimination parameters of the assessment, and how information is presented in written records and reports. This judgment will vary depending on the nature of the assessment: an evaluation for outpatient treatment will be quite different from a court-ordered assessment of whether a delinquent youth is dangerous and should be transferred to adult criminal court jurisdiction. At the outset of the evaluation, the nature of the evaluation and how the information may be used should be explained in terms developmentally appropriate to the youth, and information in written records should be worded in a way that does not provide evidence for prosecution (e.g., "gave a history of shooting at a person," rather than "shot Mr. Jones on March 13 of last year").

When treatment is mandated by the juvenile justice system, such as by a probation requirement or in a detention facility, confidentiality constraints need to be clear. Will the therapist be involved in making dispositional decisions? Will the outpatient therapist be in communication with other care providers? How much information will be given to law enforcement and correctional personnel? Given that effective intervention usually involves a multimodal approach, communication with other care providers is usually essential, but the clinician should be clear with the patient as to what sort of information will be shared and what will be kept confidential.

History of Violence

Overall, the best predictor of whether a behavior will occur in the future is whether it is occurring in the present or has occurred in the recent past (Tremblay and LeMarquand 2001). Therefore, a history of violence is key. The clinician needs to obtain both chronological detail (such as when violent behavior began and with what frequency it continued) and detailed knowledge of violent events (e.g., precipitants, emotional state during the assault, nature of the assault, feelings after). Less structured interviewing may obtain details missed by structured questioning. One useful approach for discussing a violent event with a child or adolescent is to say, "Let's suppose I was going to make a movie of what happened. Could you describe what happened in enough detail so I could do that?" Follow up with questions about the event and what led up to it, and then, once the external nature of the event is clear, go back and ask about feeling states at key points, for example, "Tell me what was in your mind when he said [or did]...."

Children and Adolescents

In addition to obtaining history of violent episodes from the child, it is important to obtain collateral history from other sources, such as parents, school, police reports, and in some cases, peers.

Diagnosis

The most common psychiatric diagnosis applied to youth with histories of violence is conduct disorder, the main criterion of which is "a repetitive and persistent pattern of behavior in which the basic rights of others or major age-appropriate societal norms or rules are violated, as manifested by the presence of three (or more) [of the listed behavioral criteria that include bullying, getting into fights, using weapons, and robbery]" (American Psychiatric Association 2000). Conduct disorder is thus a phenomenological diagnosis encompassing a wide range of antisocial behaviors. Children with the disorder typically have a history of previous ODD, a diagnosis characterized by a pattern of negativistic, hostile, and defiant behavior, but ODD does not have aggressive behavior as a criterion. The American Academy of Child and Adolescent Psychiatry has published practice parameters for the evaluation and treatment of conduct disorder (American Academy of Child and Adolescent Psychiatry 1997) and ODD (American Academy of Child and Adolescent Psychiatry 2007). Antisocial personality disorder can only be diagnosed in adults and has as one criterion that there was evidence of conduct disorder prior to age 15. ODD and conduct disorder are Axis I disorders, but when they progress to antisocial personality disorder, the condition is classified as an Axis II disorder. For intervention purposes, the construct of psychopathy, which is not included in DSM, may be useful. Psychopathy encompasses the lack of remorse and the lack of empathy components of antisocial personality but does not include the more behavioral components. The most common metric for psychopathy, the Hare Psychopathy Checklist, does have an adolescent version, the Psychopathy Checklist–Youth Version (PCL-YV; Forth et al. 2003; see discussion of rating scales later). Personality disorder has been associated with recidivism in delinquents (Steiner et al. 1999).

A comprehensive psychiatric diagnostic assessment is useful to delineate disorders that may be contributing to violence risk. Violence can be a symptom of many diagnoses in addition to conduct disorder, including pervasive developmental disorder and bipolar disorder. Conduct disorder has a very high comorbidity with attention-deficit/hyperactivity disorder (ADHD). Many violent youth give histories of exposure to violence, either as a victim or as a witness, and may meet criteria for posttraumatic stress disorder. Substance abuse is a significant risk factor, especially for preadolescents, and participation in a drug culture is likely to expose the youth to violence. Treatment of underlying conditions likely lowers violence risk.

Risk Factors and Risk Assessment Scales

Risk factors listed in Table 18–3 can provide a structure for obtaining important information. Which risk factors are especially relevant depends on the age and clinical situation. For example, biological factors appear most potent in the context of adverse parenting and are most relevant in young children; a history of bullying by a latency-age child should spur an inquiry into school attitudes and policies toward such behavior; and questions about gang membership and peer activities are especially relevant for adolescents.

There has been rather limited work on protective factors, which are thought of not simply as the absence of risk factors but as factors that *independently reduce the effect* of risk factors. Proposed protective factors include intolerant attitude toward delinquent behaviors, high IQ, and commitment to school (U.S. Department of Health and Human Services 2001), but more research needs to be done in this area.

Following work on adult actuarial risk assessment scales, efforts have been made to modify those scales to apply to adolescents (Vincent 2006). The two scales that have the most psychometric support are the PCL-YV (Forth et al. 2003) and the Structured Assessment of Violence Risk in Youth (SAVRY; Borum et al. 2005). The PCL-YV utilizes a 60- to 90-minute expert interview and provides a score but does not have cutoff values for categorical diagnosis or risk of violence. The SAVRY guides trained evaluators in a systematic assessment of risk factors associated with violence. Evaluators then make structured professional judgments in considering the applicability of each risk factor to the adolescent being evaluated. This leads to a final determination of risk as low, medium, or high. Thus far, prospective validity of these scales has not been demonstrated, but they do provide a structure for assessment. There is much weaker empirical support for structured risk assessment in girls (Odgers et al. 2005), and even assessments for case management of girls are more problematic.

Predatory Violence

It is clinically useful to distinguish between aggression that is impulsive, reactive, hostile, and affective and aggression that is predatory, instrumental, proactive, and controlled (Jensen et al. 2007; Vitiello and Stoff 1997), although many youth exhibit both. There is some evidence

Children and Adolescents | 371

that different neural pathways are involved (Blair 2004). The assessment of the child in the first case example, in which there is a clear history of past impulsive participation in group violence, will be different from the assessment of the child in the second case, for whom the key issue is the risk of an individual's acting alone in a cold-blooded, predatory manner. A youth planning predatory violence is more likely to conceal his thinking than is a youth who acts impulsively. Therefore, more indirect information is necessary. Although psychiatrists who work with youth are experienced in obtaining collateral information from parents, they are less likely to be experienced in obtaining information from peers. Yet the evaluee's friends are the most likely—more so than parents—to have heard the youth express threats, even if the friends did not take the threat seriously. One commonality in the mass school shootings by adolescents is that in each case the shooter had expressed threats toward others prior to the event (Verlinden et al. 2000). Depending on the level of risk suggested by other indicators, a youth's friends can be telephoned (with the permission of the patient) or, in higher-risk situations, questioned by law enforcement personnel. Whenever risk of predatory violence by an adolescent is a serious consideration, if at all possible some friends should be talked to.

The second key principle in assessing risk of predatory violence is to think in terms of a pathway toward violence (Borum et al. 1999). This threat assessment approach, first developed for the U.S. Secret Service (Fein and Vossekuil 1998) and later adapted to school threat assessments (O'Toole 1999; Vossekuil et al. 2002), advocates focusing less on the profile of the subject and more on whether the subject is taking steps toward targeted violence. The path begins with fantasizing about killing, progresses to beginning planning, which might involve increased interest in weapons or learning about how others have conducted mass shootings by reading on the Internet, and then moves on to more detailed preparation, such as obtaining weapons, scouting out sites, and following potential victims. The farther along this path a person is, the more risk he or she poses. It is not necessary for a person to *make* a threat in order to *be* a threat. Because an interviewee may deny intent to harm, when interviewing a potential attacker, one also looks for "leakage," such as interest in weapons and interest in other attacks, that may indicate moving on a path toward violence. It is also important to explore the motivation for the behavior that brought the subject to attention. In the case of the potential school shooter described earlier, it would be important to explore what he had in mind when he wrote the "Hit List." For cases that seem to pose medium to high threat, a team of investigators may be necessary to search for possible physical evidence or interview corroborative sources. It should be remembered, however, that the base rate of mass shootings is so low that the efficacy of this approach has not been empirically tested.

Weapons

Because of the close link between weapon carrying and the lethality of violence, a weapon assessment should be part of the evaluation of any youth being assessed for violence. In one study, the rate of firearm ownership by boys who have been in detention approaches 100%, and for girls it is about half that (Ash et al. 1996). The assessment should include a history of how and when the youth first obtained a gun, subsequently obtained weapons, and has access to non-owned guns in the home or from peers. For impulsive aggression, the issue is less one of access, because most youths can obtain a gun if they really want one, than of how frequently, for what reasons, and under what conditions the youth carries a weapon and how often and under what conditions he or she has fired at a person and demonstrates an intent to use (Ash 2002; Pittel 1998).

Formulating a Risk Assessment

Clinicians are often asked to formulate a risk assessment, as in the second example, in which the risk to the school was the referral question. The clinician should recognize that there is less research on the accuracy of predictions of dangerousness of adolescents than there is for adults. No combination of risk factors has been shown to predict with accuracy in an individual case. Therefore, the clinician should acknowledge in his or her report the limitations in prediction and limit the opinion to a risk estimate, noting which risk factors are present. It is often helpful to couch one's opinion in terms of a comparison to some group, such as youth of the same age and gender, youth in the same detention center, and so on.

Management

We have come a long way from the 1970s, when the predominant thinking was that "nothing works" in dealing with violent youth, although violent behavior remains a challenge to treat. Because violence is the product of multiple factors, the most effective treatments utilize several modalities aimed at different sources of dysfunction. These modalities vary widely depending on the nature of the clinical situation: a 4-year-old who was expelled from preschool for hitting other children will re-

Children and Adolescents

ceive different services than the adolescent in the first case example who has a long history of antisocial behavior.

Acute Management of High-Risk Youth

The first priority is protecting others from harm. In some cases this will involve hospitalization. In others, removal from the social situation in which the threat level is high, such as keeping a youth away from school by enrolling him or her in a day treatment program, will suffice.

It is important to reduce access to weapons. Brent et al. (2000) found that only one-quarter of parents were compliant with recommendations to remove guns from the home when their child was suicidal. The clinician can promote a weighing of the risks and benefits involved in carrying a handgun; highlight the penalties if a minor is caught with a handgun; and follow up to ascertain whether the advice was acted upon. Most youths justify carrying guns for protection and safety, and alternative methods of remaining safe can be discussed. Youths who carry guns and demonstrate intent to use may need civil commitment, or if control is not possible, the clinician may have a *Tarasoff* duty to protect others, depending on his or her jurisdiction.

On an inpatient unit, acute highly aggressive behavior may need to be controlled. The American Academy of Child and Adolescent Psychiatry (2002) has developed practice parameters for these difficult situations that emphasize first utilizing measures to promote a violent youth's self-control and other, less restrictive means whenever possible. When physical restraint is used on children, special attention must be paid to maintaining an unobstructed airway and ensuring that the patient's lungs are not restricted in the prone position by excess pressure on the patient's back. Staff training is a crucial factor in ensuring that seclusion and restraint will be applied in a reasonable manner. On mental health units, aggressive outbursts are usually seen as a manifestation of psychiatric problems. In juvenile detention facilities, however, such outbursts are more typically seen as volitional behavior requiring correctional action under the institution's punishment and use of force policies. In some cases, youths are receiving medication for their aggressive outbursts and may receive as-needed medications ordered for outbursts. It is important for psychiatrists working in such institutions to ensure that such discretionary use is carefully monitored.

Outpatient Psychosocial Treatment

A wide variety of treatment modalities have been tried, and a significant number are supported by some outcome studies. Most have a strong family and/or parent training component, based on the view that conduct problems and maladaptive aggression are developed and sustained by maladaptive interactions. Programs that are well supported by outcome research are listed on the Web site Blueprints for Violence Prevention (Center for the Study and Prevention of Violence 2007) and discussed in several reviews (American Academy of Child and Adolescent Psychiatry 1997; Burke et al. 2002; Cadoret et al. 1997; Connor et al. 2006).

Two programs that have demonstrated efficacy with delinquent adolescents in randomized, controlled trials are *functional family therapy*, a short-term (typically 8–15 sessions) prevention and intervention program that utilizes two-person teams to meet with the youth, families, and schools (Alexander and University of Colorado Boulder Center for the Study and Prevention of Violence 1998), and *multisystemic therapy*, in which always-on-call therapists with low case loads provide community-based multimodal treatment that addresses multiple risk factors and work to empower parents and delinquent adolescents with more adaptive coping skills (Henggeler 1998).

Medication

There is growing consensus that medication should first be used to treat any underlying disorder, such as ADHD, depression, or bipolar disorder (Connor et al. 2006; Pappadopulos et al. 2003; Schur et al. 2003). One area in which practice varies widely is the extent to which irritability in adolescents is perceived as justifying a diagnosis of possible bipolar disorder and thus the utilization of a mood stabilizer. After treating any underlying disorder, the second step is to use psychosocial approaches to manage aggressive behavior, such as cognitive-behavioral treatments, parent management training, and increasing environmental structure. Only after those approaches have failed should medication be considered for the target symptom of aggressive behavior.

In 2006, the U.S. Food and Drug Administration approved an indication for risperidone for the symptomatic treatment of irritability in autistic children and adolescents. No medications have demonstrated consistent efficacy in reducing aggression in other conditions. The most widely utilized medications are mood stabilizers and atypical antipsychotics, which appear more effective for impulsive/reactive aggression than for predatory aggression (Connor et al. 2006). Among the mood stabilizers, lithium and divalproex sodium have received the most research support. Among the atypical antipsychotics, risperidone is the best studied, and other antipsychotics have not yet been studied in randomized, placebo-controlled studies, although they are often utilized, especially in juvenile detention settings.

Environmental Interventions

Because association with delinquent peers and gangs is so central in adolescent violence, interventions that reduce peer effects or utilize them proactively have proved useful. For example, from 1991 to 1995, Boston, Massachusetts, averaged 44 street homicides of youth per year. After a community intervention beginning in 1996, that number was reduced by 63% (Kennedy et al. 2001), the so-called "Boston Miracle." Although the intervention was multipronged, the basic idea was that although in most cases the police did not know the shooter, they did know to which gang the shooter belonged, and law enforcement came down hard on all that gang's members. First, there was a community outreach effort educating gangs to the fact that following a shooting, all gang members of the presumptive shooter's gang would be prosecuted for any offense to the fullest extent possible. Police resources from the city were then concentrated on the area in which the shooter's gang operated. Law enforcement and the judiciary bought into the program, and maximum penalties were then given to that gang's members for any offense, from public drinking to assault. Those who violated probation in any manner, including such probation requirements as going to school, had their probation revoked. Because all of the gang suffered for a shooting, peer pressure rapidly began discouraging shootings.

Other interventions that strive for deterrence have been less successful. For example, after the crime wave of the early 1990s, concern for public safety led to more punitive approaches toward youth. Following the "adult crime, adult time" mantra, almost all states expanded their criteria for waiving juveniles to adult court (Sickmund 2004). The weight of the evidence now suggests that punishing juveniles as adults increases recidivism (Fagan 1996; McGowan et al. 2007). The American Psychiatric Association (2005) has called for reform of policies that punish large numbers of adolescents as adults.

Consultation

Aggression and violence in children and adolescents are among the most difficult conditions to assess and treat in child and adolescent psychiatry. Working with such youth also raises strong countertransference issues, and the imprecision of risk assessment in the context of others' lives being potentially at stake can generate considerable anxiety in the clinician. Many child psychiatrists have little experience with this population, and given the national shortage of child psychiatrists, much care is provided to adolescents by general psychiatrists and other mental health professionals. In difficult situations in which one is uncertain of what to do, it is clinically useful and prudent risk management to remember Jonas Rappeport's advice, "When in doubt, shout!" Obtain consultation from another clinician and document it.

Key Points

- The onset of serious violence is typically an adolescent phenomenon. Those whose violence begins in preadolescence have a significantly worse prognosis.
- Serious violent offending is common in high school students, but most do not continue their violent careers into adulthood.
- Many risk factors for violence have been identified, but no constellation of risk factors allows for accurate predictions of future dangerousness.
- Effective treatments for violent youth are multimodal and intervene at multiple levels. Most effective treatments include parent interventions. For adolescents, also intervening to change the patient's relationship to a delinquent peer group is important.
- The best-established use of psychopharmacology is to treat comorbid psychopathology such as ADHD or a mood disorder. No medications specifically target aggression, but mood stabilizers and atypical antipsychotics are sometimes utilized when available psychosocial treatments have not proved effective.

References

Alexander J, University of Colorado Boulder Center for the Study and Prevention of Violence: Functional Family Therapy. Blueprints for Violence Prevention. Boulder, CO, Center for the Study and Prevention of Violence, Institute of Behavioral Science, University of Colorado at Boulder, 1998

American Academy of Child and Adolescent Psychiatry: Practice parameters for the assessment and treatment of children and adolescents with conduct disorder. J Am Acad Child Adolesc Psychiatry 36:122S–139S, 1997

American Academy of Child and Adolescent Psychiatry: Practice parameter for the prevention and management of aggressive behavior in child and adolescent psychiatric institutions, with special reference to seclusion and restraint. J Am Acad Child Adolesc Psychiatry 41:4S–25S, 2002

American Academy of Child and Adolescent Psychiatry: Practice parameter for the assessment and treatment of children and adolescents with oppositional defiant disorder. J Am Acad Child Adolesc Psychiatry 46:126–141, 2007

American Psychiatric Association: Diagnostic and Statistical Manual of Mental Disorders, 4th Edition, Text Revision. Washington, DC, American Psychiatric Association, 2000

American Psychiatric Association: Adjudication of youth in the criminal justice system: position statement. 2005. Available at http://www.psych.org/edu/other_res/lib_archives/archives/200507.pdf. Accessed February 26, 2006

Ash P: Children's access to weapons, in Principles and Practice of Child and Adolescent Forensic Psychiatry. Edited by Schetky DH, Benedek EP. Washington, DC, American Psychiatric Publishing, 2002, pp 225–230

Ash P, Kellermann AL, Fuqua-Whitley D, et al: Gun acquisition and use by juvenile offenders. JAMA 275:1754–1758, 1996

Blair RJR: The roles of orbital frontal cortex in the modulation of antisocial behavior. Brain Cogn 55:198–208, 2004

Blumstein A: Youth, guns, and violent crime. Future Child 12:38–53, 2002

Borum R, Fein R, Vossekuil B, et al: Threat assessment: defining an approach for evaluating risk of targeted violence. Behav Sci Law 17:323–337, 1999

Borum R, Bartel PA, Forth AE (eds): Structured Assessment of Violence Risk in Youth. New York, Guilford, 2005

Brent DA, Baugher M, Birmaher B, et al: Compliance with recommendations to remove firearms in families participating in a clinical trial for adolescent depression. J Am Acad Child Adolesc Psychiatry 39:1220–1226, 2000

Burke JD, Loeber R, Birmaher B: Oppositional defiant disorder and conduct disorder: a review of the past 10 years, part II. J Am Acad Child Adolesc Psychiatry 41:1275–1293, 2002

Cadoret RJ, Leve LD, Devor E: Genetics of aggressive and violent behavior. Psychiatr Clin North Am 20:301–322, 1997

Caspi A, McClay J, Moffitt TE, et al: Role of genotype in the cycle of violence in maltreated children. Science 297:851–854, 2002

Center for the Study and Prevention of Violence: Blueprints for Violence Prevention. 2007. Available at http://www.colorado.edu/cspv/blueprints/index.html. Accessed March 15, 2007

Centers for Disease Control and Prevention: Physical dating violence among high school students—United States, 2003. MMWR Morb Mortal Wkly Rep 55:532–535, 2006

Centers for Disease Control and Prevention: CDC Wonder: Compressed Mortality File [author analysis]. 2007. Available at http://wonder.cdc.gov/mortSQL.html. Accessed March 30, 2007

Connor DF: Aggression and Antisocial Behavior in Children and Adolescents: Research and Treatment. New York, Guilford, 2002

Connor DF, Carlson GA, Chang KD, et al: Juvenile maladaptive aggression: a review of prevention, treatment, and service configuration and a proposed research agenda. J Clin Psychiatry 67:808–820, 2006

Elliott DS: Serious violent offenders: onset, developmental course, and termination: the American Society of Criminology 1993 Presidential Address. Criminology 32:1–21, 1994

Fagan J: The comparative advantage of juvenile versus criminal court sanctions on recidivism among adolescent felony offenders. Law Policy 18:77–114, 1996

Fein RA, Vossekuil B: Protective Intelligence and Threat Investigations: A Guide for State and Local Law Enforcement Officials (Publ. NCJ 170612). Washington, DC, U.S. Department of Justice, 1998

Foley DL, Eaves LJ, Wormley B, et al: Childhood adversity, monoamine oxidase a genotype, and risk for conduct disorder. Arch Gen Psychiatry 61:738–744, 2004

Forth A, Kosson D, Hare R: Hare Psychopathy Checklist: Youth Version. Toronto, ON, Canada, Multihealth Systems, 2003

Hann DM (ed): Taking Stock of Risk Factors for Child/Youth Externalizing Behavior Problems. Bethesda, MD, National Institute of Mental Health, 2002. Available at http://eric.ed.gov/ERICDocs/data/ericdocs2sql/content_storage_01/0000019b/80/1a/ce/6a.pdf. Accessed January 22, 2008

Hawkins JD, Herrenkohl TI, Farrington DP, et al: Predictors of Youth Violence (NCJ 179065). Washington, DC, Office of Juvenile Justice and Delinquency Prevention, 2000

Henggeler SW: Multisystemic Treatment of Antisocial Behavior in Children and Adolescents: Treatment Manuals for Practitioners. New York, Guilford, 1998

Jensen PS, Youngstrom EA, Steiner H, et al: Consensus report on impulsive aggression as a symptom across diagnostic categories in child psychiatry: implications for medication studies. J Am Acad Child Adolesc Psychiatry 46:309–322, 2007

Johnson JG, Cohen P, Smailes E, et al: Adolescent personality disorders associated with violence and criminal behavior during adolescence and early adulthood. Am J Psychiatry 157:1406–1412, 2000

Kennedy DM, Braga AA, Piehl AM, et al: Reducing Gun Violence: The Boston Gun Project's Operation Ceasefire (NCJ 188741). Washington, DC, National Institute of Justice, 2001

Levitt SD: Understanding why crime fell in the 1990s: four factors that explain the decline and six that do not. J Econ Perspect 18:163–190, 2004

Loeber R, Burke JD, Lahey BB, et al: Oppositional defiant and conduct disorder: a review of the past 10 years, part I. J Am Acad Child Adolesc Psychiatry 39:1468–1484, 2000

Marsteller FA, Brogan D, Smith I, et al: The prevalence of psychiatric disorders among juveniles admitted to DCYS Regional Youth Detention Centers: technical report. Atlanta, GA, Department of Children and Youth Services, 1997

McGowan A, Hahn R, Liberman A, et al: Effects on violence of laws and policies facilitating the transfer of juveniles from the juvenile justice system to the adult justice system: a systematic review. Am J Prev Med 32:S7–S28, 2007

Moffitt TE: Adolescence-limited and life-course-persistent antisocial behavior: a developmental taxonomy. Psychol Rev 100:674–701, 1993

Nansel TR, Overpeck M, Pilla RS, et al: Bullying behaviors among US youth: prevalence and association with psychosocial adjustment. JAMA 285:2094–2100, 2001

National Center for Health Statistics: Health, United States, 2004. DHHS Publication No. 2005–0152. Hyattsville, MD, National Center for Health Statistics, 2004

National Institutes of Health: Preventing violence and related health-risking social behaviors in adolescents: an NIH State-of-the-Science Conference. Presented at National Institutes of Health, Bethesda, MD, October 13–15, 2004

Odgers CL, Moretti MM, Reppucci ND: Examining the science and practice of violence risk assessment with female adolescents. Law Hum Behav 29:7–27, 2005

Offord DR, Lipman EL, Duku EK: Epidemiology of problem behavior up to age 12 years, in Child Delinquents: Development, Intervention, and Service Needs. Edited by Loeber R, Farrington DP. Thousand Oaks, CA, Sage, 2001, pp 95–116

O'Toole ME: The School Shooter: A Threat Assessment Perspective. Washington, DC, U.S. Department of Justice, 1999

Pappadopulos E, Macintyre JC, Crismon ML, et al: Treatment recommendations for the use of antipsychotics for aggressive youth (TRAAY), part II. J Am Acad Child Adolesc Psychiatry 42:145–161, 2003

Pittel EM: How to take a weapons history: interviewing children at risk for violence at school. J Am Acad Child Adolesc Psychiatry 37:1100–1102, 1998

Schur SB, Sikich L, Findling RL, et al: Treatment recommendations for the use of antipsychotics for aggressive youth (TRAAY), part I: a review. J Am Acad Child Adolesc Psychiatry 42:132–144, 2003

Sickmund M: Juveniles in Corrections (NCJ 202885). Washington, DC, Office of Juvenile Justice and Delinquency Prevention, 2004

Snyder HN, Sickmund M: Juvenile Offenders and Victims: 2006 National Report. Washington, DC, Office of Juvenile Justice and Delinquency Prevention, 2006

Steiner H, Cauffman E, Duxbury E: Personality traits in juvenile delinquents: relation to criminal behavior and recidivism. J Am Acad Child Adolesc Psychiatry 38:256–262, 1999

Teplin LA, Abram KM, McClelland GM, et al: Psychiatric disorders in youth in juvenile detention. Arch Gen Psychiatry 59:1133–1143, 2002

Tremblay RE, LeMarquand D: Individual risk and protective factors, in Child Delinquents: Development, Intervention, and Service Needs. Edited by Loeber R, Farrington DP. Thousand Oaks, CA, Sage, 2001, pp 137–164

Tremblay RE, Nagin DS, Seguin JR, et al: Physical aggression during early childhood: trajectories and predictors. Pediatrics 114:43–50, 2004

U.S. Department of Health and Human Services: Youth Violence: A Report of the Surgeon General. Rockville, MD, U.S. Department of Health and Human Services, 2001

U.S. Department of Health and Human Services, Substance Abuse and Mental Health Services Administration, Office of Applied Studies: National Survey on Drug Use and Health, 2005 [computer file]. ICPSR04596-v1. Research Triangle Park, NC, Research Triangle Institute [producer], 2006. Ann Arbor, MI, Inter-University Consortium for Political and Social Research [distributor], 2006-11-16. Available at http://www.icpsr.umich.edu/cocoon/SAMHDA/STUDY/04596.xml. Accessed March 26, 2006

Verlinden S, Hersen M, Thomas J: Risk factors in school shootings. Clin Psychol Rev 20:3–56, 2000

Vincent GM: Psychopathy and violence risk assessment in youth. Child Adolesc Psychiatr Clin North Am 15:407–428, 2006

Vitiello B, Stoff DM: Subtypes of aggression and their relevance to child psychiatry. J Am Acad Child Adolesc Psychiatry 36:307–315, 1997

Vossekuil B, Fein R, Reddy M, et al: The Final Report and Findings of the Safe School Initiative: Implications for the Prevention of School Attacks in the United States. Washington, DC, U.S. Department of Education, Office of Elementary and Secondary Education, Safe and Drug-Free Schools Program and U.S. Secret Service, National Threat Assessment Center, 2002

Zimring FE: American Juvenile Justice. New York, Oxford University Press, 2005

Zoccolillo M, Pickles A, Quinton D, et al: The outcome of childhood conduct disorder: implications for defining adult personality disorder and conduct disorder. Psychol Med 22:971–986, 1992

CHAPTER 19

The Elderly

Robert Weinstock, M.D.
Stephen Read, M.D.
Gregory B. Leong, M.D.
J. Arturo Silva, M.D.

Violence in geriatric patients involves many of the same factors and considerations as in younger persons. Although less frequently than younger individuals, elderly people can commit crimes, react to paranoid fears, abuse drugs, and act in revenge. Any cause of violence in a younger individual can also be a cause for violence in the geriatric population. These situations in older people generally need to be treated in similar ways, with minor modifications to account for special geriatric issues. The difference is the lower frequency of such violence as individuals mature and become less impulsive. During clinical interventions, physical and physiological changes concomitant with advancing age, such as increasing frailness and reduced metabolism and clearance, need to be taken into consideration.

However, there are specific problems that are more common in the elderly, and this chapter focuses in particular on violence as related to those factors. Elderly individuals are more likely to have memory and other cognitive problems, including dementia. Memory problems can lead to agitation when elderly individuals forget where they put things and think their possessions are stolen or forget who specific individuals in their home might be. Disorientation can lead to suspiciousness and to lashing out at "strangers" in what the patient perceives as self-defense.

Some dementias respond to clinical intervention with an emphasis on careful diagnostic assessment. Even if a diagnosis of an untreatable condition, such as progressive dementia, is found, family and caregivers can develop more realistic expectations and plans. Also, current treatments can decrease the rate of decline and diminish agitation.

As patients lose the ability to care for themselves, the development of feelings of frustration, humiliation, and helplessness can be frightening. In response to these feelings, the older patient can lash out at caregivers, which in turn can give rise in the caregivers to impatience, burnout, and other negative responses. Intervention at this juncture can make a big difference to ease the caregivers' burden.

Long-term care facilities that house the elderly may have special challenges. Patients can correctly or incorrectly feel abandoned by their loved ones when placed in such facilities. Independence is very important to such people. Well-meaning social workers sometimes can be too ready to remove patients from their homes because of relatively minor self-care deficiencies. For some such patients, independence may be worth some relatively small physical safety risk. The safest solution may not always be the best one. The values of the patient and family must be considered; otherwise, the resulting frustration can lead to violent actions.

Sexual aggression in the elderly can present problems in nursing homes and elsewhere. Individuals with Alzheimer's disease or other dementias, stroke, or other mental illnesses can develop mania or confusion that can lead to inappropriate sexual touching, paraphilias, or other unwelcome behaviors that can be perceived as aggressive. Delusional jealousy or misidentification brought on by cognitive problems can be associated with violence and inappropriate aggression.

The elderly often take multiple medications with additive side effects, drug–drug interactions, and/or resultant confusion. Reevaluating the need for each medication may be crucial because some may no longer be needed or may lead to confusion. Discontinuing some of these medications can be important, as can lowering dosages that may be excessive. Because of pharmacokinetic differences, lower dosages of many medications may be necessary. Treatment compliance remains a significant problem across all age groups but may pose a special problem among the elderly. Memory difficulties can lead to forgetting doses or taking extra ones, with resultant confusion. Organizing medications, such as with daily medication organizers, can be important and may fix the problem.

There has been an upsurge in people over the age of 60 in the prison population in recent years, but the data suggest that this is not due to an increase in offenses in that group but rather a reflection of the elderly receiving harsher sentences (Yorston and Taylor 2006). The most likely cause is mandatory sentencing guidelines, but for some crimes, such as sex offenses, elderly individuals may be punished more harshly than younger individuals. In a study of elderly forensic evaluees, most had alcohol dependence problems and nearly half had dementia (Lewis et al. 2006).

Assessment

Violent acts attract attention. One common setting in which this becomes relevant is in a general hospital. A patient can be profoundly depressed or even confused without attracting attention until the person threatens suicide—or throws a bedpan in frustration at a nurse's aide. The psychiatric attention that was being left until discharge suddenly becomes an emergency. Implicit in this scenario are two principles: that actual or threatened violence remains one of the more reliable routes to psychiatric evaluation, and that the act itself commonly occurs—and is interpreted as "crazy"—in its *perceived* inappropriateness in context.

A consequence of this scenario is that the referral for evaluation is likely to emphasize the act and its consequences—that is, how upset the victim (or potential target) is or the danger to others—more than the context. In the communicated need to "do something" urgently, the evaluator may have difficulty gaining information about the contextual issues, information that would substantially guide the "prescription"—the course of recommended response and treatment. In many circumstances the psychiatric consultant in a general hospital may not be able to perform a complete assessment (Devanand 2005; Silver and Herrmann 2004), especially in urgent circumstances. Many similar problems arise in the outpatient setting. Assessment of the problem is essential to provide appropriate management and treatment. Because any of the elements of a complete evaluation may provide the critical key to the problem, we first review the relevant portions of a complete assessment.

Chief Complaint

The patient may or may not have a "complaint"—the incident that led to the referral may have been forgotten—or the patient's complaint may be the *result* of the response of others: "Why is everyone mad at [afraid of] me?" Eliciting the patient's recall provides a valuable key to memory, insight, and lability of mood and may actually reveal the precipitant for the patient's action. In addition, in this inquiry, the consultant should note appearance, evidence for neurological or other impairments, and level of arousal and agitation.

It is necessary to understand both the violent act and the context from the point of view of others as well as the patient. The chief complaint per se will commonly originate from a caregiver, or perhaps a family member, rather than the patient. The sympathies of the caregiver, therefore, are not only important in and of themselves, but their continued commitment to the patient is also important to maintain. For example, care of dementia patients at home becomes increasingly more challenging as the dementia progresses, and in such circumstances home care generally requires increasing recourse to other services (Read 1990). It has long been recognized that the decision to place a patient elsewhere is most closely related to behavioral issues (Rabins et al. 1982). Caregivers, therefore, are likely to be the critical factors in successfully maintaining the patient's present situation or hastening the transfer to a more restrictive environment. They may also be the agents on whom one must rely for interventions to be carried out. For both patient and caregivers, it is recommended that the examiner maintain nonjudgmental sympathy to avoid prejudging, choosing sides, or activating the ever-present risk of feelings of guilt that will inhibit disclosure.

Case Example 1

Mr. M was a 74-year-old man who had retired from the U.S. Postal Service after 43 years of delivering the mail in the small town where he lived. He had married, relatively late in life, a widow he had met on his rounds whose mother had urged her daughter to pursue him. Mr. M therefore became stepfather to the widow's two children as well as a "solid citizen" who knew everyone by name and was most proud of being the greeter every Sunday prior to church services.

The police were startled one morning by his phone call: "I think I have just killed my wife." They arrived within a few minutes to find Mr. M, hammer in hand, standing by the kitchen table where his wife was slumped, clearly dead. Mr. M said, "I don't know why I did it." After his arrest and jailing, he was given a psychiatric evaluation. His psychiatric history, which he corroborated, included being hospitalized three times for severe depression. Each time, his depression had responded to antidepressant medicine, principally sertraline, with modest dosages of (different) antipsychotic medicines. His first hospitalization occurred after age 50, and the most recent had been 18 months prior to his lethal assault. This last hospitalization was precipitated by Mr. M's having appeared at the door of the police station with an axe, shouting threats and challenging the police to shoot him. Observers had agreed that Mr. M had returned to his quiet, well-behaved self after discharge. However, no psychiatric follow-up was available in his small rural community. His primary care doctor had elected to taper his medicines, and they were discontinued 2 months before the attack on his wife.

Mr. M was a modest-sized man with psychomotor retardation and a soft voice. He said at first that the events of the day of the assault were "foggy"; in fact, cognitive testing revealed modest short-term memory deficits, poor visuospatial (copying) skills, and difficulty with sequential tasks, but preserved language. He reported his mood as, "It doesn't matter" and "depressed"; to observation, he spoke mechanically, without emotional modulation, and his facial and body expressions were also very constrained.

Mr. M generated the following account of the fatal day: He had, over the 2 months since discontinuing his medicine, become increasingly withdrawn—"like I was before." His wife had begun discussions with her children about Mr. and Mrs. M moving so that the children would be able to assist with their needs and eventually, perhaps, their care. It was in this context, in fact, that Mr. M revealed that he had been orphaned early in life and that he and his sister had lived under constant fear and threat of the orphanage. Mrs. M had in fact been discussing the potential move by telephone with her daughter before Mr. M's attack. The entire narration was marked by an almost complete absence of observable or reported emotional reaction.

The psychiatric examiner's evaluation emphasized the interaction of three factors: 1) severe melancholic depression, at least approaching psychotic proportions, with relapse likely attributable to discontinued treatment; 2) cognitive disorder not otherwise specified, classifiable either as mild cognitive impairment or as mild dementia, most likely due to subcortical white matter ischemic vascular disease, consistent with findings reported on magnetic resonance imaging scan; and 3) reactive social and situational factors that, in context, had reactivated deep-seated fears of abandonment based on childhood experiences. Note that all three factors made critical contributions to the action: depression predisposed Mr. M to the most pejorative interpretation of his wife's reasonable exploration of how their future could be more secure, and it also limited his own capacity to envision this turning out well. His prior life experience may have played a critical role (the fear of abandonment is certainly fundamental) but was in fact brought to Mr. M's mind in the interview by his reflection on his homicide. Cognitive impairment (frontal systems brain impairment) was judged to have eroded impulse control and, in this situation, also to have compromised Mr. M's competence to assist with his defense in a trial.

In this example, of course, the examiner was aided by his evaluation's being at some distance in time and space from the events, but the elicitation of the content of Mrs. M's telephone call and the connection to Mr. M's deep-seated fear of abandonment based on having been orphaned—counterpoised by Mr. M's own inability to acknowledge, express, or experience the associated emotional reactions—opened an understanding of the events (sadly, of course, much too late). Note that this information, although in some sense applicable to the "chief complaint," appeared only late in the interview, after rapport had been established and following a gradual approach to the fraught circumstances of the event.

Past History

Medical/Surgical

Confusion is the term most commonly used in referrals when the diagnosis of delirium eventuates. In the elderly, in fact, delirium may commonly herald the onset of an illness such as myocardial infarction that in younger people is announced by more specific symptoms. Because of the high frequency with which mental functions abruptly decline in the elderly due to delirium related to some recent physiological challenge, the medical history is a high priority in the evaluation of the violent geriatric patient. In addition, knowledge about medical status will be vital to the choice of treatment.

The consultant should seek recent laboratory studies. Asking about recent acute illnesses or changes in the patient's status may identify, for example, a bladder infection that in an older person is associated with "confusion" more than with identifiable physical discomfort. Recent medication changes and their effects, such as the anticholinergic effects of amitriptyline commonly given to alleviate neuropathic pain, may precipitate delirium, especially in individuals with dementia. Identifying a physiological abnormality not only may lead to a specific and sometimes prompt resolution of mental derangement but also can be vital to preserving brain function.

Case Example 2

Mrs. J was a high-functioning 72-year-old woman with no personal or family history of major mental disorder who slowly became increasingly agitated over a several-week period, to the dismay of her family. Eventually, psychiatric consultation was sought, which led to voluntary psychiatric hospitalization. However, her hospital stay became involuntary after she assaulted a staff member when her husband could not be reached by phone. She was diagnosed with acute mania and started on quetiapine and lithium. She became alternately sedated and agitated as well as somewhat confused; in response to needed care interactions, she frequently responded by hitting attendants, and more than once struck other patients in a fit of irritability. At these times, she would typically be given intramuscular lorazepam and confined to the "quiet room" or restrained in her bed for several hours. She was noted to sweat pro-

The Elderly

fusely and had low-grade temperature elevation. Medications were switched to risperidone and valproic acid, but without any significant change in her clinical condition.

After 5 weeks, Mrs. J was transferred to an inpatient geropsychiatry unit; the referring doctor implied that she had a rapid-onset dementing condition. She had lost almost 30 pounds and gave the impression of hyperalertness while being sedated and of parkinsonian features of rigidity, drooling, and tremor. Neuroleptic malignant syndrome was ruled out by normal creatine phosphokinase and lactate dehydrogenase levels, but with comprehensive laboratory studies her thyroxine level was found to be 17, with a high reference level of 12.5. Vigorous treatment of her now-diagnosed Graves' disease was initiated on the geropsychiatry service by her consulting internist, with progressive calming and reduced agitation over a 3-week period. Valproic acid was discontinued and risperidone was tapered, and thus her rigidity was reduced. Temperature normalized and weight stabilized as her euthyroid state was reestablished.

This case illustrates the need for careful medical analysis and collaboration. Late-onset mania is rare. Hyperthyroidism cannot be expected to respond to "psychiatric" treatment, even when it presents "psychiatric" symptoms. A more disturbing feature of this case is that in this same time frame, after the return of euthyroid state, Mrs. J was noted to have memory impairment of which there had been no sign prior to her hospitalization, and she went on to have full-blown dementia due to Alzheimer's disease.

Alternatively, the inquiry into the mental and physical condition prior to the violent incident may lead to the identification of an emergent, not-yet-recognized dementia. A brief example is a consultation in a lovely elderly woman who lived alone. Her family stopped by to pick her up for church and found all the drawers in her kitchen had been emptied on the floor and everything scattered. After it was ascertained that this was not a break-in or robbery, she was evaluated for delirium or dementia. She presented very articulately—she was in a book club, for example—but oddly could not recall the titles of any recent books. This observation led to the demonstration of impaired short-term memory, and a history emerged of episodes of accumulating impairment during a 2-year period—and a diagnosis of Alzheimer's disease.

Case Example 3

Mr. T was a 67-year-old veteran admitted to the acute psychiatric unit from an emergency department. He had a history of depression that had been treated with fluoxetine and of very mild early dementia. He had abused crack cocaine in the past, with episodes of delusions and paranoia treated with olanzapine. His most recent hospitalization had been for pulmonary insufficiency. He was a longtime smoker and had emphysema.

He presented to the general hospital emergency department with severe agitation. He would struggle with staff when they attempted to take his vital signs or draw blood. The emergency physician decided Mr. T's problems were psychiatric and attributable to his being off medication. On admission, it could not be determined whether the patient had any family. He was medically cleared by "eyeballing" him and was sent to an acute psychiatric ward.

Because he was combative, Mr. T was placed in four-point restraints on the psychiatric ward. He was struggling with nursing staff. The medical consultant recommended giving him an intramuscular injection of haloperidol, lorazepam, and benztropine to calm him down so he could be examined. Before this was done, his blood pressure was taken and found to be 65/40, and his pulse oxygen was 78. He was sent to the intensive care unit, where he was found to be badly dehydrated with pulmonary insufficiency. Hydration cured his "psychiatric" problems. Fortunately, he had not been given the haloperidol and lorazepam, because the resultant blood pressure drop could have killed him.

This case illustrates the danger of physicians misdiagnosing an elderly patient with medical problems as having a psychiatric disorder when there is any history of psychiatric problems or dementia. Such misdiagnosis could lead to a patient's death. Fortunately, the psychiatrist and psychiatric nursing staff were alert to this possibility. Also, medical clearance by eyeballing a patient can be very risky.

Psychiatric

Psychiatric history information may be most elusive in the elderly. For example, the patient may have suppressed personal recall related to the stigma of such experiences, and family members (children) may never have been told. In addition, the patient may be delirious or demented, and hospital or nursing home staff may have no real information about prior history. Misidentification delusions in the elderly can result in violence. Substance abuse histories may also be vital but are subject to deliberate concealment or ignorance about the extent of alcohol intake, for example, which may contribute to the clinician's overlooking delirium tremens or drug-induced psychosis or affective disorder. Another caution is that a condition that today would be recognized as a major depressive episode may have been diagnosed in the early adult life of an 85-year-old as "neurosis," "schizophrenia" or other psychosis, or simply a "nervous breakdown" in older nomenclature. Elicitation of psychiatric history is usefully done in conjunction with the medical history. However, a history of prior psychiatric disorder can be critical for identifying the precipitating episode of a reemergence. As discussed above, in emergency department and medical settings, confusion and agitation can often be dismissed as psychiatric when the cause may be purely medical and physiological. A misdiagnosis or a tendency to decide that any confusion in a patient with a psychiatric history must be psychiatric can be life-threatening.

Psychosocial

Inquiry into psychosocial factors provides background information that is valuable for rapport and for identifying sources of stress (and for observing the patient's resilience and capacity to understand and appreciate such forces). Such inquiry may also reveal clues to a family illness or to an event relevant to the patient's actions. A serious issue involving a close family member, a recent bereavement, or a major financial or social decision may dominate the patient's thinking and have a greater meaning than one would expect. In addition to the direct physical and physiological effects of the patient's condition, his or her awareness of it may be a critical stressor. Whether the concern is "heart attack," "cancer," or care consequences (e.g., a lap belt used on a patient with dementia to prevent forgetful attempts to stand after hip replacement surgery), it may be experienced directly by the patient as an exacerbation of vulnerability—a perception of threat that can lead to a violent reaction to a stimulus that otherwise would not be threatening.

Mental Status Examination

Different aspects of the mental status examination will emphasize selected features likely to be especially relevant to the evaluation of a violent elderly patient. Ideally, the evaluator will be able to observe at a distance prior to direct encounter. In addition, observation at a distance may reveal the sign of a relevant general medical condition—for example, asymmetric facial or limb movements in a stroke or other focal brain injury, proptosis in Graves' disease, movement disorder, or the moon face of Cushing's syndrome. Familiarity with the expression of cognitive, mood, and behavior disorders associated with various abnormalities of brain function will also usefully inform the examination (Bogousslavsky and Cummings 2000; Strub and Black 1988).

Attentional Problems

Attentional problems are the core symptoms of delirium. The first issue is whether the patient is paying attention—that is, is able to listen to and respond appropriately to questions or requests from caregivers. Is the patient easily distracted? Can the patient reorient to the previous question after an interruption? On the other hand, can he or she then turn attention to another topic or matter on request? How much effort does this require? Is it onerous (irritating, inducing hopelessness, etc.)?

Conditions that can lead to false positives in this realm are significant hearing loss, fluency only in another language, or severe dementia. The most basic test of attention is to ask the patient to repeat single words and then phrases up to longer sentences. Copying line drawings may also reveal problems with sustaining effort and attention, and the preservation of this or other skills may suggest the presence of a language disorder, such as fluent aphasia, that can disrupt communication in a way that incorrectly suggests inattention.

It can be very helpful to describe the patient's performance over the course of the delirium. Among the several available tools, we rely on the orientation, mental control, and registration and recall sections of the Mini-Mental State Examination (MMSE) of Folstein et al. (1975). The MMSE was in fact developed as a tool to identify and give a ballpark estimation of cognitive impairment in patients seen in consultation in a general hospital setting. These items, rated over time, document performance on attentional measures more than adequately. In addition, the MMSE has gained widespread acceptance as an overall rating of the cognitive severity of dementia, and its questions tap a broader range of functions (including visuospatial skills) than many other short rating scales. Use of the MMSE therefore serves double duty in terms of its recognizability as a proxy for the overall cognitive impairments that may predate the acute illness phase or persist afterward.

Cognitive Impairment With Impaired Memory

Cognitive impairment with poor short-term memory is the core symptom complex of dementia. Impaired memory is required for a diagnosis of dementia in DSM-IV-TR (American Psychiatric Association 2000), and if the patient can repeat three words (suggesting at least a modicum of attentional capacity), his or her inability to recall those same words after several minutes signals the presence of this hallmark symptom. From the history, the consultant should have some information, at least about recent medical events, that can serve as a basis for assessing long-term memory. Other cognitive areas warrant attention, even in the initial urgent examination (for more detailed resources, see, e.g., Strub and Black 1985):

- *Language impairments* can be associated with high levels of frustration and distress and, as a practical issue, must be accounted for in developing a plan for management.

- *Visuospatial tasks,* such as copying simple drawings, can help evaluate the patient's ability to engage and focus. Abnormalities in the face of good effort are supportive evidence for dementia. Grossly disproportionate abnormalities may be associated with deficits in brain regions that organize one's sense of orientation in the most basic sense.
- *Reasoning tasks* (e.g., interpreting proverbs and idioms) may be poorly tolerated but are indicative of the level of language skill, attention, and the willingness to tolerate some degree of annoyance or perceived irrelevance. Intact responses at an abstract level are countersuggestive of dementia but may be compatible with significant encephalopathy and resulting delirium.
- *Executive functioning* as assessed by, for example, the Executive Interview (Royall et al. 1992) overlaps with and depends on attentional mechanisms but may be independently disrupted. Deficits may indicate the presence of impaired frontal lobe functions, with associated loss of empathy, judgment, and impulse control, functions that may reduce the threshold for violent, apparently impulsive reactions.

Case Example 4

Dr. F, a former surgeon and community leader, had been living at home with his wife and attending day care. He had support from his out-of-town children as well. He had been functioning as a surgeon until his memory problems became apparent. He had been cared for at home for several years after diagnosis of dementia due to Alzheimer's disease (which itself followed several years of declining short-term memory and risky financial decisions), and this home stay was supplemented by his attending adult day care. He was evaluated for nursing home placement after an emergency call about his being "agitated." Some restlessness and "agitation" had been mitigated with low-dose risperidone. However, near the end of the day care schedule, in fact within several minutes of 2:30 P.M. every day, Dr. F would suddenly transition from a relatively affable, cooperative, good-humored man into a restless, agitated, active and impatient man. He would typically claim he "needed to go [somewhere]," and he would try to push his way out toward the parking lot. Day care staff had worked out somewhat elaborate attempts to divert him, but on the day in question, he had been undeterred and had struck a staff person who finally tried to block his way physically. His wife had arrived shortly thereafter, and she also (for the first time) feared that he would be "violent."

The 2:30 P.M. transition time endured in the nursing setting. Dr. F was bright, confident, helpful, and cooperative in the morning but became impatient, demanding, and urgent from before 3:00 P.M. until past dinnertime. If staff were unable to distract or redirect him, he could become very forceful. Although this was generally limited to pushing or shoving obstructions out of his way (including staff persons or, occasionally, another patient who was unable to recognize the situation), at least the threat of more focused aggression existed. Containing his aggressive impulses was difficult—doors were "secure," but Dr. F's athleticism enabled him to get through several barriers and even to climb over the six-foot-high perimeter wall. Once out, he was also able to move very quickly.

As staff came to know him, their interventions became more effective. Organizationally, because his behavioral change was timed close to change of shift, administrative team intervention was required to ensure a continued high level of observation (instead of the distraction of completing mandated charting) and to manage the relative confusion attendant on staff comings and goings. These efforts alone remained insufficient. His behavior worsened at every attempt to reduce antipsychotic dosage, and he required doses of risperidone 2–3 mg daily, most given after lunch to maximize mid-afternoon effect and thus mute the impulse and contain the risk of aggression.

Dr. F's dementia was moderately severe at nursing home admission (e.g., MMSE score was 14/30) and continued to progress over the next 5 years. He was started on donepezil with some mild improvement. Although the diurnal pattern was unchanged, management became easier as his capabilities diminished. After surgery to repair an intertrochanteric (hip) fracture, he experienced delirium and, after recovery, was not only less mobile but also had a substantial incremental worsening of his dementia. He was also more passive, and at that point the diurnal agitation became much less marked, allowing for the tapering and discontinuation of risperidone.

Violence is common in a significant minority of Alzheimer's patients. Management of these patients requires consideration of a combination of both psychosocial milieu factors and medication.

Thought Processing

The presence of hallucinations, delusions, preoccupations, or other abnormalities may be indicative of impaired brain function and may also directly contribute to the aggressive impulse.

Disorders of Mood and Affective Regulation

Many depressive patients are irritable, which can lead to reactive hostility and, especially in the face of other damage to frontal lobe structures, to disinhibition and violence. There is evidence that aggression in the substantial minority of patients with dementia is strongly linked to the presence of depressive symptoms (Lyketsos et al. 1999). Most dementia patients in the community are not violent. If depression is factored out, dementia patients may be no more violent than other individ-

The Elderly

uals. The hyperactive, driven, grandiose manic patient may also react violently to what would otherwise be mild provocation or frustration. Attentional and cognitive deficits, as well as delusions, can be associated with both poles of mood disorder and further compromise the patient's impulse control. Because apathy can be an early sign of dementia, sometimes it is difficult to distinguish from depression in the elderly.

Case Example 5

Mrs. L was a 78-year-old woman who had been a social leader of her community and who had been married nearly 50 years to a man who continued to adore her. His devotion led him to seek assistance from every source he could find when she developed a persistent, savagely anxious depressive syndrome—and to seek an alternative if success were not promptly forthcoming.

Mrs. L had acted at nearly hysterical levels for a substantial part of every day for more than 3 years. She would throw herself into walls at times, although there was no clear attempt to commit suicide. She had torrents of tears and refused to be comforted and would at times strike at or claw at anyone who presumed to get close, including her husband and the caregivers he hired. Sleep, appetite, energy, and mental focus were all grossly deficient, and she had lost over 40 pounds in the year preceding evaluation. Although a diagnosis of depression had been made (several times), treatment had never been consistently pursued because of her own hopelessness and resistance and her husband's great concern every time someone mentioned the possibility of side effects.

Evaluation confirmed a diagnosis of severe recurrent major depression. Consultation with an internist and laboratory studies revealed no medical cause; in fact, Mrs. L remained in good health. Mr. L was involved in all phases of the assessment—with an emphasis on his accepting that the primary diagnosis was psychiatric. Once that was established, it was possible to provide realistic information about treatment options and the course of improvement that could be expected. Accordingly, Mrs. L was started on venlafaxine. Treatment response began at a dosage of 75 mg daily, with additional improvement and real symptomatic relief evident at a dosage of 150 mg daily. Each improvement, however small, was strongly reinforced both with Mrs. L and her husband. Some level of distress, agitation, and anxiety persisted with optimal doses of venlafaxine, but further improvement was achieved with the addition of small doses of risperidone and then antianxiety medication.

Mrs. L eventually returned to her primary care doctor for follow-up. Twice in 4 years she was reevaluated when symptoms returned—both times after an attempt to "stop medicine because I was better." The third relapse differed. At this point, overt difficulty with memory was seen at evaluation, and this proved to be the early finding in her developing dementia due to Alzheimer's disease. Donepezil was started, but with little effect. As her dementia progressed, she became more impaired.

In addition to increasing cognitive impairment, at every attempt to reduce mood medications, agitation and depression returned, associated at times with paranoia and agitation that could lead to her hitting caregivers or anyone else in the vicinity.

Agitation can be part of depression and can lead to violence. Depression can be an early sign of Alzheimer's but usually manifests more as apathy in such cases. Considering the persistence of the depression and the lack of response to donepezil, there most likely were two independent problems in this patient.

Treatment

Consider Acute/Emergent Treatment

At times the consultant must consider initiating treatment of violent behavior before the full evaluation process can be completed. A rapid medical response, such as restraining a patient in a bed, may be necessary to ensure the safety of the patient and others or to limit the morbidity of other responses. Two groups of medications remain the mainstays of acute calming of aggressive and violent behavior: benzodiazepines and neuroleptics. Both require careful titration and close observation but have a high safety profile in short-term use, especially when compared with the potential for injury from agitated or aggressive behavior.

"Close observation" should include frequent visualization, preferably with the patient in constant line of sight. In addition to monitoring level of agitation and aggression (i.e., the response of target symptoms), observations should include vital signs, color, any appearance of physical distress, urine output, and level of awareness. Regular notes should be made (and retained) and a supervisor and/or physician should be notified promptly of any deterioration in any parameter.

Despite the Clinical Antipsychotic Trials in Intervention Effectiveness–Alzheimer's Disease (CATIE-AD; Schneider et al. 2006) studies and recent concerns about neuroleptic medications in the elderly, most authorities continue to prefer the use of these agents in the elderly due to the greater likelihood of aggravating cognitive impairment and the risks of unsteady gait with benzodiazepines. Benzodiazepines often can also be disinhibiting. Neuroleptics may be given orally, intramuscularly, or intravenously (e.g., in an intensive care setting with established venous access), but the availability of liquid (elixir) and fast-dissolving oral preparations has greatly reduced the need for parenteral administration.

At the time of this writing there is controversy about the meaning of the CATIE-AD studies regarding the use of atypical antipsychotics in the elderly to treat agitation and aggression. It appears that these medications are effective, but this effectiveness can be negated by side effects (Schneider et al. 2006). The U.S. Food and Drug Administration (FDA) has not approved these medications for the treatment of dementia-related psychosis because of increased danger of death (Karlawich 2006). There may be a small increased risk of death (Schneider et al. 2005), but there are contradictory findings and interpretations, and many think these agents have a place and that the danger has been overblown (Barak et al. 2007; Raivio et al. 2007).

Ensure Safety of Patient and Others

Implicit in the referral will be concerns about safety, not only for the patient, but also for others. Besides understanding the context and precipitating factors for the violent act(s) that led to consultation, questioning of family and other caregivers should also gauge the commitment, skills, and resources within the existing caregiving matrix—with the consideration of whether the patient requires more intense care, either immediately or in the long run, to ensure safety. Our experience is that for the large majority, family members and caregivers remain committed to the care effort—sometimes unwisely so (e.g., failing to recognize the risk of allowing an 83-year-old woman to continue caring for her larger, more vigorous, and pathologically paranoid husband of more than 50 years—who no longer recognizes her consistently). Therefore, in this basic area, the consultant's recommendations may be the most fundamental with regard to emergency referral, acute psychiatric hospitalization, and the degree of ongoing support and structure required, whether at home or in an institutional setting (Read 1990). Use of restraints in the elderly also requires special caution. The frailness of such patients can be a risk. Confused patients can panic in restraints and might even develop a myocardial infarction. Restraints are sometimes used as an easy way to keep patients in bed or to prevent them from pulling out intravenous lines and other medical equipment. Restraints can be used also as in younger patients for out-of-control aggression.

Identify and Treat Causes of Medical Decompensation, Especially Sources of Delirium

Delirium most commonly develops over the course of hours to days. Behaviors are varied and may fluctuate over the course of the day (American Psychiatric Association 2000). Recognition of early symptoms, including memory impairment, incoherence, disorientation, disrupted sleep cycle, hallucinations, and irritability and other mood changes (de Jonghe et al. 2007) allows for mitigating their effects. These importantly include diminished immediate safety, negative impact on the patient, and the fact that prolonged delirium is associated with poor outcomes, including death and permanent brain damage. For example, in case example 2, Mrs. J's prolonged thyrotoxicosis left her with permanent memory loss, and she subsequently developed progressive dementia.

Because brain function is a sensitive marker of decompensation in the function of any major organ system—cardiac, pulmonary, hepatic, or renal—identifying the presence and cause of such dysfunction is critical. Asthma, incipient pneumonia, congestive heart failure, and electrolyte imbalance are other common illnesses for which the typical symptoms in the elderly may be "confusion" rather than specific textbook medical symptoms. An especially common cause is a bladder infection, which reliably causes confusion and abrupt decompensation in the patient with moderate to severe dementia. Delirium tremens may appear in the covertly alcoholic person. For these reasons, the consultant is urged not to dismiss the observation "she's just not herself" from a credible caregiver who knows the patient well (whether a family member, home health aide, or certified nursing assistant or nurse), because those who work closely with the patient over time will be the most sensitive to these changes.

Treat/Manage Identified Precipitants to the Violence

A major goal of the assessment process is to identify precipitants or premonitory symptoms for the violent act. In retrospect, the patient may have had pain or hunger or other discomfort; factors such as time of day or loud noises may figure in; or the actions of a caregiver or another patient, or some other clear factor, may emerge from a careful evaluation. In the obvious situation, identification by the consultant may be sufficient, and the health or social/family system will respond. In other instances, the consultant's expertise may be needed to assist with a plan or to ratify and approve a clinical approach.

The settings in which the precipitating incident occurs (e.g., skilled nursing, acute general medical floor, inpatient psychiatry, home, assisted living, day care) will bear on the range of responses available, because these locations are staffed by persons with differing levels of training and experience and are governed by differing sets of regulations. For example, in a skilled nursing facility, one can assume 24/7 availability of licensed nursing personnel, supervision of prescriptions, and a high standard of recordkeeping compared with, for example, the

The Elderly

variability of home and assisted-living settings. In a skilled nursing facility, assessments documented by means of the Minimum Data Set—a federally mandated data system that includes functional and behavioral observations and is reevaluated on at least a quarterly basis—will often assist the evaluation of context. However, in many facilities, also as a consequence of federal regulations, the consultant may find that the regulations are interpreted so as to restrict treatment and management options. The consultant who works in long-term care settings will recognize the high prevalence of mental and behavior disorders (Rovner et al. 1990) and is advised to learn the capabilities and limitations imposed by the different levels of licensure (which also vary among the different states). Useful resources are available for the specifics of behavioral management in long-term care (Katz et al. 2005; Reichman and Katz 1996; Szwabo and Grossberg 1993; see also materials available from the American Medical Directors Association [n.d.]). Although we emphasize the necessity of identifying the particularities of each case, some examples are offered.

- *Any unrecognized source of physical discomfort* can cause irritability and lead to "violent" reactions. This is perhaps especially important in assessing a demented patient who may no longer be able consciously to recognize sources of discomfort, although the "stoical" patient may not connect his or her irritability with a pain he or she was trying to ignore. The source of pain may be mechanical, such as a lumpy object left in the seat of the wheelchair, or it may be an unrecognized injury, such as an occult vertebral compression fracture or a broken hip from even a minor fall. Other "physical" sources of discomfort may be poor temperature regulation (elderly do not defend their body temperatures as effectively), hunger, or a blocked indwelling catheter. Careful systematic palpation and physical examination may be necessary to exclude a source of pain in a very demented person or someone with severe aphasia.
- *Irritating environmental stimuli* may provoke violence. Noise, bright lights, smells, a person approaching too close, or simply a harsh tone of voice can be jarring. At times the substrate will be a neurological deficit (for example, a patient [and caregivers] may not have recognized a homonymous hemianopsia, in which someone approaching is not seen until he or she suddenly appears in front of the patient—seeming, to the uninsightful patient, to have "snuck up" on him). Patients with advancing Alzheimer's disease can be observed to look straight ahead and appear to lose reactivity to peripheral vision. Patients with thalamic or other subcortical lesions may have

decreased "gating" protection from sounds or other stimuli. Recognition of these interactions guides management (one warns the hemianopic patient of an approach by talking), and the staff are prepared for a defensive "striking out" if they must tread on the patient's sensibilities. In addition, it is common for agitation to develop in the late afternoon in patients with dementia due to Alzheimer's disease (Cohen-Mansfield 2007), at which times they are likely to be more reactive to stimuli they would ignore earlier in the day, as in the case of Dr. F (case example 4).

- *Specific care needs* may also be a precipitant. Caring for a dependent elder, whether the cause is mental (dementia) or physical (paralysis after a stroke), requires the most intimate contact, and at close quarters. Family and caregivers must also be aware of other demands and are subject to fatigue themselves, and thus may become impatient or seem gruff at times. Patients may also be angry about their disability, be embarrassed, or have other causes of diminished impulse control, or there may be no specific identifiable provocation for a patient's striking out. Bathing is an especially sensitive activity. Many patients with dementia become averse to water (sometimes evoking the tired simile of "second childhood") and may become agitated while naked and slippery. The bather may lower his or her guard while attending to some sensitive detail (e.g., cleaning the perineal area), and a frightened or hurt patient at close quarters may react with a slap or punch. Adjusting bathing expectations (patients do not always require a daily bath), providing a second assistant, or finding a more congenial time of day may solve the problem. Some patients seem to manage for long periods with sponge baths in their beds only. At other times, judicious use of a short-acting antianxiety medication such as alprazolam, 0.25–0.5 mg given half an hour before commencing the activity, may be critical for allowing this kind of care to proceed. Communication problems around personal care tasks are responsible for a substantial proportion of violent incidents (Almvik et al. 2006).

Diagnose and Treat Underlying Psychiatric Disorders

Psychiatric disorders may account for a substantial part of the propensity to violent actions, either alone or by potentiating other factors. For example, the reaction to being bathed by a spouse or child is altered when the patient no longer recognizes that person, who understandably has reason to expect familiarity. Consideration of the following specific comments is important.

The Elderly

- *Coordination of team efforts, situational adjustments, and activities* all have roles in mitigating difficulties in many patients (Katz et al. 2005). Group and individual psychotherapy may be of benefit in some patients. In our opinion, the application of such efforts warrants the same critical analysis and reassessment expected for pharmacological therapy.
- *Pharmacological treatments for Alzheimer's disease* include cholinesterase inhibitors (including donepezil, rivastigmine, and galantamine) and now the NMDA (N-methyl-D-aspartate) receptor blocker memantine. Cholinesterase inhibitors partially compensate for the deficit in acetylcholine, the major neurotransmitter deficit demonstrated in Alzheimer's disease, with modest improvements in memory, attention, and clarity of thinking; benefits vary from patient to patient, and these agents do not alter the progressive course of the disease process. However, behavioral improvements are sustained in a significant percentage of patients on continuous cholinesterase inhibitor treatment, including reduced irritability, anxiety, aberrant motor behavior, delusions, and disinhibition (Aupperle et al. 2004; Gorman et al. 1993). Memantine has been shown to slow the course of progression, but short-term responses may include reduced agitation/aggression and irritability/lability (Cummings et al. 2006).
- *Alcohol and nicotine habits* can be associated with agitation and even violence in relation to the sense of urgency (craving) and confusion induced by use (presumably relative hypoxia for smokers). Naltrexone for alcohol and bupropion (sometimes with nicotine patches) for smoking have been consistently effective and reduced this nexus of distress (with the added benefit of health and safety improvement). Smoking is generally forbidden or limited in care facilities, and this can be a basis for violent attacks. As it is in younger patients, substance abuse treatment can be very important (Aradt et al. 2002).
- *Psychosis and mood disorders* may be important contributors to the diathesis leading to violence, and their treatment may be important to the control of violence. The interaction of these factors is demonstrated in the following case.

Case Example 6

Mrs. A was a wealthy, divorced 84-year-old woman originally seen in the context of a bitter and complex family struggle over property issues. In fact, this complicated situation was largely explained by Mrs. A's early dementia, which had been unrecognized. Resolution of the dementia led to conservatorship, with a commitment that she be cared for at home. Full evaluation, including single-photon emission computed tomography studies, supported a diagnosis of mixed dementia—Alzheimer's disease plus ischemic-vascular disease (Read et al. 1995).

Mrs. A was considered "spoiled," and indeed she was used to having her own way. Her major recreational activity was shopping followed by expensive lunches, but her caregivers noted problematic disinhibition: Mrs. A would yell out the car window and make vulgar gestures to others whom she perceived to be "in her way," and she was not mindful of the potential for dangerous retaliation. On other occasions she was very rude to people in restaurants. She had no appreciation for the effects of these behaviors, despite numerous discussions and illustrations; besides stigmatization of Mrs. A, the caregivers worried about her provoking physical response from an offended stranger.

Mrs. A's behaviors were mitigated with the use of donepezil and quetiapine without any evident side effects, and she was able to continue her "recreation." She was followed up at home, and it was noted that when she was "nervous," she began chain-smoking. After three cigarettes, she became slightly bluish and much more confused. She of course did not notice, experiencing her distress as the result of "company." However, with the use of nicotine patches and an agreement by conservator and caregivers, cigarettes were removed and her distress "smoothed out."

An additional piece to the puzzle was the observation that she had several-week episodes of increased motor activity, demanding behaviors, and agitation that included threats to people perceived by her as frustrating. At these times, the rapport that had been established through regular supportive discussions at monthly visits broke down. This pattern provoked review and the realization that Mrs. A was expressing the strong family history of bipolar disorder (which had also made major contributions to the original family strife). Because of her demonstrably good response to quetiapine, these periods were managed by increasing the dosage of neuroleptic rather than exposing her to possible complications of other mood-stabilizing agents.

The final challenge was how to handle a crisis—the suicide of a son, probably himself bipolar, who was beloved by Mrs. A but who had also precipitated the original crisis by defrauding her out of a large and valuable property. By this time the psychiatric consultant was familiar to all the family members, as well as caregivers and conservator, and this enabled a unified plan of management.

Empirically Evaluate Continuing Use of Medications for the Violent Patient

After treatment of specific factors as described earlier, violent behavior may continue, mandating consideration of ongoing pharmacotherapy. Unfortunately, in these days when we are exhorted to practice "evidence-based medicine," treatment of the violent elderly patient must be undertaken in the face of a paucity of data. Causes for this conundrum include the complexity of defining and monitoring treatment (including assessing outcomes); the protean heterogeneity of conditions underlying violence in the elderly; and the general neglect of studies of treatment in elderly persons. In addition, the issues evoke strong and contrary feelings, and the target patient's capacity (necessary at least, for example, for informed consent) may well be challenged by the very condition that underlies the behavior itself. Ambivalence about pharmacological treatment has also been heightened in the past 2 years by the description of safety issues related to risks that have appeared with the study of large (but heterogeneous) databases of medication use. This section emphasizes principles of treatment of the violent elderly patient, building on the assessment process described earlier.

Although not sanctioned by FDA-approved studies, neuroleptic medications (approved for the treatment of psychosis) have been the mainstay of treating agitation, aggression, and violent behaviors in the elderly in clinical practice—with an emphasis on the use of "atypical" antipsychotics (Sink et al. 2005). These medications displaced the previously widespread use of antianxiety agents, especially benzodiazepines, because of problems with unsteady gait and risk of falling, oversedation, and deteriorated cognition with benzodiazepines. Following clinical practice, we outline below an approach to use in practice.

- *Side effect profile* largely determines choice of the particular agent: olanzapine, for example, if inducing sleep and appetite are seen as beneficial side effects (in the insomniac anorectic patient); ziprasidone for the reverse situation; quetiapine or aripiprazole or risperidone if neither of those dimensions is important. An additional consideration is the route of administration and the availability of drug in elixir, intramuscular, intravenous, or rapidly dissolving forms. More rarely, depot injectable medication may be indicated.
- *Dosage is "titrated" to optimal effect,* monitoring response and side effects. Titration follows the geriatric adage "start low, go slow" (sometimes difficult to adhere to in the initial urgency created by a violent elderly patient). In addition, it is also true that some elderly patients are relatively resistant to medications—for us, the operant principle is that variability is what increases with age—and require dosages fully equivalent to, or higher than, those in younger adults. Although the biological basis for this dose–response variability is poorly understood (and in fact has been little investigated), the existence of this variability complicates the possibility of firm guidelines for dosage in complex situations such as treating violence—much less the underlying psychiatric syndromes that may have

been identified. This dose–response variability, combined with frequently medical complexity in the geriatric patient, mandates that pharmacological intervention be undertaken in a setting with knowledgeable and experienced personnel who have sufficient equipment to observe response and potential adverse effects, especially when assessing the need for further dosage increments.

- *Monitoring the response mandates targeting symptoms and keeping records.* Because the violent acts may be relatively intermittent, it is best also to monitor premonitory symptoms (e.g., irritability) in terms of timing, frequency, and intensity—and this enhances staff alertness to the overall situation.
- *The prominent side effects of concern* are extrapyramidal motor symptoms (drug-induced Parkinsonism) and autonomic instabilities, especially orthostatic hypotension. A major hazard for both of these is the risk of falling and sustaining injury. Motor symptoms should be monitored clinically, and blood pressure responses require the availability of a device and someone who knows how to use it.

Application of these principles is illustrated in the following case.

Case Example 7

An 86-year-old widow was seen for psychosis and agitation associated with the episodic delusion that the house where she lived was "not my home." This delusion appeared reliably every afternoon at 4 P.M., at which time this sweet, docile woman who enjoyed many activities became angry, anxious, and distressed and would strike out at her caregiver or anyone else who tried to reassure or correct her misperception. In fact she had run away from home twice, and consideration was being given to placing her in a care facility.

Evaluation revealed an articulate and opinionated woman with moderately severe dementia (MMSE score 14/30) fully consistent with Alzheimer's disease, as confirmed by positron emission tomography scan. The initial intervention was family education, informing them that the patient was unable to understand what was happening and did not intend her actions and that this was fully typical for midstage Alzheimer's disease, including the afternoon emergence. As a result, they arranged for a home health aide (who fortunately established good rapport with the patient). Cholinesterase inhibitor therapy was started (donepezil, titrated to 10 mg daily), together with memantine.

On this program, the patient's cognition improved modestly (MMSE rose to 17/30), and, although the afternoon psychosis continued, she was less adamant and responded better to attempts to demonstrate that the house really was her home. However, after several months, cognition again declined, and the distress and agitation and attempts to elope continued. She even threatened one evening to hit her caregiver, whom at other times she had come to call her "new daughter." At this point it was decided to add low-dose atypical antipsychotic medication, specifically quetiapine. Dosing was started at 25 mg daily at 2 P.M. and 6 P.M. She was seen 1 month later, and review of daily logs indicated there were no physical changes and that although the intensity of symptoms was less, distress still emerged in late afternoon. Dosage was slowly increased in 25-mg increments. At 100 mg twice daily, there were no reported incidents and the patient remained free of parkinsonian or metabolic side effects. She continued on this dosage without apparent adverse effects.

The use of neuroleptic medication has become more controversial in the past 2 years due to two major side effect issues: 1) treatment with antipsychotic agents potentiates (at least) the emergence of the "metabolic syndrome," which may expose patients to a higher risk of diabetes, lipid abnormalities, and cardiovascular disease; and 2) there is an increased risk of stroke. In addition, such studies as have been undertaken have provided little support for the long-term efficacy of neuroleptic treatment (in striking contrast to the perceptions of "frontline" clinicians). These concerns have culminated in adverse advisories from the FDA (U.S. Food and Drug Administration 2005), which specifically emphasizes that these medications were approved for use in schizophrenia but not for geriatric patients with dementia. These statements have been followed by "black box" warnings on the package inserts of these medications, although there is a dispute as to whether all atypical antipsychotics (or older neuroleptic medications such as haloperidol) warrant equal concern.

These difficulties have highlighted the widespread "off-label" use of these drugs in the elderly, despite a paucity of controlled studies. For these reasons, as well as poor efficacy in at least some patients, there has been interest in a variety of other medications and a corresponding large anecdotal literature (and word-of-mouth practice). Positive reports have appeared for trazodone, other serotonergic antidepressants, anticonvulsants (gabapentin, carbamazepine, and valproate), buspirone, diphenhydramine, benzodiazepines, transdermal nicotine, and estrogen (in men) (Sink et al. 2005).

At this writing, these issues remain unsettled—and unsettling. The importance of effective management and treatment of agitation and violence in elderly patients is recognized by caregivers, facilities, and the patients and families themselves in most cases. Nonpharmacological interventions that address behavioral issues and unmet needs, including those of caretakers, may be efficacious (Avalon et al. 2006). In cases where nonpsychopharmacological interventions have been insufficient, medications may enable these patients to be maintained in less restrictive settings, such as the home or an institution or assisted living facility with amenities, as opposed to a secure nursing facility.

The best approach to violence in the elderly is multifaceted. That is true also in patients with Alzheimer's disease (Lavretsky and Nguyen 2006). The clinician must, however, continually consider new evidence as it becomes available, reassess the patient's ongoing need for medication, and rely on careful informed consent.

Key Points

- Geriatric patients can be violent for the same reasons as younger individuals.
- Violence resulting from dementia and delirium with resultant confusion is more common in the elderly.
- Treatment of the underlying condition may be essential to control of violence.
- Frailness in many elderly persons may require special caution and considerations.
- Nonetheless, violence in the elderly can be serious and requires active intervention.

References

Almvik R, Rasmussen K, Woods P: Challenging behavior in the elderly monitoring violent incidents. Int J Geriatr Psychiatry 21:368–374, 2006

American Medical Directors Association: Management Tools. n.d. Available at http://www.amda.com/managementtools/index.cfm.

American Psychiatric Association: Diagnostic and Statistical Manual of Mental Disorders, 4th Edition, Text Revision. Washington, DC, American Psychiatric Association, 2000

Aradt S, Turvey CL, Flaum M: Older offenders, substance abuse, and treatment. Am J Geriatr Psychiatry 10:733–739, 2002

Aupperle PM, Koumaras B, Chen M, et al: Long-term effects of rivastigmine treatment on neuropsychiatric and behavioral disturbances in nursing home residents with moderate to severe Alzheimer's disease: results of a 52-week open-label study. Curr Med Res Opin 20:1605–1612, 2004

Avalon L, Gum AM, Feliciano L, et al: Effectiveness of nonpharmacological interventions for the management of neuropsychiatric symptoms in patients with dementia. Arch Intern Med 166:2182–2188, 2006

Bogousslavsky J, Cummings JL: Behavior and Mood Disorders in Focal Brain Lesions. New York, Cambridge University Press, 2000

Barak Y, Baruch Y, Mazeh D: Cardiac and cerebrovascular morbidity and mortality associated with antipsychotic medications in elderly psychiatric inpatients. Am J Geriatr Psychiatry 15:354–356, 2007

Cohen-Mansfield J: Temporal patterns of agitation in dementia. Am J Geriatr Psychiatry 15:395–405, 2007

Cummings JL, Schneider E, Tariot PN, et al: Behavioral effects of memantine in Alzheimer disease patients receiving donepezil treatment. Neurology 67:57–63, 2006

de Jonghe JFM, Kalisvaart KJ, Dijkstra M, et al: Early symptoms in the prodromal phase of delirium: a prospective cohort study in elderly patients undergoing hip surgery. Am J Geriatr Psychiatry 15:112–121, 2007

Devanand DP: Psychiatric assessment of the older patient, in Kaplan and Sadock's Comprehensive Textbook of Psychiatry, 8th Edition. Edited by Sadock BJ, Sadock VA. Philadelphia, PA, Lippincott Williams & Wilkins, 2005, pp 3603–3610

Folstein MF, Folstein SE, McHugh PR: "Mini-Mental State": a practical method for grading the cognitive state of patients for the clinician. J Psychiatr Res 12:189–198, 1975

Gorman DG, Read S, Cummings JL: Cholinergic therapy of behavioral disturbances in Alzheimer's disease. Neuropsychiatry Neuropsychol Behav Neurol 6:229–234, 1993

Karlawich J: Alzheimer's disease: clinical trials and the logic of clinical purpose. N Engl J Med 355:1604–1605, 2006

Katz IR, Streim JE, Datto CJ: Psychiatric aspects of long-term care, in Kaplan and Sadock's Comprehensive Textbook of Psychiatry, 8th Edition. Edited by Sadock BJ, Sadock VA. Philadelphia, PA, Lippincott Williams & Wilkins, 2005, pp 3793–3797

Lavretsky H, Nguyen LH: Diagnosis and treatment of neuropsychiatric symptoms in Alzheimer's disease. Psychiatr Serv 57:617–619, 2006

Lewis CF, Fields C, Rainey E: A study of geriatric forensic evaluees: who are the violent elderly? J Am Acad Psychiatry Law 34:324–332, 2006

Lyketsos CG, Steele C, Galik E: Physical aggression in dementia patients and its relationship to depression. Am J Psychiatry 156:66–71, 1999

Rabins PV, Mace NL, Lucas MJ: The impact of dementia on the family. JAMA 248:333–335, 1982

Raivio MM, Laurila JV, Strandberg TE, et al: Neither atypical nor conventional antipsychotics increase mortality or hospital admissions among elderly patients with dementia: a two-year prospective study. Am J Geriatr Psychiatry 15:416–424, 2007

Read SL: Community resources, in Alzheimer's Disease: Long-Term Management. Edited by Cummings JL, Miller BL. New York, Marcel Dekker, 1990, pp 235–244

Read SL, Miller B, Mena I, et al: SPECT in dementia: clinical and pathological correlation. J Am Geriatr Soc 43:1243–1247, 1995

Reichman WE, Katz PR: Psychiatric Care in the Nursing Home. New York, Oxford University Press, 1996

Rovner BW, German PS, Broadhead J, et al: The prevalence and management of dementia and other psychiatric disorders in nursing homes. Int Psychogeriatr 2:13, 1990

Royall DR, Mahurin RK, Gray KF: Bedside assessment of executive cognitive impairment: the executive interview. J Am Geriatr Soc 40:1221–1226, 1992

Schneider LS, Dagerman KS, Insel P: Risk of death with atypical antipsychotic drug treatment for dementia: meta-analysis of randomized placebo-controlled trials. JAMA 294:1934–1943, 2005

Schneider LS, Tariot PN, Dagerman KS, et al: Effectiveness of atypical antipsychotic drugs in patients with Alzheimer's disease. N Engl J Med 355:1525–1538, 2006

Silver IL, Herrmann N: Comprehensive psychiatric evaluation, in Comprehensive Textbook of Geriatric Psychiatry, 3rd Edition. Edited by Sadovoy J, Jarvik LF, Grossberg GT, et al. New York, WW Norton, 2004, pp 253–279

Sink KM, Holden KF, Yaffe K: Pharmacological treatment of neuropsychiatric symptoms of dementia: a review of the evidence. JAMA 293:596–608, 2005

Strub RL, Black FW: The Mental Status Examination in Neurology. Philadelphia, PA, FA Davis, 1985

Strub RL, Black FW: Neurobehavior Disorders: A Clinical Approach. Philadelphia, PA, FA Davis, 1988

Szwabo PA, Grossberg GT: Problem Behaviors in Long-Term Care: Recognition, Diagnosis, and Treatment. New York, Springer, 1993

U.S. Food and Drug Administration: FDA public health advisory: deaths with antipsychotics in elderly patient s with behavioral disturbances. 2005. Available at http://www.fda.gov/cder/drug/advisory/antipsychotics.htm. Accessed June 1, 2007

Yorston GA, Taylor PJ: Commentary: older offenders—no place to go? J Am Acad Psychiatry Law 34:333–337, 2006

PART VI

Special Topics

CHAPTER 20

Forensic Issues

Charles L. Scott, M.D.

Forensic expertise is often requested in situations involving a potentially dangerous person. But what does *forensic* actually mean, and how does this evaluation process differ from the provision of clinical care? The American Academy of Psychiatry and the Law (2005) provided the following definition of *forensic psychiatry* in its ethics guidelines: "Forensic Psychiatry is a subspecialty in which scientific and clinical expertise is applied in legal contexts involving civil, criminal, correctional, regulatory matters, and in specialized clinical consultation in areas such as risk assessment or employment" (p. 1).

This chapter reviews situations involving known, unknown, and deceased offenders in which a forensic evaluation may be helpful. Although clinical assessment skills are important in conducting a forensic examination, providers must be aware that having clinical expertise is vastly different from having the requisite skills to perform a forensic examination. When conducting a forensic examination, the evaluator must understand the relevant legal standard, the skills to evaluate the person in relationship to this standard, the capacity to apply information to the legal construct, and the capability to effectively translate and communicate his or her findings in the context of the legal system (Grisso 1998). Table 20–1 highlights important areas to consider when a forensic evaluation is requested.

TABLE 20–1. Forensic evaluation checklist

☐ What is the specific referral question?

☐ Is the evaluation for treatment or for legal purposes?

☐ Who is the party requesting the evaluation?

☐ Have appropriate parties been notified in advance of the evaluation?

☐ Has the evaluee or legally governing authority consented to the evaluation?

☐ Have the parameters of confidentiality been explained to the evaluee?

☐ Have appropriate collateral records been reviewed?

☐ Have appropriate third parties to interview been identified?

Forensic Evaluations of Known Offenders

Forensic evaluations are often requested of defendants involved in the criminal justice system, and the evaluator must know if any legal standard governs the particular evaluation requested. "Competency to stand trial" evaluation requests are the most common referrals for criminal forensic examinations (Rogers et al. 2001; Warren et al. 1991). The legal standard for assessing a defendant's competency was articulated in *Dusky v. U.S.* In this 1960 landmark case, the U.S. Supreme Court announced that the "test must be whether he has sufficient present ability to consult with his lawyer with a reasonable degree of rational understanding and whether he has a rational as well as a factual understanding of the proceedings against him" (*Dusky v. U.S.* 1960). Although this is less commonly requested, the forensic evaluator may also be asked to evaluate the defendant's sanity at the time of the offense and to comment on the relationship of mental illness to violent behavior. In general, the insanity defense excuses a mentally ill defendant from legal responsibility for his or her criminal behavior. The exact standard for determining a defendant's sanity varies according to jurisdiction. The majority of states in the United States use some variation of a cognitive test of insanity that determines whether the defendant, as a result of a mental disease or defect, knows or understands the nature and quality of his or her actions and/or is able to distinguish right from wrong at the time of the offense (Giorgi-Guarnieri et al. 2002). Finally, the court may also ask the psychiatrist to outline risk factors regarding a criminal defendant's risk of future

Forensic Issues

violence. Specific forensic expertise is required in assessing the risk of future dangerousness in two particular offender types: stalkers and rapists.

Case Example 1

Jill is a 47-year-old woman who has recently separated from her husband Jack after a volatile 10-year marriage. Jack has been arrested in the past for driving under the influence and has physically assaulted Jill during the course of their marriage. After Jill files for divorce, she discovers notes on her car from Jack that say she will "always be his," and he leaves numerous threatening phone calls that include both pleas to reunite and veiled threats to kill her. Jill becomes afraid and seeks out mental health counseling for advice.

Stalking

Stalking is a serious problem in the United States. All 50 states, the federal government, and the District of Columbia classify stalking as a crime. Although precise statutory definitions vary, most stalking statutes incorporate the following elements:

- A course of conduct is specified
- The conduct is directed at a specific person
- The conduct results in a reasonable person experiencing fear

Approximately 1 in 12 women and 1 in 45 men will be stalked at some point in their lifetime. Nearly 90% of stalkers are men, and the majority of female and male victims know their stalker. Women are more likely than men (59% vs. 30%) to be stalked by an intimate partner. Although the average duration of stalking is 1.8 years, the duration increases to 2.2 years when the stalking relationship involves an intimate partner. More than 70% of current or former intimate partners verbally threaten their victims with violence; 81% of women stalked by a current or prior partner are eventually physically assaulted, and more than 30% are sexually assaulted (Tjaden and Thoennes 1998).

Numerous typologies have attempted to classify stalking behavior. One of the most commonly referenced typologies was developed by Michael Zona, who initially divided stalkers into the following three categories (Zona et al. 1993):

1. *Simple obsessional:* These individuals usually have a prior relationship with the victim and are motivated by a desire to enact revenge on or to force reestablishment of the lost relationship. This group poses the greatest risk of harm to their victim.

2. *Love obsessional:* In contrast to the simple obsessional, the vast majority of these stalkers have had no prior relationship to their victim. These perpetrators may become focused on their victim after seeing him or her in the media or another public forum. They are commonly viewed by others as obsessed fans. A significant number of these individuals have a mental disorder such as schizophrenia or bipolar disorder.
3. *Erotomanic:* Stalkers in this category delusionally believe that their love object also loves them. The typical perpetrator is a female who is convinced that an older male, usually of higher status, returns her affection despite the lack of any rational evidence to support this belief.

Mullen et al. (1999) expanded the Zona typology of stalking to include five categories of stalkers, described by their primary motivation, the context in which the stalking developed, and the function of the stalker's behavior. The primary types described include the rejected, the intimacy seekers, the resentful, the predatory, and the incompetent. Characteristics of each stalker category are noted in Table 20–2.

A more recent typology classifies stalkers according to their relationship, if any, with the victim and the private versus public-figure context of their pursuit. The acronym RECON was selected for this scheme because it is both relationship (RE) and context (CON) based (Mohandie et al. 2006). The four categories of stalkers, described by the type of victim selected, are labeled "intimate," "acquaintance," "public figure," and "private stranger." An outline of this categorization scheme and the associated features are shown in Table 20–3.

The examiner should consider the possibility that a victim may make a false allegation that he or she has been stalked. Five contexts involving false claims include 1) stalkers who claim to be victims, 2) individuals who have delusions of being stalked, 3) persons who have been previously stalked and then misperceive benign acts of others, 4) persons with factitious disorder attempting to achieve the sick role, and 5) malingerers who fabricate claims for external reward such as money or to avoid criminal prosecution (Mullen et al. 2000).

Stalking can occur in a variety of circumstances and may include attempts to contact the victim directly or indirectly through the phone, mail, faxes, or personal notes left at a particular location. With the advent of electronic communication, stalkers may employ cyberspace technology and the Internet to maintain contact with their victim, either through e-mails or through gathering information about the victim by using common search engines (McGrath and Casey 2002). Text messaging or short message service via a mobile phone represents yet another

TABLE 20–2. Mullen stalker typology

Type	Characteristics
Rejected	Predominantly males who pursue an ex-intimate Goal is reconciliation or revenge Usually personality disordered rather than psychotic Frequently persistent and intrusive
Intimacy seekers	Desired attachment is usually romantic but can be to parent, child, or close relationship Believes target loves him/her and intimate relationship will occur Persists with pursuit despite responses from victim May have underlying psychotic disorder
Resentful	Targets person who stalker feels has wronged them Stalking behaviors are intended to cause fear Sense of power and control gained from stalking Feels justified as acts are retribution for misjustice
Predatory	Predominantly men who target unsuspecting women Stalking behaviors are preparation for sexual assault Pursue multiple victims over time
Incompetent	Feels entitled to relationship with person of interest Indifferent to target's preferences No insight regarding target's lack of reciprocity Persistent inept attempts

Source. Mullen et al. 1999.

developing method for the stalker to maintain communication with the victim without actual physical contact (Eytan and Borras 2005).

The degree of danger posed by a stalker depends on a variety of factors. Intervention plans to curb or stop stalking behavior should be tailored to each specific case. General recommendations noted to reduce the impact of stalking include the following (Mullen et al. 2000):

- Communicating early and clearly that any contact or attention is unwanted
- Carefully protecting personal information, to include limiting distribution of home address, telephone numbers, and cyberspace information
- Informing trusted others at home and work to prevent inadvertent disclosure of information and to protect their safety
- Contacting appropriate helping agencies such as police, victim support organizations, mental health clinics, and domestic and sexual violence programs when applicable

TABLE 20–3. RECON (relationship and context) stalker typology

Stalker type	Relationship category	Characteristics	Risk management
Intimate	Previous relationship: marriage, cohabiting, dating/sexual	Most dangerous group, with history of violence Quickly escalates Abuses alcohol and stimulants > 50% physically assault victim One-third use or threaten use of weapon > One-third have suicidal ideation or behavior	Intense probation/parole supervision Intervene to decrease risk of domestic violence before and after separation
Acquaintance	Previous relationship: employment related, affiliative/friendship, customer/client	Pursuit is sporadic but relentless Strong desire to initiate relationship One-third will assault victim or damage property	Careful diagnostic assessment Work with law enforcement and mental health
Public figure	No previous relationship; pursuit of public-figure victim	Greater proportion of female stalkers and male victims Older, with less violence history Increased likelihood of psychosis Unlikely to threaten and low violence risk	Professional protection of target Psychiatric treatment Prosecution, with forensic hospitalization as option
Private stranger	No previous relationship; pursuit of private-figure victim	Often mentally ill men 12% suicidal Communicate directly One-third are violent toward person or property	Psychiatric treatment Aggressive prosecution

Source. Mohandie et al. 2006.

Forensic Issues | 415

- Documenting and preserving all stalker contacts
- Recording all phone calls on an answering machine and keeping a separate private line for personal calls
- Obtaining self-defense training
- Avoiding all contact and confrontations

The decision to obtain a restraining order against the stalker is one that requires careful consideration, and obtaining an order may be ineffective or actually inflammatory in certain situations. In particular, Orion (1997) emphasized that restraining orders are likely to be ineffective against ex-intimates, who are heavily invested in the relationship, and erotomanic or delusional stalkers, who view legal orders as not applicable to their situation. De Becker (1997) noted that restraining orders are most likely to be effective in those situations that involve a casual acquaintance with limited emotional investment and no prior history of violence. If a decision is made to obtain a restraining order, the victim should be aware that stalkers are at higher risk to act violently during the time frame immediately following the issuance of the order, so that added precautions can be taken. A protection order should be viewed as only one component of a comprehensive plan designed to minimize risk to the victim, and such an order may not be appropriate for every case.

Rapists

Although the specific definition of *rape* varies according to jurisdiction, common legal elements of rape include the penetration of a human orifice by another person's body part or object. According to the National Crime Victimization Survey, there were more than 190,000 victims of rape or sexual assault in the United States during 1995 (Catalano 2006). The majority of rapes and sexual assaults are committed by men against women.

Groth and Birnbaum (1979) classified rapists into four main types. Two of the categories emphasize the use of sexual aggression to satisfy the rapist's need for power and the other two categories highlight the use of sexual aggression to express anger. Characteristics of each rapist subtype in this typology are outlined in Table 20–4.

A more recent typology developed by Knight and Prentky (1990), classifying rapists according to their primary motivation, includes the following four types:

TABLE 20–4. Groth rapist typology

Rapist type	Motivating factors
Power-Reassurance	Alleviate feelings of sexual inadequacy
Power-Assertive	Express potency, mastery, and dominance
Anger-Retaliation	Express rage toward women; seek revenge by degrading women
Anger-Excitation	Obtain sexual gratification from victim's suffering

Source. Groth and Birnbaum 1979.

- *Opportunistic rapists:* Offenders who commit impulsive, unplanned predatory acts to achieve immediate sexual gratification
- *Pervasively angry rapists:* Offenders who are angry in general and who seek out targets as recipients of their anger rather than to meet a sexual need
- *Sexual rapists:* Offenders who may have recurrent intrusive rape fantasies and who assault to gratify sexual needs
- *Vindictive rapists:* Offenders who are primarily angry at women and who attack to degrade and humiliate

When assessing a known rapist's risk for future dangerousness, the forensic examiner must conduct an extremely thorough interview, generally combined with structured assessments and review of collateral records. Key assessment components include the following:

- Detailed clinical interview recording the individual's account of his or her actions
- Review of key collateral records to compare victim's account and police account to alleged perpetrator's report
- Evaluation of any associated mental and/or substance use disorder
- Assessment of psychopathy and/or associated personality disorder
- Administration of standardized personality tests such as the Minnesota Multiphasic Personality Inventory
- Use of standardized questionnaires and sexual inventories
- Incorporation of actuarial risk assessment instruments and structured clinical interviews designed for the risk assessment of sexual offenders

Although physiological measures such as the penile plethysmograph or polygraph have been used to monitor treatment progress of sex offenders, they are generally not permissible in court and may not be allowed as part of the forensic examination. The recidivism risk for rapists varies according to the study conducted and the length of follow-up time measured. In their follow-up of 136 rapists, Prentky et al. (1997) found that 39% reoffended over the 25-year follow-up period. Factors associated with reoffense for rapists include the following (Prentky and Burgess 2000):

- Impulsive, antisocial behavior
- Psychopathy
- Sexual drive strength
- Sexual coercion and rape fantasies
- Number of prior sexual offenses
- Offense planning
- Attitudes (global/pervasive anger, hypermasculine/macho, seeks ways to con others, criminal)

Forensic Evaluations of Unknown Offenders

Forensic evaluators may be asked to assist law enforcement in identifying violence risk factors regarding an offender whose exact identity is yet unknown. Perhaps the most dangerous and terrifying criminal is that individual who murders multiple people yet remains undetected.

One of the most famous approaches to profiling unknown perpetrators was developed by the Behavioral Sciences Unit of the FBI Academy. FBI profilers attempt to identify a suspect by searching for specific physical and behavioral clues at the crime scene. Investigators divide crime scenes into two broad categories: organized and disorganized. *Organized crimes* are characterized by planning in advance of the offense, targeting a stranger victim, using restraints on a victim, hiding the dead body, removing the weapon and/or evidence, and general control of the crime scene. In contrast, *disorganized crimes* are described as unplanned, random, and sloppy, with minimal use of restraints, sudden violence to the victim with subsequent sexual acts, and a failure by the killer to remove the weapon or body from the crime scene. This information theoretically serves as a personality fingerprint to assist law enforcement in narrowing the field of potential perpetrators. According to the FBI profiling system, organized and disorganized crime scenes should match murderers with organized and disorganized characteristic or traits. The original data set underlying the FBI profiling system was developed by FBI agents who interviewed 36 convicted sexual murderers, 29 of whom were serial sexual killers. Profile characteristics of organized versus disorganized murderers as defined by the FBI are outlined in Table 20–5 (Ressler et al. 1988).

TABLE 20–5. Profile characteristics of organized and disorganized murderers

Organized	Disorganized
Average to above-average intelligence	Below-average intelligence
Socially competent	Socially inadequate
Skilled work preferred	Unskilled work
Sexually competent	Sexually incompetent
High birth-order status	Low birth-order status
Father's work stable	Father's work unstable
Inconsistent childhood discipline	Harsh discipline as a child
Controlled mood during crime	Anxious mood during crime
Use of alcohol with crime	Minimal use of alcohol
Precipitating situational stress	Minimal situational stress
Living with partner	Living alone
Mobility with car in good condition	Lives/works near crime scene
Follows crime in news media	Minimal interest in news media
May change jobs or leave town	Significant behavior change (e.g., drug/alcohol abuse, religiosity)

Source. Ressler et al. 1988.

Criticisms of the FBI profiling methodology have included observations that crime scene characteristics do not clearly separate organized and disorganized crimes or offenders and the concern that profile characteristics of serial murderers may not generalize to nonsexual offenders (Canter et al. 2004).

Forensic Evaluations of Deceased Persons

The circumstances surrounding a person's death are sometimes hazy, leaving an air of mystery as to why and how that person died. Consider the situation in which a wife kills her husband with a single gunshot through the heart. Was the deceased shot by a dangerous or deranged woman, was she defending herself against a brutal attack, or did her husband purposely provoke her to kill him in a veiled suicide attempt? Or consider that for many, Marilyn Monroe's death in 1962 continues to remain shrouded in mystery, with theories about her cause of death ranging from an accidental overdose to homicide committed by agents of the U.S. government.

E.S. Shneidman, co-founder of the LA Suicide Prevention Center, coined the term *psychological autopsy* to describe a posthumous evaluation process in which the examiner conducts a thorough retrospective investigation to determine the decedent's intentions and other possible causes of his or her death. Dr. Shneidman and his colleagues envisioned the use of the psychological autopsy in circumstances where the mode of death was equivocal in nature, such as drug overdoses, "suicide by cop," Russian roulette, vehicular accidents, murder-suicide, and autoerotic asphyxia (Shneidman 1981).

The evaluator conducting a psychological autopsy should carefully consider the following five concepts during retrospective investigation: 1) cause, 2) mode, 3) motive, 4) intent, and 5) lethality.

Cause explains how the person actually died. Examples of potential causes of death include a single gunshot wound to the head, a crush injury from a car accident, or a massive heart attack. Although the cause of death may be clear to the coroner, the mode of death is often more ambiguous.

Mode refers to the circumstances that led to the cause of death. When determining mode, the evaluator may find it helpful to classify the death according to the acronym NASH, which stands for Natural, Accidental, Suicide, or Homicide. In 5%–20% of death cases reviewed by the medical examiner (coroner), the mode of death is unclear (Shneidman 1981). If the mode of death is determined to be suicide, *motive* addresses why the decedent committed suicide. When determining a person's motive, the examiner attempts to understand the reasons and/or events that prompted the individual to act. In many suicides, the motive is unknown and must be inferred from the available evidence (Biffl 1996; Massello 1986). To assist in the examiner's investigation of the deceased's motive, Shneidman (1981) recommends careful review of the reasons why an individual committed suicide and why he or she chose that specific time to do it.

In contrast to motive, *intent* represents the resolve of an individual, either consciously or unconsciously, in carrying out his or her death. Understanding a person's intent is facilitated by reviewing the degree of lethality, or risk-taking, involved in the suicidal behavior (Peck and Warner 1995). Shneidman (1981) noted that *lethality* represents the probability that an individual will successfully kill him- or herself in the immediate future. He divided the degree of lethality into high, medium, low, and absent, although he did not provide precise classification criteria for these categories.

A review of the literature indicates that a variety of techniques are used to conduct psychological autopsies. Common characteristics of all techniques include a careful review of collateral records (such as the autopsy, toxicology reports, medical and mental health records, and personal diaries of the victim), interviews of survivors with a focus on the time frame immediately preceding the death, and a review of specific mental health factors such as any prior psychiatric history, prior suicide attempts, and behaviors suggesting that the person was planning to die. Suicide by cop and murder-suicide are two situations in which the forensic evaluator helps unravel the relationship of violence toward others to the offender's own death.

Case Example 2

Joe is a 48-year-old man with a long-standing history of impulsive, angry outbursts. He is extremely narcissistic and becomes aggressive whenever criticized. Because of Joe's personality, he has been unable to sustain any long-term relationships and is socially isolated. He spends a great deal of his time reading weapons magazines and fantasizes about dying while shooting others in a "blaze of glory." Because of his temper problems, he was terminated from work. He blamed his supervisor for all of his problems and decided to go to his workplace and "take out anyone and everyone."

Suicide By Cop

The phrase *suicide by cop* refers to behaviors by an individual intended to provoke a law enforcement officer to use lethal force that will result in the person's death. In a study of more than 430 exchanges of fire between police and a suspect over a 10-year period in Los Angeles County, California, researchers classified 10.5% of the cases as suicide-by-cop situations (Hutson et al. 1998). In their review of 15 deaths of suicidal persons who provoked law enforcement officers into killing them, researchers (Wilson et al. 1998) described 10 characteristics of these individuals, which are summarized in Table 20–6.

In their review of the literature, Mohandie and Meloy (2000) outlined both verbal and behavioral clues indicating risk for suicide-by-cop that may be helpful when conducting a psychological autopsy. Twelve verbal clues associated with a suicide-by-cop situation included suspects demanding authorities kill them, setting a deadline for authorities to kill them, threatening to kill or harm others, wanting to "go out in a blaze of glory," giving a verbal will, telling hostages or others they want to die, looking for a "macho" way out, offering to surrender to person in charge, indicating elaborate plans of their own death, expressing feelings of hopelessness/helplessness, emphasizing that jail is not an option, and making biblical references, particularly to resurrection and to the Book of Revelations.

Behavioral clues to suicide-by-cop risk include being demonstrative with a weapon, pointing a weapon at police, clearing a threshold in a

TABLE 20–6. Characteristics of "suicide by cop" in 15 incidents

- Incidents were perceived as life-threatening to law officers and witnesses
- 14 of the victims (i.e., suicides) were male, 13 were Caucasian, and the mean age was 32 years
- All verbally threatened homicide and resisted arrest
- Two-thirds of the victims took hostages
- All victims possessed a handgun or other weapon
- All victims posed or used their weapon during the incident
- 60% used the weapon with the intent to harm others
- 40% were intoxicated with alcohol
- 40% had documented psychiatric diagnoses, and 60% had evidence of psychiatric illness
- Depression and substance abuse were the most common psychiatric diagnoses

Source. Wilson et al. 1998.

barricade situation in order to fire a weapon, shooting at police, reaching for a weapon with police present, attaching a weapon to one's own body, giving a countdown to kill hostages with police present, assaulting or harming hostages with police present, forcing confrontation with police, advancing on police when told to stop, calling police to report a crime in progress, continuing hopeless acts of aggression even after incapacitation by gunfire, self-mutilating with police present, pointing a weapon at oneself with police present, refusing to negotiate, not making any escape demands, and getting intoxicated (Mohandie and Meloy 2000).

Murder-Suicide

Murder-suicide occurs when an individual commits suicide after taking the life of another person. In the National Violent Death Reporting System (Bossarte et al. 2006), only suicides that occur within 24 hours after a murder qualify the deaths as murder-suicide, whereas other authors extend this period to up to one week (Marzuk et al. 1992). Various labels have been used to describe the phenomenon of a murderer who subsequently takes his or her own life, including "homicide-suicide," "dyadic death," "doubly violent aggression," and "despondent killers."

Because there is no national surveillance system for murder-suicide in the United States, the exact prevalence is difficult to determine. In the majority of studies, murder-suicide rates have been reported to range from 0.2 to 0.3 per 100,000 persons (Coid 1983; Marzuk et al. 1992;

Milroy 1995), although rates as high as 0.4 to 0.5 per 100,000 persons have also been noted (Hannah et al. 1998; Hanzlick and Koponen 1994). Hanzlick and Koponen (1994) identified common precipitants for murder-suicide, as outlined in Table 20–7.

In addition to the motivators just noted, Bossarte et al. (2006), in their study of 65 murder-suicide incidents, found that a legal problem was the most common associated circumstance, experienced by one of every four perpetrators.

Marzuk et al. (1992) proposed a murder-suicide typology based on the relationship between the perpetrator and the victim. The proposed categories of murder-suicide are 1) spousal/consortial, 2) familial, and 3) extrafamilial.

Spousal/Consortial Murder-Suicides

Numerous studies indicate that the majority of murder-suicides involve male perpetrators who kill spouses or intimates (Aderibigbe 1997; Felthous and Hempel 1995; Malphurs and Cohen 2002; Marzuk et al. 1992; Milroy et al. 1997; Palermo et al. 1997) with a handgun (Malphurs and Cohen 2002). Nearly one-third of men who kill their spouse or partner will commit suicide, a statistical phenomenon not matched by females who kill intimate partners (Bossarte et al. 2006). Common psychiatric diagnoses in perpetrators of couple murder-suicides include depression (Rosenbaum 1990) and alcohol intoxication or abuse (Comstock et al. 2005).

TABLE 20–7. Thirteen suggested motivators for murder-suicide

1. Impending divorce
2. Previous divorce
3. Release or perceived loss of a nonmarital partner
4. Jealousy
5. Retaliation
6. Mercy killing
7. Altruism
8. Financial stressors
9. Family stress or dysfunction
10. Alcohol
11. Drugs other than alcohol
12. Psychiatric illness
13. Unspecified or unknown factors

Source. Hanzlick and Koponen 1994.

Marzuk et al. (1992) divided spousal/consortial murder-suicides into two subtypes: 1) amorous-jealous and 2) declining health. The amorous-jealous subtype is the most common, representing between 50% and 75% of all spousal/consortial murder-suicides. In the amorous-jealous subtype, the perpetrator is commonly a young man who kills his spouse or girlfriend with a firearm in a jealous rage during a period of actual or impending separation (Marzuk et al. 1992). More recent studies of murder-suicide in older persons also note that interpersonal conflict remains a potential trigger for these deaths, particularly in an older man married to a younger woman (Cohen et al. 1998).

In the declining-health subtype, the murderer is typically an older man (potentially in poor health) caring for his ailing wife. The perpetrator may believe his actions are altruistic and serve as a mercy suicide. Both parties may view their deaths as a dual suicide pact in which the perpetrator's actions are part of an assisted suicide.

Murder-Suicide of Other Family Members

Murder-suicides may involve a perpetrator who kills one or more family members other than a spouse or intimate partner. In an Australian study examining murder-suicides of children over a 29-year period, researchers found that when fathers killed their children, they were more likely to also kill their spouse, in contrast to mothers, who killed only their children. Furthermore, compared with men, women tended to use less violent methods to commit murder and suicide (Byard et al. 1999).

Filicide is broadly defined as the murder of a child. Three types of filicide include

1. *Neonaticide:* Murder of a child less than 1 day old
2. *Infancticide:* Murder of a child older than 1 day and less than 1 year
3. *Pedicide:* Murder of a child older than 1 year and younger than 16 years

High rates of suicide after a filicide have been noted: 16%–29% of mothers and 40%–60% of fathers take their life after murdering their child (Hatters Friedman et al. 2005; Marzuk et al. 1992; Rodenburg 1971). In a study of 30 family filicide-suicide files, the most common motive involved an attempt by the perpetrator to relieve a real or imagined suffering of the child, an action known as an "altruistic filicide." Eighty percent of the parents in this study had evidence of a past or current psychiatric history, nearly 60% having depression, 27% having psychosis, and 20% experiencing delusional beliefs (Hatters Friedman et al. 2005).

Familicide is defined as the murder of an entire family. These family annihilators are usually men with depression, intoxication, or both (Dietz 1986). Other risk factors associated with family annihilators include ongoing marital conflict and anger over separation, illness in a child, and financial stress (Hatters Friedman et al. 2005; Morton et al. 1998). In certain cases, the perpetrator believes that murdering the family members will alleviate future suffering and views his or her action as altruistic. Rare cases of depressed or psychotic adolescents have also been described in which the child kills his or her entire family prior to taking his or her own life (Malmquist 2006).

Because of the high reported rates of mental illness in parents who kill their children, evaluators should carefully consider the possibility that their depressed, suicidal, or psychotic patients who are parents may represent a potential risk of harm to their child. In addition to a standard suicide risk assessment, the clinician should explore other areas that may assist in preventing a tragic death (Hatters Friedman et al. 2005). Sample questions include

- What do you believe will happen to your child if you die or commit suicide?
- Do you have any fears or concerns that your child may be harmed by others?
- Do you have any worries regarding your child's health or unnecessary suffering?
- Are you having any thoughts about harming your child?
- Have you taken any steps to harm your child?
- If you have had thoughts of harming your child, what has kept you from doing so thus far?

Extrafamilial Murder-Suicides

Suicides after the murder of a person who is not a family member or intimate partner are relatively rare. Murder-suicides outside the family have occurred in the workplace, school settings, and public environments such as shopping malls or tourist locations. The perpetrators also have been referred to as "mass killers" or "rampage killers." Mullen (2004) proposed a classification scheme for separating types of mass killers that is defined by the relationship between the killers' intentions and their victims. This typology is described in Table 20–8.

The perpetrator of an autogenic (i.e., self-initiated) mass murder typically involves a heavily armed male who randomly shoots individuals before turning the gun on himself. The murderer may target for his

Forensic Issues | 425

TABLE 20–8. Mass killing categories

Victim-specific mass killings: deaths of the particular victims are the intended outcome.
  Family slaying
  Revenge killings
  Cult killings
  Gang killings

Instrumental mass killings: murder is a means to an end and perpetrator intends to advance a particular objective.
  Terrorist killings
  Killings incidental to other criminal activity

Massacres: murders are indiscriminate and killing people is the goal.
  Social conflict between different groups or classes resulting in civil massacres
  Autogenic massacres: individual driven by personal agenda and psychopathology

Source. Mullen 2004.

first killing a person against whom he has a grudge and subsequently expand his rampage to random victims. Such perpetrators are likely depressed and may frequently have obsessional traits with marked hypersensitivity and paranoia. Mullen (2004) found the following seven characteristics of perpetrators of autogenic massacres who survived despite their intent to commit suicide:

1. Male
2. Younger than 40 years of age
3. Socially isolated without close relationships
4. Unemployed or minimally employed
5. Bullied and/or isolated as a child
6. Fascinated with weapons
7. Collector of weapons

These murderers may also provoke law enforcement personnel to kill them after their murders—again, "suicide by cop." One study of 98 lone rampage killers in the United States found that those who were ultimately killed by police officers had the largest number of victims when compared with those who committed suicide or who were ultimately captured (Lester et al. 2005).

Key Points

Forensic evaluations of dangerousness are performed in a wide variety of situations that may involve a known, unknown, or even deceased offender. Regardless of the circumstance, forensic examiners should:

- Conduct a detailed psychiatric examination to search for the presence of mental illness, substance use disorder, and/or personality disorder
- Carefully review collateral records
- Interview individuals familiar with the offender
- Understand unique characteristics of both the offender and the potential victims when organizing a violence-prevention plan
- Be familiar with key typologies to understand underlying motivations and risk factors

References

Aderibigbe YA: Violence in America: a survey of suicide linked to homicide. J Forensic Sci 42:662–665, 1997

American Academy of Psychiatry and the Law: Ethical guidelines for the practice of forensic psychiatry, adopted May 2005. Available at http://aapl.org/pdf/ETHICSGDLNS.pdf. Accessed March 20, 2007

Biffl E: Psychological autopsies: do they belong in the courtroom? Am J Crim Law 1:123–146, 1996

Bossarte RM, Simon TR, Barker L: Homicide-suicide: characteristics of homicide followed by suicide incidents in multiple states, 2003–04. Inj Prev 12(suppl):33–38, 2006

Byard RW, Knight D, James RA, et al: Murder-suicides involving children: a 29-year study. Am J Forensic Med Pathol 20:323–327, 1999

Canter DV, Alison LJ, Alison E, et al: The organized/disorganized typology of serial murder: myth or model? Psychol Public Policy Law 10:293–320, 2004

Catalano SM: National Crime Victimization Survey: Criminal Victimization 2005 (BJS Bulletin, NCJ 214644). Washington, DC, Office of Justice Statistics, U.S. Department of Justice, 2006

Cohen D, Llorente M, Eisdorfer C: Homicide-suicide in older persons. Am J Psychiatry 155:390–396, 1998

Coid J: The epidemiology of abnormal homicide and murder followed by suicide. Psychol Med 13:855–860, 1983

Comstock RD, Mallonee S, Kruger E, et al: Epidemiology of homicide-suicide events, Oklahoma, 1994–2001. Am J Forensic Med Pathol 26:229–235, 2005

De Becker G: The Gift of Fear: Survival Signals That Protect us from Violence. London, Bloomsbury, 1997, pp 200–214

Dietz PE: Mass, serial, and sensational homicides. Bull NY Acad Med 62:477–491, 1986

Dusky v. U.S., 362 U.S. 402 (1960)

Eytan A, Borras L: Stalking through SMS: a new tool for an old behavior? Aust N Z J Psychiatry 39:204, 2005

Felthous AR, Hempel A: Combined homicide-suicides: a review. J Forensic Sci 40:846–857, 1995

Giorgi-Guarnieri D, Janofsky J, Keram E, et al: AAPL practice guideline for forensic psychiatric evaluation of defendants raising the insanity defense. J Am Acad Psychiatry Law 30(suppl):S3–S40, 2002

Grisso T: Forensic Evaluation of Juveniles. Sarasota, FL, Professional Resource Press, 1998

Groth AN, Birnbaum J: Men Who Rape: The Psychology of the Offender. New York, Plenum Press, 1979, pp 12–60

Hannah SG, Turf EE, Fierro MF: Murder-suicide in central Virginia: a descriptive epidemiologic study and empiric validation of the Hanzlick-Koponen typology. Am J Forensic Med Pathol 19:275–283, 1998

Hanzlick R, Koponen M: Murder-suicide in Fulton County, Georgia 1988–1991: comparison with a recent report and proposed typology. Am J Forensic Med Pathol 15:168–173, 1994

Hatters Friedman S, Huorda DR, Holden CE, et al: Filicide-suicide: common factors in parents who kill their children and themselves. J Am Acad Psychiatry Law 33:496–504, 2005

Hutson HR, Anglin D, Yarbrough J, et al: Suicide by cop. Ann Emerg Med 32:665–669, 1998

Knight RA, Prentky RA: Classifying sexual offenders: the development and corroboration of taxonomic models, in The Handbook of Sexual Assault. Edited by Marshall WL, Barbaree HE. New York, Plenum, 1990, pp 23–52

Lester D, Stack S, Schmidtke A, et al: Mass homicide and suicide deadliness and outcome. Crisis 26:184–187, 2005

Malmquist CP: Combined murder-suicide, in Textbook of Suicide Assessment and Management. Edited by Simon RI, Hales RE. Washington, DC, American Psychiatric Publishing, 2006, pp 495–509

Malphurs JE, Cohen D: A newspaper surveillance study of homicide-suicide in the United States. Am J Forensic Med Pathol 23:142–148, 2002

Marzuk P, Tardiff K, Hirsch CS: The epidemiology of murder-suicide. JAMA 267:3179–3183, 1992

Massello W: The proof in law of suicide. J Forensic Sci 31:1000–1008, 1986

McGrath MG, Casey E: Forensic psychiatry and the Internet: practical perspectives on sexual predators and obsessional harassers in cyberspace. J Am Acad Psychiatry Law 30:81–94, 2002

Milroy CM: The epidemiology of homicide-suicide (dyadic death). Forensic Sci Int 71:117–122, 1995

Milroy CM, Dratsas M, Ranson DL: Homicide-suicide in Victoria, Australia. Am J Forensic Med Pathol 18:369–373, 1997

Mohandie K, Meloy JR: Clinical and forensic indicators of "suicide by cop." J Forensic Sci 45:384–389, 2000

Mohandie K, Meloy JR, McGowan MG, et al: The RECON typology of stalking: reliability and validity based upon a large sample of North American stalkers. J Forensic Sci 51:147–155, 2006

Morton E, Runyan CW, Moracco KE, et al: Partner homicide-suicide involving female homicide victims: a population-based study in North Carolina, 1988–1992. Violence Vict 13:91–106, 1998

Mullen PE: The autogenic (self-generated) massacre. Behav Sci Law 22:311–323, 2004

Mullen PE, Pathe M, Purcell R, et al: A study of stalkers. Am J Psychiatry 156:1244–1249, 1999

Mullen PE, Pathe M, Purcell R: Stalkers and Their Victims. New York, Cambridge University Press, 2000, pp 187–237

Orion D: I Know You Really Love Me: A Psychiatrist's Journal of Erotomania, Stalking, and Obsessive Love. New York, Macmillan, 1997, pp 150–160

Palermo GB, Smith MB, Jenzten JM, et al: Murder-suicide of the jealous paranoia type: a multicenter statistical pilot study. Am J Forensic Med Pathol 18:374–383, 1997

Peck DL, Warner K: Accident or suicide? Single-vehicle car accidents and the intent hypothesis. Adolescence 30:463–472, 1995

Prentky RA, Burgess AW (eds): Prediction, in Forensic Management of Sexual Offenders. New York, Springer, 2000, pp 99–142

Prentky RA, Lee AFS, Knight RA: Recidivism rates among child molesters and rapists. Law Hum Behav 21:635–669, 1997

Ressler RK, Burgess AW, Douglas JE: Sexual Homicide: Patterns and Motives. New York, Lexington Books, 1988

Rodenburg M: Child murder by depressed parents. Can Psychiatr Assoc J 16:41–48, 1971

Rogers R, Grandjean N, Tillbrook CD, et al: Recent interview-based measures of competency to stand trial: a critical review augmented with research data. Behav Sci Law 19:503–518, 2001

Rosenbaum ML: The role of depression in couples involved in murder-suicide and homicide. Am J Psychiatry 147:1036–1039, 1990

Shneidman ES: The psychological autopsy. Suicide Life Threat Behav 11:325–340, 1981

Tjaden P, Thoennes N: Stalking in America: findings from the National Violence Against Women Survey. NCJ 169592. Washington, DC, Office of Justice Programs, National Institute of Justice Centers for Disease Control and Prevention, 1998

Warren JI, Fitch L, Dietz PE, et al: Criminal offense, psychiatric diagnosis, and psycholegal opinion: an analysis of 894 pretrial referrals. Bull Am Acad Psychiatry Law 19:63–69, 1991

Wilson EF, Davis JH, Bloom JD, et al: Homicide or suicide: the killing of suicidal persons by law enforcement officers. J Forensic Sci 43:46–52, 1998

Zona MA, Sharma KK, Lane J: A comparative study of erotomanic and obsessional subjects in a forensic sample. J Forensic Sci 38:894–903, 1993

CHAPTER 21

Legal Issues of Prediction, Protection, and Expertise

Daniel W. Shuman, J.D.
Britt Darwin-Looney, J.D.

Like the gift from the gods in numerous Greek myths (e.g., Midas, Pandora, Icarus), psychiatry and psychology's acquisition of the capacity to assess the risk of violence comes with burdens that may overshadow the gift. One burden of acumen in assessing risk of violence, with consequences as tragic as any visited by the mythological Greek gods, is that when violence occurs, psychiatrists and psychologists are often transformed, with the aid of the legal process, from heroes to villains for not having used their gift to prevent the violence from happening. Another burden is that when violence is legally relevant, the law expects to receive accurate prophecies from psychiatrists and psychologists, even at the expense of confidentiality and cautious science. Accordingly, a comprehensive treatment of violence necessitates a hard look at legal rules that bear on the assessment of violence. This chapter introduces those contexts and the issues they raise.

The first section of this chapter addresses an all too common legal dilemma for psychiatrists and psychologists: the impact of acumen in violence assessment and management on the rules governing therapist–patient confidentiality. Most states either recognize a statutory duty of confidentiality for psychotherapists or incorporate a professional ethics code containing a duty of confidentiality into state licensing law. If psychiatrists or psychologists have unique insights about a patient's desire to commit a violent act, should they be required to protect the victim, violate this duty of confidentiality, and reveal information about the risk of violence (acquired in a confidential relationship) to the police or an identifiable person at risk? Consider the irony of concluding that a psychiatrist may not reveal even patients' names to concerned family members or friends but may owe a duty to protect a third-party stranger who *might* be harmed as a result of the patient's violent behavior, requiring a breach of confidentiality to that person or to the police. How can the protection of confidentiality and the duty to protect coexist in a psychiatrist or psychologist's daily practice?

The second part of the chapter examines how the courts have received expert evidence assessing the risk of violence. If the law concludes that psychiatry and psychology's ability to assess violence is good enough to recognize a special relationship and impose a "duty to protect" the non-patient victim, does it follow that courts will invariably allow psychiatrists and psychologists to testify about violence assessment? Once again, there is irony in the legal recognition of a duty to protect while at the same time the legal system questions psychiatry's or psychology's acumen in cases involving violence.

Finally, no legal inquiry into violence assessment would be complete without discussing how dangerousness has shaped the nation's criminal and civil justice systems. We may question whether psychiatrists and psychologists can accurately assess the risk of violence, but a host of extant legal procedures rest on the assumption that they can (e.g., civil commitment). The decision to detain criminal defendants prior to trial or to impose capital punishment, for example, often turns on assumptions regarding the ability to assess the risk of violence.

Tarasoff's Legacy: Predicting Violence in Mental Health Patients

There are many places one could begin a legal examination of the assessment of the risk of violence. Chronologically, *Tarasoff v. Regents of the University of California* (1976) finds the debate in the courts about the ability of psychiatrists and psychologists to predict violence in full stride, with a wry twist. In civil commitment proceedings, psychiatrists, among other mental health professionals, had been touting their predictive abilities to justify preventive confinement. Rather than touting their wisdom in this case, however, the psychiatrists' and psychologists' briefs in *Tarasoff* tried to convince the courts that they are simply not that good at prediction and therefore should not be liable for getting it wrong.

Legal Issues of Prediction, Protection, and Expertise | 431

In *Tarasoff*, the parents of Tatiana Tarasoff, a U.C. Berkeley coed who was murdered by an international student who was a patient of a university psychologist, sued the psychologist, the university, and the campus police for failing to use reasonable care to protect their daughter from that patient's acts. During individual therapy sessions, the patient, Prosenjit Poddar, a spurned suitor of the victim, revealed that he was going to kill Ms. Tarasoff when she returned from vacation. The psychologist notified the campus police, advising them that his patient should be committed. However, after speaking to him, the campus police decided that the young man was rational and not dangerous and refused to confine him. When the victim returned from vacation, the patient murdered her. He was convicted of second-degree murder, which was later reversed for an erroneous jury instruction and not retried. The civil claim for negligence was filed in California state trial court, which promptly granted the defendants' motion to dismiss because the prosecution had failed to state a valid legal claim.

The trial court dismissed the claim because Tarasoff was not a patient of the psychologist and therefore the psychologist did not have a duty to protect her from his patient. An accepted principle of the common law is that one person does not have the duty to control the conduct of another, warn another of danger, or rescue another unless he undertakes that duty voluntarily or a special relationship exists that gives rise to a right of protection or a duty to control. After an appeal from the original dismissal, as well as a withdrawal of its initial opinion, the Supreme Court of California decided that either the psychologist's relationship to his patient or to his patient's victim satisfied the special relationship:

> Although, as we have stated above, under the common law, as a general rule, one person owed no duty to control the conduct of another...the courts have carved out an exception to this rule in cases in which the defendant stands in some special relationship to either the person whose conduct needs to be controlled or in a relationship to the foreseeable victim of that conduct.... Applying this exception to the present case, we note that a relationship of defendant therapists to either Tatiana or Poddar will suffice to establish a duty of care; as explained in section 315 of the Restatement Second of Torts, a duty of care may arise from either "(a) a special relation...between the actor and the third person which imposes a duty upon the actor to control the third person's conduct, or (b) a special relation...between the actor and the other which gives to the other a right of protection." (*Tarasoff v. Regents of the University of California* 1976)

The Supreme Court of California based this reasoning on a belief in the psychologist's predictive abilities. Accordingly, the court reasoned, when a psychotherapist determines, or should determine, that "his patient presents a serious danger of violence to another, he [the therapist] incurs an obligation to use reasonable care to protect the intended victim against such danger." Although the California Supreme Court obligated psychotherapists to safeguard third parties endangered by their patients, it did not address whether the defendant psychotherapist satisfied this obligation by informing the campus police and requesting confinement of his patient. Instead, the trial court dismissed the case before any evidence was presented, and the case was settled before it was tried after remand. If this same set of circumstances reached the California trial courts today, the correct answer regarding the steps to be taken by the psychotherapist would be clear. Designed to clarify when a duty arises and what fulfills it, a layer of legislation now answers these questions: "There shall be no monetary liability on the part of, and no cause of action shall arise against, a psychotherapist who, under the limited circumstances specified above, discharges his or her duty to warn and protect by making reasonable efforts to communicate the threat to the victim or victims and to a law enforcement agency" (Cal. Civ. Code § 43.92[b] [West 2007]). Whatever the *Tarasoff* court might have thought 30 years ago, the psychologist in *Tarasoff* apparently met this new statutory requirement by notifying the campus police.

Although *Tarasoff* changed California law, in our system of federalism with semiautonomous, coequal states, it did not by itself change the laws in other states. Free to choose about most elements of tort law and criminal law, however, many states have accepted *Tarasoff* in whole or in part. Many have also implemented statutes to clarify and limit the responsibility of psychiatrists and psychologists to report potentially violent patients and limit claims for breach of that duty. The vast majority of these statutes attempt to limit the situations in which reporting is required: typically, they state that the danger or threatened act of violent behavior must be imminent, although this cautionary measure is not scientifically grounded or meaningful; the potential victim must be easily identifiable from the patient's threats; and the harm to the threatened potential victim must be serious and reasonably foreseeable. For example, in New Jersey (N.J. Stat. § 2A:62A–16 [2007]) and Delaware (16 Del. C. § 5402 [2007]), a duty to protect arises only when 1) the patient has communicated to that practitioner a threat of imminent, serious physical violence against a readily identifiable individual or against him- or herself and the circumstances are such that a reasonable professional in the practitioner's area of expertise would believe the patient intended to carry out the threat; or 2) the circumstances are such that a reasonable professional in the practitioner's area of expertise would believe the pa-

Legal Issues of Prediction, Protection, and Expertise | 433

tient intended to carry out an act of imminent, serious physical violence against a readily identifiable individual or against him- or herself.

For example, if the patient revealed to the therapist that next month he or she was going to vaporize everyone in the world who had brown hair and blue eyes, this would not invoke the therapist's duty to warn or protect. Whatever *imminent* means, this is not imminent. Millions of people have brown hair and blue eyes; the patient's description of the potential victims does not make them easily identifiable. Finally, his threat to "vaporize" is not realistic or reasonably foreseeable. On the other hand, if the patient had told the therapist that tonight, with a deer hunting rifle, he or she was going to kill his neighbor with brown hair and blue eyes, then the answer would be different. The time frame is now closer and therefore less accommodating of exploring alternatives, and the victim is easily identifiable. If the threat is credible, then it would be reasonably foreseeable that the patient could use a rifle to kill the victim. Although these examples are extreme, this is the type of analysis that the statutes and courts encourage therapists to engage in when deciding how to weigh their confidential obligations to their patients against the duty to protect potential victims.

In an additional attempt to limit the duty to protect and the therapist's revelation of confidential information, some states define the individuals who may and/or must be warned of the possibility of future violent behavior. For example, if the patient's threat to kill his or her neighbor tonight is credible, the therapist must report this information to the proper authorities and the victim (but should not call the local news station or newspaper to report this threat). In California and Washington, for example, the therapist discharges his or her duty to warn and protect by making reasonable efforts to communicate the threat to the victim or victims and to a law enforcement agency (Cal. Civ. Code § 43.92[b] [West 2006]; Rev. Code Wash. §71.05.120 [2007]).

A few states, such as Texas, have rejected *Tarasoff* outright. Texas psychiatrists and psychologists are *permitted* to reveal patient threats of violence but are not *required* to do so. The Texas statute governing confidentiality provides: "A professional *may* disclose confidential information only...to medical or law enforcement personnel if the professional determines that there is a probability of imminent physical injury by the patient to the patient or others or there is a probability of immediate mental or emotional injury to the patient" (Texas Health and Safety Code 2006, emphasis added).

In *Thapar v. Zezulka* (1999), the Texas Supreme Court interpreted this statutory discretionary disclosure to be controlling in its determination or recognition of the duty to protect/warn. The surviving spouse of a person murdered by a psychiatrist's patient sued the psychiatrist, alleging negligence in diagnosing the patient's condition and in failing to warn family members or law enforcement officers of the patient's threats against his eventual victim. The Texas Supreme Court interpreted the state confidentiality statute's authorization of permissive disclosure of confidential information as a rejection of compelled disclosure, from which the court inferred a legislative rejection of *Tarasoff*. Of course, the legislature could have mentioned *Tarasoff* by name if they intended to reject it, but then again if they disagreed with *Thapar* they could have amended the law. Neither occurred.

Texas is not alone in allowing the therapist to use discretion when deciding whether to reveal the patient's violent threats. In Mississippi a therapist "*may* communicate the threat only to the potential victim or victims, a law enforcement agency, or the parent or guardian of a minor who is identified as a potential victim" (Miss. Code Ann. § 41–21–97 [2006], emphasis added). Florida law also grants the therapist substantial discretion in choosing to disclose (Fla. Stat. § 491.0147 [2006]). In both of these states, the courts have agreed that the permissive disclosure language of the statutes is inconsistent with recognition of a *Tarasoff* duty (*Boynton v. Burglass* 1991; *Evans v. United States* 1995; *Green v. Ross* 1997).

What do these differing state statutes and court interpretations demand of the best practices of psychiatrists and psychologists? They demand attention at the beginning of the relationship and the process of informed consent. Patients must be informed that confidentiality is not absolute and told what limits exist. When a psychiatrist or psychologist determines that a patient poses a risk to a third party, best practice demands attention in a consultation with colleagues and/or legal counsel to consider the risk of violence as well as the risks and benefits of alternative responses to the duty imposed. The best practice also demands that in dealing with *Tarasoff*, which is, at bottom, a negligence claim for failing to act as a reasonable psychologist would act under the circumstances, clinicians remain current in the research on assessment of the risk of violence. Of course, best practice standards also demand that psychiatrists and psychologists know the relevant laws for their states regarding what gives rise to a duty to protect third-party victims and the proper entities to notify with this information.

Daubert's Legacy: Violence and Expert Testimony

Assessment of the risk of violence is certainly not the only topic on which psychiatric or psychological expert testimony is offered. Yet it has played an important role in establishing rules for admissibility of

Legal Issues of Prediction, Protection, and Expertise | 435

expert testimony. Thus it is worthwhile to examine it for its own sake as well as for the lessons it offers about expert testimony more generally.

The approach of courts to accommodating the need for expert assistance and scientific orthodoxy has varied over time. Until the twentieth century, even on matters of science, the courts rarely demanded more than a qualified expert as a condition of admissibility, leaving the jury to determine the reliability of the method or process on which an expert's opinion rests through cross-examination and the testimony of opposing experts. Thus, for witnesses presented as experts, the sole inquiry in admissibility focused on the witnesses' education, training, or experience. Any formulas, devices, or techniques that the witness relied upon were matters of believability for the jury to decide, not matters of admissibility. That began to change with the D.C. Court of Appeals decision in *Frye v. United States* (1923). In *Frye,* a defendant charged with murder offered exculpatory evidence from an early polygraph relying on systolic blood pressure. Reasoning that the qualifications of the expert witness presenting the test results were not sufficient to justify admission without examining the accuracy of the machine itself, the decision articulated the famous "general acceptance" test to assess the admissibility of novel scientific evidence.

Frye was a refreshing recognition of the need to look at both the science and the scientist as a condition of admissibility of scientific expert testimony. However, it had its problems. It equated popularity ("general acceptance") with scientific accuracy, it left unresolved *whose* acceptance is required (polygraph examiners, psychologists, psychiatrists, or the National Academy of Sciences) and what signaled general acceptance (50%, 75%, or 90%), and it insulated the judge from scientific disputes by directing the judge to defer to scientific majority. Although the debate raged about *Frye's* merits as well as its survival under the Federal Rules of Evidence, which were intended to liberalize the admissibility of evidence, another evidentiary debate loomed over the admissibility, in capital sentencing, of predictions of violence based on a brief clinical examination. Texas was one of the states at the center of this debate, because of both its capital punishment criteria and the presence of a very persuasive psychiatric expert witness, Dr. James Grigson, who most often found himself assisting the prosecution. A critical question in Texas for a capital jury choosing whether to impose the death penalty is the risk of violence the defendant poses if not executed. In *Barefoot v. Estelle* (1983), the U.S. Supreme Court heard a constitutional challenge to imposing the death penalty based on the argument that Dr. Grigson's clinical-opinion testimony was not generally accepted as a reliable basis for a prediction of future violence, although he was very successful in persuading juries.

The Supreme Court rejected the prisoner's argument that the U.S. Constitution prohibits imposition of the death penalty based on clinical predictions regarded as unreliable by the American Psychiatric Association, among others, which filed an *amicus* brief in the case. Acknowledging problems with the accuracy of clinically based predictions, the Court refused to permit a private organization to frustrate imposition of the death penalty it had approved.

Barefoot v. Estelle (1983) presented a question of constitutional minimums—does a death sentence that rests on a clinical prediction violate due process, thus requiring a fundamental change in the criteria for the imposition of capital punishment? Because it was a state court trial and conviction, it did not specify what the Federal Rules of Evidence might demand of an expert in these circumstances above the constitutional minimums. That part of the puzzle was revealed a decade later, when the Supreme Court decided *Daubert v. Merrell Dow Pharmaceuticals, Inc.* (1993). *Daubert* was a toxic tort case, filed in California state court and removed to federal court on diversity of citizenship grounds. The plaintiff alleged that Bendectin, an anti-nausea drug manufactured by Merrell Dow Pharmaceuticals, caused limb reduction birth defects. The defendant's Motion for Summary Judgment asserted that epidemiology was the generally accepted standard for evaluating a drug's toxicity and that no published epidemiological study found a significant relationship between Bendectin and limb reduction birth defects. When the plaintiff's experts, all well-qualified research scientists with impressive credentials, offered another approach to analyzing the data, the court rejected their expert testimony, relying on *Frye*, which it assumed to be the standard applied under the Federal Rules of Evidence, and granted the defendant's motion for summary judgment.

The case made its way to the Ninth Circuit and eventually to the Supreme Court. The Court granted review to resolve the test for expert evidence under the Federal Rules of Evidence, unresolved since the rules were enacted in 1975. Examining the text of the rules, the court concluded that because nowhere in the rules was *Frye* mentioned, it could not have been intended to be the test for scientific evidence under the Federal Rules of Evidence. Instead, relying on falsifiability as the hallmark of science, the court adopted a pragmatic approach to relevance and reliability, taking into account whether the underlying methods and procedures were testable and had been tested; whether they had been subjected to peer review and publication, and if so what was the error rate and could it be controlled; and finally a rebirth of *Frye's* general acceptance test. Two other related decisions followed (*General Electric v. Joiner* [1997] and *Kumho Tire Co. v. Carmichael* [1999]) that made

Legal Issues of Prediction, Protection, and Expertise | 437

clear that these considerations were committed to the discretion of the trial court, who might apply some but not others as appropriate.

After much prognosticating about *Daubert's* likely impact on psychiatric and psychological expert testimony, the post-*Daubert* world for psychiatric and psychological experts for the most part has not differed significantly. *Daubert* was intended to ask, as a matter of admissibility, why we should believe an expert's assertion. That scrutiny has rarely occurred. For the most part, scrutiny of the methods and procedures used by psychiatric expert witnesses testifying on issues such as competence to stand trial, the insanity defense and punishment, and mental or emotional loss in personal injury claims has not changed. When the *Daubert* question is raised in the context of violence assessment in death penalty cases, courts often assume incorrectly that *Barefoot*, which addressed constitutional minimums, also disposed of the evidentiary question under *Daubert* (*Johnson v. Cockrell* 2002). It did not. Ironically, clinically based testimony is rarely challenged; rather, it is testimony based on written tests that claim an actuarial basis that more often incurs a challenge.

Where the issue is addressed and courts do not view the evidence issue as resolved by *Barefoot*, many conclude that risk assessment is not novel science to which *Frye* or *Daubert* apply (*In re detention of Thorell* [2004]). When they do apply *Frye* or *Daubert*, the written tests used in risk assessment (Static 99, Rapid Risk Assessment for Sexual Offense Recidivism, Structured Anchored Clinical Judgment–Minimum) almost always survive the scrutiny applied (*In re commitment of R.S.* [2004]). As contrasted with *Daubert's* application in toxic tort cases, its application in violence assessments and sexually violent predator commitments seems to result in less demanding scrutiny.

Violence Assessment and the Dilemma of *Daubert*

The assumption that reliable violence risk assessment is available is an unstated but central premise of numerous legal processes and procedures. As far as public safety or incapacitation is concerned, criminal punishment without reliable individual violence assessments is a blunt instrument, as reflected in judicial dissatisfaction with one-size-fits-all sentencing guidelines. Unreliable violence assessments in domestic violence cases pose frightening consequences. If the assessment of future dangerousness as required by the statutes that govern civil commitment of the mentally ill and sexually violent predators is unreliable, the resulting decision to commit is random. Necessary treatment would not reach its intended targets, and the public would be lulled into a false sense of security. The judicial system has historically relied on what it assumes to be reasonably accurate violence assessment to decide whom to incarcerate and commit.

Although criminal procedure varies from state to state, for purposes of illustration we highlight the different stages at which Texas criminal procedure calls for violence assessment. Both formal diversion (e.g., acceptance of defendant in mental health courts rather than criminal prosecution) and informal diversion (e.g., acceptance of prisoner in psychiatric emergency department rather than jail booking) turn on a violence assessment, among other things. If the defendant has been detained for a crime before guilt or innocence is decided, the court is required to address the prisoner's potential for violence to determine bail. One of the factors to be considered in setting bail is "the future safety of a victim of the alleged offense and the community" (Tex. Code Crim. Proc. Art. 17.15[5] [2006]). If society cannot otherwise be protected, bail can be denied or increased; but to operate effectively, this decision requires accurate assessment of the risk of violence.

During sentencing, evidence of "dangerousness" can be introduced as either aggravating or mitigating evidence. In capital murder sentencing, violence assessment is critical in choosing between life imprisonment and the death penalty. One of the factors that the jury must consider when determining whether to impose the death sentence in Texas for a defendant convicted of capital murder is "whether there is a probability that the defendant would commit criminal acts of violence that would constitute a continuing threat to society" (*Nenno v. State* 1998; Tex. Code Crim. Proc. Art. 7.071[2][b][1] [2006]).

As noted, predicting future violent behavior is also a foundation for civil commitment. Civil commitment is a preventative measure to provide protection from the risks some mentally ill individuals pose to themselves and society. In *O'Connor v. Donaldson* (1975), the Supreme Court held that "a State cannot constitutionally confine without more a nondangerous individual who is capable of surviving safely in freedom." If violence could not be predicted, then civil commitment could not be justified unless the state offered something "more," a justification that would presumably focus on the availability and the effectiveness of treatment, a vastly more demanding and expensive yardstick. In addition to leaving unanswered the "something more" question, the Supreme Court did not explain how "dangerousness" should be assessed, although the decision rests on the assumption that dangerousness can be reliably assessed.

Consistent with the assumption of expertise, most states have enacted statutes requiring specific mental health experts to testify in civil commitment cases. For example, in Illinois, "no respondent may be found subject to involuntary admission unless at least one psychiatrist, clinical social worker, or clinical psychologist who has examined him testifies in person at the hearing" (405 Ill. Comp. Stat. 5/3–807 [2007]). Rhode Island requires that "in determining whether there exists a likelihood of serious harm the *physician* and the court may consider previous acts, diagnosis, words or thoughts of the patient" (R.I. Gen. Laws § 40.1–5–2[7][4][2007], emphasis added). In Texas "the proof [for civil commitment] must include expert [psychiatric] testimony and, unless waived, must include evidence of either a recent overt act or a continuing pattern of behavior in either case tending to confirm the likelihood of serious harm to the person or others or the person's distress and deterioration of ability to function" (*State for Interest of P.W.* 1990).

If we are to take *Daubert* seriously and ask why we should believe what the expert is offering, how many of these assessments would survive rigorous scrutiny? Do the data support that reliable assessment techniques exist for each legally relevant context? When reliable risk assessment methods or techniques exist, how widely are they used? Here a lesson might be learned from clinical practice and its use of evidence-based medicine to encourage use of the most reliable techniques. A critical analysis of existing forensic practice resulting in research-based forensic guidelines offers the potential for greater accuracy and consistency of forensic assessments of the risk of violence.

To build these best techniques on a solid foundation and reinforce the procedures they inform, it would also be useful first to engage lawyers, judges, psychiatrists, and psychologists in an interdisciplinary dialogue to identify all of the contexts in which legal determinations turn on the risk of violence, and then to determine what the research reveals about what psychiatrists and psychologists have to contribute to the debate. In any of those contexts in which the analysis leaves us confident in the reliability of the methods used, it might be possible to recognize that concurrence so that judicial notice could be taken of the acceptance of these methods, thereby resolving the *Daubert/Frye* question. In any of these contexts in which the analysis leaves us uncomfortable with the reliability of the methods used to assess risk in this context, identification of the context should result in consideration of new assessment approaches as well as an exploration of alternative legal rules or standards (e.g., examining alternative bases for imposing capital punishment) to improve the foundation for legal decision making and avoid the temptation for psychiatrists and psychologists to answer without a scientific foundation.

Key Points

- Psychiatrists are expected by their patients and their profession to make accurate violence assessments in their clinical practice.
- Psychiatrists are expected by their patients and their profession to know what is required of them to meet their obligations to patients, those whom the patient may endanger, and society.
- Psychiatrists will be held accountable by their patients, those whom the patients harm, and society for harm that results from the failure to engage in state-of-the-art, evidence-based assessments of violence.

References

Barefoot v. Estelle, 403 U.S. 880 (1983)
Boynton v. Burglass, 590 So. 2d 446 (Fla. App 1991)
Cal. Civ. Code § 43.92(b) (West 2006)
Cal. Civ. Code § 43.92(b) (West 2007)
Daubert v. Merrell Dow Pharmaceuticals, Inc., 509 U.S. 579 (1993)
16 Del. C. § 5402 (2007)
Evans v. United States, 883 F.Supp. 124 (S.D. Miss. 1995)
Fla. Stat. § 491.0147 (2006)
Frye v. United States, 293 F. 1013 (D.C. Cir. 1923)
General Electric v. Joiner, 522 U.S. 136 (1997)
Green v. Ross, 691 So. 2d 542 (Fla. App. 1997)
405 Ill. Comp. Stat. 5/3–807 (2007)
In re commitment of R.S., 801 A.2d 219 (N.J. 2004)
In re detention of Thorell, 72 P.3d 708 (Wash. 2000), cert. denied 541 U.S. 990 (2004)
Johnson v. Cockrell, 306 F.3d 249 (5th Cir. 2002)
Kumho Tire Co. v. Carmichael, 526 U.S. 137 (1999)
Miss. Code Ann. § 41–21–97 (2006)
Nenno v. State, 970 S.W.2d 549 (Tex. Crim. App. 1998)
N.J. Stat. § 2A:62A–16 (2007)
O'Connor v. Donaldson, 422 U.S. 563 (1975)
Rev. Code Wash. (ARCW) § 71.05.120 (2007)
R.I. Gen. Laws § 40.1–5–2(7)(4) (2007)
State for Interest of P.W., 801 S.W.2d 1 (Tex. App. 1990)
Tarasoff v. Regents of the University of California, 17 Cal. 3d 425, 131 Cal. Rptr. 14, 551 P.2d 334 (1976)
Tex. Code Crim. Proc. Art. 17.15(5) (2006)
Tex. Code Crim. Proc. Art. 7.071(2)(b)(1) (2006)
Texas Health and Safety Code § 611.004(a)(2) (2006)
Thapar v. Zezulka, 494 S.W. 2d 635 (Tex. 1999)

CHAPTER 22

Sexual Violence and the Clinician

John M.W. Bradford, M.B.Ch.B., D.P.M.

Paul Fedoroff, M.D.

Philip Firestone, Ph.D.

Sexual Violence: A Review

Sexual violence is a multidimensional concept that has various definitions, depending on which professional group is using the term or the context in which it is used. Violent sexual behavior, such as a sexually motivated homicide or violent serial sexual offenses against women and children, clearly fits the definition of sexual violence. "*Any* sexual behavior against a nonconsenting partner" represents a broader definition of sexual violence and the one most commonly used. This broad definition of sexual violence would cover most sexually deviant behavior and most sexual offending behavior (Bradford 2006). It would include most of the "hands-on" paraphilias or sexual deviations (e.g., sexual sadism, pedophilia) and would exclude most of the "hands-off" paraphilias (e.g., voyeurism, fetishism, exhibitionism) (Bradford et al. 1992). Our review of sexual violence in this chapter follows this broad definition. *Sexual aggression* is a term more commonly used by mental health professionals and sexologists to cover the broad categorization of sexual violence. It is also broadly broken down into sexual aggression against women and sexual aggression against children, following the common classification of sexual offenders and sexual crimes.

Sexual violence thus includes any sexual act with nonconsenting partners. It also includes physical violence associated with a paraphilia or sexual deviation. Sexual violence includes extreme physical violence associated with coercive sexual activity. This type of violence usually involves the sexual assault and murder of adults or children as part of sadistic, sexually motivated homicides. Sexually motivated homicides are in turn classified as sadistic or nonsadistic (Gratzer and Bradford 1995). Because acts of sexual violence with nonconsenting partners are against the law, most of the perpetrators of these acts would also be classified as sexual offenders. It is important to note that the converse is not necessarily true and that not all sexual offenders have a paraphilia or sexual deviation as defined in DSM-IV-TR (American Psychiatric Association 2000). It should also be noted that sex and violence are of universal interest—as demonstrated by an Internet search using the search engine Google in which the keyword "sex" generates more than 680 million "hits" (Fedoroff, in press). A search of the major databases such as the National Library of Medicine, also using the keyword "sex," resulted in more than 4,000 journal article citations in the past 10 years, and a search on "sadomasochism" generated 148 journal articles (Fedoroff, in press). Studies of sexual violence are increasing, and interest in the subject has also been increasing in various professional groups, particularly in psychology. Psychiatrists, including forensic psychiatrists, have sadly neglected this important field even though they have many of the skill sets required to work in this area. Expertise in both the psychological and biological bases to sexual violence as well as medical and pharmacological skills for assessing and treating these individuals are critical. Most psychiatrists have these skill sets and should be involved in research as well as the assessment and treatment of sexual violence.

The consequences of sexual violence are very serious both for the perpetrators and for the victims (Fedoroff 1996). In fact, about one-third of men who molest children were sexually abused themselves and are therefore victims as well as perpetrators (Fedoroff 1996). The relationship between perpetrators and victims has led to the theoretical assumption that abuse victims may become perpetrators themselves (Fedoroff 1996). If this theoretical assumption is true, population studies on the incidence and prevalence of sexual abuse are extremely important if preventive strategies are to be put in place to reduce victimization. Various studies have shown that between 10% and 16% of males and between 20% and 27% of females have been victims of childhood sexual abuse (Finkelhor 1984; Finkelhor and Lewis 1988; Finkelhor et al. 1990). These data are critical to understanding not only the nature of pedophilia but also the degree or level of risk within the population for the

Sexual Violence and the Clinician | 443

sexual abuse of children. A Scandinavian study on population statistics reported the incidence and prevalence of sexual abuse in Denmark (Helweg-Larsen and Larsen 2005). These researchers found the average annual incidence of child sexual abuse to be 0.06 per 1,000 children under 15 years of age, using the National Patient Register as a database. When other data sets were used, for example the National Criminal Register, the incidence was found to be 0.5 per 1,000. When police reports containing comprehensive information from victims were used, the reported incidence of child sexual abuse was found to be 1.0 per 1,000 children younger than 12 years of age and 0.6 per 1,000 when exhibitionism was excluded. About 50% of intrafamilial child sexual abuse cases and about 40% of extrafamilial cases resulted in a conviction (Helweg-Larsen and Larsen 2005). Translated into North American terms, the incidence in the United States would be at least 300,000 children sexually abused in any given year and 30,000 children in Canada. Another study on childhood sexual abuse using computer-based self-administered questionnaires submitted by a national representative sample of 15- and 16-year-olds in Denmark resulted in close to 6,000 respondents. Of these, 11% reported unlawful sexual experiences (7% of boys and 16% of girls). Interestingly, these young people's interpretation of the experience was that only 1% of boys and 4% of girls felt that they had been "definitely" or "maybe" sexually abused (Helweg-Larsen and Boving Larsen 2006). This type of study is critical to understanding child sexual abuse. It also illustrates the complexity of the sexual interaction and sexual experiences of young people in recent decades. It should also focus attention on the sexual abuse of children, which should be regarded as a public health problem.

In many Western countries, programs to prevent child sexual abuse by educating children and sensitizing them to the issue have been put in place. Various programs have been developed to educate children about "good touch" and "bad touch." In addition, Western countries have instituted laws requiring the mandatory reporting of child sexual abuse as tools to prevent victimization. The actual impact of these measures on the incidence and prevalence of child sexual abuse is still a matter of debate.

In more recent years, the dramatic growth of the Internet has brought a whole new dimension to child sexual abuse. The Internet has become a new vehicle for the sexual abuse of children, requiring that new strategies be put in place to deal with this threat. The Internet has clearly become a focus of deviant sexual behavior, as demonstrated by the dramatic increase in individuals charged with the possession of child pornography. Very serious concerns have arisen about the Internet being used as a tool by pedophiles to target children. This is a worldwide phenomenon, and the concern has led to recent studies on how the Internet is being used for sexual purposes and to classify Internet offenders (Alexy et al. 2005). As the natures of perpetrators on the Internet and of the interactions that are taking place become better understood, the Internet has also become a focus for the protection of children (Mitchell et al. 2001, 2005a, 2005b, 2005c). There clearly is significant unwanted exposure to sexual solicitation and harassment of young persons (Mitchell et al. 2001). Young persons also experience considerable unsolicited exposure to pornography on the Internet (Wolak et al. 2007). The exact nature and the impact of these developments in the future is impossible to determine at this time. Studies of Internet perpetrators have shown they are quite frequently sexual offender recidivists and also have engaged in other deviant sexual offenses (Seto and Eke 2005). Individuals' use of the Internet to lure children into meeting them in order to seduce them is relatively infrequent but is of serious concern when it does occur. These perpetrators are most likely long-standing pedophilic sexual offenders using the Internet as a strategy to access children for sexual purposes. Clearly, the Internet is a new frontier for exposure to pornography by young persons as well as a vehicle for exposure to sexual solicitation by pedophiles and other Internet offenders.

Case Example: The Internet Perpetrator

Mr. S is a 52-year-old married scientist with daughters who are teenagers. He was arrested at his place of work by local law enforcement officers as part of an FBI investigation of Internet child pornography. His laptop computer at work had approximately 1,000 images of child pornography on its hard drive. Further investigation through a search warrant found 2,000 images of child pornography on his home computer, including images backed up onto compact discs. The images were carefully classified according to age groups and were all of girls 13 years of age or younger. A wide spectrum of ethnic groups was represented. Most of the images depicted young girls in sexual poses without engaging in sexual activity. About 10% of the images depicted sexual activity with an adult male, mostly performing fellatio but also including sexual intercourse in a small number of pictures. No videos were included in this child pornography collection.

Mr. S was regarded as an excellent employee; he had no criminal record, and an intensive investigation by the local child protection agency produced no evidence of his having sexually abused his own children. There was no evidence of any marital dysfunction, including no history of sexual difficulties. Mr. S was referred to a specialized sexual behaviors clinic for a pre-sentence forensic psychiatric evaluation. This included the usual psychiatric history and diagnosis but also a sex hormone profile, various sexual questionnaires (including the Bradford Sexual History Inventory; Sexual Fantasy Checklist; Derogatis Sexual Functioning Inventory; and various scales measuring pedophilic cognitive distortions, hostility, and impulsivity, as well as the Michigan Alcohol Screening Test and the Drug Screening Test), along with objective measures of sexual interest measured through penile plethysmography.

The assessment revealed that Mr. S had experienced sexual fantasies of prepubertal children during adolescence and over the years had masturbated to these fantasies but had never sexually acted out with children. On the Sexual Fantasy Checklist he endorsed moderate ongoing levels of heterosexual pedophilic fantasy. He showed mild pedophilic cognitive distortions. Objective measures of sexual interest showed an increased sexual preference toward prepubertal female children, with a Pedophile Index of 2.4. This meant that the ratio of his pedophilic arousal was 2.4 times higher than his measured arousal to consenting sex with adult females. The sensitivity of this examination is 85% and the specificity is 90%, meaning that based on a study of 100 clinical admitted pedophile subjects and 100 community control subjects, 85% of the pedophiles and 90% of the community control subjects were correctly classified by using various measures of sexual arousal. There was no evidence of any sadistic sexual preference. Mr. S immediately entered into treatment for pedophilia. His formal DSM-IV-TR diagnosis was pedophilia, opposite-sex children, nonexclusive type, mild. No other Axis I diagnoses were present. There was no evidence of significant personality disorder on Axis II. A Hare Psychopathy Checklist score of 8 was obtained on risk assessment evaluation. Formal sexual offender risk assessment using the Static-99 was not valid because he had no previous convictions for sexual offenses. His risk of future sexual offense recidivism was very low.

His treatment program consisted of psychological and pharmacological components. He was treated individually for the pedophilic cognitive distortions and attended an ongoing relapse prevention group. He was treated with selective serotonin reuptake inhibitors (SSRIs), specifically sertraline, 150–200 mg/day, to suppress the pedophilic fantasies. The pharmacological regimen was successful in eliminating the pedophilic fantasies without affecting his sexual performance. Because he was fired from his place of work, vocational counseling and rehabilitation through occupational therapy assisted him in finding alternative employment. Marital and family therapy were successful in maintaining his family unit. He received a suspended sentence and probation with a condition of treatment for 3 years. At 5-year follow-up Mr. S showed no evidence of sexual offense recidivism.

Sexual Sadism and Sexually Motivated Homicide

The operational criteria for sexual sadism in DSM-IV-TR are found under the sexual and gender identity disorders and specifically under the paraphilias. Questions have arisen as to the adequacy of the criteria and how they have been applied. At least one study of experienced forensic psychiatrists found that sexual sadism as a diagnosis was not being applied in Canadian correctional facilities as defined in DSM-IV-TR. The kappa coefficient for reliability across diagnoses was only 0.14, which is extremely poor (Marshall et al. 2002). Without reviewing all the details of this particular study, it is clear that confusion about this very significant diagnosis is evident. Confusion about the clinical aspects of sexual violence occurs even among experienced forensic psychiatrists, in part due to difficulties related to the "coercive paraphilic disorders." There was a recommendation by the Subcommittee on Sexual Disorders to include this group of paraphilias in the DSM-III-R diagnostic schema (Abel 1989; American Psychiatric Association 1987). Although there was strong empirical evidence for a diagnostic grouping of the "coercive paraphilic disorders," there was also considerable concern that the inclusion could lead to forensic psychiatric misuse of such a diagnostic classification (Abel 1989). This debate has left a gap in the diagnostic classification for males who meet the criteria for the paraphilias as well as established clinical criteria for the paraphilias (e.g., typical natural history of the paraphilias) and who are offenders against adult females. Some of these men commit rape and show a sexual preference for rape over consensual sex with adult females. The lack of an official diagnosis has led to some of these men being diagnosed as having sexual sadism and others as having paraphilia not otherwise specified. Neither of these diagnostic classifications accommodates this type of paraphilic male very well, leading to diagnostic confusion as well as forensic misuse in sexually violent predator cases in the United States.

Clinical studies of sexually sadistic homicide perpetrators are rare, mostly because this is a small group of individuals infrequently seen even in forensic psychiatric settings (Swigert et al. 1976). Two studies have looked at the offender and offense characteristics, including crime scene behavior and other factors related to sexually sadistic homicide (Dietz et al. 1990; Gratzer and Bradford 1995). Both of these studies had to review a large number of homicide perpetrators and sexual offenders before finding a relatively small number of males that met the diagnostic criteria. Dietz et al. (1990) completed an uncontrolled descriptive study of 30 sexually sadistic homicide or attempted homicide perpetrators. Intentional torture for sexual arousal was the common characteristic of this group of males. It was also clear that careful planning, including stranger victim selection, most commonly occurred. Bondage, beating, and homicide by strangulation were common offense characteristics. Gratzer and Bradford (1995) compared the Dietz et al. sample with another sample of sexually sadistic homicide and attempted homicide perpetrators and a third sample of nonsadistic sexually motivated homicide and attempted homicide perpetrators. There were many common characteristics in the sadistic homicide samples (Gratzer and Bradford 1995). Previous studies of sexually sadistic homicide perpetrators had shown that strangulation was the most common method used to perpetrate the homicide (Dietz et al. 1990; Gratzer and Bradford 1995). A well-controlled study from Finland looked at all homicides over a 7-year period in which strangulation was the cause of death (Hakkanen 2005). In contrast to previous studies, they found that there was no association between sexually sadistic homicides and strangulation as the cause of death. Although this does not mean that strangulation should be disregarded as a signature of a sadistic sexually motivated homicide, it is clear that further research is needed. The contrast between the North American studies and the Finnish study may be a cultural variation, because the chosen method of homicide does vary across different cultures. Although the North American studies point to a possible common psychopathology in sexually sadistic homicide perpetrators, there may be considerable cultural differences in this group of perpetrators.

Various studies have shown some association between sexual sadism and brain abnormality, commonly temporal lobe damage in the brain (Hucker and Stermac 1992; Langevin et al. 1988). This includes a study of sexually sadistic homicide perpetrators in which 50% of the sample was noted to have some type of neurological abnormality (Gratzer and Bradford 1995). These neuroanatomical abnormalities and their association to deviant sexuality are also supported by studies on brain activation in relation to sexual stimuli (Mouras et al. 2003; Redoute et al. 2000; Stoleru et al. 1999). More recently, a study by Briken et al. (2006b) of sexually motivated homicide perpetrators found that about one-third had obvious brain abnormalities. The sexually motivated murderers with brain abnormalities differed significantly from the group in having a higher incidence of early behavioral problems; a higher total number of paraphilias; younger victims, particularly those 6 years of age or younger; and a higher incidence of transvestic fetishism and paraphilias not otherwise specified (Briken et al. 2006b). The study strongly emphasized the need for detailed neuropsychiatric evaluation of sexually motivated homicide perpetrators. In another well-controlled study by Briken et al. (2006a) of male sexually motivated homicide perpetrators, the prevalence of XYY syndrome was examined. The prevalence was 1.8%, which is considerably higher than the prevalence in male offenders or in the general population (which would be 0.01%). In addition to the chromosome abnormality, these individuals were also diagnosed as having sexual sadism and scored in the psychopathic range on the Hare Psychopathy Checklist (Briken et al. 2006a). The higher incidence of a chromosome abnormality, particularly one involving the Y chromosome, possibly implicates androgens in the psychopathology of sexually motivated homicide. This again emphasizes the need for detailed neuropsychiatric and neurobiological evaluations as part of the forensic psychiatric workup of sexually motivated homicide perpetrators.

Although this type of homicide is a relatively rare event, the level of media coverage and the degree of psychological trauma it causes in the general public are significant, and anything that might allow us to have a better understanding of this behavior would be extremely helpful. It would also give us a stronger basis to understand and treat the condition early on in its development and therefore provide some degree of secondary prevention and protection to the public. When sexually motivated homicides are perpetrated against children, the impact on the general public is even more traumatic than if adults were involved. The degree of shock, abhorrence, and horror that occurs in any community if a child from that community is abducted, sexually assaulted, and murdered is enormous. This has often led to the misconception that pedophiles are responsible for the murder of children. To some extent this impression is based on literary work by the Marquis de Sade in the eighteenth century and factual accounts of Giles de Rais. Giles de Rais was tried for the sexually motivated homicides of 40 young boys (Brownmiller 1975; Sade et al. 1966). In actual fact, the most common perpetrators of homicides against children are the caretakers of children, and specifically the parents of children, as opposed to pedophiles. A well-controlled study completed in England confirmed this finding (Dolan et al. 2003). In this study, fathers or surrogate fathers were responsible in nearly two-thirds of the cases. Children younger than 6 months of age were the most vulnerable, and victim behavior and relationship difficulties appear to be the precipitants in more than two-thirds of the cases. By contrast, sexually motivated homicide occurred in 18.7% of the cases.

The impetus for "sexually motivated homicide" would appear to be obvious; however, there has in fact been scientific debate and controversy as to what motivates these individuals to commit their crimes. This question arguably may apply more to *serial sexual homicide,* defined as sexual homicide by perpetrators who kill three or more victims in a noncontinuous fashion using a predatory form of violence (Meloy and Felthous 2004). One hypothesis is that serial sexual homicide perpetrators are motivated by a need to achieve power and control over their victims and that sexual gratification is completely secondary. This comes from a now-dated theory of motivation for rape involving power and control (Groth et al. 1977). Crime scene examinations usually show evidence of a sexual motivation. Myers and colleagues (2006) believe that serial sexual murderers should be considered sexual offenders. They also suggest the modification of DSM criteria to accommodate this. They believe that these individuals mostly have paraphilic disorders in the sadistic spectrum and that a diagnostic classification of "sexual sadism, homicidal type" should be included as a subtype of sexual sadism (Myers 2002; Myers et al. 2006).

If sexually sadistic homicide perpetrators do have a sexual motivation, then it should be measurable by physiological methods. Sexual arousal can be measured by penile tumescence techniques known as phallometry. There is evidence both for and against the capability of this technique to discriminate between nonoffender and offender populations or between different types of offenders (Marshall and Fernandez 2000). Nonetheless, it is useful in differentiating groups of men convicted of child molesting offenses, particularly extrafamilial child sexual abuse, and in a meta-analysis on sexual offender recidivism, phallometry was found to be one of the most reliable predictors of recidivism for child molesters (Hanson and Bussiere 1998). There are several ways to measure sexual arousal, although the one favored by the lead author of this chapter (J.M.W.B.) is the use of indices reflecting relative sexual arousal or sexual preference. A calculation is made based on responses to audiotape descriptions of sex with children where the arousal to children (the numerator) is divided by the arousal to mutually consenting sex with adults (the denominator) and an index is calculated by the ratio. This means an index greater than 1 means a sexual preference in the direction of pedophilia. Indices can also be used for sexual preference in a sadistic direction. In a study of 27 child molesters who had committed or who had attempted a sexually motivated homicide, 189 nonhomicidal child molesters, and 47 community control subjects, there were clear differences between the three groups based on phallometric measures (Firestone et al. 2000a). Significantly more homicidal and nonhomicidal child molesters had pedophile indices greater than 1 compared with nonoffenders. The homicidal and nonhomicidal child molesters did not differ from each other on pedophile indices. This is not surprising, because both groups were pedophiles. However, when it came to assault indices, which measured arousal to nonsexual violence (a measurement of sadistic sexual preference), significantly more homicidal child molesters had assault indices of 1 or greater or a sexual preference for nonsexual violence, compared with the other two groups. The nonoffenders and nonhomicidal child molesters did not differ from each other on this measure (Firestone et al. 1999). This physiological evaluation was able to differentiate homicidal child molesters from nonoffenders and nonhomicidal child molesters on the basis of sexual preference. This strongly supports a sexual motivation to sexually motivated sadistic homicides.

The average psychiatrist is not likely to be asked to evaluate or treat these extremely high-risk individuals. What may occur, however, in general psychiatric practice is that individuals may present with homicidal sexual fantasies against women or children. If this presentation has been associated with any stalking of potential victims or even the urge to do this, an extreme psychiatric emergency situation exists and a referral to a forensic psychiatric subspecialist in sexology needs to occur immediately. Involuntary civil commitment to a psychiatric facility to protect the public is also indicated.

Recidivism

Understanding recidivism is fundamental to understanding sexual violence. There is a large body of scientific literature on sexual offender recidivism that covers different types of sexual offenders, and there is considerable consistency in the research findings even in studies from different countries. Recidivism studies provide information to predict subsequent risk of reoffense as well as information about treatment outcome. There are well-established and significant differences in the recidivism rates of different types of sexual offenders. The results of a task force report from the American Psychiatric Association (1999) showed that sexual assaulters of adult females ("rapists") have the highest recidivism rates, followed by extrafamilial child molesters; intrafamilial child molesters ("incest" perpetrators) have the lowest rates of recidivism. There is still evidence that recidivism rates are reflections of sexual offenses that are underreported. In order to compensate for underreporting, most recent studies include conviction rates and rearrest rates. Arguably the most accurate reflection would be a combination of conviction rates, rearrest rates, and self-reported rates of sexual offenses. Most recent studies involve a survival analysis technique. In general terms, the longer the follow-up period, the higher the reported rates of recidivism. In general, a follow-up period of at least 5 years while offenders are at risk in the community is necessary for a valid study.

A number of meta-analyses have been completed on sexual offender recidivism studies, the most significant being a study by Furby et al. (1989), followed by two by Hanson (Hanson and Broom 2005; Hanson and Thornton 1999) and a treatment outcome study meta-analysis by Alexander (1999; Furby et al. 1989; Hanson and Broom 2005; Hanson

Sexual Violence and the Clinician | 451

and Bussiere 1998). The Furby et al. (1989) study was generally regarded as a pessimistic one that was highly critical of the methodology in existing recidivism studies, but at the same time it played an important role in ensuring that future recidivism studies had improved methodology. The Hanson and Bussiere (1998) meta-analysis comprised more than 28,000 sexual offenders with a median follow-up period of approximately 4 years and included 87 studies from six different countries. The meta-analysis documented the specific factors associated with a high risk of sexual offense recidivism. The strongest predictors of sexual offender recidivism were related to sexual deviance. Phallometric measures of pedophilic sexual preference were highly correlated with the risk of future sexual offense recidivism ($r=0.32$). Prior sexual offenses ($r=0.19$); age ($r=0.13$); early onset of sexual offending ($r=0.12$); any prior offenses ($r=0.13$); and never having been married ($r=0.11$) were also strongly correlated with sexual offender recidivism. The overall recidivism rate for sexual offenses was 13.4% (Hanson and Bussiere 1998). Alexander (1999) reviewed 79 treatment outcome studies including more than 11,000 subjects. She showed that all the psychological treatments included in the study resulted in lower recidivism rates compared with an untreated group for both adults and adolescents. She also showed that mandatory treatment appeared to have a positive effect on treatment outcome compared with voluntary treatment of sexual offenders. Hanson and Broom (2005), in a follow-up meta-analysis, used different analytical techniques to examine the trends in recidivism.

Sexual offender recidivism studies have been a focus of our own research. We have completed recidivism studies of rapists, extrafamilial child molesters, incest perpetrators, and exhibitionists (Firestone et al. 1998, 1999, 2000c; Greenberg et al. 2002). The mean follow-up period for the studies was approximately 7 years, and all exceeded 5 years. The studies included phallometric data and Hare Psychopathy Checklist (PCL) scores as well as many other variables and used rearrest rates and conviction rates as a measure of recidivism taken from the Canadian Police Information Computer, a national database of arrest and conviction rates. Phallometric measures of deviant sexual preference and scores were important predictors of sexual offense recidivism, and the PCL scores were also strong predictors of violent and general recidivism. We have completed other recidivism studies as well that looked more closely at other factors related to recidivism, such as hostility (Firestone et al. 2000b, 2005b, 2006; Greenberg et al. 2000). Incest perpetrators have generally been regarded as a homogeneous group having the lowest risk of recidivism for child molesters. Some differences in recidivism risk based on victim age had been reported, and this was felt to be an important factor for future risk assessment. A study of 119 incest perpetrators consisted of a group of men ($n=48$) who had victims younger than 6 years of age compared with another group of men ($n=71$) whose victims were adolescents and more typical of incest perpetrators. Both groups showed deviant sexual preference; however, the group with the young victims had significantly more psychopathology, including substance abuse (Firestone et al. 2005a). There are also important differences in the recidivism risk for incest perpetrators whose victims are their biological daughters compared with those whose victims are stepdaughters (Greenberg et al. 2005). Deviant sexual preference was significantly lower in men who molest their biological daughters, and this crime therefore carries a lower risk of future sexual offense recidivism.

Sexual offense recidivism risk can be easily estimated by using the Static-99, developed by the Research Division of the Solicitor General of Canada (Hanson and Bussiere 1998). The ability to identify high-risk sexual offenders provides the criminal justice system with a mechanism to prevent further harm to the general public as well as a basis for sentencing of these individuals or dealing with them through civil commitment. These statistical instruments are considerable improvements over the use of unstructured clinical judgment (Hanson and Bussiere 1998). The Static-99 is scored using easily obtained information with limited training and yet provides significant accuracy in the prediction of sexual offense recidivism (Hanson and Thornton 2000; Nunes et al. 2002). It also classifies sexual offender risk levels based on scoring of the instrument as low, medium-low, medium-high, and high for sexual offense recidivism based on the potential risk. It also gives the percentage risk of future violent recidivism. This useful instrument can be utilized by the forensic or general psychiatrist not trained in specialized forensic sexology, thus providing a valid measure of future risk for sexual violence or violence in general that is considerably more accurate than unstructured clinical evaluation.

Treatment

In recent years the focus of psychological treatments has been on the cognitive-behavioral treatment spectrum. These treatments help the person with a paraphilia block or reduce thoughts of or fantasies about deviant behaviors such as child molesting. The treatments can be given on an individual basis, but in most specialized treatment programs it is performed in a group treatment setting. This not only improves the cost-effectiveness of treatment but also has a therapeutic advantage because other individuals in the group with a similar paraphilia both recognize and challenge cognitive distortions used by various members in the group. Cognitive distortions are the rationalizations used by paraphilic individuals, typically pedophiles, to justify their behavior. Covert sensitization teaches the patient to imagine the negative social consequences resulting from the deviant sexual urges to engage in paraphilic behavior. Nearly all paraphilic behavior is preceded by deviant thoughts or fantasies and urges. Individuals are taught to recognize this cycle and to interrupt it. Olfactory aversion, desensitization, satiation (masturbatory), and developing nonparaphilic interests are all techniques that are used. Without exception, psychological treatments are self-administered. Other techniques for training prosocial behaviors include social skills training, anger management training, victim empathy training, and relapse prevention. Relapse prevention in various forms is the most commonly used psychological intervention. It is an extensive framework of techniques for avoiding high-risk situations and the risk of relapse. It is based on the assumption that sex offenders make a decision to engage in treatment to stop committing deviant sexual acts but find themselves in high-risk situations frequently involving stress, interpersonal conflicts, or negative emotional states. Relapse prevention helps the patient develop strategies to prevent this sequence of events. It usually involves relapse rehearsal and a maintenance plan to avoid high-risk situations (Abel et al. 1988; American Psychiatric Association 1999).

Pharmacological treatments consist of anti-androgens, hormonal agents, and specific serotonin reuptake inhibitors. The pharmacological approach to treatment is based on the suppression of deviant sexual fantasies and urges and a reduction in sexual drive. In addition, there is evidence that deviant sexual arousal patterns measured by phallometry can also be suppressed (American Psychiatric Association 1999; Bradford 2000; Bradford and Pawlak 1993a, 1993b). The anti-androgen used in Canada is cyproterone acetate (not available in the United States). It can be given orally or intramuscularly and is a powerful blocker of intracellular androgen receptors throughout the body, including intracerebral androgen receptors in the hypothalamus. Medroxyprogesterone acetate has been widely used in the United States, and although not a true anti-androgen, it does bring about significant reductions in sexual drive by reducing circulating testosterone. Its mode of action is to induce liver enzymes to clear plasma testosterone, and it also has an antigonadotropic effect (Bradford 2000, 2001). More recently, luteinizing hormone–releasing hormone (LHRH) agonists such as leuprolide acetate have been used as pharmacological castration agents (Bradford 2000, 2001). As well, some SSRIs are used to treat paraphilic behavior by reducing sexual interest, sexual fantasies, and sexual drive. The agents most commonly used are fluoxetine hydrochloride and sertraline hydrochloride (Bradford 2001). Many of the studies of these pharmacological treatments are uncontrolled treatment outcome studies, although some double-blind studies and recidivism studies have been completed (Bradford 2000, 2001).

The lead author of this chapter has published an algorithm for the pharmacological treatment of sexual deviation (Bradford 2000, 2001). This algorithm first classifies the deviant sexual behavior into mild, moderate, severe, or catastrophic, based on a modification of DSM-III-R criteria. In addition, there is a six-level algorithm of treatment. Level 1 involves psychological treatments; level 2, the introduction of SSRIs; level 3, the combination of an SSRI and a low dose of anti-androgen treatment, either cyproterone acetate or medroxyprogesterone acetate; level 4, full oral doses of cyproterone acetate or medroxyprogesterone acetate; level 5, intramuscular cyproterone acetate or medroxyprogesterone acetate; and level 6, pharmacological castration using intramuscular cyproterone acetate or an LHRH agonist such as leuprolide acetate. Mild paraphilias would be treated at the stage one and two level; moderate at stages two and three; severe at stages four and five; and catastrophic at stage six (Bradford 2000, 2001). The introduction of SSRIs in level 2 of treatment requires a dosage level of sertraline, 150–250 mg/day, or fluoxetine, 40–60 mg/day. These SSRIs are the treatment of choice because they suppress sexual drive without causing significant problems of sexual dysfunction, particularly sexual performance. The low-dose oral anti-androgen treatment used in association with SSRIs is 50–100 mg/day of either cyproterone acetate or medroxyprogesterone acetate. Full oral anti-androgen treatment with either of these agents would have an oral dosage range of 200–400 mg/day. Intramuscular dosages of cyproterone acetate would be 100 mg every 2 weeks and of medroxyprogesterone acetate would be 400 mg every 2–4 weeks. Pharmacological castration would require leuprolide acetate, 7.6 mg intramuscularly, given monthly. Because the first 4–6 weeks of LHRH agonist treatment actually increases testosterone levels by an outpouring of LHRH from the hypothalamus, significant risk of deviant sexual acting out occurs during this time frame. This risk must be managed with the addition of an oral anti-androgen such as flutamide to cover this initial period of increased risk. The longer-term management of anti-androgen treatment requires ongoing sex hormone profile evaluations, particularly monitoring prolactin levels to avoid gynecomastia. In addition, increased risk for osteopenia and osteoporosis with long-term treatment needs to be monitored with yearly bone scans. Treatment with

Sexual Violence and the Clinician | 455

vitamin D and calcium supplements may be helpful to offset this potential risk. For a complete review of pharmacological sexual offender treatment, reference to review articles by the lead author of this chapter is recommended (Bradford 1998, 2000).

Sex is a basic biological drive, and there is considerable scientific information both from animal and human research about the neurobiological aspects of sexual behavior. Furthermore, there is considerable research showing that the actions of various pharmacological agents on hormones and neurotransmitters affect sexual behavior. Physicians, and particularly psychiatrists, are in a strong position by virtue of their training to be involved in the assessment and treatment of sexual deviation. It is unfortunate that mainstream psychiatry, including medical school training, has neglected this important area of psychiatric and medical treatment. If a major impact is to be made on child sexual abuse, psychiatrists at all levels should be more engaged in the assessment and treatment of sexual deviation. Psychology and other mental health disciplines are already strongly engaged in the assessment and treatment of sexual offenders and sexual deviation.

Key Points

- Sexual violence involves any sexual act with a nonconsenting partner and also includes physical violence associated with a paraphilia or sexual deviation.
- Various studies have shown that between 10% and 16% of males and between 20% and 27% of females have been victims of childhood sexual abuse.
- In recent years the Internet has become a vehicle for sexual offenses, usually child pornography. Studies have defined different types of Internet offenders.
- Clinical studies of sexually sadistic homicide perpetrators are rare, mostly because this condition only rarely occurs. Clinical features have been defined and an association has been found between sexual sadism and brain abnormalities.
- Sexual arousal has been shown to be one of the most reliable predictors of sexual offense recidivism. It has also been shown to discriminate between sexual offenders and nonoffenders, particularly in relation to pedophilia, and to discriminate between pedophilic homicidal perpetrators and nonhomicidal perpetrators.

- There is a large body of scientific evidence on sexual offender recidivism that shows considerable consistency even in studies conducted in different countries. Those who sexually assault adult females have the highest recidivism rates, followed by extrafamilial child molesters and lastly by intrafamilial child molesters.
- The Static-99 provides an easy way of estimating sexual offense recidivism with easily obtainable information.
- The focus of psychological treatments has been the cognitive-behavioral treatment spectrum, with a specific focus on relapse prevention.
- Pharmacological treatments include SSRIs, anti-androgens, and LHRH agonists as well as some other hormonal agents.
- An algorithm for the pharmacological treatment of sexual offenders has been developed.

References

Abel GG: Paraphilias, in Comprehensive Textbook of Psychiatry, 5th Edition. Edited by Kaplan HI, Sadock BJ. Baltimore, MD, Williams & Wilkins, 1989, pp 1069–1085

Abel GG, Mittelman M, Becker JV, et al: Predicting child molesters' response to treatment. Ann N Y Acad Sci 528:223–234, 1988

Alexander MA: Sexual offender treatment efficacy revisited. Sex Abuse 11:101–116, 1999

Alexy EM, Burgess AW, Baker T: Internet offenders: traders, travelers, and combination trader-travelers. J Interpers Violence 20:804–812, 2005

American Psychiatric Association: Diagnostic and Statistical Manual of Mental Disorders, 3rd Edition, Revised. Washington, DC, American Psychiatric Association, 1987

American Psychiatric Association: Dangerous Sex Offenders: A Task Force Report of the American Psychiatric Association. Washington, DC, American Psychiatric Association, 1999

American Psychiatric Association: Diagnostic and Statistical Manual of Mental Disorders, 4th Edition, Text Revision. Washington, DC, American Psychiatric Association, 2000

Bradford JM: Treatment of men with paraphilia. N Engl J Med 338:464–465, 1998

Bradford JM: The treatment of sexual deviation using a pharmacological approach. J Sex Res 37:248–257, 2000

Bradford JM: The neurobiology, neuropharmacology, and pharmacological treatment of the paraphilias and compulsive sexual behaviour. Can J Psychiatry 46:26–34, 2001

Bradford JM: On sexual violence. Curr Opin Psychiatry 19:527–532, 2006

Bradford JM, Pawlak A: Double-blind placebo crossover study of cyproterone acetate in the treatment of the paraphilias. Arch Sex Behav 22:383–402, 1993a

Bradford JM, Pawlak A: Effects of cyproterone acetate on sexual arousal patterns of pedophiles. Arch Sex Behav 22:629–641, 1993b

Bradford JM, Boulet J, Pawlak A: The paraphilias: a multiplicity of deviant behaviours. Can J Psychiatry 37:104–108, 1992

Briken P, Habermann N, Berner W, et al: XYY chromosome abnormality in sexual homicide perpetrators. Am J Med Genet B Neuropsychiatr Genet 141:198–200, 2006a

Briken P, Habermann N, Kafka MP, et al: The paraphilia-related disorders: an investigation of the relevance of the concept in sexual murderers. J Forensic Sci 51:683–688, 2006b

Brownmiller S: Against Our Will: Men, Women and Rape. New York, Simon and Schuster, 1975

Dietz PE, Hazelwood RR, Warren J: The sexually sadistic criminal and his offenses. Bull Am Acad Psychiatry Law 18:163–178, 1990

Dolan M, Guly O, Woods P, et al: Child homicide. Med Sci Law 43:153–169, 2003

Fedoroff J: The genesis of pedophilia: testing the "abuse to abuser" hypothesis. The Journal of Offender Rehabilitation 24:85–101, 1996

Fedoroff J: Sadism, sadomasochism, sex and violence. Can J Psychiatry (in press)

Finkelhor D: How widespread is child sexual abuse? Child Today 13:18–20, 1984

Finkelhor D, Lewis IA: An epidemiologic approach to the study of child molestation. Ann N Y Acad Sci 528:64–78, 1988

Finkelhor D, Hotaling G, Lewis IA, et al: Sexual abuse in a national survey of adult men and women: prevalence, characteristics, and risk factors. Child Abuse Negl 14:19–28, 1990

Firestone P, Bradford JM, McCoy M, et al: Recidivism in convicted rapists. J Am Acad Psychiatry Law 26:185–200, 1998

Firestone P, Bradford JM, McCoy M, et al: Prediction of recidivism in incest offenders. J Interpers Violence 14:511–531, 1999

Firestone P, Bradford JM, Greenberg DM, et al: Differentiation of homicidal child molesters, nonhomicidal child molesters, and nonoffenders by phallometry. Am J Psychiatry 157:1847–1850, 2000a

Firestone P, Bradford JM, Greenberg DM, et al: The relationship of deviant sexual arousal and psychopathy in incest offenders, extrafamilial child molesters, and rapists. J Am Acad Psychiatry Law 28:303–308, 2000b

Firestone P, Bradford JM, McCoy M, et al: Prediction of recidivism in extrafamilial child molesters based on court-related assessments. Sex Abuse 12:203–221, 2000c

Firestone P, Dixon KL, Nunes KL, et al: A comparison of incest offenders based on victim age. J Am Acad Psychiatry Law 33:223–232, 2005a

Firestone P, Nunes KL, Moulden H, et al: Hostility and recidivism in sexual offenders. Arch Sex Behav 34:277–283, 2005b

Firestone P, Kingston DA, Wexler A, et al: Long-term follow-up of exhibitionists: psychological, phallometric, and offense characteristics. J Am Acad Psychiatry Law 34:349–359, 2006

Furby L, Weinrott MR, Blackshaw L: Sex offender recidivism: a review. Psychol Bull 105:3–30, 1989

Gratzer T, Bradford JM: Offender and offense characteristics of sexual sadists: a comparative study. J Forensic Sci 40:450–455, 1995

Greenberg D, Bradford J, Firestone P, et al: Recidivism of child molesters: a study of victim relationship with the perpetrator. Child Abuse Negl 24:1485–1494, 2000

Greenberg D, Firestone P, Nunes KL, et al: Biological fathers and stepfathers who molest their daughters: psychological, phallometric, and criminal features. Sex Abuse 17:39–46, 2005

Greenberg SR, Firestone P, Bradford JM, et al: Prediction of recidivism in exhibitionists: psychological, phallometric, and offense factors. Sex Abuse 14:329–347, 2002

Groth AN, Burgess W, Holmstrom LL: Rape: power, anger, and sexuality. Am J Psychiatry 134:1239–1243, 1977

Hakkanen H: Homicide by ligature strangulation in Finland: offence and offender characteristics. Forensic Sci Int 152:61–64, 2005

Hanson RK, Broom I: The utility of cumulative meta-analysis: application to programs for reducing sexual violence. Sex Abuse 17:357–373, 2005

Hanson R, Bussiere MT: Predicting relapse: a meta-analysis of sexual offender recidivism studies. J Consult Clin Psychol 66:348–362, 1998

Hanson RK, Thornton D: Improving risk assessments for sex offenders: a comparison of three actuarial scales. Law Hum Behav 24:119–136, 2000

Helweg-Larsen K, Boving Larsen H: The prevalence of unwanted and unlawful sexual experiences reported by Danish adolescents: results from a national youth survey in 2002. Acta Paediatr 95:1270–1276, 2006

Helweg-Larsen K, Larsen HB: A critical review of available data on sexual abuse of children in Denmark. Child Abuse Negl 29:715–724, 2005

Hucker SJ, Stermac L: The evaluation and treatment of sexual violence, necrophilia, and asphyxiophilia. Psychiatr Clin North Am 15:703–719, 1992

Langevin R, Bain J, Wortzman G, et al: Sexual sadism: brain, blood, and behavior. Ann N Y Acad Sci 528:163–171, 1988

Marshall WL, Fernandez YM: Phallometric testing with sexual offenders: limits to its value. Clin Psychol Rev 20:807–822, 2000

Marshall WL, Kennedy P, Yates P: Issues concerning the reliability and validity of the diagnosis of sexual sadism applied in prison settings. Sex Abuse 14:301–311, 2002

Meloy J, Felthous A: Introduction to this issue: serial and mass murder. Behav Sci Law 22:289–290, 2004

Mitchell KJ, Finkelhor D, Wolak J: Risk factors for and impact of online sexual solicitation of youth. JAMA 285:3011–3014, 2001

Mitchell KJ, Finkelhor D, Wolak J: The Internet and family and acquaintance sexual abuse. Child Maltreat 10:49–60, 2005a

Mitchell KJ, Finkelhor D, Wolak J: Protecting youth online: family use of filtering and blocking software. Child Abuse Negl 29:753–765, 2005b

Mitchell KJ, Wolak J, Finkelhor D: Police posing as juveniles online to catch sex offenders: is it working? Sex Abuse 17:241–267, 2005c

Mouras H, Stoleru S, Bittoun J, et al: Brain processing of visual sexual stimuli in healthy men: a functional magnetic resonance imaging study. Neuroimage 20:855–869, 2003

Myers WC: Juvenile Sexual Homicide. San Diego, CA, Academic Press, 2002

Myers WC, Husted DS, Safarik ME, et al: The motivation behind serial sexual homicide: is it sex, power, and control, or anger? J Forensic Sci 51:900–907, 2006

Nunes KL, Firestone P, Bradford JM, et al: A comparison of modified versions of the Static-99 and the Sex Offender Risk Appraisal Guide. Sex Abuse 14:253–269, 2002

Redoute J, Stoleru S, Gregoire MC, et al: Brain processing of visual sexual stimuli in human males. Hum Brain Mapp 11:162–177, 2000

Sade DAF, Wainhouse A, Seaver R: The Marquis de Sade: The 120 Days of Sodom and Other Writings. New York, Grove Press, 1966

Seto MC, Eke AW: The criminal histories and later offending of child pornography offenders. Sex Abuse 17:201–210, 2005

Stoleru S, Gregoire MC, Gerard D, et al: Neuroanatomical correlates of visually evoked sexual arousal in human males. Arch Sex Behav 28:1–21, 1999

Swigert VL, Farrell RA, Yoels WC: Sexual homicide: social, psychological, and legal aspects. Arch Sex Behav 5:391–401, 1976

Wolak J, Mitchell K, Finkelhor D: Unwanted and wanted exposure to online pornography in a national sample of youth Internet users. Pediatrics 119:247–257, 2007

CHAPTER 23

Violence Toward Mental Health Professionals

William R. Dubin, M.D.

Autumn Ning, M.D.

The idea that a clinician can be the target of violence by a patient is an inconceivable one to most caregivers. Yet clinicians are at significant risk for being assaulted. According to the Department of Justice's Crime Victimization Survey for 1993–1999 (Duhart 2001), the annual rate for nonfatal violent crime (rape and sexual assault, robbery, and aggravated and simple assault) for all occupations was 12.6 per 1,000 workers. For physicians, the rate was 16.2, and for nurses, it was 21.9. However, for psychiatrists, the rate was 68.2 per 1,000; for mental health custodial staff, it was 69.0; and for other mental health workers, it was 40.7. Of psychiatrists who have responded to surveys, the rate of assault ranges from 3% to 40%, with an average of 40% (American Psychiatric Association 1993; Davies 2001; O'Sullivan and Meagher 1998). Among psychiatric residents, the percentage of respondents reporting being assaulted ranges from 19% to 64% (American Psychiatric Association 1993; Black et al. 1994; Coverdale et al. 2001; Schwartz and Park 1999), with a high rate of repeat assaults that ranges from 10% to 31% (Chaimowitz and Moscovitch 1991; Fink et al. 1991; Milstein 1987).

Nonpsychiatric residents also experience a high rate of assaults. Twenty percent of surgical residents have reported being assaulted (Barlow and Rizzo 1997); other studies report that 16%–40% of internal medicine residents who responded to surveys were assaulted (Coverdale et al. 2001; Milstein 1987; Paola et al. 1994; VanIneveld et al. 1996).

The emergency department may be the most dangerous place to work in a hospital. Emergency departments are open to the public and are accessed by an unscreened patient population. Police bring potentially violent patients to the emergency department on a daily basis, and the number of drug-abusing patients who present has also increased. Studies have documented the alarming incidence of weapons brought into the emergency department (Goetz et al. 1991; Thompson et al. 1988) and the high incidence of violence against staff (Foust and Rhee 1993; Jenkins et al. 1998; Lavoie et al. 1988; Pane et al. 1991; Wyatt and Watt 1995). Of psychiatric patients seen in psychiatric emergency services or an emergency department, 4%–17% have been reported to have weapons (Anderson et al. 1989; Goetz et al. 1991; McNeil and Binder 1987).

Statistics regarding the homicide rate within the medical profession are not available from either the American Medical Association or the American Psychiatric Association. There are no aggregate studies addressing homicide against physicians. Data of such events are either in case or media reports (American Psychiatric Association 1993; Dubin and Lion 1996; Ladds and Lion 1996). Fatal assaults occur in a range of settings, including private outpatient offices, community mental health centers, academic centers, hospitals, and even military installations, perpetrated by patients with a variety of psychiatric diagnoses. Homicides have been committed by patients using guns, knives, blunt instruments, and physical assault.

Case Examples

Case Example 1: Violence in the Psychiatric Emergency Service

Mr. A, a 30-year-old man, was brought to the psychiatric emergency service by police at his own request after he told them he was depressed and suicidal and wanted to go to the hospital. He was using $200 worth of cocaine per day and reported symptoms of major depression. He stated, "I am hopeless and feel like I might hurt myself or others." Mr. A had presented a month earlier with a similar complaint and had been referred to outpatient treatment. The managed care company reported the patient had a long history of drug and psychiatric treatment related to his drug use. He had never followed up with outpatient treatment, even with a case manager.

In the psychiatric emergency service the patient was labile and easily agitated and could only with effort be redirected. He was temporarily placed in an open seclusion room in view of the nurses' station while waiting to be seen by the psychiatric resident. He was observed to pace in the room. When the resident approached the patient, the patient became calmer and cooperative. He denied the history reported by the managed care company, stating he did not know what they were talking about, that he had not had treatment recently and had not sought help in a year. The physician confronted the patient with the fact that he had a record of the patient presenting in the past month. The patient became agitated and shouted, "Who the f*** cares? I'm suicidal NOW." The physician began to explain to Mr. A in a quiet tone that there was a note in the patient's records from the insurance company regarding the many presentations he had had. The patient then kicked the physician twice in the abdomen before staff was able to restrain him.

This patient had a known history of drug use, was labile, easily agitated, and was seen pacing in the seclusion room. The resident chose to confront the patient and, in essence, called the patient a liar, violating the dynamic of violence by humiliating this already labile patient. Rather than focusing on affect management, the resident chose to give a rational explanation to the patient about the documented history of drug treatment and his history of noncompliance. The resident instead should have addressed the affect, considered medication, and, most importantly, had additional staff present with him during the interview.

Case Example 2:
Failure of a Risk Assessment in an Outpatient Office

Mr. B, in his early 30s, held his psychiatrist hostage for 90 minutes, threatening to beat him up and to destroy the property in the psychiatrist's private home office. When the patient had initially called for an appointment, the psychiatrist learned that Mr. B had a history of violent episodes and paranoid responses to psychiatrists. Mr. B stated on the phone that he was an impossible case but that his initial response to this psychiatrist was positive. During the first four treatment sessions, Mr. B had continually pressed the psychiatrist to demonstrate an interest in him. After the fourth session he had called the psychiatrist at 11 P.M. and asked to meet with him to discuss a crisis. The psychiatrist responded that he could not meet him and that he would see him at the next scheduled time. At the next appointment Mr. B walked into the office, locked the door, and began his threatening behavior. Mr. B screamed and verbally abused the psychiatrist for 90 minutes, pushing him around and knocking diplomas off the wall. Although angry and fearful, the psychiatrist talked to the patient in a calming manner. The psychiatrist did not challenge Mr. B but calmly pointed out possible repercussions. The patient finally left the office and never returned or contacted the psychiatrist. The psychiatrist acknowledged his own sense of grandiosity and vanity had been enhanced when the patient made positive comments about him on the phone and that this further strengthened his denial of the risk of aggression that this patient posed.

This patient had a risk profile that suggested he was at risk for violence—that is, a history of violence and conflicts with previous psychiatrists. The psychological defense of denial resulted in the psychiatrist's minimizing the risk and treating the patient in his home office. The psychiatrist should have either treated this patient in a more secure setting or declined to take this patient into treatment at the initial phone interview.

Case Example 3: Threats of Violence Toward a Surgeon

Mr. C was a 30-year-old man with no formal psychiatric diagnosis who was seeing a resident plastic surgeon in the clinic to be evaluated for a rhinoplasty. He had a history of stalking behavior and threatening with a gun, which was not known until after the incident. After multiple elective rhinoplasties, the patient became violent in the clinic and was removed and told never to return. The resident surgeon on the patient's first rhinoplasty completed his residency and moved to another state, where the patient found him through the unwitting participation of the residency department. Mr. C began to write letters to the surgeon, calling her a "butcher" and stating "you won't be able to operate again." She notified the police, the FBI, and the postal authorities, who told the patient that it was unlawful to write threatening letters. The patient continued to write threats on the outside of envelopes. The doctor was informed that because these weren't actual letters, there was no way to press charges. The threats continued, but at a lessened frequency, and eventually ceased.

Unknown in this case is the degree to which the department physicians and staff were attuned to the risks attendant in the specialty of plastic surgery and whether they had a methodology for psychologically assessing patients and risks. Also unknown is how they handled requests by patients regarding information about residents who graduated. The physician in this case acted quickly and decisively and may have deterred more aggressive action by the patient by enlisting law enforcement officers to speak with the patient.

Case Example 4: Violence as a Result of Psychotic Transference in an Outpatient Setting

Ms. D, a woman in her late 30s, walked into her psychiatrist's private office in his home and pulled out a knife. According to the psychiatrist, Ms. D was having a positive transference reaction and believed that the psychiatrist was the object of her desires, which she could not control. The psychiatrist saw the threat as her way of destroying him in order to free herself from this predicament. The psychiatrist noted that he had compounded the problem: because Ms. D was a physically small woman, he had failed to interpret a previous acting-out episode in which she had thrown an ashtray at him. He had never told her that such behavior was dangerous and unacceptable.

The psychiatrist responded to Ms. D in a calm, clear voice, saying that it was not acceptable to threaten him with the knife, that she did not have to do this to relieve her pain, and that he would not hurt her. As he talked, he grabbed her wrist and bent it forward, and she released the knife. Changes in treatment included active interpretation of the patient's fears of closeness, as well as stricter limit setting. The psychiatrist's belief that he could overpower the patient led to his denial of the discomforting anxiety one usually feels when a psychotic transference develops in a therapeutic relationship.

Because of the patient's size and possibly her gender, this psychiatrist used denial and minimized the risk by failing to set limits with the patient after the first aggressive incident. After that first episode the psychiatrist also should have reevaluated the safety of treating this patient in his home office. Grabbing the patient's wrist to take away the knife was a questionable strategy and risked possible injury to the psychiatrist or the patient. It would have been preferable to continue the talk-down strategy.

Facilitating Clinician Safety

Risk Assessment

The most effective strategy for enhancing clinician safety is to anticipate potential aggression. Tardiff (1996) suggested certain clinical, psychological, and historical variables that increase a patient's potential for violence (Table 23–1). Although there is no specific combination or number of these risk factors that can predict violence, their presence alerts the clinician that the patient poses a risk. The clinician who is aware of these risk factors has the opportunity to develop treatment strategies to minimize the potential for violence. Several important risk factors for violence are outlined in Table 23–1.

For psychiatrists with offices in their homes or in office buildings, all new patients should have at least a 15- to 20-minute interview on the phone that includes a risk assessment for violence. A risk assessment evaluation should include intent to harm self or others, possession or access to a weapon, recent violence, formulation of a definitive plan of violence, drug and alcohol use, adherence with aftercare and medication management, and associated psychiatric or medical conditions (Petit 2005). Other components of a risk assessment include present illness, past psychiatric history, military history, legal history, and a mental status examination (Buckley et al. 2003). Patients with a history of violence or paranoia, or who have borderline personality disorder with little impulse control, should not be interviewed initially in a private office (Berg

TABLE 23–1. Risk factors for violence

- A past history of repetitive violence
- Agitation, anger, disorganized behavior
- Poor compliance during the interview
- A detailed or planned threat of violence
- Available means for inflicting injury, such as ownership of a weapon
- History of childhood physical or sexual abuse
- Presence of organic disorder
- Presence of psychotic psychopathology, especially delusions or command hallucinations
- Presence of borderline or antisocial personality disorder
- Presence of alcohol or drug use
- Belonging to a demographic group with an increased prevalence of violence: young, male, lower socioeconomic group

Source. Adapted from Tardiff 1996.

2000). If possible, such patients should be interviewed the first time in a more secure setting such as an outpatient department, a crisis service, or an emergency department. For unknown patients who are making their first visit, appointments should be scheduled for the middle of the day when numerous staff are present as opposed to early morning or late evening. Sessions may be scheduled so that other staff is immediately available in the vicinity of the office or in the interview room during the appointment. For high-risk patients in hospital settings, the clinician may choose to leave the office door open during the interview, with staff or security present, or interview the patient in a conference room where a large table can provide a barrier between the clinician and patient.

A major impediment to the effective management and treatment of a violent patient is the psychological defense of denial. Denial allays the clinician's anxiety by disavowing thoughts, feelings, or external reality factors that are consciously intolerable. Therefore, clinicians ignore clinical data or behavior that suggests a patient may become violent. For example, rather than acknowledging anxiety and fear, the psychiatrist may project an image of false machismo, fearlessness, and confidence. Other manifestations of denial are failure to obtain pertinent data regarding a patient's previous history of violence or arrests and failure to question a patient about current aggressive behavior. A risk assessment begins to neutralize the potent psychological defense of denial in the clinician. Anticipation of violence leads to preventive treatment planning and can significantly enhance safety.

Dynamics of Violence

The successful management of violence is predicated on an understanding of its dynamics. Violence is a reaction to feelings of passivity and helplessness. A patient's threatening behavior is commonly an overreaction to feelings of impotence, helplessness, and perceived or actual feelings of humiliation. A clinician who encounters a threatening patient should avoid becoming verbally or physically aggressive toward the patient. Psychiatrists who respond to threatening patients with physical or verbal aggression are significantly more likely to be injured or have property destroyed than those who acknowledge their fear but also express a desire to help the patient (Dubin et al. 1988). The strategy of a nonthreatening offer to provide help is reassuring to the patient and is the centerpiece for intervention with a potentially violent patient.

The Prodrome of Violence

Aggression rarely occurs suddenly and unexpectedly. Generally there is a prodromal syndrome consisting of increasing tension and anxiety, escalating verbal stridency and abuse, and increasing motor activity usually characterized by pacing behavior. Intervention using talk-down strategies during this period of escalation will frequently avert violent behavior. In such an escalating situation, the clinician must be sure that the patient can hear and respond. A patient who is under the influence of alcohol or drugs is not a good candidate for talk-down techniques. By using a soft, assertive voice and short sentences, the clinician can rapidly determine if the patient if paying attention (Maier 1996). Volume, tone, and rate of speech should be lower than the patient's, although if too low, the patient may perceive it as a threat (Berg et al. 2000). The clinician should talk down a patient by agreeing with him or her and not arguing (Maier 1996). It is important not to respond to the content of the patient's speech. The patient should be "overdosed" with agreement (Maier 1996). An escalating patient should be approached from the front or side, because an approach from behind is extremely threatening. The clinician should also never turn his or her back to the agitated or threatening patient (Berg et al. 2000).

Affect Management

The main strategy for de-escalating a potentially violent patient is affect management. Patients who are affectively aroused will need to ventilate their history, and the clinician should not overly intrude into the interview (Eichelman 1995). Often the patient who is overwhelmed with angry affect intimidates the clinician, who then responds with logical and rational explanations. This type of intervention only inflames the patient. Affect management involves acknowledging the patient's affect, validating the affect when appropriate, and encouraging the patient to talk about his or her feelings. For instance, the clinician might say, "I can see how angry this makes you. If I were given medication against my will I would be as angry as you are. Let's talk more about your feelings." Phrases such as "ventilate," "talking it out," "getting it off your chest," or "catharsis" are colloquialisms that refer to the process of allowing a person to discharge his or her affect. Addressing the affect serves several purposes. It teaches the patient to reduce his or her internal state of tension by verbalizing feelings and teaches that it is not necessary to hit someone or destroy furniture to feel better. Giving the patient the opportunity to ventilate affect often defuses an escalating patient and averts a more violent confrontation.

Additional Management Techniques

Emotionally distraught patients require an active response from a clinician. Active eye contact and body language that signal attentiveness and connectedness to the patient will reduce the probability that the patient will need to explode or assault to get his or her point across (Eichelman 1995). However, prolonged or intense direct eye contact can be perceived as menacing by the patient (Petit 2005). Eichelman (1995) described interventions that are effective in aggression management. The use of active listening techniques, such as paraphrasing to the patient in brief, encapsulated form the content of his or her statements, helps to convey that the clinician understands what the patient is experiencing. It is important to be honest and precise when responding to patients. Dishonesty may set the clinician up for either retribution or a tenuous therapeutic relationship. Eichelman (1995) further recommended that in all situations the clinician keep a proper physical distance from the patient. Assaultive patients have a larger body buffer zone, and a rule of thumb is to keep two quick steps or at least an arm's distance from the patient. A personal space can be visualized as an oval zone extending 4–6 feet all around (Berg et al. 2000). If the patient is standing, the clinician should stand. If the patient is sitting, the clinician should also sit down and not stand over the patient during the interview. If the patient is pacing, the clinician can model for the patient by walking with the patient but at a much slower pace. Berg et al. (2000) recommended that the clinician take a posture that makes him or her appear small and thus less threatening. This can be done by holding the hands at waist level with palms up and open or assuming the *Thinker* stance (one forearm crosses the chest, the opposite elbow rests on it with the index finger touching the cheek or chin).

Limit Setting

At times clinicians react to escalating or agitated behavior with punitive threats, in an attempt to set limits. A threatening intervention, however, is contrary to the dynamics of violence because it evokes feeling of impotence or humiliation in the patient and increases the risk of violence. Overt anger or hostility should never be expressed toward an agitated patient (Petit 2005). Limit setting can be therapeutic and avert violent behavior. Green et al. (1988) described the basic philosophy behind limit setting, which is to contain and counteract maladaptive behavior that interferes with therapy and threatens the safety of the clinician. Green et al. (1988) further note that effective limit setting involves clear identification of the specific behaviors that need to be altered and precise articulation of the consequences that will follow if the inappropriate behavior persists. If the therapist lacks clarity in his or her thinking or communications to the patient concerning inappropriate behavior, the intervention may confuse and disorganize the patient. Whenever possible, interpretive interventions should precede the imposition of limits, because this affords the patient greater flexibility in exercising his or her own autonomy and discretion.

Successful limit setting is most effective when this sequence is followed (Green et al. 1988):

1. The patient is told of the behavior that is unacceptable.
2. The patient is told why the behavior is unacceptable.
3. The patient is offered several alternative treatment interventions.

For example, a clinician can say to a patient, "You cannot yell, curse, or threaten other patients in the day room. They are afraid of you, and they think that you will harm them. Therefore, you can go to your room and listen to the radio until you feel calmer, or we can walk to the seclusion room and I will give you some medication." Given several options, the patient will usually accept whichever is preferred. If given a choice, the patient will pause to consider the options, and each pause decreases the amount of energy behind the anger. As this process continues, the patient will slowly regain self-control (Maier 1996). Offering only one option invites the patient to argue and negotiate, which leads to further escalation and frequently culminates in an assault against the clinician or restraint of the patient.

Thackrey (1987) described several important clinical caveats regarding limit setting. Alternatives regarding both expected and prohibited behaviors must be stated concretely and in terms of actions that can be performed immediately. Whenever possible, directives or alternatives should be expressed in positive terms ("Do this," which describes acceptable behavior) rather than negative terms ("Don't do that," which describes no acceptable alternatives). The best limits are absolute rather than relative (e.g., "Don't bang on the windows" rather than "Don't bang on the windows so hard"). An essential part of limit setting is for the clinician to determine whether the patient is capable of responding. In general, the greater the degree of cognitive impairment, the less able the patient is to understand or respond to limit setting. In these instances, and depending on the location of the threat, the clinician should call for help or leave the interview office immediately if no one else is available to assist in the management of the patient.

Safety in the Psychiatric Emergency Service and Inpatient Unit

There are certain environmental variables that can be modified to decrease the potential for violence, especially in emergency departments or inpatient units. They include shortening the waiting time, decreasing stimuli by offering the patient a comfortable chair in an office or an option to lie down, and offering the patient a cup of water or juice or some food (Petit 2005).

When interviewing patients who have been violent or who have the potential for violence, especially in an emergency department or inpatient unit, the clinician should remove his or her glasses, if possible (Tardiff 1996). Neckties should be removed or tucked in, and jewelry such as necklaces and earrings should be removed (Tardiff 1996). The physician may want to consider tightly securing long hair. Clinicians should always consider that running away from a patient may become necessary and should always wear shoes that will make running easier.

Clinicians should leave when a situation seems totally uncontrollable (Bowie 1989). Before leaving, the clinician should consider what must be done to escape and identify the nearest safe place, how far it is, and the best way to get there (Bowie 1989). The clinician should not run as a panic reaction but should leave as a positive action. The clinician should run toward a place of safety and not just away from danger. Once beginning the escape, the clinician should not hesitate or stop until he or she is free and clear.

Threat Management

Overview

A neglected area in clinician safety is threat management. Unfortunately, there is a paucity of research in this area. There are no data detailing the clinical context in which most threats occur or of the outcome of threats. Threats can take many forms. They can be verbal, written, by phone, or relayed by a third party. Patients can threaten the clinician in an impulsive, emotional outburst; by a calm, serious statement; in a joking, flippant manner; or through vague innuendos (Tardiff 1996). Threats can be in the form of property damage, visits to a therapist's home, or loitering around a therapist's office on days when there is no appointment (Jenkins 1989). The sending of love letters, pornographic materials, or vacation pictures can represent threats (Jenkins 1989). Threats can also take the form of veiled comments that show a patient is involved in the clinician's personal life (Maier 1996). Such comments might include knowledge of the clinician's car or home address or the names of the clinician's children. These statements are made as a way of showing interest in the clinician but are usually out of proportion to the therapeutic relationship (Maier 1996).

Threats to clinicians can occur in a variety of settings, including clinical settings such as the emergency department, inpatient unit, outpatient clinic, or private office. They can occur in custody hearings, disability evaluations and hearings, forensic evaluations and hearings, competency hearings, and in nonpsychiatric medical settings, or they may come from spouses of patients.

Dynamics of a Threat

Threats are a means by which a patient tries to gain control of others through manipulation (Maier 1996). When patients make manipulative comments, they are often of such a nature that the clinician is not encouraged to share them with his or her peers. For instance, a patient may ask a female clinician if she is pregnant or has her period. He may tell a male clinician that he looks hung over or make some comment about the clinician's sexual identity. The interplay between positive comments and personal judgments can provide for effective manipulation, resulting in the clinician's behavior becoming predictable and thus usable by the patient against the clinician at some future time. In this process, the patient establishes a secret relationship with the clinician, binding the clinician to the patient, governing the clinician's conduct, and distorting his or her judgment (Maier 1996). Sharing the secret with a colleague is the first step in managing this process.

Types of Threats

Brown et al. (1996) described two types of threat situations: situational and transferential threats. A *situational threat* occurs when a psychiatrist acts as an administrator, usually on an inpatient unit or emergency department. For example, a psychiatrist frustrated a patient's wish by denying a request to go out on a pass to get more medication. The patient threatened the psychiatrist, an emergency code was called, the patient was restrained or escorted from the hospital, and the threat situation ended with no psychiatrist being injured.

A *transference threat* occurs within the context of ongoing psychotherapy. The threats to therapists described by Brown et al. (1996) were often insidious and in several instances continued for many years. Although no psychiatrists who were the targets of transference threats were physically injured, the threats were very disruptive, both to the psychiatrists and to their families. The treating psychiatrist who initially viewed the threat as an issue to be resolved in therapy often tolerated transference threats. The threat situation often continued for many months before the psychiatrist recognized the inherent danger. Rather than diluting the transference by disengaging from the patient, many of the therapists intensified the transference by increasing the frequency of treatment sessions. Therapists often have difficulty disengaging from a patient. Such situations may be compared with the problem of marital separation when two parties are locked in a pathological relationship (Lion 1995). By the time the treating psychiatrist in this example sought consultation from a colleague, the clinician was so enmeshed in the patient's distorted or psychotic transference that the resolution of the threat situation was complicated, if not impossible. When a clinician is threatened or perceives a threat, he or she should initially seek expert consultation.

Monitoring Threats

Psychiatrists must pay close attention to any changes in either transference or countertransference feelings as they arise in the therapy situation. Any changes in behavior or affect, either by the therapist or the patient, should alert the clinician to a potential change in the therapeutic relationship. Such behavior might include patient requests for more therapy sessions, frequent phone calls or messages on the answering machine, notes or gifts between sessions, increased and frequent flattery, or increased anger, hostility, or withdrawal. Therapists who treat more primitive character disorders or paranoid or psychotic patients run a certain risk as closeness develops (Lion 1995). This is a risk that must be continuously assessed and dealt with. Often, subtle actions, such as the patient's moving back his or her chair, defensive posturing, or tardiness late in the course of therapy, should alert a clinician to a problem in the transference (Lion 1995). In such situations, immediately reviewing the case with a colleague is a prudent first step toward understanding the change in the therapeutic relationship, assessing whether a threat exists, and if one does exist, the level of risk. Similarly, a clinician should also monitor his or her countertransference. Feelings of increasing attraction, dread, anxiety, or anger toward a patient might signal the beginning of a distorted transference.

Managing Threat Situations

When a threat is made, a clinician should act decisively and immediately. Threats are messages and require comment (Lion 1995). To ignore them is to indicate that the clinician is indifferent to suffering and does not care. When a clinician is threatened, direct confrontation such as "You're scaring me with your threat" or "Why do you have to go around scaring me and others with your threats? Is this the only way that you can relate to people, to be scary?" is often effective (Lion 1995). If the clinician has any alliance with the patient, interpretive statements can facilitate understanding and resolution of the threat (Lion 1995). Examples of interpretive comments include, "Why do you go around threatening and alienating people?" or "Do you have any positive feeling about our therapy?" The therapist may try to clarify the meaning of the threat, but a patient's failing to respond to reasonable interventions and continuing to make threats are considerations for termination of therapy. Rather than intensifying the transference by continuing to engage the patient in therapy, the therapist should focus on diluting the transference by establishing distance and separation from the patient.

A written threat must be preserved with a minimal disruption of the physical evidence. Envelopes and all packaging materials must be saved, only minimally handled (preferably with cotton gloves touching the extreme edges), and stored in a plastic bag (Dietz 1990). Telephone threats that are on tape should be saved, and under no circumstances should the tape be erased. If a threat is by telephone or in person, an attempt should be made to reconstruct the conversation verbatim and to immediately record as much detail as possible (Dietz 1990).

For clinicians who work in institutional settings, diluting the transference can be done by involving the chief clinical administrator. In developing a response to a threat, it can be very useful and reassuring to meet with departmental representatives from security, legal affairs, administration, employee health, human affairs, the director of clinical services, and a psychiatric consultant familiar with violence management techniques (Tardiff 1996). This group can provide various perspectives on evaluating different options, from legal to therapeutic, in responding to threats.

A designated administrator should notify the patient that the administrator is aware of the threat situation and that it will not be tolerated. Furthermore, the patient should be informed that the threatened clinician will not accept phone call or letters or have any further interaction with the patient. The administrator should offer to help the patient find another therapist should he or she wish to continue therapy. Legal assistance should be concomitantly obtained. The hospital legal staff should unambiguously convey to the patient that threatening a staff clinician is behavior that will not be tolerated and that he or she will be prosecuted if the threats continue.

For psychiatrists in private practice, involving the district attorney is more effective than obtaining help from the family lawyer. Consultation with a colleague, especially one with experience in dealing with such situations, is extremely valuable. Threats must be dealt with decisively and without ambivalence.

When threats persist despite the interventions discussed, additional steps should be considered. If the patient is told not to return to the therapist's office, security guards or doormen should be alerted not to allow the patient entrance and to notify the therapist if the patient tries to enter the building. A description of the patient should be given to the security staff. If security staff or doormen are not available, the local police precinct should be notified immediately if the patient is seen on the premises. While the threat is ongoing, the therapist should alter his or her schedule and not leave the office at night alone or come in early in the morning alone. The therapist should park near the office, in as public a location as possible. The therapist should avoid parking in isolated, dark areas where there is little traffic and where there are places for a patient to hide. If threats are severe and ongoing, the therapist should consider varying daily routines and travel routes. Although this can be disruptive to the therapist's life, it also increases his or her safety.

Stalking

There are various definitions of *stalking* (Meloy 1998). From a clinical perspective, stalking is obsessional pursuit, harassment, and intimidation by a person who has a significant personal relationship (or believes one to exist) with the object of the unwanted attention (Miller 2001). Stalking of clinicians is a behavior representative of a pathological attachment or deranged transference, or it may be the result of a dissatisfying outcome (Lion and Herschler 1998). Eight percent of adult American women and 2% of adult American men have been stalked sometime in their lives (Meloy 1998). At least half of stalkers may explicitly threaten their victims, and the frequency of violence toward their objects ranges from 25% to 35% (Meloy 1998). The homicide rate among victims of stalking is less than 2% (Meloy 1998). Physicians and mental healthcare staff are at even greater risk of being stalked than the general population, particularly by their patients. Recent studies have found that 11% of mental health professionals responding to a survey had been stalked, with psychologists and psychiatrists more likely to experience longer periods of stalking (Galeazzi et al. 2005). Sandburg et al. (2002) reported that 53% of inpatient clinical staff were stalked, threatened, or harassed at some point during their career. Gentile et al. (2002) found that 10% of psychologists had been stalked at least one time, and Ashmore et al. (2006) found that 50% of responding mental health nurses had been stalked.

Although violence is obviously the most disturbing potential outcome of stalking, this phenomenon also deserves close attention because most victims of stalking experience major life disruptions and psychological disturbance, including anxiety, depression, or symptoms of trauma (Meloy 1998). Lion and Herschler (1998) presented cases of psychiatrists who have been threatened or stalked and spent enormous amounts of time and money on protective measures and legal fees; some had to relocate their families and practices to other parts of the country.

Immediate management of stalking is imperative and does not differ significantly from the management of threats. Meloy (1997) recommended 10 guidelines for the clinical management of stalking, covering the following points: a team approach, personal responsibility for safety, documentation and recording, no initiated contact, protection orders, law enforcement and prosecution, treatment if indicated, segregation and incarceration, periodic violence risk assessment, and the importance of dramatic moments, which are events that shame or humiliate the perpetrator. Lion and Herschler (1998) further suggested being attuned to early inappropriate behaviors and boundary violations and considering the risk that such violations will escalate over time to the point of physical danger. Clinicians should seek legal and forensic consultation early—preferably prior to an intervention.

The Armed Patient

If a patient appears in a treatment setting with a weapon, as few staff as possible should be exposed to the risk of injury (Tardiff 1996). Staff should retreat to an office. The clinician should acknowledge the obvious—"I see you have a gun" (Tardiff 1996). He or she should be calm and not become counteraggressive or threatening. The clinician should encourage the patient to talk during the initial phases and repeat the patient's concerns. The firearm is almost invariably an expression of feelings of inadequacy and fear (Dubin 1995). The clinician should try to speak to the underlying psychological issues. It is important to identify areas in which the patient's viewpoint is correct rather than initially trying to demonstrate the areas in which the patient's viewpoint is wrong. The alliance can be enhanced if the clinician can identify similarities between him- or herself and the patient.

If a short time passes without the patient's actually firing the gun, the likelihood of its eventual use is diminished. Initially, however, the clinician should comply with whatever demand the patient may make and take special care to avoid further upsetting the patient. There should be no attempt to take the weapon from the patient. A suggestion should be made to have the patient put the weapon down gently (Tardiff 1996). One should not reach for the gun or tell the patient to drop the gun, because it might discharge (Tardiff 1996).

Office Safety

The most problematic issue is the individual clinician who practices alone. Office safety requires planning and persistence, and clinicians should be cognizant of safety issues. Ideally, offices should have two doors, one into the reception room and another locked door that leads into the actual treatment office. This second door should have a peephole so that the clinician can see who is in the outer office. Ideally, a clinician may wish to have two entrances to his or her office so that if a threatening patient comes into the reception area, there is another means of exit. If a clinician does not have a receptionist, he or she should consider a panic alarm or buzzer system to notify either building security or police in the event of a threatening or aggressive patient.

Institutional outpatient sites should be constructed so that there is a physical and personal buffer for the clinician. Offices in outpatient clinics should have panic buttons or an organized strategy to notify a receptionist, other staff, or even the police of a threatening situation. A protocol should be developed to train office staff to recognize patients who are at risk for violence. Strategies should be put in place so that the office staff can notify the clinical staff or, if necessary, the police without alarming the patient when he or she begins to escalate or presents to the office in a threatening manner. For instance, a simple code such as "Dr. Smith, can you see Mr. Jones immediately?" may be a signal that Mr. Jones is demonstrating behavior that puts him at risk for violence. This nonthreatening phone call then allows the clinician to implement other strategies, such as calling the police or mobilizing other clinic staff to help contain the patient. A different code should be developed to alert staff that an armed patient is in the waiting area. Such an alarm should be simple and not threatening, for example, "Is room 22 available?" Direct alarm systems to the police should also be considered, especially for the situation in which a patient has a weapon or is suspected of having a weapon. Such a system should be inconspicuous so as not to alert the patient that an alarm is being sounded.

There are certain architectural features that can further enhance safety. An office should be decorated in a manner consistent with the type of patient that the clinician is treating. If a clinician is treating psychotic patients or patients with a history of aggression, or if he or she frequently evaluates new patients, there are specific office safety issues that should be considered. Safe offices will have heavy furniture that cannot be lifted or used as a weapon. Offices, especially in emergency departments or inpatient units, should not have hard, sharp objects such as small ashtrays, artwork, lamps, or other decorations that can be thrown or used as weapons. All office doors should swing out into a hall and not into an office. This prevents a patient inside the office from blocking the therapist's egress by leaning against the door. Berg et al. (2000) recommended several strategies for enhancing safety in emergency departments and clinics. Having windows in the doors of the examining rooms allows privacy while lending a sense of the possibility of being monitored for unacceptable behavior. Security cameras also provide a sense that behavior is being monitored, and posting rules makes it clear that violence will not be tolerated and has consequences.

Key Points

Managing aggressive, violent patients is a clinical challenge. However, if the clinician periodically reviews the key points of clinical management, most encounters with a violent patient can have a satisfactory outcome. The fundamental management strategies include:

- Performing a risk assessment on all new patients.
- Not evaluating or treating patients at risk for violence alone or in an isolated office.
- Remembering that violence is a response to feelings of helplessness, passivity, and perceived or actual feelings of humiliation.
- Using nonthreatening talk-down strategies and using affect management as the centerpiece of the intervention.
- Setting limits by offering the patient two options, with one being the preferred option.
- Being cognizant of the different manifestations of a threat, because threats take many forms.
- Monitoring transference and countertransference and evaluating any change in the context of a developing threat situation.
- Immediately seeking consultation if a threat is perceived or if the clinician questions whether a patient's behavior is a threat.
- Immediately initiating threat management strategies without hesitation or ambivalence.
- Anticipating the potential for stalking and immediate and early consultation with a forensic expert.
- Responding in a nonthreatening manner to an armed patient and offering help and understanding.
- Periodically evaluating offices and patient areas and implementing changes that will enhance safety.

References

American Psychiatric Association: Clinician Safety: Report of the American Psychiatric Association Task Force on Clinician Safety. Report No. 33. Washington, DC, American Psychiatric Association, 1993

Anderson AA, Ghali AY, Bansil RK: Weapon carrying among patients in a psychiatric emergency room. Hosp Community Psychiatry 40:845–847, 1989

Ashmore R, Jones J, Jackson A, et al: A survey of mental health nurses' experiences of stalking. J Psychiatr Ment Health Nurs 13:562–569, 2006

Barlow CB, Rizzo AG: Violence against surgical residents. West J Med 167:74–78, 1997

Berg AZ, Bell, CC, Tupin J: Clinician safety: assessing and managing violent patients. New Dir Ment Health Serv 86:9–29, 2000

Black KJ, Compton WM, Wetzel M, et al: Assaults by patients on psychiatric residents at three training sites. Hosp Community Psychiatry 45:706–710, 1994

Bowie V: Coping With Violence: A Guide for the Human Services. Sydney, Australia, Karibuni Press, 1989

Brown GP, Dubin WR, Lion JR, et al: A preliminary classification of threats against clinicians. Bull Am Acad Psychiatry Law 24:367–376, 1996

Buckley PF, Noffsinger SG, Smith DA, et al: Treatment of the psychotic patient who is violent. Psychiatr Clin North Am 26:231–272, 2003

Chaimowitz GA, Moscovitch A: Patient assaults against psychiatric residents: the Canadian experience. Can J Psychiatry 36:107–111, 1991

Coverdale J, Gale C, Weeks S, et al: A survey of threats and violent acts by patients against training physicians. Med Educ 35:154–159, 2001

Davies S: Assaults and threats on psychiatrists. Psychiatr Bull 25:89–91, 2001

Dietz PE: Defenses against dangerous people when arrest and commitment fail, in Review of Clinical Psychiatry and the Law, Vol 1. Edited by Simon RI. Washington, DC, American Psychiatric Press, 1990, pp 205–219

Dubin WR: Assaults with weapons, in Patient Violence and the Clinician. Edited by Eichelman BS, Hartwig AC. Washington, DC, American Psychiatric Press, 1995, pp 53–72

Dubin WR, Lion JR: Violence against the medical profession, in Creating a Secure Workplace: Effective Policies and Practices in Health Care. Edited by Lion JR, Dubin WR, Futrell DE. Chicago, IL, American Hospital Publishing, 1996, pp 3–14

Dubin WR, Wilson SJ, Mercer C: Assaults against psychiatrists in outpatient settings. J Clin Psychiatry 49:338–345, 1988

Duhart DT: Violence in the Workplace, 1993–1999. Bureau of Justice Statistics Special Report, NCJ 190076. Washington, DC, U.S. Department of Justice, 2001

Eichelman BS: Strategies for clinician safety, in Patient Violence and the Clinician. Edited by Eichelman BS, Hartwig AC. Washington, DC, American Psychiatric Press, 1995, pp 139–154

Fink DL, Shoyer B, Dubin WR: A study of assaults against psychiatric residents. Acad Psychiatry 15:94–99, 1991

Foust D, Rhee KJ: The incidence of battery in an urban emergency department. Ann Emerg Med 22:583–585, 1993

Galeazzi GM, Elkins K, Curci P: The stalking of mental health professionals by patients. Psychiatr Serv 56:137–138, 2005

Gentile SR, Asamen JK, Harmell PH, et al: The stalking of psychologists by their clients. Prof Psychol Res Pr 33:490–494, 2002

Goetz RR, Bloom JD, Chenell SL, et al: Weapons possession by patients in a university emergency department. Ann Emerg Med 20:8–10, 1991

Green SA, Goldberg RL, Goldstein DM, et al: The art of limit setting, in Limit Setting in Clinical Practice. Edited by Green SA, Goldberg RL, Goldstein DM, et al. Washington, DC, American Psychiatric Press, 1988, pp 1–13

Jenkins MG, Rocke LG, McNicholl BP, et al: Violence and verbal abuse against staff in accident and emergency departments: a survey of consultants in the UK and the Republic of Ireland. J Accid Emerg Med 15:262–265, 1998

Jenkins PL: Harassment, in Hazards of Psychiatric Practice: A Clinical and Legal Guide for the Therapist. Chicago, IL, Year Book Medical Publishers, 1989, pp 14–25

Ladds B, Lion JR: Severe assaults and homicide within medical institutions: epidemiologic issues, in Creating a Secure Workplace: Effective Policies and Practices in Health Care. Edited by Lion JR, Dubin WR, Futrell DE. Chicago, IL, American Hospital Publishing, 1996, pp 15–24

Lavoie FW, Carter GL, Danzi, DF, et al: Emergency department violence in United States teaching hospitals. Ann Emerg Med 17:1227–1233, 1988

Lion JR: Verbal threats against clinicians, in Patient Violence and the Clinician. Edited by Eichelman BS, Hartwig AC. Washington, DC, American Psychiatric Press, 1995, pp 43–52

Lion JR, Herschler JA: The stalking of clinicians by their patients, in The Psychology of Stalking: Clinical and Forensic Perspectives. Edited by Meloy JR. New York, Academic Press, 1998, pp 163–173

Maier GJ: Managing threatening behavior: The role of talk down and talk up. J Psychosoc Nurs Ment Health Serv 34:25–30, 1996

McNeil DE, Binder RL: Patients who bring weapons to the psychiatric emergency room. J Clin Psychiatry 48:230–233, 1987

Meloy JR: The clinical risk management of stalking: "Someone is watching over me..." Am J Psychother 51:174–184, 1997

Meloy JR: The psychology of stalking, in The Psychology of Stalking: Clinical and Forensic Perspectives. Edited by Meloy JR. New York, Academic Press, 1998, pp 1–23

Miller MC: Stalking. Harv Ment Health Lett 17:5–6, 2001

Milstein V: Patient assaults on residents. Indiana Med 80:753–755, 1987

O'Sullivan M, Meagher D: Assaults on psychiatrists: a three-year retrospective study. Ir J Psychol Med 15:54–57, 1998

Pane GA, Winiarski AM, Salness KA: Aggression directed toward emergency department staff at a university teaching hospital. Ann Emerg Med 20:283–286, 1991

Paola F, Malik T, Qureshi A: Violence against physicians. J Gen Intern Med 9:503–506, 1994

Petit JR: Management of the acutely violent patient. Psychiatr Clin North Am 28:701–711, 2005

Sandberg DA, McNiel DE, Binder RL: Stalking, threatening, and harassing behavior by psychiatric patients toward clinicians. J Am Acad Psychiatry Law 30:221–229, 2002

Schwartz TL, Park TI: Assaults by patients on psychiatric residents: a survey and training recommendations. Psychiatr Serv 50:381–383, 1999

Tardiff K: Assessment and Management of Violent Patients, 2nd Edition. Washington, DC, American Psychiatric Press, 1996

Thackrey M: Therapeutics for Aggression. New York, Human Sciences Press, 1987

Thompson BM, Nunn J, Kramer I, et al: Disarming the department: weapon screening and improved security to create a safer emergency department environment. Ann Emerg Med 17:419, 1988

VanIneveld CH, Cook DJ, Kane SL, et al: Discrimination and abuse in internal medicine residency. J Gen Intern Med 11:401–405, 1996

Wyatt JP, Watt M: Violence towards junior doctors in accident and emergency departments. J Accid Emerg Med 12:40–42, 1995

CHAPTER 24

Intimate Partner Violence and the Clinician

Susan Hatters Friedman, M.D.
Joy E. Stankowski, M.D.
Sana Loue, Ph.D., J.D., M.P.H.

Intimate partner violence (IPV) can take any of several forms, including emotional, physical, and/or sexual abuse. This chapter focuses specifically on the physical and sexual abuse inflicted by one individual against his or her intimate partner, who may be a spouse, a live-in partner, or a date of the opposite or same sex. It should be recognized, however, that emotional abuse and physical violence are often related. The physical violence may take numerous forms, including battering or beating, rape, murder, or forced suicide; may be effected through the use of fists, feet, sexual organs, poisoning, drowning, hanging, fire, electrical shocks, knives, guns, and/or other weapons (Loue 2001b); and can occur in a variety of settings, not just the home. The violence may be perpetrated for various proffered reasons, including economic pressures and dissatisfaction with the partner's attitudes or behavior.

Incidents of physical abuse may occur only intermittently, but an abusive partner may use emotional abuse to gain and retain control during the interim periods (Dutton and Golant 1995). This "cycle of

---

This research was supported in part by National Institute of Mental Health grant R01 MH63016.

violence," as it has been referred to, consists of three phases. The first, or tension-building, phase is characterized by verbal, emotional, and sometimes physical abuse of lesser severity. Often the victim will attempt to alleviate the situation by placating the batterer. The second, or acute battering, phase represents the discharge of built-up tension. Although the victim may be blamed for "triggering" the abuse, the actual cause of the violence is often a stressor external to the relationship (such as difficulties at work) or internal to the abuser. Acute battering episodes are often unpredictable. During the third, or "honeymoon," phase, the abuser attempts to apologize for his or her actions through apologies, gifts, helpfulness, and increased emotional closeness with the victim. It is during this phase that the bond between the abuser and his or her victim is intensified, because the victim now experiences the positive aspects of the relationship and comes to believe in the partner's voiced commitment to the relationship. This intensified emotional closeness and commitment increases the difficulty of leaving the abusive relationship (Walker 2000).

In the United States, the lifetime prevalence of physical assault by an intimate partner against women in a population not defined by mental illness has been found to range from 9% to 30% (Bureau of Justice Statistics 1998; Tjaden and Thoennes 2000), and the prevalence of rape by an intimate is approximately 8% (Tjaden and Thoennes 2000). The range of estimates is due, in part, to variations across studies in the methods used to collect data (e.g., personal interviews, telephone interviews, written surveys); the sampling methods used (e.g., hospital patients, general population, clinic outpatients); and definitions of partner violence.

Previous research has identified the following risk factors for partner violence in the United States: younger age, urban residence, lower levels of education, and lower income (Sorenson et al. 1996). Prior history of abuse, including childhood abuse (Friedman and Loue 2007), may also increase risk. Female victims of IPV have been found to be more likely to use multiple substances (alcohol, cigarettes, and illegal drugs) than are nonvictims (Martin et al. 1996). Pregnancy has also been established as a risk factor for IPV victimization (Miller and Finnerty 1996). Pregnant women especially at risk for battering during their pregnancies are those who have been battered prior to pregnancy (McFarlane et al. 1992). Homicide is a leading cause of death during pregnancy (Frye 2001). Research indicates that homicide is more likely to occur among couples of lower socioeconomic status and those in which the wife is significantly younger than the husband (Chimbos 1998). It has been hypothesized that the homicide may be related to partner concerns about paternity or changing role expectations.

Various theories have been advanced in an attempt to understand and explain why partner violence occurs. These theories are outlined in Table 24–1. Some theories focus on why the violence occurs, whereas others attempt to understand why battered women remain in the abusive relationship.

Intimate Partner Violence and Severe Mental Illness

Specific diagnoses, including schizophrenia, depression, anxiety disorders, substance use disorders, and personality disorders, may elevate the risk of victimization from IPV (Bergman and Ericsson 1996; Briere et al. 1997). Limited reality testing, impaired judgment, impaired executive function, and difficulty with social relationships may potentially increase a person's vulnerability to abusive or coercive relationships (Goodman et al. 1995). Social isolation and the stigma of mental illness, which make some women eager to please, also may increase their risk (Gearon and Bellack 1999). Women may be unable to distinguish between the physical closeness that signifies emotional intimacy and the physical closeness associated with assaultiveness, and thus they may not remove themselves from potentially dangerous situations (DeNiro 1995).

There is a well-established association between IPV and posttraumatic stress disorder (PTSD), depression, and substance abuse (Coker et al. 2005; El-Bassel et al. 2003; Houry et al. 2005; Mueser et al. 1998). Symptoms of mental illness may worsen with victimization (Campbell 2002). Victimization from IPV or other traumas may act as a stressor, further increasing symptomatology. Among battered women in treatment for depression or anxiety, the majority believed that the battering had worsened their symptoms (Weingourt 1990).

Evidence suggests that IPV victimization may increase the already elevated suicide risk among the mentally ill. Studies have found that more than one-third of battered women have attempted suicide (Dienemann et al. 2000; Golding 1999). Similarly, up to 44% of suicide attempts may have abuse as a precipitating factor. A study of outpatients with depression or anxiety found that those who had been physically assaulted were three times more likely to attempt suicide (Kaplan et al. 1995).

Case Example

Marta [all names used in the case example are fictitious] is a Hispanic woman in her mid-30s who was diagnosed with major depression some years ago. Marta moved from Puerto Rico to the mainland United States at a relatively young age. Both her brother and an uncle repeatedly

TABLE 24–1. Theories of causation of intimate partner violence

Theory	Description
Why the violence occurs	
Culture of violence (Wolfgang and Ferracuti 1967)	Subcultures develop norms that permit the use of physical force or violence.
Ecological theory (Belsky 1980)	Risk of assault is a function of the interplay between factors at the macrosystemic, exosystemic, microsystemic, and ontogenetic levels of the environment.
Evolutionary theory (Lenski and Lenski 1970; Rohner 1975; Wilson and Daly 1993)	1. Obedience is valued in societies with a hierarchically organized structure; violence may be used as a means of securing obedience. 2. Partner violence is evolutionary and occurs as a mechanism to ensure the male partner's sexual dominance and reproductive advantage. 3. Sexual proprietariness is a psychological adaptation of the human male; the jealousy and related violence are directly tied to women's reproductive value.
Exchange theory (Gelles 1983)	People use violence to obtain their goals as long as the benefits outweigh the costs.
Theory of marital power (Cromwell and Olson 1975)	Those who lack power will be more likely to physically abuse their partners.
Patriarchy theory (Dobash and Dobash 1979)	Wife assault is a systematic form of domination and social control of women by men; assault is committed by men who believe that patriarchy is their right; the use of violence to maintain male dominance is acceptable to society.
Resource theory (Blood and Wolfe 1960; Goode 1971)	Decision-making power within a family derives from the value of the resources that he or she brings to the relationship. The more external control one has of resources outside of the family, the less likely he or she will be to use violence as a means of control.
Social learning theory (O'Leary 1988)	Family violence arises due to a constellation of factors, including individual characteristics, couple characteristics, and societal characteristics.

TABLE 24–1. Theories of causation of intimate partner violence *(continued)*

Theory	Description
Why people stay	
Investment theory (Rusbult 1980)	One's willingness to remain in a relationship increases as the balance of the rewards over costs from staying in the relationship exceeds the balance of rewards over the costs in alternative relationships or arrangements.
Traumatic bonding theory (Dutton and Painter 1981, 1993)	Over time, the imbalance of power within a relationship increases as the dominant party develops an inflated self-image and the subordinate person feels increasingly negative about him- or herself and becomes increasingly dependent on the abusive partner.

sexually abused her as a young child. Marta was raised in the Roman Catholic faith and more recently became a member of the religious community known as Mita y Aaron, founded by a Puerto Rican woman. Although Marta has been involved in several relationships, she has never married and has no children.

Marta has not used any substances for approximately 7 years, but during her prior relationship with Jorge, she was dependent on alcohol and heroin. Jorge was physically abusive, but Marta believed that, as a good woman, she was responsible for her partner's happiness. She described his abuse thus:

> One day we were walking down the street when he punched me on my jaw. He accused me of looking at a man sitting on his porch.... I felt dizzy, and he started yelling at me and calling me a bitch. I could not wake up before him because he would beat me. I had to lay there and look at the ceiling. That is the worst feeling in the world. You stare at the walls and ceiling and think about your life a lot.... He would put his arm around me to make sure I would not go anywhere.

Marta explained why she tolerated the abuse, which included rape:

> One day he got crazy, and he kicked me out of the apartment because his sister was telling him bad things about me. He took me close and threw me down the steps. For a day I slept in the hallway. Then [he] said he called the cops and the cops told me I needed to leave his place. I could not say anything because the apartment was under his name only.... He would tell me what I was thinking, and he was right. It was my job to sexually satisfy him, so he continued to have anal sex with me.

One incident finally convinced Marta to leave Jorge:

> He was asking me for money for drugs. I didn't want to give it to him.... He would buy clothes and spend all of his money, and then he would want my half of the money. On that day he told me to withdraw all the money, and I told him I was not going to withdraw all the money.... After he beats me he starts to cry on top of me and tells me he loves me. After that he tells me to get up and tells me to go with him on Broadway so I can sell my body. Never in my life I've done something like that, honest to God.... He hits me and takes me over there. He tells me to get dressed and he cuts my leg with a knife. He said if I didn't give him the money I was going to have to sell myself. Well, he takes me and on the way there he beats me.... On Broadway he gave me a big beating. It was a beating like you could not imagine....
>
> ...I didn't want to sell my body so I resisted. Well he took me back to the house and told me to get dressed because we were going to the bank. I said to myself I can take no more beatings anymore

Intimate Partner Violence and the Clinician

so I'm going to give him the money. He took me to a bridge where there was a lady doing drugs.... She had AIDS. Then, he asked her for the needle.... I wanted that money to leave him and then he takes me under the bridge.... Because he didn't clean it and that needle automatically would give him hepatitis. He automatically would get hepatitis. For sure he got it. I knew afterwards. I got hysterical and wanted to leave but he didn't let me leave.

Well, he started hitting me...and the girl would tell him look she is a nice girl don't hit her.... I started to run...he hit me. He stabbed me with the needle on my hands and thighs. When I felt him stabbing me I thought about the lady he shared the needle with. I thought of her and how I would get AIDS.... I'm fucked up now.... I lost my mind and I told God I did not deserve this. Everything went through my mind.... I was struggling so he would stop. I threw dirt in his eyes; I tried to defend myself. I fell on the floor and there was glass on the floor. I started to cut myself. Because I said to myself I'm already sick. I had no hope. I gave my life to him.... A lot of things went through my mind. It was like I was going to die. I left a good man and I started to cut my venas [veins]. Well when he saw me cutting myself he said, "Ah, you want to die," so he began to hit me on my head. He didn't cut himself; he took me back to the house we stayed at. He makes me take a bath and get dressed.

After this incident, Marta attempted suicide with an overdose of pills and was hospitalized for 3 months. After discharge, she had the courage to leave Jorge and continued her treatment for depression and addiction. She resides with her current partner, Humberto, and his child from a previous marriage in a large urban city on the mainland.

This unfortunate case demonstrates multiple issues for the clinician regarding IPV. Marta had depression and self-esteem difficulties and a childhood history of abuse as well as IPV victimization. IPV can occur not just at home but also in public (including some carryover to the workplace). Her victimization did not merely occur in solitude but also in front of others and on the street, and she was victimized with multiple methods. Suicidality, such as Marta experienced, is relatively frequent among IPV victims. Her thoughts and decisions about staying in the relationship or leaving are illustrative as well.

Assessment

Assessing Abuse

Partner victimization is more common than many of the symptoms that are routinely brought up during psychiatric visits, and yet it is infrequently discussed. Often women do not report victimization to their therapists (Hilberman and Munson 1987; Jacobson and Richardson 1987) even when directly asked. However, IPV victimization should often be a consideration on the differential diagnosis.

Reasons for the reluctance of victims to discuss their abuse are numerous. Victims may come to accept the victimization, may be ashamed, or may not even conceptualize their own experiences as abuse or assault. Male victims may be especially reluctant to reveal abuse perpetrated on them by either a female or a same-sex partner. As a consequence, many physicians do not know that their patients are victims (Sahay et al. 2000). PTSD among those with serious mental illness is also frequently undetected (Cusack et al. 2006; Salyers et al. 2004), although it is a frequent consequence of victimization.

Given the frequency and consequences of IPV, physicians should consider integrating into their practice careful, specific, routine inquiries into experiences of victimization (Carlile 1991; Carlson et al. 2003). Questioning about violence can be approached with a discussion about decision making in relationships (Jacobson and Richardson 1987). Normalizing statements regarding the frequency of victimization can introduce inquiry (Friedman and Loue 2007). Women can be asked about fears of being harmed or of their children being harmed. Abuse screening measures also exist (Soeken et al. 1998). Direct specific inquiry into present and past traumatic experiences can be fruitful. Practitioners should also explore the possibility of violence by same-sex partners and by women.

Because many women seek care primarily from family practitioners or obstetrician-gynecologists, these professionals may be the first to detect IPV during routine screening. IPV can have serious psychiatric consequences (exacerbating underlying conditions or triggering new ones), so a referral to psychiatry should be considered. The psychiatrist can then provide evaluation, monitoring, and, if necessary, treatment for comorbid mental illness. The psychiatrist can also obtain a victimization history, which can be critical in medication management, discharge planning, and safety planning.

Assessing for the Commission of Abuse

It is equally important that clinicians conduct an assessment to determine a patient's risk of *committing* partner violence. In one study of 375 men screened in three family medicine clinics, 8.5% (32) had committed acts of physical violence against their intimate partners during the preceding year (Oriel and Fleming 1998).

As in many areas of violence, the strongest predictor of IPV perpetration is past violence, especially before adulthood (Moffitt et al. 2001). Other risk factors associated with the commission of IPV by men include parental rejection or shaming behavior, physical assault by a mother, fear of abandonment, trauma symptoms, the use of alcohol or drugs to deal with pain, a tendency to blame others, frequent anger, and mood swings. Male batterers have also been found to have antisocial personality traits, to act out their hostility, to need an excessive amount of control, to experience tremendous insecurity, to have high levels of jealousy, and/or to have low self-esteem (Dutton and Golant 1995; Jacobson and Gottman 1998). Although it is popularly believed that men are more likely to batter their partners than are women, more recent studies suggest that the rate of violence committed by female partners against their male intimates may equal that committed by men against their female partners (Straus 1993). Male batterers, however, are responsible for most acts of the more serious and egregious forms of physical violence, such as choking, punching, and the use of weapons (Gormley 2005).

Questions to ascertain whether an individual is at risk of committing violence may initially focus on his or her relationship with a partner and can become progressively more specific about techniques that are used by the couple to handle anger. Certain disorders have been found to be associated with the commission of violence in general: personality disorders, some types of schizophrenia, mood disorder, and impulse control disorders (Ferris et al. 1997). A physician diagnosing one of these disorders may, in the presence of other indicators, wish to address the issue of perpetration of partner violence. Men with substance use disorders and women with histories of self-harm or suicide attempts are also common among batterers (Buttell and Carney 2006).

Treatment and Management

The Victim

It is notable that Minnesota Multiphasic Personality Inventory–2 profiles of abused women may be quite similar to those of inpatients with schizophrenia or borderline personality disorder (Khan et al. 1993). A patient who is an IPV victim may feel unsafe in her own home without being "paranoid." Similarly, the inability to sleep may be self-protective. Psychiatrists should be careful in evaluating these symptoms. Pharmacotherapy choice can reflect consideration of IPV. For example, sedating medications could decrease the ability to escape from or respond to dangerous situations.

Mistrust, emotional isolation, and impaired self-esteem in IPV victims are fodder for psychotherapy (Hilberman and Munson 1987). Role-playing may be a useful method (Gearon and Bellack 1999). Cognitive-behavioral therapy may address symptoms of anxiety and depression.

Psychiatrists should be able to refer their patients either directly to shelters, services, and crisis management services or to someone familiar with these resources. In addition, the development of a safety plan and available legal options should be considered. A patient's decision to leave a violent relationship is not made lightly. The patient may be ambivalent, fear for his or her children, fear being alone, fear retaliation, have religious beliefs about staying in the marriage, or have significant financial difficulties and be isolated from his or her support group.

The Assaultive Partner

Male batterers are not a homogeneous group and may differ in their personality style (moody and emotional, cold and calculating, or insecure and jealous [Hamberger and Hastings 1988]). Abusive females may be compulsive, histrionic, and/or narcissistic (Buttell and Carney 2006). Accordingly, treatment must consider the characteristics of the individual. Batterers' physiological responses to their own violence (cold and remorseless or reactive and threatened) are also important. Many batterers receive treatment through court-mandated batterer intervention programs, which use multiple sessions of cognitive-behavioral therapy to reduce batterer aggression. The effectiveness of these programs is questionable, however—possibly because they offer a single approach to dealing with a multidimensional problem (Buttell and Carney 2006).

Couples or family therapy is another means of treating batterers. Although some therapists advise a victim to leave the relationship, others believe that advising this is unethical and encourages passivity in the victim. In cases of severe violence where the victim is not psychologically competent, the therapist may be ethically bound to intervene. In cases of lower-severity mutual violence, however, the therapist might best adopt the principle of neutrality, respecting both victim and batterer as autonomous individuals (Wilcoxen 1985).

Legal Issues

Protection and the Reporting of Intimate Partner Violence

In some instances in which the healthcare provider believes that a patient may be a danger to his or her intimate partner, the provider may have a duty to protect the potential target, according to a line of court cases that began in 1976 with *Tarasoff v. Regents of the University of California* (see also Chapter 21). The court held that when a patient "presents a serious danger…[the therapist] incurs an obligation to use reasonable care to protect the intended victim against such danger." That obligation could be satisfied by warning the intended victim of the potential danger, by notifying authorities, or by taking "whatever other steps are reasonably necessary under the circumstances." Some version of a *Tarasoff* duty, whether through case law or statute, has been adopted in many states and may provide immunity to the psychiatrist for the breach of confidentiality in cases of violence risk.

Most, if not all, states have laws mandating the reporting by healthcare providers of elder abuse, including violence inflicted by an intimate partner (Loue 2001a). As of 2000, seven states (California, Colorado, Kentucky, Mississippi, Ohio, Rhode Island, and Texas) had laws requiring providers to report IPV injuries (Houry et al. 2002), but these laws vary drastically. California and Colorado notably further require that healthcare providers report instances of injury resulting from partner violence to law enforcement, whereas Mississippi and Kentucky providers report to the department of public welfare. In Ohio, physicians must have documented IPV injuries in the record, whereas Rhode Island requires injuries to be reported for data collection purposes only. Texas requires documentation, shelter referral, and informing patients that IPV is a crime. Twenty-three states had statutes in 2000 requiring reporting of injuries received from crimes (and IPV is a crime in these states) (Houry et al. 2002). However, many physicians are unaware of these reporting statutes or may be aware yet still not report (Houry et al. 2002). Arguments *against* mandatory IPV reporting, in addition to those involving the exception to confidentiality, include that a reporting requirement may increase risk for retaliatory abuse, may deter victims from seeking care, and may create expectations that the system might not be able to meet. Arguments *for* mandatory reporting include that it would increase detection of abuse and potentially improve victim safety while not deterring most victims from seeking medical care (Houry et al. 2002; Sachs and Rodriguez 2000).

Separation and the pursuit of legal remedies may actually increase a woman's risk of harm (Jordan 2004). Fewer than half of IPV incidents are reported (Tjaden and Thoennes 2000), and arrest rates vary. Intimate partners who assault or rape are less likely to be arrested than other individuals committing similar acts. Over a quarter of those who are arrested re-assault prior to trial (Jordan 2004). Civil Protection Orders (CPOs; also known as restraining orders) may be helpful but do not guarantee safety; CPOs are violated approximately 40% of the time and may even elevate the woman's risk (Spitzberg 2002). Considerations regarding the seeking of CPOs include offender's employment or social standing, severity and persistence of the violence, length of relationship, presence of children, and living situation (Jordan 2004).

The Psychiatrist as Expert

"Self-defense" as an affirmative legal defense usually requires an objective, honest, reasonable belief that one's life is in immediate danger. "Imperfect self-defense," in contrast, lowers the severity of the charge and usually requires that the belief be subjectively reasonable. A woman in an abusive relationship may believe that she is in acute danger related to specific circumstances and may act to kill her aggressor, whereas a "reasonable man" (without a history of victimization) in the same situation might not have perceived the same risk. "Battered women's syndrome" has been used to explain this type of "imperfect self-defense."

Battered women's syndrome is not a DSM diagnosis but rather a term used in the legal arena. The concept derives from the theory of learned helplessness, which holds that individuals will not attempt to escape abusive situations where they have learned from previous experiences that all such efforts will be futile (Seligman 1975). The concept of the syndrome has been criticized because of the lack of an agreed-upon definition, the underlying assumption of pathology in the victim, and the application of the term to partner violence only in situations involving the commission of a crime, such as the killing of the abusive intimate (Dutton 2006). In addition, it has been erroneously asserted that in order to claim a battered-woman defense, a woman who kills her male partner in self-defense must have been suffering from PTSD.

Expert testimony regarding battered women has been used in the United States, Canada, Australia, New Zealand, and the United Kingdom (Schuller and Rzepa 2002; Tang 2003). Since the landmark American case of Beverly Ibn-Tamas, in 1979, expert evidence about battered women's syndrome may be allowed in the courtroom (*Ibn-Tamas v. United States* 1979). However, some courts require what is known as a *Daubert* hearing (*Daubert v. Merrell Dow Pharmaceuticals* 1993) to determine whether there is sufficient scientific validity to go forward with the theory. If the defense fails to establish the scientific validity of the theory at the time of this hearing, they will not be permitted to present this evidence to the jury at the time of the trial. It is critical to note here that the term *scientific validity* in the legal context carries a different meaning than it does in the context of scientific research (see Chapter 21).

Intimate Partner Violence and the Clinician

The expert can provide information regarding the context or framework for the woman's violence, the woman's belief in the reasonableness of her actions, why women stay in these relationships, the use of excessive force, the impact of the abusive relationship, the learned helplessness model, psychological effects of battering, and the cyclical pattern of violence, including the potential contrition ("honeymoon") phase (Dutton 2006; Schuller and Rzepa 2002; Walker 2000). However, the expert must be careful not to mislead the court into believing that learned helplessness is the only appropriate pattern of victim response to IPV. Other women cope differently with IPV victimization, and the expert should use caution not to create a prejudice against women who do not fit the pattern. One study (Schuller and Rzepa 2002) asked Canadian undergraduates ($N=200$) about a hypothetical case of a battered woman who killed her abuser. They found that the student mock jurors showed greater leniency when presented with expert testimony (primarily with a nullification instruction) and presented with a passive response history for the woman.

Key Points

- Intimate partner violence (IPV) can be perpetrated by men against women, by women against men, or by same-sex partners.
- Severely mentally ill women may be at increased risk of IPV.
- IPV may exacerbate existing symptoms of mental illness.
- Patients may not disclose IPV to their care providers out of fear, shame, and embarrassment.
- Responses to IPV may mimic symptoms of mental illness. For instance, a woman may appear to be disorganized and paranoid when she may actually be living in fear of severe injury.
- Psychiatrists and other health professionals may perform an assessment to determine if their patient fears for his or her safety because of IPV or if the patient may be likely to perpetrate violence against a partner.
- Healthcare providers may be required by law to warn the potential victim if they believe that a patient is likely to perpetrate IPV and/or to report to designated authorities the occurrence of IPV.

References

Bergman B, Ericsson E: Family violence among psychiatric inpatients as measured by the Conflict Tactics Scale (CTS). Acta Psychiatr Scand 94:168–174, 1996

Belsky J: Child maltreatment: an ecological integration. Am Psychol 35:320–335, 1980

Blood RO, Wolfe DM: Husbands and Wives: The Dynamics of Married Living. Glencoe, IL, Free Press, 1960

Briere J, Woo R, McRae B, et al: Lifetime victimization history, demographics, and clinical status in female psychiatric emergency room patients. J Nerv Ment Dis 185:95–101, 1997

Bureau of Justice Statistics: Bureau of Justice Statistics Sourcebook of Criminal Justice Statistics, 1997. Washington, DC, U.S. Department of Justice, 1998

Buttell FP, Carney MM: Women Who Perpetrate Relationship Violence. Binghamton, NY, Haworth Press, 2006

Campbell JC: Health consequences of intimate partner violence. Lancet 359:1331–1336, 2002

Carlile JB: Spouse assault on mentally disordered wives. Can J Psychiatry 36:265–269, 1991

Carlson E, McNutt LA, Choi DY: Childhood and adult abuse among women in primary health care: effects on mental health. J Interpers Violence 18:924–941, 2003

Chimbos PD: Spousal homicides in contemporary Greece. Int J Comp Sociol 39:213–223, 1998

Coker AL, Weston R, Creson DL, et al: PTSD symptoms among men and women survivors of intimate partner violence: the role of risk and protective factors. Violence Vict 20:625–643, 2005

Cromwell RE, Olson DH: Power in Families. New York, Wiley, 1975

Cusack KJ, Grubaugh AL, Knapp RG, et al: Unrecognized trauma and PTSD among public mental health consumers with chronic and severe mental illness. Community Ment Health J 42:487–500, 2006

Daubert v. Merrell Dow Pharmaceuticals, 509 U.S. 579 (1993)

DeNiro DA: Perceived alienation in individuals with residual-type schizophrenia. Issues Ment Health Nurs 16:185–200, 1995

Dienemann J, Boyle E, Baker D, et al: Intimate partner abuse among women diagnosed with depression. Issues Ment Health Nurs 21:499–513, 2000

Dobash RE, Dobash R: Violence Against Wives. New York, Free Press, 1979

Dutton DG, Painter SL: Traumatic bonding: the development of emotional attachments in battered women and other relationships of intermittent abuse. Victimology 1:139–155, 1981

Dutton DG, Painter SL: Emotional attachments in abusive relationships: a test of traumatic bonding theory. Violence Vict 8:105–120, 1993

Dutton MA: Intimate partner violence: 25 years of expert testimony. Presentation at the annual meeting of the American Academy of Psychiatry and the Law, Chicago, IL, October 2006

Dutton MA, Golant SK: The Batterer: A Psychological Profile. New York, Basic Books, 1995

El-Bassel N, Gilbert L, Witte S, et al: Intimate partner violence and substance abuse among minority women receiving care from an inner city emergency department. Womens Health Issues 13:16–22, 2003

Ferris LE, Norton PG, Dunn EV, et al: Guidelines for managing domestic abuse when male and female partners are patients of the same physician. JAMA 278:851–857, 1997

Friedman SH, Loue S: Incidence and prevalence of intimate partner violence by and against women with severe mental illness: a review. J Womens Health 16:471–480, 2007

Frye V: Examining homicide's contribution to pregnancy-associated deaths. JAMA 285:1510–1511, 2001

Gearon JS, Bellack AS: Women with schizophrenia and co-occurring substance use disorders: an increased risk for violent victimization and HIV. Community Ment Health J 35:401–419, 1999

Gelles RJ: An exchange/social theory, in The Dark Side of Families: Current Family Violence Research. Edited by Finkelhor D, Gelles RJ, Hotaling GT, et al. Beverly Hills, CA, Sage, 1983, pp 151–165

Goode W: Force and violence in the family. J Marriage Fam 33:624–636, 1971

Goodman LA, Dutton MA, Harris M: Episodically homeless women with serious mental illness: prevalence of physical and sexual assault. Am J Orthopsychiatry 65:468–478, 1995

Golding JM: Intimate partner violence as a risk factor for mental disorders: a meta-analysis. J Fam Viol 14:99–132, 1999

Gormley B: An adult attachment theoretical perspective of gender symmetry in intimate partner violence. Sex Roles 11/12: 785–795, 2005

Hamberger LK, Hastings J: Characteristics of male spouse abusers consistent with personality disorders. Hosp Community Psychiatry 39:763–770, 1988

Hilberman E, Munson K: Sixty battered women. Victimology 2:460–470, 1987

Houry D, Sachs CJ, Feldhaus KM, et al: Violence-inflicted injuries: reporting laws in the fifty states. Ann Emerg Med 39:56–60, 2002

Houry D, Kaslow NJ, Thompson MP: Depressive symptoms in women experiencing intimate partner violence. J Interpers Viol 20:1467–1477, 2005

Ibn-Tamas v. United States, 407A.2d 626 (1979)

Jacobson A, Richardson B: Assault experiences of 100 psychiatric inpatients: evidence of the need for further inquiry. Am J Psychiatry 144:908–913, 1987

Jacobson NS, Gottman JM: When Men Batter Women: New Insights into Ending Abusive Relationships. New York, Simon and Schuster, 1998

Jordan CE: Intimate partner violence and the justice system. J Interpers Viol 19:1412–1434, 2004

Kaplan ML, Asnis GM, Lipschitz DS, et al: Suicidal behavior and abuse in psychiatric outpatients. Comp Psychiatry 36:229–235, 1995

Khan FI, Welch TL, Zillmer EA: MMPI-2 profiles of battered women in transition. J Pers Assess 60:100–111, 1993

Lenski G, Lenski J: Human Societies: An Introduction to Macrosociology. New York, McGraw Hill, 1970

Loue S: Elder abuse and neglect in medicine and law: the need for reform. J Leg Med 22:159–209, 2001a

Loue S: Intimate Partner Violence: Societal, Medical, Legal and Individual Responses. New York, Plenum, 2001b

Martin SL, English KT, Clark KA, et al: Violence and substance use among North Carolina pregnant women. Am J Public Health 86:991–998, 1996

McFarlane J, Parker B, Soeken K, et al: Assessing for abuse during pregnancy: severity and frequency of injuries and associated entry into prenatal care. JAMA 267:3176–3178, 1992

Miller LJ, Finnerty M: Sexuality, pregnancy, and childbearing among women with schizophrenia-spectrum disorders. Psychiatr Serv 47:502–506, 1996

Moffitt TE, Caspi A, Rutter M, et al: Sex Differences in Antisocial Behavior: Conduct Disorder, Delinquency, and Violence in the Dunedin Longitudinal Study. Cambridge, United Kingdom, Cambridge University Press, 2001

Mueser KT, Goodman LB, Trumbetta SL, et al: Trauma and posttraumatic stress disorder in severe mental illness. J Consult Clin Psychol 66:493–499, 1998

O'Leary KD: Physical aggression between spouses: a social learning theory perspective, in Handbook of Family Violence. Edited by Hasselt VB, Morrison RL, Bellack AS, et al. New York, Plenum, 1988, pp 31–55

Oriel KA, Fleming MF: Screening men for partner violence in a primary care setting: a new strategy for detecting domestic violence. J Fam Pract 64:393–398, 1998

Rohner RP: They Love Me, They Love Me Not: A Worldwide Study of the Effects of Parental Acceptance and Rejection. New Haven, CT, HRAF Press, 1975

Rusbult CE: Commitment and satisfaction in romantic situations: a test of the investment model. J Exp Soc Psychol 16:172–186, 1980

Sachs CJ, Rodriguez MA: Should Physicians be required to report domestic violence to the police? West J Med 173:225, 2000

Sahay S, Piran N, Maddocks S: Sexual victimization and clinical challenges in women receiving hospital treatment for depression. Can J Commun Ment Health 19:161–174, 2000

Salyers MP, Evans LJ, Bond GR, et al: Barriers to assessment and treatment of posttraumatic stress disorder and other trauma-related problems in people with severe mental illness: clinician perspectives. Community Ment Health J 40:17–31, 2004

Schuller RA, Rzepa S: Expert testimony pertaining to battered woman syndrome: its impact on jurors' decisions. Law Hum Behav 26:655–673, 2002

Seligman MEP: Helplessness: On Depression, Development, and Death. San Francisco, CA, WH Freeman, 1975

Soeken KL, McFarlane J, Parker B, et al: The abuse assessment screen, in Empowering Survivors of Abuse: Health Care for Battered Women and Their Children. Edited by Campbell JC. Thousand Oaks, CA, Sage, 1998, pp 195–203

Sorenson SB, Upchurch DM, Shen H: Violence and injury in marital arguments: risk patterns and gender differences. Am J Public Health 86:35–40, 1996

Spitzberg BH: The tactical topography of stalking victimization and management. Trauma Violence Abuse 3:261–288, 2002

Straus MA: Physical assaults by wives: a major social problem, in Current Controversies in Family Violence. Edited by Gelles RJ, Loseke DR. Newbury Park, CA, Sage, 1993, pp 67–87

Tang K: Battered woman syndrome testimony in Canada: its development and lingering issues. Int J Offender Ther Comp Criminol 47:618–629, 2003

Tarasoff v. Regents of the University of California, 17 Cal. 3d 425, 131 Cal. Rptr. 14, 551 P.2d 334 (1976)

Tjaden P, Thoennes N: Full report of the prevalence, incidence, and consequences of violence against women: findings from the National Violence Against Women Survey. Washington, DC, U.S. Department of Justice, 2000

Walker LEA: The Battered Woman Syndrome, 2nd Edition. New York, Springer, 2000

Weingourt R: Wife rape in a sample of psychiatric patients. Image J Nurs Sch 22:144–147, 1990

Wilcoxen M: A Handbook for Health Professionals, Education Wife Assault. Toronto, ON, Canada, 1985

Wilson M, Daly M: An evolutionary psychological perspective on male sexual proprietariness and violence against wives. Violence Vict 8:271–294, 1993

Wolfgang ME, Ferracuti F: The Subculture of Violence: Toward an Integrated Theory of Criminology. London, England, Tavistock, 1967

CHAPTER 25

Workplace Violence and the Clinician

Ronald Schouten, M.D., J.D.

Workplace violence has been a major concern for the American workplace and public in recent decades. Although international terrorism has been the focus of foreign policy and the media, workplace violence has continued to be a leading concern of employers (Pinkerton Consulting and Investigations 2003). The term *workplace violence* conjures up images of disgruntled, armed employees wreaking havoc, killing and injuring coworkers, and in most cases killing themselves or being killed in the process of apprehension by police. Contrary to public perception and media portrayals, such stereotypical workplace violence episodes have decreased in frequency since 1994 (Bureau of Labor Statistics 2006a), as has the overall rate of violent crime in the United States. Much more common is an array of behaviors that are justifiably included under a broad definition of workplace violence or aggression: nonfatal assaults, bullying, harassment (both sexual and nonsexual), verbal abuse, threats from both known and anonymous sources, and hoaxes. Acts of terrorism with conventional or chemical, biological, radiological, or nuclear weapons can also be included as incidents of workplace violence, given that workplaces are common targets of terror attacks (Schouten et al. 2004).

The need to understand and manage acts of violence in the workplace has given rise to multiple theories, proposed methods for identifying potentially violent employees, and prevention measures. Although some, but by no means all, acts of workplace violence are perpetrated by individuals with Axis I disorders, all such actions represent abnormal behavior. Therefore psychiatrists and other mental health professionals are called upon for assistance in understanding, assessing, managing, and preventing workplace violence. This chapter explores some of the more common areas of workplace violence, with an emphasis on traditional concerns relating to fatal and nonfatal acts of interpersonal aggression and the challenges entailed in scientifically studying them. It examines some of the popular myths and misconceptions relating to workplace violence, reviews approaches to preventing and managing these events, and discusses the roles that mental health professionals can play in this area.

Case Example

ABCD Corporation, based in the northeastern United States, is a manufacturer and distributor of consumer electronics. Over the past 5 years, ABCD has been gradually outsourcing its manufacturing operations, service centers, and distribution networks. As a result, its U.S.-based workforce has shrunk by 30% over 2 years, with rumors of additional cuts in the near future. Most recently, plans were announced to move the entire customer service operation to Bangalore, India, over the next year. The U.S. customer service representatives have been offered the option of transferring to ABCD's manufacturing plant in Arkansas, taking an early retirement package, or working until such time as the U.S. operation is closed.

Six weeks after the announcement that the customer service operation would be outsourced, a large envelope bearing excess postage and addressed to the Chief Executive Officer (CEO) arrived in the mail. ABCD's corporate security director took possession of the envelope and turned it over to the local hazardous materials team for screening prior to opening. The envelope was opened when no indication of toxic substances was found. Inside were digital photographs of the CEO's wife and children leaving their home on the way to school. Appropriate security measures were put in place and a full-scale investigation was opened by law enforcement. No suspicious behavior was observed near the CEO's home, and the investigation turned up no useful leads that could tie the mailing to anyone in the community or at ABCD.

Word of the mailing spread quickly among ABCD employees. Employees began wondering what might happen next and speculated who among them might have done this. Some commented that they were certain something else would happen, given how the company had "screwed all of us." Several commented that the CEO was getting what he deserved and that although they did not want to see anyone hurt, he had a good scare coming to him, given the terror he was causing the employees by sending their jobs overseas.

Three weeks after the mailing, graffiti began appearing in the men's restroom. Obscene and graphic, and written in an awkward hand, the graffiti made direct threats of violence toward the CEO and ABCD. Police investigation, including interviews with a number of employees who used that restroom, yielded little. Through the interviews, police and ABCD security learned that fear among employees, as well as anger at ABCD for the downsizing and for failing to deal with the threats, was growing. There was discussion of installing video cameras in the men's room and the hall leading to it, but corporate counsel advised that these were prohibited by state privacy laws. Employees' concerns increased when they began to discover pieces of office equipment inexplicably broken.

The list of suspects who might possibly be responsible for the letter, graffiti, and sabotage was long. No one at ABCD was happy about the employment situation. The economy was poor, good jobs were scarce in the region, and most of the employees had families with young children.

Among the employees, the gossip was that **James Wilson** was a likely suspect. James, a programmer in the information services division, was slated to have his job eliminated when the outsourcing began. Thirty years of age, James was regarded as a loner, did not socialize with coworkers, and lived with his elderly parents. He took advantage of the company flextime policy, often coming to work late and staying until the early morning hours. James's sole known recreational activity was computer fantasy games, with which he was rumored to be "obsessed." An employee with whom James had attended high school told colleagues that James had owned a handgun in high school.

Gossip about James preoccupied the plant, much to the detriment of productivity. The gossip increased when another letter arrived with a note threatening that "If I go down, you all go down." James was interviewed by police and corporate security and denied involvement in any of the events. As rumors about James continued, and employees began complaining to human resources that he seemed "odd" and they were afraid of him, a decision was made to send him for a fitness-for-duty evaluation, even though his job performance had remained good. The psychiatrist retained to perform the evaluation, **Dr. Anderson,** was told that James was being referred because he "fit the profile" of someone who might commit an act of workplace violence.

Dr. Anderson found James to be an anxious young man with symptoms of obsessive-compulsive and avoidant personality disorders. There was no indication of psychosis, mood disorder, or other mental disorders, nor was there any indication of hostility toward ABCD or his coworkers. Interviews with James's supervisor revealed that he was quiet and diligent, was irritable at times and avoided other employees, but had never been threatening or violent. His personnel record was unremarkable; his criminal background check was clean. The expressions of concern from coworkers were vague, unsubstantiated, and based on their perception that he was "odd" and had a history of mental illness. The psychiatrist concluded that James did not pose a risk of harm to ABCD or its employees and found him fit for duty. Upon his return, a number of coworkers complained to Human Resources that they did not care what the evaluator said, they were still concerned. Several threatened to not come to work. ABCD decided to eliminate James's position ahead of schedule and offered him the standard severance package.

Three weeks after the evaluation was completed, ABCD announced the timetable for transitioning customer service operations to Bangalore. One week later, a customer service representative visited the director of Human Resources and hesitantly reported that one of her colleagues, **Bill Smith,** had flown into a rage when he received the announcement of the timetable by e-mail. Sitting in his cubicle, he had begun cursing ABCD and the CEO, stating that he just was "not going to take it." At lunch, he told colleagues that he was "fed up with the B.S." from ABCD and talked about how losing his job was going to destroy his family. The Smiths' son had multiple medical problems, his wife stayed home to care for the child, and he had no idea what they would do for healthcare coverage when he lost his job. He talked about taking out a substantial life insurance policy "just in case something happened" to him. The coworker also talked about how Bill muttered that "ABCD ain't seen nothing yet" and that the "fun" was just about to begin.

A background investigation of Bill revealed that he was a 48-year-old married father of two children, ages 10 and 12, and a college graduate. Bill had no record of criminal charges, although local police had been called to the home on two occasions related to domestic disputes. Colleagues commented that Bill had drunk excessively at company events over the previous year. In addition, his personnel file contained a verbal and a written warning for verbally abusive behavior toward coworkers.

A meeting was called of ABCD's security director, Human Resources director, and the company attorney to decide how to proceed. A decision was made to question Bill Smith, who confessed that he was responsible for all of the incidents and explained that he had acted only after becoming severely depressed over the upcoming changes. Bill told the security director that he felt he had nothing to lose and that this last-ditch effort might get ABCD to at least reconsider what it was doing. In the meantime, James Wilson had retained an attorney, who filed a disability discrimination complaint with the appropriate agency on his behalf as well as a civil suit alleging defamation.

This case example, a composite of actual cases, represents a range of behaviors that fall within the parameters of workplace violence. Although definitions of workplace violence vary, a commonly used definition is the one offered by the National Institute of Occupational Safety and Health, which defines *workplace violence* as "violent acts, including physical assaults and threats of assault, directed toward persons at work or on duty" (National Institute of Occupational Safety and Health 1996). The case example contains multiple events that would be considered acts of workplace violence under this definition: the threat contained in the mailing, the graffiti, and Bill's implied threats contained in his statements to coworkers. Broader definitions tend to use the term *workplace aggression* and would encompass Bill's verbal abuse of coworkers and the sabotage (Griffin and Lopez 2005; Neuman and Baron 1998).

Inclusive definitions of workplace violence are useful in that they convey the continuum along which acts of workplace aggression lie and raise awareness of the impact of nonviolent aggressive behavior. However, they can also cause confusion when it comes to conducting and reading research in the field and developing response strategies (Waddington et al. 2005).

The Knowledge Base for Workplace Violence

Prevalence

The Bureau of Labor Statistics (BLS) of the U.S. Department of Labor has maintained statistics on both fatal and nonfatal workplace injuries for many years. BLS data going back to 1992 indicate that workplace homicides peaked in 1994 and have declined overall since then (Bureau of Labor Statistics 2006a). Overall, in 2004 and 2005, workplace homicides dropped from third to fourth place among the most common causes of workplace death, behind motor vehicle accidents, falls from high places, and being struck by an object (Bureau of Labor Statistics 2006a). It should be kept in mind that the BLS database counts individual homicides rather than incidents. Thus a single event in which five people die (four victims and the perpetrator) would be counted as five homicides, meaning that the 567 workplace homicides reported by BLS for 2005 actually represent a lower number of individual incidents.

Workplace violence is divided into four types (University of Iowa Injury Prevention Research Center 2001). *Type I* violence includes all incidents committed by individuals who have no connection to the workplace. These events primarily occur in the course of robberies or other crimes, but also include acts of terrorism such as the attacks of September 11, 2001. Those workplace homicides were not, however, included in the CFOI data for 2001 (Bureau of Labor Statistics 2006a) because of their unique characteristics.

Type II violence includes acts perpetrated by customers or clients. This includes, for example, assaults by patients on clinicians, by clients on lawyers, and by bank customers on tellers. The events that garner the most attention—assaults by current and former coworkers—fall within *Type III*. Finally, *Type IV* acts are those carried out in the workplace by relatives, current and former spouses or partners, and other acquaintances. These incidents primarily include domestic violence situations in which the perpetrator seeks out the victim in the workplace.

This category has been getting increased attention as awareness of the significance of domestic violence grows.

Since BLS began keeping its Census of Fatal Occupational Injuries data in 1992, Type I incidents have constituted the overwhelming majority of workplace homicides. From 1997 to 2005, Type I events accounted for 78% of workplace homicides. Type II events accounted for 5%, Type III for 10%, and Type IV for 7% (Bureau of Labor Statistics 2007). The Bureau of Justice Statistics has estimated that approximately 1.7 million individuals are directly affected by acts of workplace violence annually, although this is likely an underestimate (Duhart 2001). Compared with workplace homicides, which are reported to law enforcement, estimates of nonfatal acts of violence or aggression in the workplace are more difficult to obtain. According to the Bureau of Justice Statistics, as many as 27% of individuals who are physically assaulted at work never report it to anyone, and 52% never report the event to law enforcement. Like homicides in the workplace, the incidence of nonfatal assaults declined across all occupations from 1993 to 1999, with decreases of 51% for medical workers and 28% for mental health workers (Duhart 2001).

Nonfatal workplace assaults appear to be distributed among the four types in proportions somewhat different from workplace homicides. A study of nonfatal workplace violence incidents reported to a police department by Scalora et al. (2003) found that 53% of the incidents were Type I, occurring at the hands of external sources. Type II (customers, clients, or patients) accounted for 13.8% of the sample, and Type III (coworkers) accounted for 11%. Type IV incidents (related individuals) composed 22% of the sample.

In a study of workplace violence prevention focusing on 2005, BLS surveyed 7.4 million employers in the United States, covering 128 million employees in private industry and state and local governments (Bureau of Labor Statistics 2006c). The survey gathered information on a number of aspects of workplace violence, including 1) fatal and nonfatal workplace violence incidents of all types, as defined by physical assaults, threats of assault, harassment, intimidation, or bullying; 2) the impact of such incidents; 3) steps taken in response to the incidents; and 4) the existence of workplace violence policies and procedures.

The BLS study found that 5.3% of all employers reported a violent incident in 2005, although almost 50% of the largest employers (with more than 1,000 employees) reported an incident. Only 4.8% of all private employers reported an incident, whereas 32% of state government and 14.7% of local government respondents reported at least one incident (Bureau of Labor Statistics 2006c). Approximately equal percentages

Workplace Violence and the Clinician | 507

(2%) of private industry establishments reported incidents in Type I–III categories, with a smaller percentage (0.8%) reporting a Type IV incident. Among state employers, Type III incidents were reported by 17.5% of employers, Type II by 15.4%, Type I by 8.7%, and Type IV by 5.5.%. Among local government employers, however, the distribution was somewhat different: Type II, 10.3%; Type III, 4.3%; Type I, 3.7%; and Type IV, 2.1% (Bureau of Labor Statistics 2006c). The explanation for these disparities is open to speculation.

From a slightly different perspective, it is worth noting that of all the nonfatal occupational injuries and illnesses resulting in lost days from work in private industry, assaults and violent acts accounted for 1% of the total in 2005 (Bureau of Labor Statistics 2006b). This represented a decrease of 18% from 2004. The vast majority (96%) of these occurred in service-providing establishments; 67% occurred in the healthcare industry and were primarily Type II (patient or client) incidents (Bureau of Labor Statistics 2006b).

In the case example, ABCD is confronted with threats and potential assaults that cannot be categorized when they first occur. References to the employment situation strongly suggest that the source is internal, that is, Type III. However, until more investigation is done, it would be premature to rule out the possibility that the threat was coming from an outside source, such as a member of the community who might be angry about ABCD's plans (Type I), a customer or client (Type II), or a family member of an employee who will be affected by the changes (Type IV).

Legal Risks Associated With Workplace Violence

Like physicians, employers are concerned with legal liability. Workplace violence is an area fraught with legal risks, ranging from the requirements of regulatory agencies to civil and criminal liability. A brief summary of these legal risks is in order.

The General Duty Clause of the Occupational Safety and Health Act (OSHA) requires that employers maintain a workplace that is free of safety hazards that are known, or should be known, to the employer (Occupational Safety and Health Act of 1970). State laws impose similar requirements. Regulations promulgated under OSHA also require that employers have a disaster plan in place (Occupational Safety and Health Standards 2001). In the case example, failure to respond to any of the potential threats could result in civil penalties if actual harm occurred or if other OSHA violations, such as a lack of a disaster plan, were detected.

Employers are responsible for providing workers' compensation benefits to employees who suffer injuries arising from work-related activities. In many states, this includes stress-related injuries and illnesses. If ABCD employees were to be disabled from work due to anxiety related to the threat situation, ABCD's workers' compensation carrier would likely have to provide benefits to the affected employees. Although this is not a liability issue per se, ABCD could find its workers' compensation insurance premiums increasing as a result.

Traditional common-law negligence claims may pose the biggest risk to employers in this area. These could take the form of premises liability (*Kohler v. McCrory Stores* 1992), negligent hiring (employment of a violent individual whose potential was known or easily could have been known), negligent retention (retaining a violent employee after the propensity is known), negligent supervision, or vicarious liability (Brakel 1998; Elzen 2002).

Individuals wrongly suspected or accused of threats or violent acts may also bring suit against the employer under a variety of theories. These can include actions for defamation (*Morgan v. Bubar, et al.* 2006), violation of privacy and other civil rights (*Pettus v. Cole* 1996), and disability discrimination. The Americans with Disabilities Act and analogous state statutes prohibit disparate treatment of individuals on the basis of a current disability, past history of a disability, or the perception that they have a disability (Americans With Disabilities Act 1990). In the case example, James could allege that ABCD eliminated his position prematurely because he was perceived as having a mental disability and therefore posed a risk of violence (Laden and Schwartz 2000). The Americans with Disabilities Act does not protect individuals with disabilities from discipline if they violate workplace rules, even if the violation was the result of the disability (*Hamilton v. Southwestern Bell* 1998; *Mammone v. President and Fellows of Harvard College* 2006; *Palmer v. Circuit Court of Cook County* 1998). Thus, Bill can be terminated for his actions, even if he could prove that his behavior was somehow linked to a disability, such as depression. Employers may require their employees to meet certain qualification standards, and these can include a requirement that the employee not pose a direct threat to the health or safety of other individuals in the workplace (Americans With Disabilities Act 1990; *Jones v. American Postal Workers Union* 1999).

Risk Factors for Workplace Violence

Efforts to study the causes, perpetrators, and victims of workplace violence have been hampered by a number of methodological problems.

Workplace Violence and the Clinician | 509

First, there are a limited number of cases of workplace homicides to study. Second, nonfatal workplace assaults are underreported. Third, there is a shortage of perpetrators to study, because they are either unwilling to participate or unavailable due to death by suicide or in the course of apprehension. Fourth, the quality of information available from individual events is not of uniformly high quality. Much of it comes from sensationalized media reports that are often premature in their analysis or from court documents that necessarily reflect biased adversarial views of the perpetrator (e.g., opposing experts testifying on the mental state of the perpetrator in pursuit of an insanity defense). Fifth, organizations affected by acts of workplace violence strive to maintain their confidentially and tend not to make themselves available for post hoc analysis. Finally, prospective controlled studies of employee and organizational characteristics, with random assignment to intervention strategies, are virtually impossible to conduct due to ethical and legal considerations.

Considerable attention has been given to "profiles" of workplace violence perpetrators that would allow individuals who pose a risk of violence to be identified in advance and either excluded from the workplace or subjected to specific interventions to prevent violence. The problems with these profiles are well known and recognized by legitimate experts in the field, yet the fact that a given individual "fits the profile" is a common basis for concern by employers and coworkers (American Society of Industrial Security 2005; Association of Threat Assessment Professionals 2005; Federal Bureau of Investigation 2002). The fundamental problem with the profiling approach to workplace violence is the same as that encountered when mental health professionals attempt to predict violence of any type, including suicide. Specifically, when there is a low-incidence phenomenon, even a highly sensitive test will result in an unacceptably high level of false positives—in effect, many individuals will be falsely identified as being at risk (Rosen 1954). A related problem is that none of the proffered profiles of workplace violence perpetrators has ever been empirically tested; that is, proposed traits have not been assessed for their base rate among perpetrators as well as in a matched control group of non-perpetrators.

In addition to the false-positive problem, profiles also create a problem with false negatives that mistakenly rule out true positives. This problem is apparent in the case example: the traditional profile that focuses on whether an individual has a mental illness (often translated as being "odd" in the eyes of his coworkers), is a "loner," lives with his parents, and may have owned a weapon made James the primary suspect and object of concern. Indeed, had Bill's coworker not come forward to report his threatening behavior, James might have remained the primary suspect. Action taken against an employee based on the employee's fitting a profile can provide a basis for a discrimination claim, as in James's case, where the action arises from the belief that the person has a mental disability and fails to undertake an individual analysis under the direct-threat provision (Laden and Schwartz 2000).

The absence of a reliable profile that allows for prospective identification of those who have engaged in acts of violence or are likely to do so has been demonstrated in two excellent studies conducted under the auspices of the U.S. Secret Service. These studies, which looked at would-be and actual assassins (Fein and Vossekuil 1999) and school shooters (Vossekuil et al. 2000), revealed the diversity of individuals who engaged in such activities, amply demonstrating the absence of a set profile.

Identified Risk Factors

As outlined, there are limitations to the profiling approach and to the research on workplace violence. Nevertheless, research studies of nonfatal workplace aggression have identified characteristics of individuals who engage in aggressive acts in the workplace. Similar studies have been conducted of the characteristics of organizations that are victims of such acts. Importantly, these studies, summarized here, do not purport to identify the base rate of similar characteristics in the community. As a result, these studies do not address the false-positive problem and the difficulties that arise from it. A partial listing of identified risk factors is provided in the following discussion.

Individual Risk Factors

Individual and organizational risk factors for nonfatal Type III aggression have been identified in a number of studies. Greenberg and Barling (1999) found that a past history of aggression and quantity of alcohol consumed were positively correlated with aggression against coworkers, whereas perceptions of unjust treatment and workplace surveillance were related to aggression against supervisors. Their findings regarding the role of perceived victimization and injustice have been confirmed by other researchers (Ambrose et al. 2002; Aquino and Bradfield 2000; Aquino and Douglas 2003; Baron et al. 1999; Dupre and Barling 2006; Jockin et al. 2001; Skarlicki and Folger 1997). Other individual risk factors for workplace aggression include trait anger (Chen and Spector 1992; Douglas and Martinko 2001); threat to identity (Aquino and Douglas 2003); hostility, low frustration tolerance, and reactivity to stress (Chen and Spector 1992; Jockin et al. 2001; Storms and Spector 1987); negative affectivity (Penney and Spector 2005); thinking that revenge is justified and having a tendency to blame others for personal problems (Douglas and Martinko 2001); and a history of antisocial behavior (Jockin et al. 2001; Warren et al. 1999). It has also been suggested that extremes of temperature and resultant changes in adrenaline level may be related to workplace aggression (Simister and Cooper 2005).

Various environmental factors and acute stressors, some of which are contained in the case example, have been associated with workplace aggression. These include pay cuts or freezes (Baron and Neuman 1996), termination (Allen and Lucero 1998), and low level of control over one's job (Storms and Spector 1987). Among individuals with mental illness, Haggard-Grann et al. (2006) found an increased risk of criminal violence in relationship to suicidal ideation or parasuicide within 24 hours before the violent event, hallucinations, acute conflicts with others, and being denied psychiatric care within 24 hours before the event. Notably, violent ideation did not appear to be associated with increased risk, and paranoid ideation was associated with a small and statistically nonsignificant risk.

The relationship between mental illness and violence is explored in detail elsewhere in this volume. It is worth noting here that to date, no empirical studies have identified severe mental illness as a risk factor for workplace homicide specifically. Nevertheless, the presence of such illnesses among some perpetrators of workplace violence is evidenced by case review and my personal experience. Recent research on violence and mental illness indicates that active psychotic illness, coupled with symptoms of paranoia and a past history of either conduct disorder or antisocial personality disorder, increases the risk of violent behavior (Brennan et al. 2000; Hodgins 2006; Swanson et al. 2006). In a community sample, examination of associations between psychotic-like experiences and interpersonal violence in individuals without severe mental illness revealed that such experiences are associated with an increased risk of assault with intent to harm, intimate partner violence, and arrests for assault, with paranoid ideation and unusual experiences such as visions serving as particular risk factors (Mojtabai 2006). Substance abuse has also been identified as a major risk factor for violence among individuals with and without Axis I disorders (Chen and Spector 1992; Jockin et al. 2001; Pastor 1995).

Organizational Risk Factors

Some of the organizational risk factors for workplace violence appear to include pay cuts or freezes, use of part-time employees, changes in management, reengineering, budget cuts, deteriorating physical workplace environment (Baron and Neuman 1996), low work group harmony (Cole et al. 1997), and failure to discipline aggressive employees (Allen and Lucero 1998). Again, some of these are found in the case example. Karl and Hancock (1999) proposed that organizations are at increased risk of workplace aggression if they conduct terminations with more than one supervisor present or on a Monday or Tuesday.

Classification of Factors as Static or Dynamic

The risk factors for workplace violence can be broadly divided into factors that are *historical* or *static*—that is, unchangeable—and those that are *dynamic*—that is, fluctuating and potentially modifiable (Douglas and Skeem 2005; Mills 2005; Philipse et al. 2006). Historical features include individual risk factors such as trait anger and history of antisocial behavior. Dynamic features can include organizational characteristics, life stressors, and illness. This characterization of risk factors is of importance in the process of assessing potential threatening situations and managing them.

Threat Assessment in Workplace Violence

Psychiatrists and other mental health professionals may be called upon to assess the risk of violence in a specific work-related situation. These consultations most commonly involve assessment of risk posed by an identified current or former customer or client (Type II), an identified current or former employee (Type III), or a person related to an employee, usually through a domestic relationship (Type IV). Less frequently, the consultant may be asked to assess risk posed by an anonymous threatener or to assist in identifying an anonymous threatener.

As in any other consultation, the prospective consultant should first define the exact consultation question and objectively determine whether she or he is qualified to fulfill the request. Violence risk assessment involving mental illness is a common feature of psychiatric residency and clinical psychology training, and much of mental health clinical practice revolves around this activity. It is important to keep in mind, however, that workplace violence risk assessments are not standard clinical evaluations. They differ from the clinical task in 1) their purpose, 2) the party to whom responsibility is owed, 3) the database that may be available, and 4) the range of options available. Each of these elements is discussed in greater detail below.

Workplace violence risk assessments are forensic consultations, requested by and for the benefit of third parties—not clinical evaluations conducted for the benefit of the evaluee. Ideally, the evaluation will have a beneficial impact on all parties involved, but the goal is not to diagnose and provide treatment, or even a treatment referral, for the evaluee. The goal is to determine the level of risk to which the referring party is exposed and to assist in managing that risk. Although clinicians have a duty to behave in an ethical manner no matter what their role, the fiduciary duty that arises from the doctor–patient relationship to act only in the best interests of the patient is owed not to the evaluee but to the party requesting the assessment (Schouten 1993; Strasburger et al. 1997). The evaluating clinician has a duty to the evaluee to disclose information to the employer only with consent (American Academy of Psychiatry and the Law 2005), although the employer may make participation in the evaluations and release of information a contingency of any future employment. Even so, the evaluating clinician should only disclose information on a need-to-know basis and should be aware of the extent to which Health Insurance Portability and Accountability Act privacy requirements apply to these evaluations (Gold and Metzner 2006).

The databases available in workplace violence consultations and clinical evaluations differ, with each more limited and more complete in certain ways. Clinical evaluations occur in person, whereas the workplace violence consultant may never meet the subject face to face. On the other hand, the consultant will ideally have more comprehensive information from a wider range of sources than is available to the average clinical evaluator. In clinical settings, the primary sources of information are generally limited to the patient him- or herself and perhaps family members. Time and location permitting, the outpatient evaluator may have access to the evaluee's medical records. In contrast, the workplace violence consultant will often make the risk determination on the basis of background information, interviews with collateral sources, review of documents and other communications, and often comprehensive background checks, which can provide the basis for a structured assessment based on actuarial risk factors.

It is also important to keep in mind that in workplace violence risk assessments, only a small proportion of subjects will have identifiable Axis I or even Axis II disorders. Thus, options available to the clinical evaluator may not be accessible to the consultant. For example, voluntary or involuntary hospitalization may be available for an individual who is engaging in threatening behavior as a result of a mental illness. In the absence of such an illness, or sufficient risk of harm to justify involuntary commitment, alternative solutions to maintaining safety must be found. This may require a decision as to whether the matter should be referred to law enforcement or if a legal action, such as a restraining order, should be pursued.

The Threat Assessment Process

Psychiatry is a solitary profession. Although clinical teams are responsible for treatment in institutional settings, psychiatrists continue to be trained in a largely dyadic model in which the primary interactions are between doctor and patient or several patients in group therapy. Even when the clinician is working on a team, the other team members tend to be other mental health professionals. When called upon to render an opinion regarding risk of violence in a workplace setting, we tend to fall back into the familiar practice of attempting to solve the problem presented to us by relying on our individual skills and experience.

Those who would provide consultation on workplace violence consultations are well advised to abandon the traditional individualistic approach and to seek the input of team members from diverse backgrounds (Schouten 2003, 2006). Mental health professionals are most effective in this regard when they serve as members of or consultants to threat management teams established by organizations to handle crises that may arise. These teams are also referred to as "threat assessment" or "crisis management" teams, and they are common elements of workplace violence policies—where such policies exist. BLS has reported that 70% of establishments had no workplace violence policies as of 2005 (Bureau of Labor Statistics 2006c). Commonly composed of individuals from corporate security, human resources, and legal departments, threat management teams are ideally on call around the clock, 365 days a year, and are responsible for implementation of policies, liaison with law enforcement, and investigation and management of incidents (American Society of Industrial Security 2005; Schouten 2003). The team is designed in such a way that consultants such as mental health professionals can be called in as needed (Schouten 2003).

The role for mental health professionals on the team will vary depending on the sophistication of the team and the experience of the consultant. In some cases, the psychiatrist or other mental health professional who possesses the necessary knowledge and experience will take the lead; in others, the process will be led by experienced corporate security or law enforcement professionals. It has been my experience that the best results and most satisfying experiences are the product of a group process in which individuals from different disciplines, with mutual respect for each other, share their knowledge and perspectives.

Invariably, the rest of the team looks to the mental health expert for an assessment of the subject's level of risk. It is up to the expert to undertake an assessment involving a variety of factors, both historical and dynamic, that may increase or mitigate risk. In this setting, as in traditional clinical settings, it is important to keep in mind that violent behavior is the product of interactions among three sets of factors: 1) individual factors, 2) triggers, and 3) environmental factors—that is, whether the environment encourages or dissuades potential violence (Borum et al. 1999; Fein and Vossekuil 1995). A number of such factors were discussed earlier in this chapter, as was the distinction between historical and dynamic factors. Thus, in conducting the risk assessment and advising the team, the consultant is examining a broad array of information, much of which comes from sources other than the evaluee.

The ideal threat assessment includes not only a broad range of information from background investigation and collateral sources but also an opportunity to interview the subject of concern and to apply a structured or semistructured approach, utilizing available instruments where applicable. This approach, which combines actuarial and clinical risk assessment models, is both flexible and more likely to be accurate (Association of Threat Assessment Professionals 2005; Borum et al. 1999). The risk assessment itself will be framed in terms of relative risk, as opposed to percentage of likelihood.

Once the risk assessment is conducted, the consultant may be called upon to utilize skills that are more closely linked to clinical skills, such as understanding the motivation and behavior of the subject of concern and suggesting ways in which the situation can be managed to decrease the likelihood of harm to all concerned. As with other situations in which psychiatrists are applying their clinical skills in the interests of third parties rather than the person being evaluated, there are ethical concerns that must be considered (Arboleda-Florez 2006; Janofsky 2006; Sen et al. 2007).

The consultant who undertakes these consultations, such as Dr. Anderson in the case example, can avoid ethical transgressions by following a few basic principles. These include limiting disclosure of previously unknown information to need-to-know situations or those where there is no expectation of privacy on the part of the subject; modeling respectful behavior for all individuals; combating stereotypes of mental illness; discouraging discrimination; and pursuing solutions that protect the client requesting the consultation without unnecessary harm to the individual of concern.

Assuming in the case example that a consultant finds that Bill Smith poses a moderate risk of violence under the existing circumstances, the challenge is to design an intervention that decreases the immediate risk of violence, protects ABCD, and decreases the risk going forward. This would likely include consultation with security staff on protective measures for ABCD and individual employees. Whether to discharge Bill

Smith will be a business decision that takes into consideration not only risk issues but also the impact of retaining Mr. Smith when his behavior is known to other employees. From a violence risk management standpoint, however, all parties may be best served by a mandatory medical leave, possible short-term disability, and ongoing provision of health insurance benefits. In the event that Mr. Smith is to be discharged, a severance package that includes severance pay and ongoing health benefits can decrease the stress of termination, especially in a situation like his where family health issues constitute an ongoing stressor.

Key Points

- Workplace violence is a subject that has captured the imagination of the public and the media due to the human drama and tragedy involved.
- Because this type of violence is about abnormal behavior, psychiatrists and other mental health professionals will continue to be called upon to provide risk assessments, develop prevention strategies, and suggest methods to mitigate risks.
- As mental health professionals, we have much to offer in terms of workplace risk assessment, prevention, and mitigation. Individuals who choose to pursue this rewarding professional activity can do so effectively so long as they undertake the proper training, understand the tasks ahead of them, and stay within the boundaries of knowledge, skill, and professional ethics.

References

Allen R, Lucero M: Subordinate aggression against managers: empirical analyses of published arbitration abstracts. The International Journal of Conflict Management 9:234–257, 1998

Ambrose ML, Seabright MA, Schminke M: Sabotage in the workplace: the role of organizational injustice. Organ Behav Hum Decis Process 89:947–965, 2002

American Academy of Psychiatry and the Law: Ethics Guidelines for the Practice of Forensic Psychiatry. Bloomington, CT, American Academy of Psychiatry and the Law, 2005

American Society of Industrial Security: Workplace Violence Prevention and Response Guideline. Alexandria, VA, American Society of Industrial Security, 2005

Americans With Disabilities Act, 42 U.S.C. § 12113(b) (1990)

Aquino K, Bradfield M: Perceived victimization in the workplace: the role of situational factors and victim characteristics. Organization Science 11:525–537, 2000

Aquino K, Douglas S: Identity threat and antisocial behavior in organizations: the moderating effects of individual differences, aggressive modeling, and hierarchical status. Organ Behav Hum Decis Process 90:195–208, 2003

Arboleda-Florez JE: The ethics of forensic psychiatry. Curr Opin Psychiatry 19:544–546, 2006

Association of Threat Assessment Professionals: Violence Risk Assessment Guideline: Standard Considerations for Assessing the Risk of Future Violent Behavior. Huntington Beach, CA, Association of Threat Assessment Professionals, 2005

Baron R, Neuman J: Workplace violence and workplace aggression: evidence on their relative frequency and potential causes. Aggress Behav 22:161–173, 1996

Baron RA, Neuman JH, Geddes D: Social and personal determinants of workplace aggression: evidence for the impact of perceived injustice and the Type A behavior pattern. Aggress Behav 25:281–296, 1999

Borum R, Fein R, Vossekuil B, et al: Threat assessment: defining an approach for evaluating risk of targeted violence. Behav Sci Law 17:323–337, 1999

Brakel SJ: Legal liability and workplace violence. J Am Acad Psychiatry Law 26:553–562, 1998

Brennan PA, Mednick SA, Hodgins S: Major mental disorders and criminal violence in a Danish birth cohort. Arch Gen Psychiatry 57:494–500, 2000

Bureau of Labor Statistics: National Census of Fatal Occupational Injuries in 2005. Washington, DC, U.S. Department of Labor, 2006a

Bureau of Labor Statistics: Nonfatal Occupational Injuries and Illnesses Requiring Days Away from Work, 2005. Washington, DC, U.S. Department of Labor, 2006b

Bureau of Labor Statistics: Survey of Workplace Violence Prevention, 2005. Washington, DC, U.S. Department of Labor, 2006c

Bureau of Labor Statistics: Census of Fatal Occupational Injuries: Occupational Homicides by Selected Characteristics, 1997–2005. Washington, DC, U.S. Department of Labor, 2007

Chen P, Spector P: Relationships of work stressors with aggression, withdrawal, theft and substance use: an exploratory study. Journal of Occupational and Organizational Psychology 65:177–184, 1992

Cole L, Grubb P, Sauter S, et al: Psychosocial correlates of harassment, threats and fear of violence in the workplace. Scand J Work Environ Health 23:450–457, 1997

Douglas KS, Skeem JL: Violence risk assessment: getting specific about being dynamic. Psychol Public Policy Law 11:347–383, 2005

Douglas SC, Martinko MJ: Exploring the role of individual differences in the prediction of workplace aggression. J Appl Psychol 86:547–559, 2001

Duhart DT: Violence in the Workplace, 1993–1999 (Report No.: NCJ 190076). Washington, DC, U.S. Department of Justice, 2001

Dupre KE, Barling J: Predicting and preventing supervisory workplace aggression. J Occup Health Psychol 11:13–26, 2006

Elzen WL: Workplace violence: vicarious liability and negligence theories as a two- fisted approach to employer liability. Is Louisiana clinging to an outmoded theory? La Law Rev 62:897–928, 2002

Federal Bureau of Investigation: Workplace Violence: Issues in Response. Quantico, VA, U.S. Department of Justice, 2002

Fein RA, Vossekuil B: Threat Assessment: An Approach to Prevent Targeted Violence. Rockville, MD, National Institute of Justice, 1995

Fein RA, Vossekuil B: Assassination in the United States: an operational study of recent assassins, attackers, and near-lethal approachers. J Forensic Sci 44:321–333, 1999

Gold LH, Metzner JL: Psychiatric employment evaluations and the Health Insurance Portability and Accountability Act. Am J Psychiatry 163:1878–1882, 2006

Greenberg L, Barling J: Predicting employee aggression against coworkers, subordinates and supervisors: the roles of person behaviors and perceived workplace factors. Journal of Organizational Behavior 20:897–913, 1999

Griffin RW, Lopez YP: "Bad behavior" in organizations: a review and typology for future research. J Manage 31:988–1005, 2005

Haggard-Grann U, Hallqvist J, Langstrom N, et al: Short-term effects of psychiatric symptoms and interpersonal stressors on criminal violence: a case-crossover study. Soc Psychiatry Psychiatr Epidemiol 41:532–540, 2006

Hamilton v. Southwestern Bell, 136 F.3d 1047 (5th Cir. 1998)

Hodgins S: Crime and violence by persons with mental illness: new evidence requires new mental health policies and practices. Neuropsychiatrie 20:7–14, 2006

Janofsky JS: Lies and coercion: why psychiatrists should not participate in police and intelligence interrogations. J Am Acad Psychiatry Law 34:472–478, 2006

Jockin V, Avery R, McGue M: Perceived victimization moderates self-reports of workplace aggression and conflict. J Appl Psychol 86:1262–1269, 2001

Jones v. American Postal Workers Union, 192 F.3d 417 (4th Cir. 1999)

Karl K, Hancock B: Expert advice on termination practices: how expert is it? Public Pers Manage 28:51–62, 1999

Kohler v. McCrory Stores, 615 A.2d 27 (Pa. 1992)

Laden VA, Schwartz G: Psychiatric disabilities, the Americans with Disabilities Act, and the new Workplace Violence Account. Berkeley Journal of Employment and Labor Law 21:246–270, 2000

Mammone v. President and Fellows of Harvard College, 276 N.E.2d 847 (Mass. 2006)

Mills JF: Advances in the assessment and prediction of interpersonal violence. J Interpers Violence 20:236–241, 2005

Mojtabai R: Psychotic-like experiences and interpersonal violence in the general population. Soc Psychiatry Psychiatr Epidemiol 41:183–190, 2006

Morgan v. Bubar, et al. Conn. Super. 1828 (2006)

National Institute of Occupational Safety and Health: Violence in the Workplace: Risk Factors and Prevention Strategies. DHHS (NIOSH) Publication No. 96-100. Cincinnati, OH, National Institute of Occupational Safety and Health, 1996. Available at http://www.cdc.gov/niosh/violcont.html. Accessed July 15, 2007

Neuman JH, Baron RA: Workplace violence and workplace aggression: evidence concerning specific forms, potential causes, and preferred targets. J Manage 24:391–419, 1998

Occupational Safety and Health Act of 1970. 29 U.S.C. § 654 (5)(a) (1970)

Occupational Safety and Health Standards, Subpart E—Means of Egress. 29 C.F.R. § 1910.38 (2001)

Palmer v. Circuit Court of Cook County, 351 F.3d 117 (7th Cir. 1997) cert denied, 522 U.S. 1096 (1998)

Pastor LH: Initial assessment and intervention strategies to reduce workplace violence. Am Fam Physician 52:1169–1174, 1995

Penney LM, Spector PE: Job stress, incivility, and counterproductive work behavior (CWB): the moderating role of negative affectivity. Journal of Organizational Behavior 26:777–796, 2005

Pettus v. Cole, 57 Cal.Rptr.2d 46 (Calif. Court Appeals 1996)

Philipse MWG, Koeter MWJ, van der Staak CPF, et al: Static and dynamic patient characteristics as predictors of criminal recidivism: a prospective study in a Dutch forensic psychiatric sample. Law Hum Behav 30:309–327, 2006

Pinkerton Consulting and Investigations: Top Security Threats and Management Issues Facing Corporate America. Parsippany, NJ, Pinkerton Consulting and Investigations, 2003

Rosen A: Detection of suicidal patients: an example of some limitations in the prediction of infrequent events. J Consult Psychol 18:397–403, 1954

Scalora MJ, Washington DO, Casady T, et al: Nonfatal workplace violence risk factors: data from a police contact sample. J Interpers Violence 18:310–327, 2003

Schouten R: Pitfalls of clinical practice: the treating clinician as expert witness. Harv Rev Psychiatry 1:64–65, 1993

Schouten R: Violence in the workplace, in Mental Health and Productivity in the Workplace. Edited by Kahn JP, Langlieb AM. San Francisco, CA, Jossey-Bass, 2003, pp 314–328

Schouten R: Workplace violence: an overview for practicing clinicians. Psychiatr Ann 36:790–797, 2006

Schouten R, Callahan MV, Bryant S: Community response to disaster: the role of the workplace. Harv Rev Psychiatry 12:229–237, 2004

Sen P, Gordon H, Adshead G, et al: Ethical dilemmas in forensic psychiatry: two illustrative cases. J Med Ethics 33:337–341, 2007

Simister J, Cooper C: Thermal stress in the USA: effects on violence and on employee behaviour. Stress and Health 21:3–15, 2005

Skarlicki D, Folger R: Retaliation in the workplace: the roles of distributive, procedural, and interactional justice. J Appl Psychol 82:434–443, 1997

Storms P, Spector P: Relationships of organizational frustration with reported behavioural reactions: the moderating effect of locus of control. Journal of Occupational Psychology 60:227–234, 1987

Strasburger LH, Gutheil TG, Brodsky A: On wearing two hats: role conflict in serving as both psychotherapist and expert witness. Am J Psychiatry 154:448–456, 1997

Swanson JW, Swartz MS, Van Dorn RA, et al: A national study of violent behavior in persons with schizophrenia. Arch Gen Psychiatry 63:490–499, 2006

University of Iowa Injury Prevention Research Center: Workplace Violence: A Report to the Nation. Iowa City, University of Iowa Injury Prevention Research Center, 2001

Vossekuil B, Reddy M, Fein R: Safe School Initiative: An Interim Report on the Prevention of Targeted Violence in School. Washington, DC, U.S. Secret Service, 2000

Waddington PAJ, Badger D, Bull R: Appraising the inclusive definition of workplace "violence." Br J Criminol 45:141–164, 2005

Warren J, Brown D, Hurt S, et al: The organizational context of non-lethal workplace violence: its interpersonal, temporal, and spatial correlates. J Occup Environ Med 41:567–581, 1999

CHAPTER 26

Vehicular Crashes and the Role of Mental Health Clinicians

Alan R. Felthous, M.D.

Thomas M. Meuser, Ph.D.

Thomas Ala, M.D.

By virtue of their training, experience, and practice, mental health professionals are often in a good position to identify and assess conditions that may impair fitness to drive an automobile. There is much current debate regarding whether clinicians should be expected to identify which individuals, because of mental disorder, cannot safely drive and, if clinicians make such an assessment, what reasonable protective measures they should be expected to take.

Through its position statement on the topic, the American Psychiatric Association (1993) maintains that thorough assessment of driving functions does not lie within the scope or abilities of psychiatrists. In their practice, psychiatrists should not be expected to make assessments of driving competence per se but rather to show awareness and concern for how certain conditions may affect fitness to drive. Rather than assume any protective responsibilities of a coercive or disclosing nature, psychiatrists can foster safe driving through patient education and monitoring. Psychiatrists can tell their patients how some symptoms of their disorder can affect driving safety, especially concerning well-researched conditions such as dementia. They should explain that certain medicines can impair a person's alertness and coordination when driving, especially if combined with alcohol. Finally, the American Psychiatric Association encourages psychiatrists to preferentially prescribe medications less likely to interfere with driving for their patients who are expected to drive.

Vehicular crashes[1] are responsible for untold morbidity and mortality in the United States, especially those involving teenage and young adult drivers. Most mentally disordered individuals, like nearly everyone else, drive and probably do so safely. Also like other drivers, the mentally disordered are quite capable of being in a crash, even causing it, without mental disturbance contributing in a causal sense. Then again, sometimes a crash *is* related to a disturbed mental state.

Mental disorder can cause an individual to crash either deliberately or accidentally (Felthous 2006). A mentally disordered individual may decide to crash to commit suicide, to kill unknown victims, or both. An accidental crash can be due to the mental disorder directly, such as when an individual with bipolar disorder drives fast and recklessly during a manic episode. Other neurological conditions of concern include epilepsy and other disorders of consciousness, such as narcolepsy. Conditions with poor regulation of emotional and behavioral control such as intermittent explosive disorder, borderline personality disorder, and antisocial personality disorder can all motivate risk-taking behaviors that may elevate crash risk.

Intoxication with alcohol is an all too common cause of vehicular crashes, even without the presence of other serious mental illness. Individuals already at risk due to mental disorder can increase their risk by ingesting intoxicating substances. Physicians may prescribe medications that are sedating or have other properties that impair mentation and driving competence; on the other hand, some medications and performance-enhancing substances can improve driving ability. Situational distraction, distress, and especially drowsiness can compromise safe driving in normal individuals. A cup of caffeinated coffee can help the weary driver safely finish a long haul. Stimulants may restore narcoleptic individuals to safe driving capability, and the same may be true for anticonvulsants in epileptics, antipsychotic medications in drivers with psychotic disorders, mood stabilizers in those with bipolar disor-

---

[1] In this discussion the term *accident* is used selectively, not generically, because not all crashes are unintended.

ders, and antidepressants in depressed individuals. Empirical evidence demonstrates that when depressed patients are treated with antidepressant medication, their driving competence and safety parameters improve (Ärzte-Zeitung 2007). Although safe clinical practices emphasize appropriate warnings and precautions for medications that can compromise safe driving, the tremendous value of medication in enhancing driving skill and safety when prescribed appropriately must not be overlooked.

Obviously, a great variety of illnesses, medical conditions, and physical disabilities can impair driving skill and increase the risk for a crash. Here we focus on several mental and neurological disorders that can adversely affect driving and that mental health clinicians are likely to encounter. The categorical conditions included are psychosis and schizophrenia, depression, dementia, and disturbances in consciousness, particularly seizures or epilepsy and narcolepsy. Legal responsibilities of treating physicians are considered by using case examples; however, the clinician is best advised to refer to jurisdictional, especially controlling statutory, law regarding reporting requirements.

Mental Disorders

Psychosis and Schizophrenia

A literature review conducted by the National Highway Traffic Safety Administration (Dobbs 2005) concluded that individuals with untreated psychotic disorders and, overall, those with schizophrenia, depressive or anxiety disorders, alcoholism, and personality disorders are at greatest risk for motor vehicular crashes. Studies of schizophrenic drivers show a relationship to crash rates if correction is made for exposure to driving. (Those with serious mental impairments spend less time driving than their unafflicted counterparts.) There is general agreement that one should not drive during the acute phase of a psychotic illness (American Psychiatric Association 1995; Austroads 1998; Canadian Medical Association 2000).

Little is written, however, on how to determine when a condition is sufficiently acutely psychotic that driving should be restricted. This is presumably because current psychotropic medications have shortened the duration of acute psychotic exacerbations—and therefore of periods when driving should be restricted. Moreover, the customary standard of practice is to hospitalize the individual who is acutely psychotic, thus minimizing for that period that individual's exposure to driving and potential for causing a crash.

Not everyone who is competent and willing to consent to hospitalization meets criteria for emergency involuntary hospitalization. Threats, preparatory acts, and attempts to seriously harm self or others, especially if psychotically driven, simplify the decision and the legal justification for emergency hospitalization. The evaluator asks about current thoughts and past acts of self-harm, suicide, and homicide.

An example of a psychotic driver who causes a crash comes from the landmark legal case *Naidu v. Laird* (1988).

Case Example 1

Mr. Hilton Putney had been hospitalized numerous times, had failed to take prescribed medication in the community, had attempted suicide on several occasions, and had deliberately crashed his car on two occasions. Immediately after he was discharged from Delaware State Hospital, Mr. Putney stopped taking medication and did not keep his outpatient appointment. He deliberately crashed his car into another, killing the other driver, Mr. George Laird. Mr. Putney was charged with manslaughter and found not guilty by reason of insanity. The lawsuit against Dr. Naidu and other hospital psychiatrists resulted in a $1.4 million verdict. The Supreme Court of Delaware, referring to the *Tarasoff* duty of therapists to protect third persons from foreseeable harm caused by their patients, upheld the cause of action.

Vehicular crashes by psychotically disturbed individuals cannot always be anticipated by threats. They are not necessarily preceded by an expressed plan or intention. Worrisome signs include prior history of crashes, especially if associated with destructive thoughts, disorganized thought, or agitation. The most effective prevention is probably hospitalization while the patient is acutely psychotic and close monitoring after discharge to ensure medication compliance and mental stability, exercising early intervention when signs of decompensation appear. Where hospitalization is not practical but psychotic symptoms and significantly impaired concentration cause concern, the patient should be discouraged from driving. Family members can sometimes be helpful in supporting the patient's transportation needs.

Depression

Most authorities would agree that depressed individuals may drive if their mood is stable and any medications are regulated (American Psychiatric Association 1995; Austroads 1998). Austroads (1998) advised against driving while medications are being adjusted, whereas the American Psychiatric Association (1995) recommended that the physician warn the patient that any newly prescribed medication can affect driving ability. There is general agreement that individuals who are profoundly depressed with impaired concentration should not drive (American Psychiatric Association 1995; Austroads 1998; Canadian Medical Association 2000). Although controversy exists over the number of crashes caused by suicidal drivers (Dobbs 2005), practiced mental health clinicians are familiar with individual patients who have thought of making a suicidal crash while driving or have actually attempted this.

Case Example 2

Mr. Tony Marconi,[2] a 60-year-old retired fireman, reported at the hospital emergency department that he was thinking of committing suicide by drug overdose or vehicular crash. Diagnoses included major depressive disorder and cocaine dependence. Although he took antidepressant medication as prescribed, he still felt depressed, so he tried to self-augment with cocaine. Even this extra measure did not assuage his depression. When interviewed the day after admission to the hospital inpatient psychiatric service, Mr. Marconi denied having had a specific method of suicide in mind: he stated that he came to the hospital only to obtain help with depression and said he was thinking of suicide but without a method or plan in mind. When asked specifically about drug overdose, he acknowledged having attempted suicide by drug overdose several years ago but denied that this was a recent consideration.

When asked about suicide by vehicular crash, Mr. Marconi said this had occurred to him just before a prior hospitalization about 3 weeks earlier. While he was driving on a busy interstate highway and feeling hopeless about his unrelenting depression and insuperable cocaine addiction, it suddenly occurred to him that he could at that very moment steer his car into another vehicle and end his misery once and for all in a fatal crash. When asked if he had concern about the other driver, Mr. Marconi said this did occur to him as a secondary consideration. The thought of harming another person importantly constrained him from a disastrous turn of the steering wheel and impelled him to drive straight to the hospital to obtain help.

The case of Mr. Marconi illustrates a general challenge in suicide assessment and a specific challenge where the would-be method of suicide is by crash. While in the hospital emergency department, a patient will sometimes express a method for committing suicide and then the following day will deny having entertained the same plan. He may have cited the method initially in order to gain hospital admission and

---

[2] For this and the subsequent case examples, information is altered to obscure identification and resemblance to any particular individual.

then denied it in order to be released or to have suicide precautions lifted. There are obviously other possible explanations for such a discrepancy. In any event, description of such a method is associated with the thought, regardless how strong or weak the intent. Without contravening evidence of insincerity, such specific methods should be taken seriously at the time, especially when availability of this patently lethal method is established.

With further assessment, Mr. Marconi's self-reported spontaneous impulse to commit suicide by crash was convincing. This example illustrates a challenge in preventing suicide by crash. In contrast to firearms, for example, people rely on driving cars for personal mobility, access to services, productive employment, and living comfort, so exposure is high. Yet the impulse to commit suicide by crash can occur impulsively and with no advance warning. After the patient with such impulses is no longer acutely suicidal and can be discharged, he or she should be cautioned against driving after taking illegal drugs and when feeling hopeless and depressed. Even before suicidal thoughts resurface, if these conditions arise it is time to call upon mental health services.

Case Example 3

> Ms. Lilian Quen is a 35-year-old woman who was admitted to the hospital with major depressive disorder. She had been feeling hopeless and having suicidal thoughts of killing her children as well as herself. Although not psychotic, she could not bear the thought of her children not being raised and cared for by herself. Two methods occurred to her: poisoning by overdosing with medicine and driving her car with both children inside into a river. She seriously thought of the latter method recurrently over several years. Several times she made initial preparations by placing her children in the car and driving to a riverbank. Noticing that she was distraught, her children asked what was the matter, gave solace to their mother, and in so doing interrupted Ms. Quen's fatal intentions.

This would have been a crash of another kind, driving the car into the river in a combined homicide-filicide. It serves as another example of the importance of assessing suicide and homicide risk by obtaining a detailed history of prior thoughts, preparatory acts, and attempts and by asking the details of the method(s) considered in addition to asking about desperate thoughts. The suicide-homicide prevention plan involves the child protective authorities, aggressive treatment of depression, careful discharge planning before hospital release, and close monitoring afterward. Extended restriction of driving should be a part of the prevention plan.

Dementia

For patients diagnosed with a progressive dementia such as Alzheimer's disease, it is not a matter of *if* retirement from driving will be necessary but *when*. Alzheimer's disease differs from other conditions reviewed in this chapter because current treatments cannot restore driving fitness in those already impaired. Whereas patients with early, mild forgetfulness and a safe driving record may retain sufficient ability to drive for a time, those with more advanced impairment (i.e., deficits in divided attention, visuospatial skills, and/or executive functioning) are likely to pose a hazard on the road (Carr et al. 2006). The American Psychiatric Association (1997) recommends that patients with moderate dementia be required to stop driving for reasons of individual and public safety. The American Academy of Neurology argues that even those at the mild stage have sufficient deficits to warrant driving cessation (Dubinsky et al. 2000).

In a landmark study by Linda Hunt and colleagues at Washington University (Hunt et al. 1997), patients evaluated as clinically normal and as being in the early stages of dementia were administered a detailed on-road performance evaluation. Patients were characterized as either very mildly demented or mildly demented by use of the Clinical Dementia Rating (CDR; Morris 1993), 0.5 and 1 levels, respectively. Overall ratings of "safe," "marginal," or "unsafe" were assigned to each older driver. The majority (97%) of those judged to be clinically normal (CDR 0) were found to be safe or marginal drivers. This number dropped to 81% for very mildly demented (CDR 0.5) drivers and 59% for mildly demented (CDR 1) drivers. As many CDR 1 drivers were found to be unsafe as safe—41% in both cases. Subsequent testing over time revealed that the majority of these demented drivers moved from safe/marginal to unsafe categories over a 2-year period, with mildly demented (CDR 1) individuals showing the steepest decline (Duchek et al. 2003).

Based on these and other findings, it is reasonable to consider the transition from CDR 0.5 to CDR 1 stages of dementia (i.e., very mild to mild) as the *critical period* for driving-related assessment, discussion of driving retirement, and implementation of a cessation and alternative transportation plan (Meuser et al. 2006). Primary care and specialist physicians, including psychiatrists, can play important evaluative and counseling roles in this process, according to the American Medical Association's Older Drivers Project (American Medical Association 2003; Wang and Carr 2004). In-office interview and screening procedures are sufficient, in many cases, to "risk stratify" patients into likely safe or unsafe categories. Advancing impairment and evidence of on-road problems (e.g., reports of near misses, accidents, traffic tickets) would support a recommendation to stop driving.

Few physicians have the time, confidence, or expertise to make an independent decision on driving fitness. The American Medical Association encourages patient referrals for on-road evaluation (which are typically provided by a certified driver rehabilitation specialist or trained occupational therapist), mobility counseling to develop an alternative transportation plan (often provided by a counselor or social worker), and consultation with local support organizations (e.g., the Alzheimer's Association, the area Council on Aging). It often takes a community of health and service professionals, working together with the patient and family, to implement an effective driving retirement plan.

In contrast to other conditions reviewed in this chapter, dementia is one for which it is recommended that the psychiatrist participate in the driving assessment/retirement process (American Psychiatric Association 1997). Protection of individual and public safety warrants such involvement. Crash risk is doubled in persons with dementia, ranging from an 8% to 10% crash rate per year (Brown and Ott 2004). Along with family members, clinicians are often the first professionals to become aware of changes in physical health and cognitive status that may affect fitness to drive. Early intervention can reduce exposure to accidents for the driver with dementia, his or her passengers, and others on the road. Under ideal circumstances, the demented driver will accept medical advice to stop driving and move into driving retirement willingly. Under less optimal circumstances, the clinician and family may need to build a case for retirement. Often with physician input and family persistence, driving retirement can be achieved even in patients who lack insight. However, some patients may need to be forced via a formal report to the state driver licensing authority—the Department of Motor Vehicles in most states—to trigger a formal review and de-licensing process.

The *Physician's Guide to Assessing and Counseling Older Drivers* (American Medical Association 2003) provides step-by-step guidance for the assessment and counseling process, culminating in state reporting for challenging cases where loss of awareness, denial, or stubbornness obstruct prudent decision making. In dementia, fitness to drive is not a one-time clinical concern but something that must be approached with both sensitivity and care over a period of time (Meuser et al. 2006). A number of recommendations for practice flow from this concept and are applicable to psychiatric care.

- Driving retirement is appropriate for discussion soon after the diagnosis of progressive dementia is made. A sufficient body of research

is available on Alzheimer's disease to indicate that retirement from driving is an inevitable endpoint for most patients (Carr et al. 2006; Meuser et al. 2006). Individualized assessment is necessary to determine when retirement is prudent on a per-case basis. Psychiatrists (as well as other physicians) should encourage dementia patients and their families to review transportation needs and actively plan for driving cessation to occur within 1–3 years, or sooner if individual circumstances warrant more immediate action.
- When safety concerns are identified, psychiatrists should refer demented patients for on-road driving evaluation and use other referral options to support the assessment and retirement planning process. Not all communities have such referral options, however, and referral to the state authorities may be the only viable option in some cases.
- For those who demonstrate intact driving skills, repeat evaluations are suggested on a yearly basis until the inevitable decision to retire must be made (see discussion in Duchek et al. 2003).
- Driving is a complex task involving many individual and environmental variables that cannot be assessed fully or controlled. The determination of a safety risk due to medical or psychiatric health is a clinical activity involving reasoned judgment based on available data. This can be challenging when conflicting data exist, and the American Medical Association recognizes that thoughtful professionals can disagree.
- In terms of legal protection, psychiatrists and other physicians who act in the best interests of their demented patients, encourage reasoned decision making concerning driving safety, and document their actions should be protected from liability if a patient causes an accident. As a recent position statement of the American Academy of Neurology points out, however, this is a gray area for all practicing physicians today due to differences in state laws and imperfect evaluation methods (Bacon et al. 2007). For physicians aware of a driving fitness problem in a demented patient, the riskiest course from legal and ethical standpoints would be to do nothing. Each physician should be aware of the specific reporting laws in his or her state and request legal counsel for any policy or practice in regard to reporting clientele.
- Ultimately, it is the responsibility of state government (or other governmental entities outside of the United States) to evaluate and de-license drivers in response to medical fitness or other safety concerns. A few states, such as California, mandate that persons diagnosed with Alzheimer's disease be reported (California Department of Motor Vehicles Health and Safety Code, Section 103900), but most

make reporting a voluntary process. Psychiatrists and other physicians can do their part by facilitating reasoned decisions about driving in their demented patients and formally reporting those who refuse to stop driving when the time has come. See the American Medical Association's (2003) *Physician's Guide* for a review of laws in all 50 states and suggestions for how to make a report.

Case Example 4

Mrs. Burns has very mild Alzheimer's disease (CDR 0.5) and lives by herself in a rural area. Her closest family member lives an hour away and visits weekly to check on her well-being. Her family handles all of her finances and housekeeping and sets up her weekly pillbox to assist with medication administration. Mrs. Burns and her family report that her driving ability remains unimpaired. Her daily routine is to drive into town 3 miles to socialize and to have her main meal of the day. Her friends do not drive, and visiting them requires her to operate a motor vehicle. In addition, she is reluctant to leave the home she has enjoyed for the past 30 years.

Case Example 5

Mr. Young has moderate Alzheimer's disease (CDR 2) and lives with his wife in a suburban area. Mrs. Young has never driven. They go out regularly to run errands, shop, go to restaurants, and visit friends and family. Mrs. Young has vetoed all recommendations that Mr. Young have a driving performance test, because they would then be isolated if he should fail. She states that he drives well, but she does add that she has to tell him where to turn and when to stop.

In both cases, the family believes the person with dementia to be a safe driver. In the first case, the family is aware of Mrs. Burns' driving and supportive of it continuing. We are led to assume that no on-road incidents or problems have occurred. These should be inquired about by the clinician.

This cannot be assumed in the case of Mr. Young, however, because his wife clearly has secondary motives for keeping him on the road. At the moderate stage of disease, he is past the critical period for driving-related assessment and retirement planning. The fact that she must serve as his "copilot," prompting him on where to go, is another concern. In this case, unless Mr. Young's driving ability can be confirmed through an on-road evaluation, it may be necessary to submit a report to the state Department of Motor Vehicles. A viable alternative transportation plan could help ease Mrs. Young's concerns about isolation. Should Mr. Young refuse to stop driving, some creative efforts may be necessary to stop his driving altogether. Such efforts may include filing down his ignition key or disabling the car so that it is inoperable. Just having a car in the driveway may satisfy some patients, especially those with more advanced memory loss. The vehicle could also be sold.

Disturbances in Consciousness

Two neurological conditions involving sudden, unpredictable loss of consciousness are seizures and narcolepsy. Other conditions with loss of consciousness, such as syncope and sleep apnea, create similar concerns about driver safety, but this discussion is limited to neuropsychiatric conditions. A seizure can occur once in a lifetime or it can be recurrent, depending on the etiology. An underlying neurological disorder as well as electroencephalographic abnormalities predicts seizure recurrence (Berg and Shinnar 1991). Epilepsy by definition involves recurrent loss of consciousness and the function of other faculties, depending on the nature of the disorder. Most states in the United States withhold or withdraw the epileptic person's license until a specific period of time has elapsed without a seizure. The length of this seizure-free period varies between states and ranges from 3 months to 2 years (Dobbs 2005). While the epileptic is at risk for a seizure, other activities to be avoided include operating heavy machinery, swimming, being in the immediate vicinity of an open fire or a body of deep water, and other obviously perilous situations.

Falling asleep behind the wheel is thought to be a common cause of vehicular accidents. Narcolepsy and sleep apnea are of special concern because sudden attacks of drowsiness and sleep are not easily controlled by those afflicted. Narcolepsy symptoms include catalepsy, hallucinations, and sleep paralysis. Emotions can induce a spontaneous loss of muscle strength known as catalepsy, which, in addition to "sleep attacks," puts the narcoleptic driver at risk. A narcoleptic individual should not drive as long as the risk of sudden sleep remains. The Canadian Medical Association (2000) recommends no vehicular driving if a cataleptic episode has occurred within the past 12 months.

Legal Duties of Clinicians to Prevent Vehicular Crashes

The common law principle of non-responsibility to third parties would normally protect a clinician for liability when her or his patient harms another in a crash. After all, clinicians should not be responsible for all that their patients do, intentionally or accidentally. In a number of cases, however, appellate courts have upheld causes of action against physicians, even for harm inflicted on third persons, if the physician should have taken some reasonable preventive measure (Felthous 1989a).

This liability is more likely to occur if the patient/offending driver had been hospitalized and then released or discharged with incomplete symptom control. In *Tarasoff*-like jurisprudence, such cases can be classified as involving the "foreseeable rule," where the crash can reasonably be anticipated even if the other specific individual victims cannot be identified in advance (see Felthous 1989b).

In *Schuster v. Altenberg* (1988) the Supreme Court of Wisconsin upheld a claim wherein the driver, Edith Schuster, was a psychiatric outpatient with manic-depressive illness. She was killed in the accident, and her daughter was left with both legs paralyzed. Causes of action included negligent diagnosis and treatment, failure to seek civil commitment, and "failure to warn the patient's family of her condition and its dangerous implications" (p. 4). *In dicta*, the court equated warning the patient with treating the patient: "Warning a patient of risks associated with a condition and advising the patient as to appropriate conduct constitutes treatment as to which the physician must exercise ordinary care" (p. 6). The court's approach to this case raises the question of which disorders would require such a warning (Felthous 1989b). Today, despite the *Schuster* decision, it is not likely that the standard of practice would be to warn bipolar patients generally of the risk of driving once they are deemed safe enough to be treated as outpatients.

Clinicians have a duty to inform their patients about material side effects of the medicines they prescribe. This can include the potential side effect of drowsiness and a warning not to drive or operate heavy machinery until the patient becomes accustomed to the drug and aware of its effects. If the patient is not so informed, takes the prescribed sedating or otherwise mind-altering drug, and then, because of the drug's side effect, loses control of his or her vehicle, resulting in an accident, the physician can be held liable for injuries that the patient sustained from the accident or, in some jurisdictions, injuries inflicted on others.

An oft-cited case example of this type of liability with corresponding legal duty of the clinician to inform the patient is *Gooden v. Tips* (1983). The plaintiff, who was struck and injured, argued that the physician who prescribed Quaalude was negligent for failing to warn her against driving while taking this medicine. The holding for the Court of Appeals of Texas found the petition to be sufficient. Likewise, in *Kirk v. Michael Reese Hospital and Medical Center* (1985), an Illinois court found that such a duty to warn a patient of adverse effects of a medication can "extend to cover members of the public who may be injured as a proximate cause of the failure to adequately warn" (p. 911).

If the patient already knows of the risk, however, liability may not necessarily extend to a prescribing physician who did not give such a warning. A psychiatrist and psychologist in Connecticut were sued with the claim that they failed to warn a patient not to drive her vehicle while she was taking medication that altered her sleep cycle (*Weigold v. Patel* 2004). The medication caused her to fall asleep at the wheel, it was claimed, and to strike another car, resulting in the death of the other driver. Because the driver/patient knew that her driving was impaired, she, not her treaters, created the proximate cause by driving anyway. The clinicians could not control the patient's behavior, and therefore their failure to warn the patient not to drive was not the proximate cause of the victim's death. The court concluded that the psychiatrist and psychologist had no duty to warn the patient not to drive.

Regardless of what jurisdictional law requires in the way of informing patients of the side effects of medication and the risk of driving when sedated, such information is reasonable to convey. By the same token, the benefits of a medicine should also be shared with patients, including the likelihood that a medication or combination of medicines can improve driving performance. Psychotically disorganized patients can be expected to be at greater risk for an automobile accident because of their mental disorder. Antipsychotic medicines improve symptoms of psychosis and disorganized thinking, and thus driving competence should also be restored. Anticipating the sedative potential of antidepressant medications, pharmaceutical companies include warnings of driving risk in the package inserts of many such agents. Yet empirical evidence demonstrates that when depressed patients are treated with antidepressant medication, their driving competence and safety parameters improve (Ärzte-Zeitung 2007).

Clinicians have also been held liable for failing to diagnose a condition that could risk a vehicular crash and for not informing the patient of the risk. In Iowa, a driver lost control of a vehicle during a seizure and ran into a pedestrian. The injured pedestrian sued the driver's physician, claiming failure to diagnose the seizure, to determine its cause, to advise the patient not to drive, and to warn the patient of the risk associated with driving. Moreover, it was claimed that the physician negligently assured the driver that he could drive. On appeal, the Supreme Court of Iowa held that the plaintiff's petition with the above claims stated a cause of action against the physician (*Freeze v. Lennon* 1973).

Conclusion

It is impossible to estimate the number of vehicular crashes attributable to a mental or neurological disorder. Crashes are generically and colloquially referred to as "accidents" even when the cause of apparent human error is unknown. A death from a gunshot wound will be investigated as a possible homicide, suicide, or accident, but so many vehicular crashes appear to have been accidents that, beyond determining alcohol and drug levels, in many cases greater scrutiny and suspicion are unlikely to accurately distinguish intentional from accidental crashes after the fact. Yet mental health clinicians have, at least from experience, knowledge of suicidal or homicidal thoughts, preparation and acts involving motor vehicles, and psychological and neurological deficits that can result in a vehicular crash.

For psychiatrists and psychologists inexperienced in evaluating driving competence, preventing vehicular crashes may be an unwelcome but necessary challenge, especially where progressive dementia is concerned. This aspect of risk management has received far less attention than, say, the clinician's legal duty to warn or protect in regard to a patient's risk of harming others following a threat. Even when such a risk is first registered by a serious verbal threat, clinicians regard themselves as service providers to individuals, not protectors of the public. Yet clinicians must routinely make interventional decisions, such as whether to hospitalize (involuntarily when this is needed and justified), based on apparent risk of harm to self or others. The movement away from hospital treatment toward community treatment has probably increased, not decreased, the risks of mentally and neurologically disordered individuals being involved in vehicular crashes. Independent of such public policy changes, the demographically aging population, with far more demented and otherwise disordered drivers in the future, increases the magnitude of the challenge.

Clinicians are expected to conduct competent diagnosis and risk assessment for personal violence, which should include potential for intentional violence with a motor vehicle. Management of such risks can be handled as is done for violence risk management when, for example, a firearm is involved: with education and counseling; hospitalization if mental disorders and risk are acute; proper treatment; alliance and cooperation with significant others; reduced access and driving exposure; and selection and titration of specific risk control measures needed by the patient. When the risk is due to a neurological condition with impaired driving abilities or risk of disturbed consciousness, some gross attempt to rate the risk is recommended: low risk, educational measures; high risk, interventional restrictive measures (e.g., a responsible family member secures the car keys); intermediate risk, refer for neuropsychological and/or driving competency assessment. For specific legal reporting duties, clinicians should refer to controlling jurisdictional law.

Key Points

- Medications are double-edged swords: they can impair or improve driving competence, depending on how they are used.
- Risk assessment interviews should be informed by the possibility of suicide or homicide by vehicular crash.
- For patients with Alzheimer's disease, it is not a matter of *if* retirement from driving should occur but *when*.
- Laws or protective duties for clinicians regarding the risk of vehicular crashes are variable and jurisdiction-specific.

References

American Medical Association: Physician's Guide to Assessing and Counseling Older Drivers. Chicago, IL, American Medical Association, 2003

American Psychiatric Association: Role of the Psychiatrist in Assessing Driving Ability: Position Statement (APA Document Reference No. 930004). Approved by the Board of Trustees, December 1993, Approved by the Assembly, November 1993. Washington, DC, American Psychiatric Association, 1993

American Psychiatric Association: Position statement on the role of psychiatrists in assessing driving ability. Am J Psychiatry 152:819, 1995

American Psychiatric Association: Practice guidelines in the treatment of Alzheimer's disease. Am J Psychiatry 154(suppl):1–39, 1997

Ärzte-Zeitung: Autofahren Klappt bei Depressiven mit Antidepressiva besser als ohne, 2007. Available at http://www.aerztezeitung.de/docs/2006/02/03/020a0401.asp?cat=/medizin/depression-65K-. Accessed January 24, 2006

Austroads: Assessing Fitness to Drive. Austroads Guidelines for Health Professionals and Their Legal Obligations. Sydney, Australia, Superline Printing, 1998

Bacon D, Fisher RS, Morris JC, et al: American Academy of Neurology position statement on physician reporting of medical conditions that may affect driving competence. Neurology 68:1174–1177, 2007

Berg AT, Shinnar S: The risk of seizure recurrence following a first unprovoked seizure: a quantitative review. Neurology 41:965–972, 1991

Brown LB, Ott BR: Driving and dementia: a review of the literature. J Geriatr Psychiatry Neurol 17:232–240, 2004

California Department of Motor Vehicles Health and Safety Code, Section 103900. Available at http://www.dmv.ca.gov/pubs/vctop/appndxa/hlthsaf/hs103900.htm. Accessed January 23, 2008

Canadian Medical Association: Determining Medical Fitness to Drive: A Guide for Physicians. Ottawa, Canada, Canadian Medical Association, 2000

Carr D, Duchek J, Meuser T, et al: The older driver with cognitive impairment. Am Fam Physician 73:1029–1034, 2006

Dobbs BM: Medical Conditions and Driving: A Review of the Literature (1960–2000). Washington, DC, National Highway Traffic Safety Administration, 2005

Dubinsky RM, Stein AC, Lyons K: Practice parameter: risk of driving and Alzheimer's disease (an evidence-based review). Report of the Quality Standards Subcommittee of the American Academy of Neurology. Neurology 54:2205–2211, 2000

Duchek JM, Carr DB, Hunt LA, et al: Longitudinal driving performance in early stage dementia of the Alzheimer type. J Am Geriatr Soc 51:1342–1347, 2003

Felthous AR: The duty to warn or protect to prevent automobile accidents, in Review of Clinical Psychiatry and the Law, Vol 1. Edited by Simon RI. Washington, DC, American Psychiatric Press, 1989a, pp 221–238

Felthous AR: The Psychotherapist's Duty to Warn or Protect. Springfield, IL, Charles C Thomas, 1989b

Felthous AR: Personal violence, in Forensic Psychiatry. Edited by Simon RI, Gold L. Washington, DC, American Psychiatric Publishing, 2006, pp 471–500

Freeze v. Lennon, 210 NW.2d 576 (1973)

Gooden v. Tips, 651 SW.2d 364 (Tex. App. 1983)

Hunt LA, Murphy CF, Carr D, et al: Environmental cueing may effect performance on a road test for drivers with dementia of the Alzheimer type. Alzheimer Dis Assoc Disord 11(suppl):13–16, 1997

Kirk v. Michael Reese Hospital and Medical Center, 483 NE.2d 906 (Ill. App. 1 Dist. 1985)

Meuser TM, Carr DB, Berg-Weger M, et al: Driving and dementia in older adults: implementation and evaluation of a continuing education project. Gerontologist 46:680–687, 2006

Morris JC: The Clinical Dementia Rating (CDR): current version and scoring rules. Neurology 43:2412–2414, 1993

Naidu v. Laird, 539 A.2d 1064 (1988)

Schuster v. Altenberg, Wisconsin Supreme Court, No. 87–0115, 1988

Wang C, Carr D: Older driver safety: a report from the Older Drivers Project. J Am Geriatr Soc 52:143–149, 2004

Weigold v. Patel, 840 A.2d 19 (Conn. App. 2004)

Recommended Readings

Felthous AR: The duty to warn or protect to prevent automobile accidents, in Review of Clinical Psychiatry and the Law, Vol 1. Edited by Simon RI. Washington, DC, American Psychiatric Press, 1989, pp 221–238

Meuser TM, Carr DB, Berg-Weger M, et al: Driving and dementia in older adults: implementation and evaluation of a continuing education project. Gerontologist 46:680–687, 2006

CHAPTER 27

School Violence

Carl P. Malmquist, M.D., M.S.

In dealing with school violence, one persistent impression is of confusion and overlap in defining the topic. Some confine it to high schools, whereas others include middle schools as well as violence at the college level. A second source of confusion is that some restrict the discussion to lethal violence, whereas others include all levels of nonfatal victimization, including violations of school discipline. The focus of violence presents a third complication. Some focus on students as the victims of violence, ranging from those who restrict the topic to mass levels of violence with multiple victims to those who focus on a single episode with one perpetrator and one victim. However, faculty and nonstudents may also be victims. A fourth difficulty in defining the topic is variations in the scope of violence. If the violence occurs on the playground during school hours, it would likely be included, but not necessarily if it occurs after school hours or involves students driving away from school in cars. A fifth source of difficulty is that the categories of individuals involved can be a mixture: students as victims and perpetrators, nonstudents in the school as perpetrators, ex-students, outside adults, and so on.

What these situations suggest is that the data on school violence, let alone the reported incidence of crimes, may often be underestimated and unreliable. This would hold not only for data from law enforcement agencies but also that from school systems, which may not regularly report such data to the public. Some school systems report "student crime" to state departments of education, but there is a lack of consistency within districts and states. Although part of this may be poorly functioning systems, there may also be an element of trying to minimize such data to protect the image of school districts. The National Research Council and Institute of Medicine (2003) used the following criteria for lethal school violence: taking place in or associated with schools, committed by students of the school, and resulting in multiple victimizations in a single incident. Note that this approach is narrowed to students committing lethal acts, but it does not specify which level of schools (such as colleges or lower grades), and the incident can be either in or "associated with" schools.

Assessment of the Extent of School Violence

Background

Violence in school settings is not a new phenomenon. Historical evidence reveals it existed in ancient civilizations back to 2000 B.C.E. Thereafter, four types receive mention: rebellious clashes, focused anger with an agenda, student protests, and random acts of violence (Midlarsky and Klain 2005). Nor is it only recently that students brought weapons to schools. Interestingly, school violence became more widespread in the United States after compulsory education was adopted. By 1900, 31 states had made education compulsory, with the goal of disseminating "Americanism," and saw an accompanying increase in violence (Crews and Counts 1997).

During the economic depression in the 1930s, school violence was minimal, but after 1950 the momentum accelerated. Students became active in social movements and in various protests, such as those concerned with school segregation and racial equality. In the 1960s, clashes over civil rights, racism, and the Vietnam War were reflected in school violence. The period from 1964 to 1968 saw the number of assaults on teachers increase from 253 to 1,801, and weapons offenses in schools increased from 396 to 1,508 (Beavan 1970). Diverse ideas arose as to why different types of violence occurred in schools, varying from a macro perspective on communities to a focus on individual predispositions, and looking at issues such as the use of corporal punishment (in schools and at home), bullying, violence in the community, weapons availability, media violence, use of psychoactive substances, and personality difficulties.

Current Situation

In 1977 the federal government published a revealing study on school crime (National Institute of Education 1977). It found that although teenagers spend only 25% of their time in school, 40% of robberies and

36% of physical attacks on them occurred there. A 1995 survey of students ages 12–18 years reported 2.5 million students were victims of some type of crime at school. Serious crimes accounted for 186,000 victims in schools (through rape, aggravated assault, sexual assault, and robbery); 47 of these resulted in school-associated deaths, including 38 homicides (Kaufman et al. 2001).

The U.S. Department of Education and the U.S. Department of Justice conduct an annual survey reported as "Indicators of School Crime and Safety." They draw on a variety of sources, such as national surveys of students, teachers, and principals, and data collected from federal departments and agencies. The 2006 report indicated that in the school year 2005–2006 for youths ages 5–18 there were 28 school-associated violent deaths—21 homicides and 7 suicides—and 48 school-associated deaths when staff and nonstudent school associates were included—37 homicides, 9 suicides, and 2 legal interventions (Dinkes et al. 2006).

Data from the "Indicators" report for all school-age youth during the 2003–2004 academic year indicated 1,418 overall homicides, with 19 occurring at school, and 1,282 suicides, with 3 occurring at school. From 1992 through the 2004–2005 school years, the range was from 11 to 34 homicides at school per year. Any year with a mass school shooting elevates the incidence for that year. It is often stressed that homicides of school youths are more frequent outside of school than in school. The limitation of such a statistic is that children spend only 6–7 hours at school, 5 days a week, for 8–9 months compared with the entire remaining time period outside school in a year. Interestingly, the annual survey for 2004 found students ages 12–18 experienced about 1.4 million "nonfatal" crimes at school, which included 583,000 violent crimes (simple assault and serious violent crime) and 863,000 thefts—a victimization rate of 33 thefts and 22 violent crimes per 1,000 students.

Larger schools are more likely to have violent incidents and to report them to police than are smaller ones. Secondary schools are also more likely to do so than the lower grades. Ninety percent of schools with more than 1,000 students report a violent incident. Similarly, urban districts are more likely than rural or suburban districts to experience crime and make reports to police. A contrast is that rampage school shootings, although much rarer, are likely to occur in suburban or rural settings.

The Centers for Disease Control and Prevention (CDC; 2008) has analyzed data from the School-Associated Violent Death (SAVD) study. The SAVD study dealt with "school-associated" student homicides: those occurring in public or private elementary and secondary schools, on the campus or on the way to or from classes or school-sponsored events. The study found 116 school-associated homicides of students, associated with 109 homicide events, from July 1999 through June 2006. Seventy-eight percent of the homicides occurred on school campuses. A reported 65% included gunshot wounds, 27% included stabbings or cuttings, and 12% included beatings, indicating some overlap. The report noted that although homicide is the second leading cause of death among those ages 5–18 years in the United States, school-associated homicides represent less than 1% of all homicides of school-age children. A major limitation of the SAVD study is that the cases were identified from news media reports, which would result in underestimation.

Bullying

Bullying is cited so often as a link to school violence, if not shootings, that it merits a detailed discussion. Some go so far as to argue that if bullying were dealt with, school violence would be dealt with as well. Given the American school system, this is not likely to happen. A problem is that bullying encompasses a large number of students, which includes many acquiescent observers. The "Indicators" report defined victimization by bullying as including 1) being made fun of, called names, or insulted; 2) being subjected to rumors; 3) being threatened with harm; 4) being pushed, shoved, tripped, or spit on; 5) being made to do things one does not want to do; 6) being excluded from activities or a group on purpose; and 7) purposeful destruction of property. Some would restrict its meaning to repeated, negative acts by a child or group against another. Although the acts may be physical, the usage encompasses verbal taunts or manipulative behavior to exclude others. Implicit is a power game that is played out with different scenarios.

Surveys of students reveal that 16% of children say they have been bullied during a current school term, and about 30% of sixth- through tenth-graders say they have been involved as a bully or a target (Nansel et al. 2001). Adverse consequences of such behavior, reported on both sides, include more physical and psychological problems, persistence in the role of victim, a shift from victim to perpetrator, and problems with self-esteem and depression (Van der Wal et al. 2003). The causal relationship between school bullying and psychopathological behavior has been debated in terms of which comes first. Psychopathological behavior, such as social problems, aggression, and externalizing behavior problems, may be the consequence of bullying experiences rather than the cause (Kim et al. 2006). Explanations for bullying are also being sought from neuroscience research involving limbic activation, varying levels of autonomic arousal, and temperamental variations from integrity of prefrontal/executive regulatory capacities (Sugden et al. 2006).

School Violence

Newman (2004) employed a social causation model for school shootings, utilizing multiple sources of information. Rampage shootings in schools were explained in terms of boys feeling inferior in existing school hierarchies, especially when their masculinity was threatened. Newman also posited movies, television, music, and news reports as "scripts" for how masculinity can be asserted. Widespread availability of guns and the increasing inability of school administrators to identify and assist disturbed or troubled youths were also noted. This failure is parallel to the ineffectual procedures in courts and communities trying to deal with disturbed youths. There is also the problem of bullying in those school settings where adult supervision is minimal, such as at recess or on playgrounds.

Court decisions also limit the discipline and authority of public school personnel. Inability to share information among schools, social agencies, and the police due to confidentiality and privacy restrictions is a factor. There is a catch-22 in that school administrators are legally restricted in responding to student misbehavior, yet may be sued by parents of victims for failing to respond to early warning signals. Of course, the key question that remains is whether cognizance of bullying and other disturbing behavior can predict violence and lead to intervention so that serious violence or killing will not occur.

Notable Cases of School Shootings

There are a host of cases of school shootings, and each could merit a discussion or book on its own. These cases reveal a diversity that calls into question any attempt to create a profile from factors such as being a loner, being a bully, or being bullied. Below is a list of recent highly publicized cases, followed by a discussion of three in more detail.

1. *1996, Lynville, Tennessee:* A teenager fired a rifle in a school hallway, killing a teacher and a student.
2. *1996, Moses Lake, Washington:* A junior high school student on the honor roll used a high-powered rifle to shoot and kill two students and a math teacher.
3. *1997, Pearl, Mississippi:* A 16-year-old boy killed his mother and then went to his high school, where he shot and killed two students and wounded seven.
4. *1997, Paducah, Kentucky:* A 14-year-old opened fire with a .22-caliber pistol on a prayer group in the lobby of his high school, killing three students and wounding five.
5. *1998, Edinboro, Pennsylvania:* At an eighth-grade graduation party,

a 14-year-old shot and killed a science teacher and wounded another teacher and two students.
6. *1998, Fayetteville, Tennessee:* During graduation week, an 18-year-old honor student shot a classmate in the school parking lot because the victim was dating the shooter's ex-girlfriend.
7. *1998, Jonesboro, Arkansas:* Two boys, ages 11 and 13 years, set off a school fire alarm and then shot at students who were exiting the building, killing four students and a teacher and wounding ten.
8. *1998, Springfield, Oregon:* A 15-year-old killed his parents at home, then went to his high school, where he killed two people and wounded twenty.
9. *1999, Notus, Idaho:* A tenth-grader came to school with a shotgun and blasted it in the hallway.
10. *1999, Littleton, Colorado:* Two high school students at Columbine High School shot and killed twelve students and one teacher and wounded twenty others before committing suicide.
11. *1999, Conyers, Georgia:* A month after Columbine, a 15-year-old did a copycat shooting, wounding six students with a .22-caliber rifle after twelve shots. He then pulled out a .357 magnum, fired three more shots, and put the handgun in his mouth but hesitated and was taken into custody.
12. *2000, Mount Morris Township, Michigan:* A 6-year-old shot a girl in his first grade class when they quarreled.
13. *2001, Santee, California:* A boy said to be bullied shot and killed two students in the schoolyard.
14. *2003, New Orleans, Louisiana:* Four teenage gang members in a gang-related event shot and killed a 15-year-old and wounded three other students.
15. *2003, Cold Spring, Minnesota:* A 15-year-old shot and killed one student and wounded another at his high school.
16. *2003, San Diego, California:* There were two consecutive school shootings in one year by marginalized and socially ostracized shooters (Palinkas et al. 2003).
17. *2004, Washington, D.C.:* During a confrontation between students, one student was shot to death in their high school.
18. *2005, Red Lake, Minnesota:* A 16-year-old boy on an Indian reservation shot and killed his grandfather and the grandfather's companion and then proceeded to his high school, where he shot and killed a security guard, a teacher, and five students and wounded seven other students.
19. *2006, Nickel Mines, Pennsylvania:* A 32-year-old male milk delivery truck driver killed five Amish schoolgirls and injured five others in an execution-style killing in a one-room schoolhouse.

20. *2007, Blacksburg, Virginia:* A 23-year-old college student at Virginia Polytechnic Institute and State University shot and killed 32 students and faculty and then committed suicide. This was classified as the worst peacetime shooting in U.S. history.

Although such lists are revealing, they provide almost no knowledge of what motivated the killings and the background scenario. Because many of the actors committed suicide, it is often an ex post facto attempt to reconstruct the situation relying on media sources, relatives, and past medical/psychological records if these are made available. Appraisal of three well-known cases illustrates the diversity.

Focused Discussion of Three Diverse Cases

Columbine

The shootings at Columbine High School in Littleton, Colorado, by Eric Harris, age 18, and Dylan Klebold, age 17, in April 1999 garnered nearly endless publicity (Malmquist 2006). In their shooting spree, 12 students and one teacher were killed, and 20 students were left wounded. Planning had begun up to a year beforehand. One bomb was planted a few miles away as a diversionary tactic. Other bombs were placed in cans to discharge while the boys were in the school, but these failed to go off. Upon arriving at school on the day of the killings, the boys had two 20-pound propane bombs that they planted in the cafeteria, but only one went off.

The onset of the shooting was in the school parking lot, where two students were killed and eight wounded. Observers reported that the two boys were yelling "Go! Go!" upon entering the school. Later, there was an exchange of fire with the police. A teacher who spotted the boys was shot in the back and killed. The boys proceeded to the second floor, shooting along the way, and then entered the library, where one student was killed. Intended victims were first taunted. The boys then returned to the cafeteria and tried to detonate the failed bomb, which only caught on fire. The finale occurred back in the library, where the boys exchanged gunfire with law enforcement before both committed suicide by gunshots to the head.

Investigation revealed that their goal had been to kill hundreds and to be remembered as the greatest mass murderers of all time. An FBI analysis did away with several myths connected to the shootings (Cullen 2004). Some of the myths were that they were targeting athletes and Christians, that they were part of a "trench coat Mafia" group, and that they were outcast Goths. The fact is that they were out to have the highest possible body count, and no one was specifically targeted.

The shootings were not impulsive, nor did they appear to be an act of revenge against students and teachers per se, except in the sense that the victims were now under their control, vulnerable and helpless. Investigation revealed that the boys resented the possibility that they might later be seen as "petty school shooters." To avert this, the goal was to amass the largest possible number of deaths, and if the bombs had been wired correctly, about 600 deaths would have occurred. In terms of personality characteristics, the two were quite different. Klebold was hotheaded, depressed, and suicidal. Harris had more psychopathic traits—"nice" on the surface but actually cold, calculating, and homicidal. He was described as someone who took pleasure in lying and was contemptuous of others. Without Harris, it is doubtful that Klebold alone could have carried out such a mission.

Jonesboro, Arkansas

In a quite different type of case, Andrew Golden, age 11 and in sixth grade, and Mitchell Johnson, age 13 and in seventh grade, carried out a partnership shooting at Andrews Middle School on March 24, 1998. Much of the background material on this event is taken from the case study by the National Research Council and Institute of Medicine (2003). The outcome was four students and one teacher dead and nine students and one teacher wounded. Just after recess, Andrew was seen by other students pulling the handle on the fire alarm and exiting the school. Students responded to the alarm and marched outside to the playground.

On a hillside 100 yards away, the two boys, dressed in camouflage shirts, opened fire. Police arriving at the top of the hill 10 minutes later were stunned by how young the shooters were. When apprehended, the boys had 11 guns (Remington rifles, Smith and Wesson pistols, derringers, and semiautomatics) and several hundred shells that belonged to Andrew's father and grandfather. The shooting clearly had been planned, because they had a van full of provisions, including sleeping bags and pillows, a load of junk food, and a map to a remote hunting area where they planned to hide.

The boys had driven to the school area in Mitchell's stepfather's van, which Mitchell barely knew how to handle. Nine weeks earlier they had planned what to do if it was raining and students did not come out to the playground if there was a fire alarm drill. Ballistics reports revealed that Mitchell killed at least one but probably two people and wounded at least three. Andrew, a more skilled shot, fired 25 shots, killing three and wounding at least two others in the course of 5 minutes. Although all but one of the victims shot were female, it remains conjectural whether anyone was specifically targeted.

Many students did not know that the two boys knew each other beyond a casual level. Mitchell had arrived in Arkansas only 2 years earlier after being raised in Minnesota, where his parents had gone through a heated divorce. His mother was a correctional officer, and after the divorce she first took a job in a federal prison in Kentucky. Two sons were born in the marriage: Mitchell and a younger brother. Prior to the divorce Mitchell's father was described as a hard drinker, a disciplinarian, mean-tempered, and explosive. In addition, when Mitchell was 8 years old, an older boy had begun to rape him, and later his younger brother, repeatedly. The mother married again for a third time to a man who had served prison time on a drug charge, but they had settled down and the family was living in a trailer camp.

Mitchell presented a mixed picture. Some saw him adjusting well as a new student, being polite and singing in a church choir. However, his dark side was seen in belligerent, boastful, and bullying behavior. A few weeks before the shooting he had been disciplined for wearing a baseball cap in school. He was both furious about this and unrepentant. He wrote a paper stating he had some squirrels he wanted to kill, which led the teacher to give the paper to the school principal. Although adults saw Mitchell as a troubled boy, his peer group saw him as a moody boy with a temper who was seeking some place in the social pecking order.

Andrew Golden was younger, but about half of the people interviewed saw him as the leader. He came from a gun-owning family, the guns used were from his family, and he was a marksman. An only child, he was seen by others as belligerent, although his parents saw him as doing no wrong. School behavior was erratic, varying from class clown to "chip off the old block," similar to the way his father had been at the same school as a boy.

Psychiatric reports on the two boys described Andrew as the more troubled, and in contrast to Mitchell, he never spoke to anyone about the incident, nor did his family. Observations in the juvenile facility where the boys resided for several years after the trial reflect wide differences. Mitchell was cooperative, repentant, and liked by staff; Andrew remained silent and kept to himself. An insanity defense was raised for Andrew, but the court ruled a juvenile was not entitled to such a defense, a decision upheld by the Arkansas Supreme Court. Because the boys were not yet 14 years of age, they could be detained only until they reached 21, which left many in the community incredulous.

Virginia Tech

There have been earlier notable cases of lethal violence at a college level that are sometimes ignored in discussions of "school shootings" (Simon 1996). Charles Whitman at the University of Texas in 1966 killed his wife and mother and then, from a tower on the campus, shot 13 people to death and wounded 31 others before he committed suicide. Gan Lu, an astrophysicist at the University of Iowa, shot and killed a physics professor and a rival who won an award Lu had hoped to receive; he then killed five other faculty members and wounded another person before committing suicide. In 1993 Wayne Lo, an 18-year-old student at Simon's Rock College in Massachusetts, used a high-powered assault rifle to kill a professor in his car and a student in the library and then wounded four others. Perhaps it is stretching school shootings to include Ted Kaczynski, the Unabomber, but he was a one-time college professor who sent bombs through the mail that killed 3 persons and wounded 23 others over 17 years. The victims were either university professors or worked in technology.

The mass killing at Blacksburg, Virginia, on April 16, 2007, by a 23-year-old college student is a recent picture of a troubled young male who stumbled along until the fatal day. Seung-Hui Cho murdered 32 people and wounded 17 and then committed suicide, in the worst peacetime shooting in American history. Many factors remain elusive. That morning he went to a dormitory and killed a male and female student whose selection remains a puzzle. Cho then mailed off a manifesto to NBC News with pictures of himself posing with guns and video clips and making a rambling verbal attack on wealthy people. In an essay found in his room, he blamed practically everyone except himself for what he was doing—women, religion, the wealthy, debauchery, and "deceitful charlatans" ("The Virginia Tech Massacre" 2007).

Almost a 2-hour gap occurred before Cho then appeared in a classroom building half a mile away. He locked the doors with chains so that those inside could not escape and proceeded into various classrooms, trying to kill everyone in them with two semiautomatics: a Glock 9 mm and a Walther P22. Those who survived said he was silent as he went about shooting students and faculty at close range, putting two or three bullets in each to make sure they died. When police burst into the building, he shot himself.

Before any name was released by officials, some classmates guessed that the shooter was Cho. He had rarely spoken to anyone, referred to himself as "Question Mark," hid behind sunglasses, and was seen as intimidating. In a creative writing class, the themes of his papers involved money, fury, sex, religion, and overbearing adults. In 2005, two female students complained to police that Cho was stalking them but did not press charges. At that time a district court found him "mentally ill and an imminent danger to self and others," but he never received any treatment. His situation later exposed the flaws in a labyrinthine mental health system (Schulte and Jenkins 2007). A court had committed him for "involuntary outpatient commitment," which exists in many states as a category of civil commitment. The problem is in the follow-up and the lack of clarity as to who assumes responsibility for ensuring that the individual receives treatment. Is it the court system, some agency, or the individual himself? In Cho's case, no one assumed responsibility.

Discussion

There is a distinction between the pervasive problem of "school violence" and lethal school (rampage) shootings. The former is closer to the problems of juveniles with ongoing conduct problems and is the more classic picture of juvenile offenders in which a subset become violent. Social and family disorganization are relevant. Lethal school shootings present a different set of problems. Attempts are often made to create profiles from these rampage killers' characteristics, such as being a loner and avoiding people, or to propose psychiatric diagnoses in retrospect. A major limitation is that such profiles include a great many youths with personality characteristics and social difficulties similar to those of the few who carry out such acts.

Consider the contrasting personalities of Golden and Johnson in their joint act at Andrews Middle School in Arkansas, or contrast them with that of Cho at Virginia Tech. A major obstacle to knowledge about school killers is the lack of psychiatric and psychological data on the perpetrators, either because they have committed suicide or because such data are kept private. Hence, our knowledge is often based on newspaper reports or police statements. One approach tried to systematize such offenders within four operant styles: adaptive, conservative, integrative, and expressive (Fritzon and Brun 2005). The *adaptive* offender targets specific individuals; the *conservative* is affected by an external trigger in which self-esteem is threatened; the *integrative* targets others whom he identifies with his internal conflicts, and then commits suicide; and the *expressive* is randomly violent.

The U.S. Secret Service developed a profile of 41 school shooters from 37 school incidents (Vossekuil et al. 2000). The most frequent motive was revenge, with about three-fourths of the perpetrators threatening suicide before an attack. Although the report concluded there was no evidence the shootings were the result of a mental disorder, the perpetrators were described as feeling extremely depressed or desperate. Two-thirds felt persecuted, and three-fourths were dealing with a major change in a relationship or a loss of status.

This profile was consistent with a report by Meloy et al. (2001) of adolescent mass murderers (not all in schools) in which a precipitating event of personal loss or status threat had occurred. In 75% of the cases, the shooters had communicated threats beforehand. The report emphasized bullying and the frequent motive of revenge. McGee and DeBernardo (1999) described 12 shooting incidents in middle and high schools of "classroom avengers." Again it was stated the shooters did not show overt signs of a mental disorder, yet had a significantly depressed mood. On reviewing these reports, the depression theme recurs often enough to raise the question of whether those in contact with adolescents are sufficiently adept at detecting depressive states.

An FBI report focused on the "myths" connected to school shootings (O'Toole 2000). Among the myths examined were links to revenge, anger about being bullied, unresolved anger about other matters, gun availability in the homes of the perpetrators, the impact of violent video games, and being a loner. The study argued against the idea that the shooters shared these attributes. The debate as to whether the shooters were mentally ill or had "mental problems" continued to intrude in all these studies. Although the brooding ruminations of Cho suggest a serious mental illness, other shooters may simply be referred to as having a prominence of strong emotions whose ascendancy takes over their decision making.

The FBI focus was on threat assessment, and they employed the concept of "leakage." The student intentionally or unintentionally "leaks" a cry for help by way of feelings, thoughts, fantasies, or intentions about an impending violent act. The clues may be subtle threats, boasting, innuendoes, or predictions that can appear in stories, diaries, essays, letters, and drawings. The leakage may involve "jokes" about violence or destruction that are then retracted with "I was just joking." At times there are efforts to get friends or classmates to help with preparations for a violent act.

A troublesome question deals with unshared information that was available in the communities before such shootings. If such suspicions are shared, a question arises as to how wide the sharing should be. A retrospective study of 253 school-associated violent deaths in the United States found more than half the perpetrators had signaled the future event by notes, threats, or journal entries (Anderson et al. 2001). However, unless we opt for a society with a norm of routinely inform-

School Violence

ing on each other, with every suspicion being investigated within schools or by some agency, looking for and sharing such information is not likely to be a practical solution, especially given adolescents' devotion to secrecy.

In response to public concern about school shootings, Congress asked the National Research Council of the Institute of Medicine to study school shootings that had occurred in a 2-year period (National Research Council and the Institute of Medicine 2003). Shootings in urban and suburban communities were distinguished. Shootings in an urban environment involved grievances between individuals known in their communities. In the suburban milieu there was an overall low level of crime and violence, with the boys being seen as alienated, associating with delinquents, and having a recent change in behavior, unrecognized mental health problems, and easy access to guns. In five of the six communities studied, there had been rapid social change, with parents and teachers having a poor understanding of the impact this had on adolescents. The study report emphasized that understanding school shootings requires recognizing a conjunction of three things: a person with some predisposing potential for violence, a situation with elements that create a risk of violent events, and, usually, a triggering event. The emphasis was on using a narrative approach for an explanation of particulars and societal structural factors that make violence more likely. Focusing on situational factors, perhaps altering one link in the chain of events could have deflected the ultimate act.

Prevention

None of the measures proposed in this section will eliminate the occasional rampage homicidal shooting in schools. However, it is possible that intervention at earlier stages might head off problems that could eventuate in serious school violence. Such primary prevention of shootings could operate silently if intervention is successful. Two overriding policy questions arise with increased preventive efforts. One is whether families and children are willing to lose some liberties by greater intrusions into their lives when the payoff may be low. The second is whether the public is willing to assume the additional costs that such measures require.

A striking feature of writings on prevention of "school violence" is the contrasting emphasis by those in clinical fields compared with those in education. Clinically oriented writers focus on serious assaultive episodes, whereas educators are more concerned about the daily prevalence of various types of violence that intrude on educational processes.

Educators' concerns are with the patterns of victimization that permeate some schools, such as thefts, verbal abuse, bullying, vandalism, fights, punching, grabbing, and sexual taunts. Prevention in this context means a school milieu where students and faculty are not assaulted and do not live in a state of fear. Tracking is difficult and often subjective, so the focus is on physical acts.

Diverse attempts to control such actions have had varying degrees of success. Students with conduct disorders or emerging personality disturbances may be referred for medications or taught cognitive-behavioral techniques to foster better self-control. Alertness to detect students with interpersonal difficulties related to various types of violence is important. The linchpin is screening for susceptible students with whom to intervene and having the right personnel available to connect. Even then, as in psychotherapy, some students resist participation. Similar difficulties arise when troubled students end up in court proceedings that are plagued by loopholes and by inadequate follow-up if therapeutic approaches are ordered, as occurred with Cho.

Various interventions are being tried, such as social skills training, anger management, empathy training, and training in moral reasoning. Some schools have introduced conflict resolution programs, but these are based on the assumption that students want to be safe and free from conflict; the reality is that in some schools, carrying a gun or being willing to fight is not only seen as masculine but as a way to be safe.

Similar dilemmas arise in programs intended to control bullying. One assumption is that asking students and faculty not to go along with bullying will get a positive response and that those in authority will take action in confronting such behavior. If those in authority do not respond, or prefer other solutions, the student is left doubly exposed—from the bullying itself and the failure of responsible adults (Hunter et al. 2004). A dual approach is needed, which means intervening with the bully and supporting the victim. Failure often reflects a lack of application and enforcement from a majority of the participants. In some schools, prevention may have to include guarding the school entrance. Metal detectors have become an approach in such settings, with school security checking bathrooms, monitoring groups loitering near the school, and using video surveillance devices. An extension of this approach has been legislation prohibiting possession of a weapon within so many feet of school property.

Conclusion

Those who work with adolescents and families have knowledge of what may prevent some violence in schools. To what extent various risk factors are dealt with so that some future act of violence is thwarted may never be known. It is often a matter of trying to intervene with a focus on risk factors (MacNeil 2002). An important area of potential risk is the adolescent's social environment, such as income level, availability of drugs and alcohol, and family disorganization. A second area is the psychological and neuropsychiatric aspects of an individual in terms of impulse control, beginning conduct problems, and possible psychiatric disorders. A third area of risk focuses on the psychological milieu of the adolescent. This includes family conflict, inconsistent or overly harsh punishments, and failing or changing educational performance.

The key is connecting with those adolescents most in need of intervention and then taking action and involving people with sufficient expertise. In cases like Columbine, Jonesboro, and Virginia Tech, the trouble was in either no one detecting the individual or too many people ignoring what they saw and heard. An approach of trying to predict who might engage in a mass shooting is wasteful because it bypasses approaches that may thwart such a later outcome. It may be helpful to zero in on high-risk students for intervention, first through implementing better sharing of records and ideas within school systems and among teachers, then by extending this to clinicians and the juvenile justice system. As noted, this approach necessitates caution about violations of privacy and also requires a sensitive person in charge to exercise wise judgment in sharing information about students.

Key Points

The following preventive measures are recommended to lessen the likelihood of school violence:

- Increased security measures—more security officers, metal detectors, electronic devices, and photographic devices in and around schools
- Greater sensitivity to signs and symptoms that indicate a troubled student, or one communicating harm, such as by "leakage." This is superior to attempts to profile "school shooters."

- Better training for teachers in normal and abnormal adolescent psychology
- Availability of competent professional personnel to assess, and possibly treat, students seen as needing assistance
- Greater sharing of records among schools, police, courts, and community agencies, which requires clarification of roles and confidentiality issues
- Efforts to counter the "macho" or hypermasculine milieu that permeates many schools, based on an athletic culture and bullying, by offering rewards for other models and activities; this should involve inquiry into a student culture where bullying is tolerated by the majority.
- Zero tolerance in schools not only for weapons but also for behavior such as pushing, shoving, and intimidation. Threats raise issues of free speech.
- Better integration among schools, courts, and mental health facilities for follow-through to avoid the type of situation that occurred with Cho at Virginia Tech

References

Anderson M, Kaufman J, Simon TR, et al: School-associated violent deaths in the United States, 1994–1999. JAMA 286:2695–2702, 2001

Beavan K: School violence on the increase. New York Times Educational Supplement, February 12, 1970, p 16

Centers for Disease Control and Prevention: School-associated homicides—United States, 1992–2006. MMWR Morb Mortal Wkly Rep MMWR 57(2):33–36, January 18, 2008

Crews GA, Counts MR: The Evolution of School Violence in America. Westport, CT, Praeger, 1997

Cullen D: The depressive and the psychopath: at last we know why the Columbine killers did it. Slate, April 20, 2004. Available at http://slate.msn.com/id/2099203. Accessed April 20, 2004

Dinkes R, Cataldi EF, Kena G, et al: Indicators of School Crime and Safety: 2006. U.S. Departments of Education and Justice. Washington, DC, U.S. Government Printing Office, 2006

Fritzon K, Brun A: Beyond Columbine: a faceted model of school-associated homicide. Psychology, Crime and Law 11:53–71, 2005

Hunter L, MacNeil G, Elias M: School violence: prevalence, policies, and prevention, in Juvenile Justice Sourcebook. Edited by Roberts AR. New York, Oxford University Press, 2004, pp 101–125

Kaufman P, Chen X, Choy S, et al: Indicators of School Crime and Safety, 2001. Washington, DC, U.S. Government Printing Office, 2001

Kim YS, Leventhal BL, Koh Y, et al: School bullying and youth violence. Arch Gen Psychiatry 63:1035–1041, 2006

MacNeil G: School bullying: an overview, in Handbook of Violence. Edited by Rapp-Paglicci I, Roberts AR, Wodarski J. New York, Wiley, 2002, pp 247–261

Malmquist CP: Homicide: A Psychiatric Perspective. Washington, DC, American Psychiatric Publishing, 2006

McGee JP, DeBernardo CR: The classroom avenger: a behavioral profile of school based shootings. The Forensic Examiner 8:16–18, 1999

Meloy JR, Hempel AG, Mohandie K, et al: Offender and offense characteristics of a nonrandom sample of adolescent mass murderers. J Am Acad Child Adolesc Psychiatry 40:719–728, 2001

Midlarsky E, Klain HM: A history of violence in the schools, in Violence in Schools: Cross-National and Cross-Cultural Perspectives. Edited by Denmark F, Krauss HA, Wesner RC, et al. New York, Springer, 2005, pp 37–57

Nansel T, Overpeck M, Pilla R: Bullying behavior among U.S. youth: prevalence and association with psychosocial adjustment. JAMA 285:2094–3100, 2001

National Institute of Education: Violent Schools, Safe Schools: The Safe Schools Study Report to the Congress, Vol 1. Washington, DC, U.S. Government Printing Office, 1977

National Research Council and Institute of Medicine: Deadly Lessons: Understanding Lethal School Violence. Edited by Moore MH, Petrie CV, Braga AA, et al. Washington, DC, National Academies Press, 2003

Newman KS: Rampage: The Social Roots of School Shootings. New York, Basic Books, 2004

O'Toole ME: The School Shooters: A Threat Assessment Perspective. Quantico, VA, Critical Incident Response Group, National Center for Analysis of Violent Crime, 2000

Palinkas LA, Prussing E, Landsverk J, et al: Youth-violence prevention in the aftermath of the San Diego East County school shootings: a qualitative assessment of community explanatory models. Ambul Pediatr 3:246–252, 2003

Schulte B, Jenkins CL: Cho didn't get court-ordered treatment. Washington Post, May 7, 2007, p A01

Simon RI: Bad Men Do What Good Men Dream: A Forensic Psychiatrist Illuminates the Darker Side of Human Behavior. Washington, DC, American Psychiatric Press, 1996

Sugden SG, Kile SJ, Henderson RL: Neurodevelopmental pathways to aggression: a model to understand and target treatment in youth. J Neuropsychiatry Clin Neurosci 18:302–317, 2006

Van der Wal M, Cees AM, Hirasing R: Psychosocial health among young victims and offenders of direct and indirect bullying. Pediatrics 111:1312–1317, 2003

The Virginia Tech massacre. The Economist, April 21, 2007, pp 27–29

Vossekuil B, Reddy M, Fein R, et al: Safe School Initiative: An Interim Report on the Prevention of Targeted Violence in Schools. Washington, DC, U.S. Secret Service, 2000

CHAPTER 28

Clinically-Based Risk Management of Potentially Violent Patients

Robert I. Simon, M.D.

The goal of violence risk management is to eliminate or decrease the chance of another person's injury or death resulting from actions by a patient, as well as the potential legal liability. Risk management principles usually represent ideal or best practices, whereas the legal standard of care requires only the provision of ordinary or reasonable, prudent care (Simon 2005). Risk management decisions based solely on the clinician's defensive desire to avoid malpractice liability or to provide a defense against a malpractice claim can increase liability exposure by engendering worst practices.

Clinically-based risk management principles are patient centered, supporting the treatment process and the therapeutic alliance (Simon 2004). Clinically-based risk management upholds the ethical principle of "first do no harm." A working knowledge of the legal regulation of psychiatry assists the practitioner in managing clinical-legal dilemmas that frequently arise in the treatment and management of potentially violent patients, while also preventing disruption of the doctor–patient relationship.

Defensive practices can be divided into the preemptive and the avoidant. *Preemptive practices* utilize procedures and treatments aimed at preventing or limiting liability—for example, hospitalizing a patient at low to moderate risk of violence who could be effectively treated as an outpatient. *Avoidant practices* forego necessary procedures or treatments based on the fear of being sued, even though the potentially violent patient would benefit from the interventions—for example, failing to involuntarily hospitalize a litigious patient at high risk for violence who is refusing voluntary hospitalization, or involuntarily hospitalizing a patient primarily as a risk management measure.

Potentially violent patients frequently confront the clinician with complex diagnostic, treatment, and management issues, most often in outpatient, inpatient, and emergency department settings. They can also create judgment-numbing anxiety in the clinician. Consultation with a colleague is always an option. The clinician should "never worry alone" (T.G. Gutheil, personal communication, December 2002). Consultation supports good clinical care while also providing a "biopsy" of the standard of care. Clinically-based risk management puts the patient's well-being first, avoiding defensive practices that can harm both the patient and the clinician.

Some of the issues that potentially violent patients present to the clinician are illustrated in the following hypothetical case.

Case Example

Dan, a 36-year-old married man, enters treatment with a psychiatrist for depression, insomnia, and anxiety. His symptoms arise from longstanding marital strife. The psychiatrist agrees to see the patient once a week for psychotherapy and medication management. Within a month after beginning treatment, Dan begins to suspect that his wife is having an affair. He finds "racy" e-mails sent to his wife by a coworker. A near-violent confrontation occurs. She adamantly denies having an affair. He leaves the home, goes to a hotel, and calls his psychiatrist.

The patient's psychiatric condition rapidly worsens over the next week. He is unable to sleep. He ruminates about killing his wife. He admits to having guns at home. The psychiatrist sees the patient more frequently, adjusts medications, and explores Dan's potential for violence toward his wife. Dan has a history of violent rages, although he has never harmed his wife or anyone else. He intends to break into his house, get his guns, and threaten to kill his wife.

The psychiatrist informs the patient that psychiatric hospitalization is necessary. The patient refuses. The psychiatrist performs and documents a careful violence risk assessment, which indicates that Dan is at acute, high risk for violence. If he does not enter the hospital voluntarily, the psychiatrist will be forced to involuntarily hospitalize him. Dan reluctantly agrees to hospitalization. With his permission and in his presence, the psychiatrist calls Dan's wife and informs her of the violent threats by her husband. She is not surprised. She is told that Dan is going directly to the hospital. The locks on her house are changed. A security system is installed after she speaks with the police.

The psychiatrist tells Dan's wife to remove all guns and ammunition from the home and secure them in a place unknown to the patient. She is asked whether guns might be kept in a car, at work, or anywhere else. The psychiatrist asks for a callback from the patient's wife once the guns and ammunition are removed, which he receives within an agreed-upon time.

Dan shows rapid improvement while on the psychiatric unit. He is seen daily by his psychiatrist. His medications are adjusted. The treatment team provides valuable input regarding the patient's behaviors. No violent outbursts or threats occur. Depression and agitation moderate.

With the patient's approval, the psychiatrist arranges for a meeting with the patient and his wife together on the inpatient unit. With the psychiatrist present, Dan is able to express his anger appropriately and safely. His wife openly expresses her disappointments with the marriage, stating that she has had the entire burden of caring for their three children. The meeting is very emotional but frank and productive. The psychiatrist recommends marital counseling, which both accept. They continue to talk by phone.

After performing and documenting a careful violence risk assessment, the psychiatrist determines that Dan's risk of violence is now low. As agreed upon during the inpatient meeting, the doctor and the patient will inform the patient's wife about the date and time of discharge. Dan agrees to enter the hospital's partial hospitalization program on the day after his discharge. The couple remains separated.

Initially, the psychiatrist sees Dan three times a week to ensure stabilization of his condition. Dan and his wife continue marital therapy. By mutual agreement, the couple have no other direct contact with each other. The patient is grateful for the psychiatrist's care during the crisis. The therapeutic alliance is strengthened.

Outpatients: Duty to Warn and Protect

In *Tarasoff v. Regents of the University of California* (1976), the California Supreme Court recognized that a duty to protect third parties from patient violence was imposed only when a special relationship existed between a foreseeable victim, the individual whose conduct created the danger, and the defendant. A doctor–patient relationship creates a special relationship that supports a duty to exercise reasonable care to protect others from a patient's acts of violence. In most states, a psychotherapist has a duty, established by case law or statute, to act affirmatively to protect an endangered third party from a patient's violent or dangerous acts. Although some courts have declined to find a *Tarasoff* duty in a specific case, a number of courts have recognized some variation of the original *Tarasoff* duty. Very few courts have limited or rejected the *Tarasoff* doctrine (*Evans v. United States* 1995; *Green v. Ross* 1997). Most courts have not found a duty to warn or protect absent a foreseeable victim.

The *Tarasoff* court did not use the phrase "imminent danger." "Imminent" appears frequently in the mental health literature. It is common parlance among clinicians. It is also a legal term of art found in civil commitment statutes; in duty to warn and protect statutes and case law, usually under the rubric of dangerousness; and in seclusion and restraint policies. "Imminence" of violence is another word for the short-term prediction of violence, for which no standard of care exists. "Imminent" violence should not be a substitute for comprehensive violence risk assessment. It is a myth firmly entrenched in both psychiatry and the law (Simon 2006).

Clinicians have found that the duty to protect provides more latitude for treatment interventions than the original duty-to-warn doctrine. Except in states with immunity statutes limiting the responsibility of therapists for the patients' violent acts, no hard-and-fast rules have been created requiring clinicians to employ specific interventions to warn and protect endangered third parties. In jurisdictions where no duty to warn or protect currently exists, case law from other states may be applied in deciding suits that allege such a duty.

Generally, courts have held that the therapist's control over an outpatient is not sufficient to establish a duty to protect without a foreseeable victim. In treatment of an outpatient, the *Tarasoff* duty applies when there is evidence, through either threats or acts, that the patient is potentially violent to a specific, foreseeable victim. The dangers must be substantial, involving serious bodily harm or death. If no threats or violent acts are uncovered after careful clinical evaluation, liability is unlikely even if violence should occur.

The duty to warn does not obviate implementing other clinical interventions that may be more effective. Simply warning an endangered third party is rarely sufficient by itself. Other clinical interventions are usually required—for example, seeing the patient more frequently, adjusting medication, or hospitalization.

When the clinician decides to issue a warning, the warning should take place, if possible, in the presence of the patient and with the patient's consent. In an emergency, however, the clinician does not need the patient's consent. With few exceptions, a legal problem arising in psychiatric treatment can be successfully addressed through good clinical practice and a clear understanding of the relevant legal requirements. Thus, warning should be used after other clinical interventions have been tried and failed or in conjunction with other clinical interventions.

Generally, if the clinician decides to warn, an interview may be arranged or a phone call made so that the potential victim can ask questions. Language difficulties between the clinician and the endangered person may contribute to tragic consequences unless detected and clarified. Sometimes, a trusted bilingual third party may act as a go-between. The warning should be made clearly.

How a warning is given is the crucial factor (Simon and Shuman 2007). When the clinician discusses the warning with the patient prior to giving it, the result for therapy and the alliance can be positive. Not discussing the warning with the patient usually turns out badly for the therapeutic alliance and the therapy. Warning a potential victim of patient violence must be done with discretion. If the potential victim feels that evasive action can be taken and that the therapist is genuinely concerned and acting responsibly, the warnings are received positively. When a potential victim sees no options for evasion and the therapist is perceived as not behaving responsibly, a profound negative reaction can occur. The threatened individual may take preemptive violent action against the patient.

With the advent of e-mail and the teleconference, clinicians are treating and managing psychiatric patients at a distance. Treating a patient by e-mail or teleconference creates a doctor–patient relationship with an unabridged duty of care. Active case management of a potentially violent patient should not be attempted in this mode. An in-person, face-to-face examination of the patient is necessary.

In the duty to warn and protect endangered third parties from patient violence, a number of risk management steps should be considered (see Table 28–1).

Inpatient Discharge

Although the *Tarasoff* duty was originally applied to the outpatient setting, the same legal duty to protect individuals and society from harm by mental patients arises for the release of violent inpatients. Generally, the duty to warn is of narrower scope than the duty not to discharge a violent patient. In outpatient cases that involve failure to warn and protect an endangered third party, the threat of violence is serious, violence is foreseeable, and usually the victim is identifiable. The duty not to discharge a violent inpatient has a broader scope because the patient may not express specific threats toward persons or groups, thus posing a threat to the general public. In hospital discharge cases, the clinician's duty extends beyond that owed to readily identifiable victims. Psychiatrists face greater liability exposure for the release of potentially violent hospital patients than in outpatient cases alleging a *Tarasoff* duty (Simon 1992).

In inpatient release cases, the courts have held that there is a duty to control, with or without a foreseeable victim. The duty to evaluate the

TABLE 28–1. Duty to warn and protect: risk management

- Perform and document comprehensive violence risk assessments that inform treatment and management interventions. Evaluate and document effectiveness of interventions.
- Perform violence risk assessments at critical junctures (e.g., on admission to and discharge from an inpatient unit; when making outpatient decisions to warn and protect).
- Violence risk assessment is a process, not an event. Document each risk assessment.
- Obtain prior patient records. Courts have held clinicians responsible for not knowing important information contained in the patient's prior records.
- Document decision-making rationale and risk-benefit assessment (e.g., risks and benefits of continued outpatient treatment versus risks and benefits of hospitalization).
- Consult with another clinician and/or attorney when confronted by clinical-legal uncertainty in the management of a potentially violent patient.
- Issue appropriate warnings to potentially endangered third parties, if clinical interventions fail. Warnings should be issued even when the endangered third party is aware of the potential violence by the patient.
- Avoid reflexive warning that can harm the patient by unnecessarily breaching confidentiality and exposing the patient to a preemptive act of violence by the endangered third party. Also recognize that warning, by itself, is usually insufficient.
- Hospitalize—voluntarily or involuntarily—patients at acute, high risk for violence, whether or not an individual or the general public is endangered.
- Implement clinical interventions, including involuntary hospitalization, in the best interest of the patient and for the safety of others, rather than as a defensive action to avoid perceived liability.
- Consider first the duty to protect, rather than the duty to warn, allowing the practitioner to exercise clinical options that also preserve patient confidentiality. It may be necessary to invoke both options.

patient for the risk of violence according to usual professional standards would obviate a *Tarasoff* duty because the continued high risk of violence would require further hospitalization. Litigation involving release of potentially violent patients who harm others will turn on whether the clinician was negligent in evaluating the patient prior to discharge. If the court releases a patient deemed dangerous by the clinician, the clinician should go on record with his or her concern about the patient's potential for violence. The judicial decision to release insulates the psychiatrist from liability (Simon and Shuman 2007).

Risk management principles applicable to discharge from an inpatient facility are noted in Table 28–2.

Clinically-Based Risk Management

TABLE 28–2. Patient discharge from inpatient facilities: risk management

- Obtain records of previous treatments and hospitalizations. The past is prologue.
- Document thoroughly the decision-making process regarding discharge planning (e.g., note risks and benefits of continued hospitalization versus risks and benefits of discharge).
- Systematically assess and document the patient's risk of violence, including the treatment and management interventions informed by the violence assessment. Evaluate the effectiveness of interventions.
- Conduct violence risk assessments regularly to determine the current level of risk. Violence risk assessment is a process, not an event. Document each risk assessment.
- Consider obtaining a consultation from a clinician and/or attorney regarding complex clinical-legal issues surrounding the discharge of patients at risk for violence.
- Utilize input from the treatment team in discharge decision making. The staff has observed and treated the patient 24 hours a day, 7 days a week.
- Inform the person previously threatened by the patient of the patient's impending discharge. The warning should be made even when the clinician is certain that the person is aware of the patient's discharge and the potential danger.
- Arrange a meeting with the patient's spouse, partner, and family (if available) to discuss issues relating to the patient's impending discharge. Preferably, significant others should be seen individually initially to determine if a meeting is workable. Determine if significant others will support or destabilize the patient.
- Structure after-care planning for maximal adherence to treatment by the patient.
- Patients should be seen for outpatient treatment as soon as possible after discharge. Patients should be provided written instructions regarding postdischarge treatment and management.
- Discuss with the patient who to contact or where to go for help, if he or she fears a loss of control over violent impulses. Provide resources and telephone numbers. Be sure that the telephone numbers are correct.
- Do not discharge patient solely based on denial of insurance benefits or for other financial reasons.
- Educate the patient and significant others about the patient's mental disorder and the necessity for continued treatment.
- Involuntarily hospitalize patients at acute, high risk for violence who refuse voluntary hospitalization.

Patients With Access to Guns

All patients at risk for violence must be asked if there are guns at home or easily accessible elsewhere, or if they intend to purchase a gun. Patients who have a gun at home usually have more than one gun. Persons with guns in the home are at greater risk of dying from a homicide than those without guns in the home (Dahlberg et al. 2004). Gun safety management requires a collaborative plan between the clinician, the patient (if possible), and a designated person responsible for removing guns from the home. The designated person should be told that all guns must be removed, even if he or she does not believe the patient will use a gun to harm others. Denial may doom the gun removal plan.

A callback to the clinician from the designated person is requisite to confirm that guns and ammunition have been removed and secured according to the agreed-upon plan. Verification is essential to gun safety management. The verification principle in gun safety management applies to outpatients, inpatients, and patients evaluated in emergency departments, although its implementation may vary according to the clinical setting. Document the gun removal plan and verification (Simon 2007; see also Table 28–3).

Documentation

Documentation is an essential part of good patient care. It encourages the clinician to sharpen clinical focus and to clarify decision-making rationale (Simon 2004). The record is an active clinical tool, not just an inert document. The clinician treats the patient, not the chart. Documentation is a risk management measure that also supports good clinical care.

For patients at risk for violence, it is necessary to document clinical interventions and the rationale for clinical decisions. Documentation should specifically address what was done, the reason(s) for doing it, and the rationale for rejecting alternative interventions and treatment (Slovenko 2002). Violence risk assessment should be contemporaneously documented. If a malpractice claim is made against the psychiatrist, contemporaneous documentation assists the court in considering the many clinical complexities and ambiguities that exist in the assessment, treatment, and management of patients at risk for violence.

Clinically-Based Risk Management

TABLE 28–3. Gun safety management

- Ask patients at risk for violence about guns at home or elsewhere (e.g., car, office, or workplace). Patients who have a gun at home usually have more than one gun.
- Consider invoking the emergency exception to consent (see Chapter 21) if a patient who is at high risk for committing violence toward others withholds consent to contact the patient's significant others.
- Designate a willing, responsible individual, usually a family member or partner, to follow through with the gun removal plan as instructed by the clinician. The patient should be included in gun safety planning, if possible.
- Confirm that all guns and ammunition were separated and removed from the home and safely secured in a location unknown to the patient. There is no safe storage at home.
- Obtain a callback from the responsible, designated person confirming that the gun(s) and ammunition have been removed and safely secured.
- Document that the gun removal plan was implemented by the designated individual and that a callback was received from that individual confirming the removal of guns according to the plan.
- Verification is the essence of gun safety management. Merely asking a significant other to remove the gun(s) from the home without a confirming callback can end tragically. Family members may not follow through with removal of gun(s) from the home due to denial and for other reasons (see Simon 2007).

Key Points

- Clinically-based risk management principles are patient centered, supporting the treatment process and the therapeutic alliance. Unduly defensive risk management practices based on the clinician's fear of being sued or the need to provide a legal defense if sued may subvert good patient care and invite a lawsuit.

- Risk management principles usually represent ideal or best practices. The legal standard of care requires only the provision of ordinary or reasonable care.

- No standard of care exists for the prediction of violence. There is no research that supports the ability of the clinician to predict who will or will not be violent. The purpose of violence risk assessment is to identify treatable and modifiable risk and protective factors that will inform the clinician's treatment and management of the patient.

- The clinician's treatment and management of the potentially violent patient often requires a team approach that includes significant others, as well as consultation with other mental health professionals, inpatient staff, lawyers, law enforcement officials, and the judicial system. Never worry alone.

- The duty to protect endangered third parties from patient violence should be considered a national standard of care for all mental health professionals.

- A working knowledge of the legal regulation of psychiatry assists the practitioner in managing the clinical-legal dilemmas that often arise in treating and managing potentially violent patients, while also preserving the doctor-patient relationship.

- Active case management of a potentially violent patient should not be attempted by e-mail or video conference.

- Documentation is an essential aspect of good patient care and clinically-based risk management.

References

Dahlberg LL, Ikeda RM, Kresnow MJ: Guns in the home and risk of violent death in the home: findings from a national study. Am J Epidemiol 160:929–936, 2004

Evans v. United States, 883 F.Supp 124 (5D Miss. 1995)

Green v. Ross, 691 502d.542 (Fla. App. 1997)

Simon RI: Clinical Psychiatry and the Law, 2nd Edition. Washington, DC, American Psychiatric Press, 1992

Simon RI: Assessing and Managing Suicide Risk: Guidelines for Clinically Based Risk Management. Washington, DC, American Psychiatric Publishing, 2004

Simon RI: Standard of care testimony: best practices or reasonable care. J Am Acad Psychiatry and Law 33:8–11, 2005

Simon RI: The myth of "imminent" violence in psychiatry and the law. Univ Cincinnati Law Rev 75:631–644, 2006

Simon RI: Gun safety management with patients at risk for suicide. Suicide Life Threat Behav 37:518–526, 2007

Simon RI, Shuman DW: Clinical Manual of Psychiatry and Law. Washington, DC, American Psychiatric Publishing, 2007

Slovenko R: Psychiatry in Law/Law in Psychiatry. New York, Brunner-Routledge, 2002

Tarasoff v. Regents of the University of California, 17 Cal. 3d 425, 131 Cal. Rptr. 14, 551 P.2d 334 (1976)

Index

*Page numbers printed in **boldface** type refer to tables or figures.*

AA (Alcoholics Anonymous), 155
AASI (Abel Assessment of Sexual Interest), 71–72
Abandonment, 330
    fear of, among elderly persons, 382, 385
    purposeful, targeted, defensive violence in reaction to, 171
    targeted, impulsive violence in reaction to, 172
    violence related to perception or fear of, 177–179
Abel Assessment of Sexual Interest (AASI), 71–72
Acamprosate, for alcoholism, 153
Access of patient
    to potential victim, 7
    to weapons, 6, 372, 373, 557
Acetaldehyde, 153
Acetaldehyde dehydrogenase, 153, 154
Acetylcholine, in Alzheimer's disease, 399
Acquaintance stalkers, 412, **414**
Acquired immunodeficiency syndrome (AIDS), 196, 489
Active listening, 468
Actuarial violence risk assessment, 3–4, 17–31, 46, 59. *See also* Structured violence risk assessment
    compared with clinical risk assessment, 3–4, 17–21, **28**
    on continuum of structure, 17–18
    implications for clinical intervention, 19
    in outpatient settings, 237–238
    psychological testing and, 59–60
    reliance on static risk factors, 19
    role of clinical judgment in, 18
    of sexual offender evaluation, 70
    time frame for validity of, 18–19

Acute confusional state, 197
Acute dystonic reaction to lorazepam and haloperidol, 302, 305, 309
Addiction, 149–155. *See also* Substance abuse disorders
    definition of, 149
    as disease, 155
    identification of, 151–152
    media dramatization of, 151
    modafinil for patients with, 150
    neurobiology of, 149
    treatment of, 152–155
        in elderly persons, 399
        evidence-based strategies for relapse prevention, 152
        patient–treatment matching for, 155
        pharmacological, 152–154
        psychotherapy, 154–155
        12-Step facilitation therapy, 155
        12-Step programs, 152, 155
Addiction (television series), 151
ADHD (attention-deficit/hyperactivity disorder), 150, 374
    conduct disorder and, 369
    Tourette's syndrome and, 195
Adolescents, 359–376
    adaptive functions of aggression in, 211
    antidepressant effects on suicide risk in, 90
    attention-deficit/hyperactivity disorder in, 369
    bullying and, 361, 540–541, 545
    conduct disorder in, 360, 363, 369
    controlling access to weapons, 372, 373
    dating violence among, 361–362
    depression in
        abuse or neglect and, 79–80

Adolescents *(continued)*
  depression in *(continued)*
    bullying and, 79
    deliberate self-harm and, 87
    maternal depression and, 78
    passive exposure to domestic violence and, 78
    as predictor of violence, 83
  developmental trajectories toward violence in, 362–364, **363**
  differences between violence in adults and, 360, **361**
  epidemiology of violence among, 360–362
  gangs and, 359, 362, 365, 375
  gender and violence among, 359, 360–361
  homicide rates in, 359, 362
  inhalant use by, 9
  intermittent explosive disorder in, 216
  juvenile justice system for, 359, 367–368
  management of violence in, 372–376
    acute management of high-risk youth, 373
    consultation, 375–376
    environmental interventions, 375
    outpatient psychosocial treatment, 373–374
    pharmacotherapy, 374–375
    waiving juveniles to adult court, 375
  mental health interventions for, 359–360
  myths about youth violence, 37
  passive exposure to parental violence, 78
  peer effects and violence in, 363, 364, 365, 375
  prevalence of violence among, 359, 360–362
  Psychopathy Checklist–Youth Version for, 62
  rehabilitation of, 367
  risk factors for violence in, 364–365, **366**, 370
  school violence and, 79, 359, 365, 371, 537–552
  self-injurious behaviors among, 225–226
  substance abuse among, 364, 369–370
  Surgeon General's report on youth violence, 37
  violence among, 11, 22, 23
  violence risk assessment in, 365–372
    consent and confidentiality for, 367–368
    dimensions of, **367**
    formulating a risk assessment, 372
    history of violence, 368–369
    for predatory violence, 370–372
    psychiatric diagnosis, 369–370
    risk factors and risk assessment scales, 364–365, **366,** 370
    setting for, 366–367
    weapon assessment, 372
Adoption studies, 364
β-Adrenergic blockers, 200, **203**, 316
Affect management, 463, 465, 467–468
Affective recognition, 330
Affective regulation disorders, in elderly persons, 392–394
African Americans, 35
  alcohol-related intimate partner violence among, 145
  arrests for aggravated assaults, 37
  culturally appropriate assessment in psychiatric setting, 46
  culturally appropriate assessment of intimate partner violence in, 52–53
  myths about youth violence among, 37
  overdetermination of dangerousness, 38
  risk for violence or homicide, 37
  seclusion and restraint of, 38
  serial killing by, 38
  women
    spiritual/religious support for, 81

Index

as victims of intimate partner violence, 80, 81
Aftercare, 13, 14
Age. *See also* Adolescents; Children; Elderly persons
　at first violent episode, 35
　suicide risk and, 89
　violence risk and, 11, 22, 23
Aggression
　adaptive functions of, 211
　anger and, 212
　antidepressant effects on, 84
　biology of
　　in mood disorders, 92–93
　　serotonin, 92–93, 215
　bipolar disorder and, 83, 84
　categories of, 212
　continuum of severity of, 211–212
　definition of, 68, 212
　dementia and, 185–187
　depression and, 83, 84
　drug-induced, 9
　hostility and, 212
　impulsivity and, 68, 211–228 (*See also* Impulsive aggression)
　instruments for assessment of, 68
　intent and, 212
　neurochemistry of, 215–216
　pharmacotherapy for, 84–85, 253–254, 301–318
　premeditated, 212–213, 262, 312
　psychotherapy for, 325–337
　schizophrenia and, 10
　serotonin transporter polymorphisms and, 93
　as stress management strategy in animal models, 211
　theoretical models of, 212–213
Aggression Questionnaire, 68, 212
　Anger subscale of, 67
　Hostility subscale of, 68
Aggression replacement strategies, 201
Agitation, 5
　brain tumors and, 194
　cocaine-induced, 9, 198
　de-escalating emotion in patients exhibiting, 265

in dementia, 186–187
emergency psychiatric services for, 279–280, 284–285
inpatient assaults and, 260
medication-induced, 198
pharmacotherapy for, 84–85, 253–254, 301–318
after traumatic brain injury, 187, 188
AIDS (acquired immunodeficiency syndrome), 196, 489
Akathisia, 10, 198, 200, 301
　lithium for, 315
Alaska Natives
　arrests for aggravated assaults, 37
　risk for violence or homicide, 37
　substance abuse and suicidality among, 144
Alcohol Use Disorders Identification Test (AUDIT), 151
Alcohol use/abuse, 7–9, 13, 27, 141–146
　child abuse and, 144–145
　date rape and, 143
　disinhibition induced by, 9
　early-onset, 148
　elder abuse and, 145
　fetal exposure to, 213
　gangs and, 146
　genetic vulnerability to, 152
　head injury and, 149
　intimate partner violence and, 82–83, 145–146
　intoxication due to, 6, 9
　　homicide and, 142
　　vehicular crashes and, 522, 534
　neurobiology of alcohol, 143
　prevalence of, 141, 151
　psychiatric comorbidity with, 148–149
　　bipolar disorder, 85
　　intermittent explosive disorder, 85, 217
　　posttraumatic stress disorder, 133
　　pyromania, 219
　rape and, 143
　screening for, 151
　suicide and, 89, 146

Alcohol use/abuse (*continued*)
  suicide and (*continued*)
    spousal/consortial murder-suicide, 422
  treatment for dependence on, 152–155
    for at-risk heavy drinkers, 151–152
    in elderly persons, 399
    guidelines for primary care physicians, 151, 152
    patient–treatment matching for, 155
    pharmacological, 152–154
      acamprosate, 153
      disulfiram, 153–154
      naltrexone, 152–153, 399
      topiramate, 154
    psychotherapy, 154–155
    12-Step facilitation therapy, 155
    12-Step programs, 152, 155
  violence and, 107, 141–146, 250
    case examples of, 141–142
    factors associated with, 142
    mechanisms of link between, 143
  withdrawal from, 133
    benzodiazepines for, 133, 305
    delirium during, 9
    pharmacotherapy for violence during, 302
Alcohol–disulfiram reaction, 153–154
Alcoholics Anonymous (AA), 155
Alkyltin exposure, 197
Alprazolam, before care activities for elderly dementia patient, 398
Alzheimer's disease, 186–187, 382, 387, 391–392, 393–394, 397–398. *See also* Dementia
  acetylcholine deficit in, 399
  cholinesterase inhibitors for, 392, 393, 399, 402
  driving safety and, 527–531
American Academy of Child and Adolescent Psychiatry, 369
American Academy of Neurology, 527, 529

American Academy of Psychiatry and the Law, 409
American Board of Forensic Psychology, 28, 29
American Indians
  arrests for aggravated assaults, 37
  risk for violence or homicide, 37
  substance abuse and suicidality among, 144
American Medical Association's Older Drivers Project, 527–528
American Psychiatric Association
  position on driving safety, 521–522, 527
  practice guideline for posttraumatic stress disorder, 124
  recognition of structural racism, 36
  task force report on restraint and seclusion, 341–342, **342**, 343, 348
Americans with Disabilities Act, 508
γ-Aminobutyric acid (GABA), 215
Amok, 44, **45**
Amphetamine, 9, 198
Amputation of extremities, 225
Anabolic steroids, 9, 198
Androgens, 92, 448
Anger, 5, 212
  depression and attacks of, 252, 254
  distinction from hostility, 68
  instruments for assessment of, 67–68, 72
  in posttraumatic stress disorder, 124, 132, 134
  in schizophrenia, 10
Anger management programs, 25, 216
  for youth at risk for school violence, 550
Anger-excitation rapists, **416**
Anger-retaliation rapists, **416**
Anti-androgen treatment, 335, 453–455
  monitoring for adverse effects of, 454–455
Anticholinergic delirium, 198
Anticonvulsants, 84–85, 253, 303, 314–315, 334. *See also specific drugs*
  for aggressive elderly patients, 403
  for chronic aggression, 200, **203**

Index

combination treatment with
  antipsychotics, 314–315
  driving safety and, 522
Antidepressants, 384
  for aggressive elderly patients, 403
  driving safety and, 523, 524–525, 533
  effect on aggression, 84
  effect on suicide risk, 90, 92
  for psychotic depression, 285
  use on 72-hour extended
    observation unit, 287
Antipsychotics, 84, 85, 199–200, 302–314. *See also specific drugs*
  for aggressive/agitated elderly
    persons, 401–403
    acute/emergent treatment, 394–395
    administration routes for, 394, 401
    case example of, 402–403
    choice of drug for, 401
    controversy about, 403
    dosage of, 401–402
    metabolic syndrome due to, 403
    monitoring response to, 402
    risk of death in elderly dementia
      patients, 200–201, 395, 403
    side effects of, 401, 402
  anti-hostility effects of, 313
  combination therapy with mood
    stabilizers, 314–315
  driving safety and, 522, 533
  electroconvulsive therapy and, 316
  long-term treatment with, **202,** 312–314
  in psychiatric emergencies, 280, 294, 295, 302–305
    intramuscular administration of,
      303–311, **304, 306–307**
  suicidal patient, 295
  for psychotic depression, 285
  racial differences in administration
    of, 38
  second-generation, 312
  side effects of, 401, 402
    agitation, 198
    akathisia, 301–302
    use on 72-hour extended
      observation unit, 287
    for violent psychotic inpatients, 114, 253–254, 267
    for violent youth, 374–375
Antisocial behaviors
  in combat veterans with
    posttraumatic stress disorder,
    125–126
  in conduct disorder, 369
  intellectual disability and, 220
  intimate partner violence and, 491
  prenatal risk factors for, 213–214
  self-injurious behaviors and, 226
Antisocial personality disorder, 11, 13, 23, 107, 181
  conduct disorder and, 363, 369
  driving and, 522
  purposeful, instrumental violence
    and, 168–169
  purposeful, noninstrumental
    violence and, 170
  schizophrenia, violence and, 250–251
  substance abuse and, 148
  workplace violence and, 511
Anxiety/anxiety disorders
  in assault victims, 80
  intermittent explosive disorder and, 217
  rage and, 334
  self-injurious behaviors and, 226
Anxiolytics, 198
Apathy, in dementia, 393, 394
Appearance of patient, 5–6
Aripiprazole
  for aggressive elderly patients, 401
  intramuscular, **304,** 305, **307,** 310–311
    adverse effects of, 310
    combined with lorazepam, 310
    dosage of, **304,** 310
    indications for, 310
    transition to oral administration, 311
  long-term treatment with, 312–314
Armed patient, 476
Arrest reports, 5

Arsenic exposure, 197
Arsonists, 218–219. *See also* Pyromania
ASD. *See* Autism spectrum disorder
Asian Americans, 35
    arrests for aggravated assaults, 37
    culturally appropriate assessment of interpersonal violence in, 49–50
        barriers to, 50, **51**
    risk for violence or homicide, 37
Assaults
    by brain-injured patients, 187
    classification of, 109–111, 113, **264**
    on clinicians, 248–249, 254, 259, 461–478 (*See also* Violence toward clinicians)
    by elderly person on day care staff, 391–392
    ethnicity and arrests for, 37
    by inpatients, 109–118, 259–272
        on clinicians, 470
        criminal prosecution for, 269–270, **271**
        elderly persons, 383, 386
        environmental risk factors for, 114–115, 260–261
        gender and, 260
        impulsive vs. premeditated, 262
        instrumental vs. reactive, 109–110, 262–263
        long-term risk factors for, **261**
        management of, 113–118
        measures of control for, 264, **266**
        mental states associated with, 109
        motivations for, 109, 113, 261–270
        on nursing staff, 259, 263–265
        patient characteristics associated with, 109, 259–260
        prediction of, 113, 114
        prevention of, 114
        reactive vs. instrumental, 109–110, 262–263, **264**
        research on classification of, 110–111
        short-term risk factors for, 260
        staffing ratios, ward atmosphere and, 261
        threatening behaviors before, 112
        videotape recording of, 111–112, 262
    paranoia and, 107
    psychiatric disorders in victims of, 80
    psychotic, 110–111, 262–263, **264, 266–267**
        indicators of impending assault, **267**
        strategies for prevention of, 267
    by psychotic patients in the community, 116
    in schools, 539
    sexual (*See* Sexual assault/rape; Sexual violence)
    against stalking victims, 411
    substance abuse among victims of, 80, 82
    suspiciousness and, 107–108
    of "warn" category, 112
    in workplace, 506
Assertive Community Treatment, 284
Assessment instruments
    Aggression Questionnaire, 67, 68, 212
    Alcohol Use Disorders Identification Test, 151
    Balanced Inventory of Desirable Responding, 69
    Barratt Impulsivity Scale, 68–69, 72, 214, 224
    Brief Psychiatric Rating Scale, 315
    Buss-Durkee Hostility Inventory, 215, 224
    Child Behavioral Checklist, 214
    Classification of Violence Risk, 18, 23–26, **28**, 30
    Clinical Dementia Rating scale, 527
    Cook-Medley Hostility Inventory, 68
    HCR-20, 21–23, **28,** 30, 39, 46, 240–241
    InterSept Scale for Suicidal Thinking, 295
    Mental Health Triage Scale, 283

Index

Millon Clinical Multiaxial
  Inventory–3, 63, 64, 65, 163
Mini-Mental State Examination,
  285, 390, 392, 402
Minnesota Multiphasic Personality
  Inventory–2, 28, 63–65, 67, 72,
  163, 416
National Triage Scale, 283
Novaco Anger Scale, 67, 72
Overt Aggression Scale, 7, **8,** 188,
  199, 215
Paulhus Deception Scales, 69–70
Personality Assessment Inventory,
  63, 64, 65, 163
Positive and Negative Syndrome
  Scale, 313, 314
Psychopathy Checklist, 62–63
Psychopathy Checklist–Revised, 27,
  62–63, 213
Psychopathy Checklist–Youth
  Version, 62, 369, 370
Rapid Risk Assessment for Sexual
  Offender Recidivism, 29, 437
Rorschach Inkblot test, 29, 66–67, 72
Standard Family Violence Index,
  127
State/Trait Anger Expression
  Inventory, 67
Structured Assessment of Violence
  Risk in Youth, 370
Structured Guide for the
  Assessment of Violence, 285
Violence Risk Appraisal Guide, 18,
  26–27, **28,** 30
  for youth, 369, 370
Athletes, anabolic steroid use by, 9
Ativan. *See* Lorazepam
Attentional problems, assessing
  elderly persons for, 389–390
Attention-deficit/hyperactivity
  disorder (ADHD), 150, 374
  conduct disorder and, 369
  Tourette's syndrome and, 195
Attitudes
  dysfunctional, deliberate self-harm
    and, 88
  racially based, of clinicians, 36

AUDIT (Alcohol Use Disorders
  Identification Test), 151
Autism spectrum disorder (ASD), 221–
  222, 227
  case example of, 221
  in DSM, 221
  prevalence of, 221
  self-injurious behaviors and, 225
  types of aggression associated with,
    222
Autoimmune deficiency encephalitis,
  193
Available means of inflicting harm, 6–7
Avoidant personality disorder
  nontargeted, impulsive violence
    incidental to emotional escape
    and, 176
  purposeful, targeted, defensive
    violence and, 171
  targeted, impulsive violence and,
    172, 174

Balanced Inventory of Desirable
  Responding, 69
Baltimore Epidemiologic Catchment
  Area Follow-Up study, 216
Barbiturates, 198
Barefoot v. Estelle, 435–436, 437
Barratt Impulsivity Scale, 68–69, 72,
  214, 224
Bathing, of patient with dementia, 398
Battered women's syndrome, as legal
  defense, 494. *See also* Intimate
  partner violence
Beck Depression Inventory, 88
Behavioral disinhibition, 68
  alcohol-induced, 9
  benzodiazepine-induced, 317
  neurocorrelates in dementia, 187
Behavioral disturbances
  brain tumors and, 194
  in brain-injured patients, 187
  of children
    parental substance abuse and,
      78–79
    passive exposure to parental
      violence and, 78

Behavioral disturbances (*continued*)
  in dementia, 185
  in systemic lupus erythematosus, 198
  in Tourette's syndrome, 196
Behavioral Sciences Unit of the FBI Academy, 417
Behavioral treatments for aggression, 201, 204
Belligerence, 9, 106. *See also* Aggression; Anger
Benzodiazepines, 331
  abuse of, 82, 268
  for aggression, 199–200, **203**, 316, 317
  for agitated/aggressive elderly patients, 401, 403
    acute/emergent management, 394
    before care activities for dementia patients, 398
  for alcohol withdrawal, 133, 305
  for escalating anxiety, 334
  long-term treatment with, 316
  in psychiatric emergencies, 302, 303
  as quenching agents, 334–335
  during seclusion and restraint, 352
  side effects of, 198
  tolerance to, 305, 316
  withdrawal from, 305, 316
Benzoylecgonine, 147
Benztropine, 388
  for acute dystonic reaction, 302
Binswanger's disease, 196
Bipolar disorder, 25, 301
  in adolescents, 374
  deliberate self-harm and, 88–89
  driving safety and, 522, 532
  ethnicity and diagnosis of, 35
  in genesis of violence, 83–86
    in elderly dementia patient, 400
  legal problems associated with, 84
  multiple sclerosis and, 196
  pharmacotherapy for aggression/agitation in, 302–303
  prevalence of, 90
  pyromania and, 219
  self-injurious behaviors and, 225

  sex offenses and, 84
  substance abuse and, 84, 85, 251
  suicide in, 90–91
    lithium to reduce risk for, 91, 92
  after traumatic brain injury, 187
  violence prevalence in, 107, 250
BLS (Bureau of Labor Statistics), 505–506, 514
Blueprints for Violence Prevention, 374
Borderline personality disorder, 11, 13, 26, 166, 252
  childhood abuse and, 214
  driving safety and, 522
  nontargeted, impulsive violence incidental to emotional escape and, 175–176
  patient dependency on therapist in, 331
  purposeful, instrumental violence and, 168–169
  self-injurious behaviors in, 226
  targeted, impulsive violence and, 172
  violence related to perceived/feared loss or abandonment and, 178
"Boston Miracle" in assault reduction, 375
Bouffée delirante, 44, **45**
Bradford Sexual History Inventory, 445
Bradycardia, olanzapine-induced, 308
Brain
  correlates of aggression in dementia, 187
  effects of prenatal substance exposure on development of, 214
  encephalitis, 192–194
  minimal brain dysfunction, 196
  neurobiology of addiction, 149–150
  neurobiology of aggression
    in mood disorders, 92–93
    role of serotonin, 92–93, 215
  neurobiology of alcohol, 143
  regions of dysfunction associated with aggression and impulsivity, 214–215

Index

sexual sadism and abnormalities of, 447
traumatic injury of, 187–188, 196, **204**, 214–215
tumors of, 194, 196
white matter disorders, 196
Brief Psychiatric Rating Scale, 315
Bullying, 79, 110, 115, 173, 359, 361, 365
  control of, 550
  in schools, 540–541, 545
Buprenorphine maintenance treatment, 154
Bupropion, for smoking cessation, 399
Bureau of Justice Standards, 506
Bureau of Labor Statistics (BLS), 505–506, 514
Buspirone, for aggressive elderly patients, 403
Buss-Durkee Hostility Inventory, 215, 224

Cafard, **45**
Caffeine and driving safety, 522
Calcium, during anti-androgen therapy, 455
Cambodians, 35
  culturally appropriate assessment of interpersonal violence in, 51–52
Cannabis, 86, 148, 150, 335
  bipolar disorder and, 85
  prevalence of use, 107
Capital punishment cases, 430, 435–436, 438
Carbamazepine, **203**, 315
  for aggressive elderly patients, 403
Carbon monoxide exposure, 197
Cardiovascular effects of antipsychotics
  olanzapine, 308
  ziprasidone, 308
Caregivers
  assuring safety of, 395
  behavioral strategies for, 201
  of dementia patients, 185–186
  elderly persons lashing out at, 382
  interviewing of, 384

Castration, 225
  pharmacological, 453–455
Catalepsy, driving safety and, 531
Catastrophic reactions, poststroke, 189
Cathard, **45**
CATIE (Clinical Antipsychotic Trials of Intervention Effectiveness), 107–108
CATIE-AD (Clinical Antipsychotic Trials of Intervention Effectiveness–Alzheimer's Disease), 394–395
Caucasians
  arrests for aggravated assaults, 37
  risk for homicide, 37
  serial killing by, 38
CDR (Clinical Dementia Rating) scale, 527
Centers for Medicare and Medicaid Services (CMS), requirements for use of seclusion and restraint, 341, 344–345, 351
Central nervous system infections, 192–194
Central nervous system tumors, 194
Cerebral glucose metabolism, 214
Cerebrovascular accident, 188–189, 196, 389
  antipsychotics and, 403
Chart review, 5
Chemical restraint, 351
Child Behavioral Checklist, 214
Child custody cases, 168, 175
Child pornography on Internet, 444–445
Childhood abuse or neglect, 23
  alcohol-related, 144–145
  deliberate self-harm and, 87, 92, 226
  impulsive aggression and, 214
  mood disorders related to, 79–80
    parental substance abuse and, 78
    physical abuse, 79
    prevention of, 82
    sexual abuse, 79–80
    verbal and emotional abuse, 79
  posttraumatic stress disorder in veterans and, 126
  racial reporting bias for, 38

Childhood abuse or neglect (*continued*)
self-injurious behaviors and, 226
sexual abuse, 87, 214, 545
among adult perpetrators of sexual violence, 442
convictions for, 443
deliberate self-harm and, 87
incest perpetrators, 450, 451–452
Internet as tool for, 443–445
mood disorders related to, 79–80
prevalence of, 442–443
programs for prevention of, 443
and risk for sexual victimization as adult, 79, 82–83
suicide and, 80, 214, 223
treatment of adults with history of, 82
Children, 359–376. *See also* Adolescents
aggression related to prenatal substance exposure of, 213–214
bullying and, 79, 540–541
conduct disorder in, 363
developmental trajectories toward violence in, 362–363, **363**
epidemiology of aggression in, 360
gender and aggression in, 360
inhalant use by, 9
maladjustment of, 22, 27
oppositional defiant disorder in, 363, 369
parental murder of, 448
murder-suicide, 423–424
passive exposure to parental violence, 78, 80
of substance-abusing parents, 78–79
temper tantrums in, 216
trauma exposure and later aggression in, 214
as victims of sexually motivated homicide, 448
Cho, Seung-Hui, 546–547, 550
Cholinesterase inhibitors, for Alzheimer's disease, 392, 393, 399, 402
Christians, 35
Citalopram, 316
Civil commitment, 430
expert testimony at hearing for, 438–439
for imminent risk of violence, 244–245
involuntary outpatient commitment, 547
predicting future violence and, 438–439
Civil Protection Orders (CPOs), in cases of intimate partner violence, 493–494
Classification of Violence Risk (COVR), 18, 23–26, **28,** 30
case examples of use of, 25–26
classification tree methodology of, 23–24
clinician review of, 24
combining risk factors for, 23–24
generating final risk estimate with, 24
predictive validity of, 23
selecting and measuring risk factors for, 23
Clinical Antipsychotic Trials of Intervention Effectiveness (CATIE), 107–108
Clinical Antipsychotic Trials of Intervention Effectiveness–Alzheimer's Disease (CATIE-AD), 394–395
Clinical Dementia Rating (CDR) scale, 527
Clinical violence risk assessment, 3–14, 19–20, 46
case examples of, 12–13
clinicians responsible for, 3
collateral sources of information for, 4
compared with actuarial or structured risk assessment, 3–4, 17–21, **28,** 30
documentation of, 14
factors in, **5,** 5–12, 14
alcohol and drug use, 7–9
appearance of patient, 5–6
available means, 6–7
demographic characteristics, 11–12
intent, 6

Index

past history of violence or
    impulsive behaviors, 7, **8**
personality disorders, 11
presence of violent ideation and
    degree of planning/
    formulation, 6
psychosis, 10
treatment noncompliance, 11
implications for clinical
    intervention, 19
in outpatient settings, 237–239
preventive interventions based on,
    3, 14
principles of, 4–5
professional subjective judgment
    for, 19
questions for, 4
reassessments, 14
reliance on dynamic risk factors, 19
research on validity of, 19–20
time frame for validity of, 4, 18
for violence in the short term, 3, 4

Clinicians
active listening by, 468
anxiety about therapy with suicidal
    patients, 327–328
assessment of patients' driving
    competence by, 527–530, 534
comfort in dealing with potential
    violence, 249
on crisis management teams in
    workplace, 514–515
duty to warn and protect potential
    victims, 246, 247, 269, 333–334,
    373, 430–434, 524, 557–559, **560**
expert testimony of, 430, 434–439
eye contact with violent patient, 468
honesty of, 468
inexperience with violent patients,
    326–327
irrational fear of violent patients,
    332–333
legal duties to prevent vehicular
    crashes, 531–534
legal responsibility for a patient's
    violent act, 247
limit setting by, 469–470

pathological attachment to, 332
patient dependency on, 331
physical distance and posture with
    violent patient, 468
racial and cultural differences
    between patients and, 39
racially biased attitudes of, 36
responsibility for violence risk
    assessment, 3
risk management of potentially
    violent patients, 555–564
safety of, 248–249, 254, 332
threats against, 471–475
treatment guidelines for patients
    who drink too much, 151, 152
violence toward, 461–478
    additional management
        techniques for, 468–469
    affect management for, 463, 465,
        467–468
    anticipation of, 466
    assessing risk for, 465–466, **466**
    dynamics of, 467
    in emergency settings, 462–463,
        470
    on inpatient unit, 470
    limit setting and, 469–470
    in outpatient settings, 248–249,
        332, 463–464
    prevalence of, 461
    prodrome of, 467
    psychiatrist's denial of risk for,
        464, 465, 466
    as result of psychotic
        transference in outpatient
        setting, 464–465
    threats toward a surgeon, 464
Clonazepam, **203**, 316
Clozapine, 114, 253–254, 267, 303, 312–
    313
    anti-hostility effects of, 313
    for intermittent explosive disorder,
        317
CMS (Centers for Medicare and
    Medicaid Services), requirements
    for use of seclusion and restraint,
    341, 344–345, 351

Cobalamin deficiency, 196
Cocaine, 9, 13, 39, 147, 150, 268, 525
  agitation induced by, 9, 198
  crack, 9, 362, 387
  disulfiram for addiction to, 154
  fetal exposure to, 213, 214
  topiramate for addiction to, 154
Cognitive distortions of sexually violent persons, 453
Cognitive impairment
  in elderly persons, 381–382
    assessment of, 390–392
  in persons with Intellectual disability, 189–190, 219–221, 227
Cognitive-behavioral therapy
  for aggression, 317
  for alcoholism, 155
  for depression and posttraumatic stress disorder resulting from violence exposure, 82, 132–133, 135
  for sexually violent persons, 452
  for students at risk for school violence, 550
  with violent youth, 374
"Cold" threats, 268–269
Collateral sources of information about patient, 4, 13
College students
  date rape among, 143
  substance abuse and suicidality among, 143
Columbine High School shootings, 543–544
Command hallucinations, 108–109, **267**, 267–268, 295
Community Mental Health Act, 277
Community psychiatric emergency services, 289–291
  crisis residence, 289
  crisis respite, 290
  crisis response services, 289–290
  mobile crisis intervention team, 290–291
Community violence and mood disorders, 81
Competency to stand trial, 410

Comprehensive Psychiatric Emergency Programs (CPEPs) (New York), 278
Computed tomography, of aggression in dementia, 187
Conduct disorder
  antisocial personality disorder and, 363, 369
  attention-deficit/hyperactivity disorder and, 369
  oppositional defiant disorder and, 363, 369
  schizophrenia, violence and, 250–251
  serious violence and, 108
  serotonin transporter polymorphisms and, 93
  workplace violence and, 511
  in youth, 360, 363, 369
Confidentiality, 429
  breach of, 241–242
    to protect potential victims, 246, 247, 429–434, 493 (*See also* Duty to warn and protect potential victims)
    to seek additional sources of information, 241
  of interview with adolescent, 367–368
  vs. safety concerns, 241
Confusion
  amphetamine-induced, 9
  in delirium, 197
  in elderly persons, 386
  in systemic lupus erythematosus, 198
  after traumatic brain injury, 187
Congenital brain disorders, 189–190. *See also* Intellectual disability
Consultation for violence risk management, 556
  in youth, 375–376
Cook-Medley Hostility Inventory, 68
Correctional facilities, structured risk assessment for violence after discharge from, 4
Corticosteroids, 198
Cortisol secretion, childhood abuse, and trauma exposure, 78

Index

Cortisone, 198
Countertransference, 332–333
  monitoring of, 472, 473
  racism and, 40
  in treatment of children and adolescents, 375
Couples therapy, 557
  for intimate partner violence, 492
  for pedophilia, 445
  for posttraumatic stress disorder, 134, 137
Court-mandated treatment
  for batterers, 492
  psychotherapy, 327
Covert sensitization, for paraphilias, 453
COVR. *See* Classification of Violence Risk
CPEPs (Comprehensive Psychiatric Emergency Programs) (New York), 278
CPOs (Civil Protection Orders), in cases of intimate partner violence, 493–494
Crack cocaine, 9, 362, 387. *See also* Cocaine
Criminal behavior, 5, 7
  alcohol consumption and, 142
  among combat veterans with posttraumatic stress disorder, 124
  drop in violent crime rates, 362
  among elderly persons, 381
  mania and, 84
  motivations for, 109
  prenatal tobacco exposure and, 214
  prosecution for inpatient assaults, 269–270, **271**
  by psychotic men, 109
  in schools, 538–539
Criminal defendants, 430
  forensic evaluations of, 409–426
  preventive confinement of, 430
  state requirements for violence risk assessment of, 438
Crisis management teams for workplace violence risk assessment, 514
Crisis residence, 289

Crisis respite, 290
Crisis response services, 289–290
  for victims of intimate partner violence, 492
Crisis stabilization unit, 286–287
Culturally competent violence risk assessment, 35–54. *See also* Ethnicity/race
  cross-cultural validity of assessment instruments, Psychopathy Checklist, 63
  culturally appropriate assessment, 42–43
    culture-bound syndromes, 44, **45**
    DSM-IV-TR Outline for Cultural Formulation, 43–44, **44**
    in psychiatric setting, 44–46
  denial of racism by majority culture, 46
  interpersonal violence, 41–42
    culturally appropriate assessment of, 47–53
  problems in assessing violence risk in people of color, 37–41
    case examples of, 39–41
    groups at greatest risk for violence or homicide, 37–38
    overdetermination of dangerousness, 38–39
    youth violence, 37
Culture
  definition of, 42
  effect on symptom expression, 42
  protective effect on mental health, 43
Culture of violence, intimate partner violence and, **486**
Culture-bound syndromes, 44, **45**
Cushing's syndrome, 389
Cyproterone acetate, for paraphilias, 453, 454

Dangerousness
  civil commitment and, 438–439
  dependence of judicial system on assessment of, 430, 437–438
  minimization of, 4

Dangerousness (*continued*)
  overdetermination in people of color, 38–39
  of rapist, 416
  sentencing and, 438
  of stalker, 413
Date rape, 143
Dating violence, 361–362
Daubert v. Merrell Down Pharmaceuticals, Inc., 436–437, 439, 494
DBH (dopamine-β-hydroxylase), 154
de Rais, Giles, 448
DEA (Drug Enforcement Agency), 133
Death penalty, 430, 435–436, 438
"Decade of the Brain," 151
Deceased persons, forensic evaluations of, 418–425
  murder-suicide, 421–425, **422, 425**
  suicide by cop, 420–421, **421**
Decelerative techniques, 201
De-escalation techniques, 265, **266**
  affect management, 463, 465, 467–468
  eye contact, 468
Defensiveness, assessment of, 69–70
Deinstitutionalization, 221
Deliberate self-harm (DSH), 86–89, 92. See also Self-injurious behaviors; Suicide
  among adolescents, 87
  childhood abuse and, 87, 92
  definition of, 86
  depression and, 86–88
  dysfunctional attitudes and, 88
  among elderly persons, 87–88
  impulsive acts of, 87
  by poisoning, 87
  risk factors for, 86
  suicide and, 86, 92
  vs. suicide attempt, 222
Delirium, 197, **197**, 388, 395–396
  during alcohol withdrawal, 9
  anticholinergic, 198
  assessment of, 390
  early signs of, 395–396
  in elderly persons, 386, 395–396
  phencyclidine-induced, 9
  in systemic lupus erythematosus, 198

Delusional disorder, 10
Delusions
  during alcohol withdrawal, 9
  of being stalked, 412
  crimes motivated by, 109
  of elderly patients, 382, 388
  illicit drug–induced, 9
  in mania, 10
  murder-suicide and, 423
  paranoid, 10, 12, 64, 118, 265–266, **267,** 284
  persecutory, 10, 108, 266, **267**
  in schizophrenia, 10, 12, 265–266
  violence associated with, 107–108, 109, 251–252
    in dementia, 187
    emotional charge associated with, 251–252
    among inpatients, 266–267, **267**
    substance abuse and, 149
Dementia, 185–187, 381–382
  aggression in, 185–187
  acute/emergent treatment of, 394–395
  case example of, 391–392
  cholinesterase inhibitors for, 392, 393, 399, 402
  depression and, 392–394
  environmental stimuli and, 397–398
  managing precipitants of, 396–398
  mutifaceted approach to, 404
  neurological correlates of, 187
  nursing home placement due to, 186
  pharmacotherapy for, 400–404
  physical discomfort and, 397
  predictors of, 187
  sexual aggression, 382
  specific care needs and, 398
  treating underlying psychiatric disorders in, 398–400
  apathy in, 393, 394
  atypical antipsychotics and risk of death in elderly patients with, 200–201

Index

cognitive and memory impairment
in, 381–382, 390–392
depression and, 393–394
driving safety and, 522, 527–531
identification of, 388
with Lewy bodies, 186, 198
prevalence of, 185
rapid-onset, 387
in rheumatological diseases, 198
Demographic characteristics
of suicidal patients, 89
of violent patients, 11–12
Denial of risk by clinician, 464, 465, 466
Dependent personality disorder
nontargeted, impulsive violence
incidental to emotional escape
and, 176
purposeful, targeted, defensive
violence and, 171
targeted, impulsive violence and,
172, 174
Depression, 25, 284
in adolescents, 374
maternal depression and, 78
anger attacks in, 252, 254
in assault victims, 80
biology of aggression in, 92–93
among combat veterans, 81
deliberate self-harm and, 86–88
driving safety and, 523, 524–526,
533
in elderly persons, 392–394
in genesis of violence, 83–86
in elderly persons, 384–385, 399
as goal of treating violent patients,
328
intimate partner violence and, 41,
80–81, 127, 485, 488
mixed, 84
murder-suicide and, 422, 423, 424
postpsychotic, 329
poststroke, 189
posttraumatic stress disorder and,
128, 129
psychotic, 285
public fear of violence due to, 148
self-injurious behaviors in, 226

serotonin level and, 93, 215
suicide and, 89–90, 223, 224
treatment approaches for violence
in, 81–83
violence in genesis of, 77–83
community violence, war, and
terrorism, 81
direct abuse or neglect, 79–81
adult assault, 80
intimate partner violence, 41,
80–81
physical abuse, 79
sexual abuse, 79–80
verbal and emotional abuse,
79
passive exposure, 77–79
parental substance abuse, 78–
79
witness to domestic violence,
77–78
violence prevalence in, 106
Derogatis Sexual Functioning
Inventory, 445
Desensitization, for paraphilias, 453
Developmental disorders, 189–190,
219–221. *See also* Intellectual
disability
Diabetes mellitus, 106
*Diagnostic and Statistical Manual of
Mental Disorders* (DSM-IV-TR)
autistic disorder in, 221
culture-bound syndromes in, 44, **45**
impulse-control disorders in, 218
intermittent explosive disorder in,
216
mental retardation in, 219
Outline for Cultural Formulation,
43–44, **44**, 46, 54
pyromania in, 218
Diagnostic Interview Schedule, 107
Dialectical behavior therapy, 317
Dietary supplementation, during anti-
androgen therapy, 455
Diphenhydramine
for aggressive elderly patients, 403
for dystonic reaction, 302
Disability discrimination, 504, 508

Discharge from inpatient facilities, 13, 14, 559–560, **561**
　Classification of Violence Risk for, 25–26
Discrimination, racial, 36
Disorganized and organized crime scenes, FBI profiling of, 417–418, **418**
Disorientation, in elderly persons, 381
Dissociation, in culture-bound syndromes, **45**
Disturbances in consciousness, driving safety and, 531
Disulfiram
　for alcoholism, 153–154
　for cocaine dependence, 154
Divalproex. *See* Valproate
Documentation, 562
Domestic violence, 41–42. *See also* Intimate partner violence
　childhood mood disorders associated with passive exposure to, 77–78
　escalating pattern of, 7
　parental substance abuse and, 78
　screening for, 41
Donepezil, for Alzheimer's disease, 392, 393, 399, 402
Dopamine, 215
Dopamine-β-hydroxylase (DBH), 154
Driving safety, 7, 521–535
　dementia and, 527–531
　depression and, 524–526
　disturbances of consciousness and, 531
　intoxication and, 522
　legal duties of clinicians to prevent vehicular crashes, 531–534
　Physician's Guide to Assessing and Counseling Older Drivers, 528–530
　psychosis, schizophrenia and, 523–524
　suicidal drivers, 522, 524–526
　warning patients about medication effects on, 522–523, 532–533
Droperidol, intramuscular, **304**

Drug abuse. *See* Alcohol use/abuse; Substance abuse disorders
Drug Enforcement Agency (DEA), 133
Drug Screening Test, 445
DSH. *See* Deliberate self-harm
DSM-IV-TR. *See Diagnostic and Statistical Manual of Mental Disorders*
Dusky v. U.S., 410
Duty to warn and protect potential victims, 246, 247, 269, 333–334, 373, 430–434, 524, 557–559
　best practices for, 434, 558
　inpatient discharge and, 559–560
　from intimate partner violence, 492–494
　issuing a warning, 558–559
　language barriers and use of translator, 558–559
　risk management steps for, 559, **560**
　state allowances for therapist discretion in, 433–434
　vs. therapist–patient confidentiality, 246, 247, 429–430
Dynamics of violence, 467
Dysarthria, 6

Eating disorders, self-injurious behaviors and, 224, 226
Ecological theory of intimate partner violence, **486**
ECT (electroconvulsive therapy), 316
Elderly persons, 381–404
　alcohol-related abuse of, 145
　assessment in, 383–394
　　chief complaint, 383–386
　　in inpatient setting, 383
　　mental status examination, 389–394
　　　attentional problems, 389–390
　　　cognitive and memory impairment, 390–392
　　　disorders of mood and affective regulation, 392–394
　　　thought processing, 392

Index

past history, 386–389
    medical/surgical, 386–388
    psychiatric, 388–389
    psychosocial, 389
referral for, 383
atypical antipsychotics and risk of death in, 200–201
causes of violence among, 381–382
criminal behavior in, 381
deliberate self-harm among, 87–88
delirium in, 386
delusions of, 382, 388
effects of memory and cognitive deficits in, 381–382
incarcerated, 382–383
inpatient assaults by, 383, 386
lashing out at caretakers, 382
long-term care facilities for, 382
medication-related problems in, 382, 386
physiological changes in, 381
sexual aggression in, 382
treatment of violent behavior in, 394–404
    acute/emergent treatment, 394–395
    for causes of medical decompensation, especially delirium, 395–396
    ensuring safety of patient and others, 395
    for identified precipitants of violence, 396–398
    pharmacotherapy, 400–404
    for underlying psychiatric disorders, 398–400
    use of restraints, 395
Electroconvulsive therapy (ECT), 316
Electroencephalogram, 214
Emergency settings, 12, 277–296. *See also* Psychiatric emergency services
extended psychiatric observation services, 285–289
managing violent patients in, 13
    with posttraumatic stress disorder, 130–131
patient refusal to comply with intake procedures of, 6
pharmacotherapy for acute agitation/aggression in, 302, 303–311, **304, 306–307**
psychiatric decision making in, 278
psychiatric emergency room, 280–284
safety in, 13, 14, 281, 282, 291, 462–463, 470
seclusion and restraint in, 13, 280, 291–295, 340–341
violence in, 462
violence risk assessment in, 3
violence toward clinicians in, 462–463, 470
weapons search in, 46, 249, 462
Emotional abuse during childhood
mood disorders related to, 79
and risk of adult sexual victimization, 79, 82–83
Emotional lability
alcohol intoxication and, 9
in bipolar disorder, 83
Empathy, 252
intrinsic derangement of, 330
Empathy training, for students at risk for school violence, 550
Employee assistance programs, 134
Employment problems, 22, 23. *See also* Workplace violence
Encephalitis, 192–194
autoimmune deficiency, 193
herpes simplex, 192–193
lethargica, 192
other types of, 192–193
paraneoplastic, 193
β-Endorphin, alcoholism and, 152
Environmental factors and violence, 11–12, 253
design of psychiatric emergency room, 281
design of seclusion room, 280, 350
among elderly dementia patients, 397–398
among inpatients, 114–115, 260–261
interventions for youth, 375

Environmental factors and violence (*continued*)
    safety of clinician's office, 248–249, 332, 463–464, 465–466, 476–477
    in workplace, 511–512
Epidemiologic Catchment Area study, 106, 148
Epilepsy, 190–192
    driving safety and, 522, 531
    ictal aggression in, 191
    interictal aggression in, 191
    postictal aggression in, 191
Epinephrine secretion, childhood abuse, and trauma exposure, 78
Erotomanic stalkers, 412
Escalating pattern of violence, 7, 265
Escitalopram, for chronic aggression, **202**
Estrogen therapy, for elderly men, 403
Ethnicity/race. *See also* Culturally competent violence risk assessment
    alcohol-related intimate partner violence and, 145
    antipsychotic administration and, 38
    arrests for aggravated assaults related to, 37
    child abuse reporting bias related to, 38
    "color line" in U.S., 36
    dearth of information in mental health literature on, 36
    discrimination based on, 36
    "monocultural ethnocentrism," 36
    myths about youth violence related to, 37
    overdetermination of dangerousness in people of color, 38–39
    problems in assessing violence risk in people of color, 37–41
    psychiatric diagnosis and, 35
    racial and cultural differences between patients and clinicians, 39
    as risk marker for violence, 37, 38
    seclusion and restraint of minority patients, 38
    structural racism, 36
    substance abuse and, 35
    suicide risk and, 89
    Surgeon General's report on mental health and, 36
    transference, countertransference and, 40
    treatment interventions and, 38–39
    violence or homicide risk and, 37
        intimate partner violence, 80
Euphoria
    cocaine-induced, 9
    in intermittent explosive disorder, 217
Evolutionary theory of intimate partner violence, **486**
Exchange theory of intimate partner violence, **486**
Executive functioning, assessing in elderly persons, 391
Exhibitionism, 441, 443
Expert testimony, 430, 434–439
    Barefoot vs. Estelle, 435–436, 437
    at civil commitment hearing, 438–439
    Daubert v. Merrill Dow Pharmaceuticals, Inc., 436–437
    Federal Rules of Evidence and, 435, 436
    Frye v. United States, 435, 437
    "general acceptance" test for admissibility of, 435
    history of admissibility of, 435
    regarding battered women, 494–495
    reliability of assessments used for, 437, 439
Exposure therapy, for posttraumatic stress disorder, 132
Extended psychiatric observation services, 285–289
    admission criteria for, 285–286
    benefits of, 285
    case example of, 287
    crisis stabilization unit, 286–287
    length of stay in, 285
    72-hour observation bed, psychiatric, 288–289

Index

23-hour observation bed, psychiatric, 286
Extrapyramidal symptoms, 402
Eye contact with violent patient, 468
Eye enucleation, 225
Eyeball pressing, 225

Factitious disorder, false allegations of stalking due to, 412
Familicide, 424
Family. *See also* Caregivers
 disruption of, 11
 domestic violence within, 41–42
 incest perpetrators in, 450, 451–452
 informing about institutional policies and practices on use of seclusion and restraint, 346
 interviewing of, 4
  about past episodes of violence, 7
 intimate partner violence within, 41–42, 80–81, 483–495 (*See also* Intimate partner violence)
 murder-suicide within, 422–424
 removing guns from patient by, 6
Family therapy
 for delinquent adolescents, 374
 for intimate partner violence, 492
 for pedophilia, 445
Fantasies
 sexual, 445
 violent, 23
Federal Bureau of Investigation (FBI)
 profiling of organized and disorganized crime scenes, 417–418, **418**
 report on myths about school shootings, 548
Federal Rules of Evidence, 435, 436
Fetal alcohol syndrome, 219
Fetal substance exposure, 213
Fetishism, 441
"Fight, flight, or freeze" responses, in posttraumatic stress disorder, 124
Fighting. *See also* Aggression; Assaults
 amphetamine-induced, 9
 antisocial personality disorder and, 11
 in childhood and adolescence, 360–361
 impulsive suicide and, 224
 reactive, 110
 schizophrenia and, 10
Fight-or-flight response, 215
Filicide, 448
Filicide-suicide, 423, 526
Finger biting, 225
Fire setting. *See* Pyromania
Fluoxetine, 316, 387
 for paraphilias, 454
 for posttraumatic stress disorder, 132
Fluphenazine decanoate, 117
Flutamide, 454
Forgiveness therapy, 82
Forensic evaluations, 409–426
 checklist for, **410**
 of deceased persons, 418–425
  murder-suicide, 421–425, **422, 425**
  psychological autopsy, 418–420
  suicide by cop, 420–421, **421**
 of known offenders, 410–417
  for competency to stand trial, 410
  to determine risk for future violence, 410–411
  for insanity defense, 410
  Internet child pornographers, 444–445
  rapists, 415–417, **416**
  stalkers, 411–415, **413, 414**
 skills for performance of, 409
 of unknown offenders, 417–418
  FBI profiling of organized and disorganized crime scenes, 417–418, **418**
Forensic psychiatry, defined, 409
Frustration, 109
 in elderly persons, 382
 impulsive aggression and, 213
 low tolerance for, in brain-injured patients, 187
Frye v. United States, 435, 437

GABA (γ-aminobutyric acid), 215
Gabapentin, for aggression, 82, 253
 in elderly patients, 403

Gait abnormalities, 6
Galantamine, for Alzheimer's disease, 399
Gang activity, 359, 365, 375
　alcohol and, 146
　youth homicide and, 362
Gas exposure, 197
Gasoline inhalation, 9
Gender and violence risk, 11, 23, 253
　childhood sexual abuse, 442
　in children and adolescents, 359, 360–361
　among inpatients, 260
　intellectual disability and, 220
　intermittent explosive disorder, 216
　murder-suicide, 422
　pyromania, 218
　rape, 415
　sexual sadism, 446
　stalking, 411
　suicide, 89, 223
Genetics
　depression, aggression, and serotonin transporter polymorphisms, 93
　twin and adoption studies of violence, 364
Gilles de la Tourette syndrome, 195–196
　attention-deficit/hyperactivity disorder and, 195
　self-injurious behaviors in, 225
Glue inhalation, 9
Golden, Andrew, 544–545, 547
Gooden v. Tips, 532
Gordis, Enoch, 155
Grandiosity
　in bipolar disorder, 83
　cocaine-induced, 9
　violence and, 108
Graves' disease, 387, 389
Grigson, James, 435
Group therapy
　for paraphilias, 452–453
　prison-based, 325
Guided imagery, for posttraumatic stress disorder, 132

Gun safety management, 6, 372, 373, 557, 562, **563**
Gun-related violence, 6
　among adolescents, 79, 362, 365, 372, 373
　controlling patient access to weapons, 6, 372, 373, 557, 562, **563**
　management of armed patient, 476
　mass murder, 424–425
　murder-suicide, 422
　posttraumatic stress disorder and, 128, 129, 133
　school shootings, 79, 359, 365, 371, 541–549, 551
　　Columbine High School, 543–544
　　FBI report on myths about, 548
　　Jonesboro, Arkansas, 544–545
　　managing threats or predictions of, 548–549
　　National Research Council report on, 549
　　notable cases of, 541–543
　　operant styles of perpetrators of, 547
　　profiles of perpetrators of, 547–548
　　social causation model of, 541
　　Virginia Tech, 546–547
　suicide, 85

Hallucinations, 284
　during alcohol withdrawal, 9
　command, 108–109, **267**, 267–268, 295
　violence and, 108–109
　and violence in schizophrenia, 10
Hallucinogens, 9
Haloperidol, 12
　anti-hostility effects of, 313
　for chronic aggression, **202**
　intramuscular, 13, 294, 302, **304**, 305
　　combined with lorazepam, 302, 305, 388
　during seclusion and restraint, 351
　for violent inpatients, 114, 254
Harassment, 60

Index

Hare Psychopathy Checklist (PCL), 62–63
   cross-cultural validity of, 63
   in perpetrators of sexual violence, 445, 448
      recidivism risk, 451
   screening version of, 62
Harris, Eric, 543–544
HCR-20, 21–23, **28**, 30, 39, 46
   case example of use in outpatient setting, 240–241
   combining risk factors for, 22
   generating final risk estimate with, 22–23
   predictive validity of, 21
   Psychopathy Checklist–Revised and, 62
   selecting and measuring risk factors for, 22
   use in clinical practice, 28, 29
Head banging, 225
Head injury. *See* Traumatic brain injury
Health Insurance Portability and Accountability Act, 513
Helping Patients Who Drink Too Much: A Clinician's Guide, 151, 152
Helplessness, 213, 331
   of elderly persons, 382
   learned, of victim of intimate partner violence, 495
Hepatolenticular degeneration, 195
Herpes simplex virus (HSV) encephalitis, 192–193
Hispanics, 35
   culturally appropriate assessment of interpersonal violence in, 52
   myths about youth violence among, 37
   risk for violence or homicide, 37
Histrionic personality disorder, 252
Homicide, 7, 12, 39
   of abuser by victim of intimate partner violence, 494–495
   alcohol intoxication and, 142
   cocaine and, 147
   by elderly persons, 384–385
   ethnicity and, 37–38
   FBI profiling of organized and disorganized crime scenes, 417–418, **418**
   intermittent explosive disorder and, 217
   mass murder, 11, 37–38
   murder-suicide, 421–425
   patients' disavowal of tendencies toward, 327
   against physicians, 462
   during pregnancy, 484
   random but purposeful, 177
   in schools, 79, 359, 365, 371, 539–549
      (*See also* School violence)
   serial killing, 38
   sexually motivated, 447–450
      brain abnormalities in perpetrators of, 447
      child victims of, 448
      impetus for, 448–449
      measuring sexual arousal in perpetrators of, 449–450
      serial killings, 448–449
      sexual sadism and, 442, 445–450
      XYY syndrome in perpetrators of, 447–448
   by strangulation, 446, 447
   studying autopsy reports of victims of, 327
   suicide and, 91–92, 328–329
   targeted, impulsive, 173–174
   in workplace, 501, 505, 506, 509
   youth, 37, 359, 362, 375, 539
Honesty in responding to patients, 468
Hopelessness, 284
   suicidality and, 87, 90, 525, 526
Hormonal therapy, 335
Hospitalization. *See also* Inpatients
   assaults by psychotic patients during, 109–118
   decision for admission to, 3, 13
   of high-risk youth, 373
   involuntary, 430
      for acute psychosis, 523–524
      expert testimony at hearing for, 438–439

Hospitalization (*continued*)
involuntary (*continued*)
for imminent risk of violence, 244–245
predicting future violence and, 438–439
management of violent psychotic patients during, 113–118
patient transfer from outpatient therapist to, 336
risk management for discharge from, 13, 14, 559–560, **561**
for risk of imminent violence, 244
violence among intellectually impaired patients during, 189–190
Hostility, 212
antipsychotic effects on, 313
distinction from anger, 68
instruments for assessment of, 68
HSV (herpes simplex virus) encephalitis, 192–193
Huntington's disease, 195, 204–205
Hydrocarbon inhalants, 9
5-Hydroxyindoleacetic acid, 92
Hyperarousal, 109
Hyperthyroidism, 387
Hypervigilance, 335
Hypoglycemia, 198
Hypotension, antipsychotic-induced, 402
aripiprazole, 310
olanzapine, 308
Hypothalamic-pituitary-adrenal axis
effects of childhood abuse and trauma exposure on, 78
mood symptom, violence and, 92
Hypoxia, 196

Ibn-Tamas v. United States, 494
Ictal aggression, 191
IED. *See* Intermittent explosive disorder
Iich'aa, **45**
Imminence of risk, assessment of, 244–245
Impatience, 6

Impulsive aggression, 68, 211–228
in autism, 221–222
in borderline personality disorder, 11
drinking and, 144
etiology of, 213–216
childhood trauma, 214
neurochemistry, 215–216
prenatal development, 213–214
traumatic brain injury and brain dysfunction, 214–215
by inpatients, 262
in intermittent explosive disorder, 216–217
neuropsychological testing of persons with, 213
in personality disorders
nontargeted, impulsive violence incidental to emotional escape, 174–176
targeted, impulsive violence and, 172–174
in persons with intellectual disabilities, 219–221
in posttraumatic stress disorder, 124
in pyromania, 217–219
reactive assaults due to, 110
in schizophrenia, 10
self-injurious behaviors due to, 224–226
suicide, 222–224
treatment of, 253
Impulsivity, 252
instruments for assessment of, 68–69, 72
past history of, 7
phencyclidine-induced, 9
Incarcerated persons, 326
elderly, 382–383
group therapy for, 325
posttraumatic stress disorder in, 126
substance abuse and mental illness among delinquent youth, 364
Incest perpetrators, 450, 451–452
Incoherence, amphetamine-induced, 9
Incompetent stalkers, **413**
Infanticide, 423, 448

Index

Informed consent
  and confidentiality for interview of adolescent, 367–368
  for pharmacological treatment of elderly patients, 401
  for treatment during 72-hour hold, 288
Inhalant abuse, 9
Inpatients. *See also* Hospitalization
  acute management of high-risk youth, 373
  aftercare for, 14
  assaults by, 109–118, 259–272
    criminal prosecution for, 269–270, **271**
    environmental risk factors for, 114–115, 260–261
    gender and, 260
    impulsive vs. premeditated, 262
    long-term risk factors for, **261**
    motivations for, 109, 113, 261–270
    on nursing staff, 259, 263–265
    patient characteristics associated with, 109, 259–260
    prevention of, 114
    reactive vs. instrumental, 109–110, 262–263, **264**
    research on classification of, 110–111
    short-term risk factors for, 260
    staffing ratios, ward atmosphere and, 261
    threatening behaviors before, 112
    videotape recording of, 111–112, 262
  cold threats by, 268–269
  discharge of, 13, 14, 559–560, **561**
    Classification of Violence Risk for, 25–26
  ensuring safety of, 13, 14, 113, 115
  management of violent behavior among, 113–118
    case examples of, 116–118
    criteria for, 113
    interpersonal interactions, 115–116
    least restrictive environment for, 113
    pharmacological, 113, 114
    physical space, 114–115
    predicting violence, 113, 114
    principles of, 113–114
    seclusion and restraint, 113–114, 259
    treatment team for, 113
  managing threats against clinicians by, 473–474
  measures of control for, 264, **266**
  protecting personal property of, 115
  violence among intellectually impaired patients, 189–190
Insanity defense, 410, 524
Institute of Medicine, 538, 549
Instrumental violence, 109–110
  among adolescents, 370–372
Intellectual disability, 189–190, 219–221, 227
  and aggression in institutional vs. community settings, 189–190, 220–221
  case example of, 219
  definition of, 219
  in DSM, 219
  gender and aggression in, 220
  negative effects of aggression in persons with, 220
  prevalence of aggression in persons with, 220
  self-injurious behaviors and, 225
  skill deficits and probability of aggression in, 221
  types of aggressive behavior associated with, 220
Intensive Case Management, 284
Intent to harm, 6
Interictal aggression, 191–192
Intermittent explosive disorder (IED), 11, 13, 216–217, 227, 317
  age distribution of, 216
  aggressive episodes in, 217
    frequency and duration of, 217
    physical and affective symptoms of, 217

Intermittent explosive disorder (*continued*)
  alcohol abuse and, 217
    bipolar disorder and, 85
  case example of, 216
  diagnostic criteria for, 216
    concerns about validity of, 217
  driving and, 522
  DSM classification of, 216
  gender and, 216
  helping patients recognize origins of rage in, 329
  pharmacotherapy for, 317
  prevalence of, 216, 317
  psychiatric comorbidity with, 217
Internet
  child sexual abuse and, 443–444
    case example of, 444–445
  pornography on, 444
  stalking and, 412
Interpersonal violence, 37–38, 41–42. *See also* Aggression; Assaults; Fighting
  definition of, 41
  ethnicity and risk for, 37–38
  among inpatients, 115–116
    case studies of, 116–118
  intimate partner violence, 41–42, 47–53, 80–81
  as means of control, 48
  posttraumatic stress disorder and, 124
    among combat veterans, 125
InterSept Scale for Suicidal Thinking, 295
Interviews
  to assess short-term potential for violence, 4, 13
  with caregivers, 384
  in outpatient settings, 238–239
  of significant others, 4, 13
  telephone, 465
Intimacy-seeking stalkers, **413**
Intimate partner violence (IPV), 41–42, 80–81, 327, 483–495
  alcohol-related, 82–83, 145–146
  assessing risk for commission of, 490–491
  assessment for victims of, 489–490
  case examples of, 41–42, 47, 82–83, 485–489
  couples or family therapy for, 492
  crisis management for, 492
  culturally appropriate assessment of, 47–53
    A–E model for, 48, **49**
    in African Americans, 52–53
    in Asian Americans, 49–50, **51**
    in Cambodians, 51–52
    case example of, 47
    in Latinos, 52
    in Muslims, 47
    in Somalis, 48–49
    in Vietnamese, 50–51
  in cultures that consider women to be inferior, 48
  cycle of violence in, 483–484
  definition of, 41
  depression in victims of, 80–81, 485, 488, 489
  emotional abuse, 483–484
  ethnicity and, 80
  exposure of children to, 78, 80
  factors affecting patient's decision to leave violent relationship, 489, 492
  forms of physical abuse, 483
  in gay couples, 41
  health consequences of, 41
  helping patients recognize origins of, 329
  legal issues related to, 492–495
    arrests, 493
    battered women's syndrome as legal defense, 494
    protection and reporting, 492–494
    psychiatrist as expert, 494–495
    restraining orders, 493–494
  perpetrated by veterans with posttraumatic stress disorder or depression, 127
  posttraumatic stress disorder in victims of, 80, 485
  during pregnancy, 41, 484
  prevalence of, 41, 80, 484

Index

rape, 484, 488
risk factors for, 484, 491
screening for, 41, 490
settings for, 489
severe mental illness and, 485–489
spousal/consortial murder-suicide, 422–423
stalking and, 411
suicidality and, 80–81, 82, 485, 489
theories of causation of, **486–487**
treating assaultive partner in, 492
treating victims of, 82, 489, 491–492
victims' reluctance to discuss, 490
women as perpetrators of, 491, 492
Intimate stalkers, 412, **414**
Intoxication
alcohol, 9
impaired judgment due to, 9
inhalant, 9
murder-suicide and, 422, 424
phencyclidine, 9
self-injurious behaviors and, 225
signs of, 6
vehicular crashes due to, 522
violence, personality disorders and, 167, 171, 173, 178
Investment theory of intimate partner violence, **487**
Involuntary hospitalization, 430
for acute psychosis, 523–524
expert testimony at hearing for, 438–439
for imminent risk of violence, 244–245
predicting future violence and, 438–439
Involuntary outpatient commitment, 547
IPV. See Intimate partner violence
Irritability
in adolescents, 374
anabolic steroid use and, 9
antipsychotic-induced, 200
brain tumors and, 194
in brain-injured patients, 187, 188
hypoglycemia and, 198
inpatient assaults and, 260

in intermittent explosive disorder, 217
in mood disorders, 83
in posttraumatic stress disorder, 132
sleep deprivation and, 198

Johnson, Mitchell, 544–545, 547
Joint Commission for the Accreditation of Healthcare Organizations (JCAHO), regulations for use of seclusion and restraint, 339–340, 341, 344, 346, 351, 353
Jonesboro, Arkansas, school shootings, 544–545, 547
Judgment impairment during intoxication, 9
Judicial system, 5, 430. See also Legal issues
dependence on accurate assessment of dangerousness, 430, 437–438
for juveniles, 359, 367–368
waiving juveniles to adult court, 375

Kaczynski, Ted, 546
Kirk v. Michael Reese Hospital and Medical Center, 532
Klebold, Dylan, 543–544
Klüver-Bucy syndrome, 193

LA Suicide Prevention Center, 418
Lack of remorse, 11, 40, 61
Lamotrigine, 253, 303, 315
Language impairments, in elderly persons, 390
Latinos. *See* Hispanics
Lead exposure, 197
Least restrictive environment, 113
Legal issues, 326, 429–440
civil commitment, 430, 438–439
consent and confidentiality for interview of adolescent, 367–368
criminal prosecution for inpatient assaults, 269–270, **271**
duties of clinician to prevent vehicular crashes, 531–534

Legal issues *(continued)*
　duty of clinicians to warn and protect potential victims, 246, 247, 269, 333–334, 373, 430–434, 524, 557–559, **560**
　expert testimony of clinicians, 430, 434–439
　forensic evaluations, 409–426
　insanity defense, 410, 524
　juvenile justice system, 359, 367–368
　legal responsibility and violence associated with personality disorder, 165
　legal risks associated with workplace violence, 507–508
　legal standard for competency to stand trial, 410
　related to intimate partner violence, 492–495
　related to potential violence, 246–247
　restraining orders against stalkers, 415
　seclusion and restraint, 353
　structured risk assessment for violence after discharge from treatment facility, 4
　waiving juveniles to adult court, 375
Lesch-Nyhan syndrome, 345
Leuprolide acetate, for paraphilias, 453, 454
Lewis, Kurt, 239
Lewy body dementia, 186, 198
LHRH (luteinizing hormone–releasing hormone) agonists, for paraphilias, 453, 454
Licensed independent practitioner (LIP), to initiate and monitor seclusion and restraint, 344
Limbic system, in alcohol effects, 143
Limit setting by clinician, 469–470
Lithium, 314, 374
　for akathisia, 315
　antisuicide effect in bipolar disorder, 91, 92
　combination therapy with antipsychotics, 315
　for elderly patients, 386

Lo, Wayne, 546
Long-term care settings, 186, 382, 392, 396–397
　managing identified precipitants of violence in, 396–398
Long-term violence risk
　actuarial risk assessment of, 18
　psychological testing for assessment of, 61
Lorazepam
　abuse of, 268
　for alcohol withdrawal, 305
　for chronic aggression, **203**
　intramuscular, 13, 302, **304**, 305, 386
　　advantages and disadvantages of, 305
　　combined with aripiprazole, 310
　　combined with haloperidol, 302, 305, 388
　withdrawal from, 316
Loud patients, 5, 106
Love obsessional stalkers, 412
Lu, Gan, 546
Luteinizing hormone–releasing hormone (LHRH) agonists, for paraphilias, 453, 454

MacArthur Violence Risk Assessment Study, 23, 28, 38, 67–68, 69
Mal de pelea, **45**
Malingering, false allegations of stalking due to, 412
Manganese exposure, 197
Mania, 13, 25. *See also* Bipolar disorder
　aggression and, 84–86
　deliberate self-harm and, 88
　in elderly persons, 386, 393
　legal problems associated with, 84
　multiple sclerosis and, 196
　poststroke, 189
　psychosis in, 10
　subtypes of, 84
Marijuana. *See* Cannabis
Marital power theory of intimate partner violence, **486**
Marital status and suicide risk, 89
Marital/couples therapy, 557

Index

for intimate partner violence, 492
for pedophilia, 445
for posttraumatic stress disorder, 134, 137
Marquis de Sade, 448
Mass murder, 11, 37–38
  categories of, 424, **425**
  characteristics of perpetrators of, 424–425
  instrumental, **425**
  massacres, **425**
  school shootings, 79, 359, 365, 371, 541–549, 551
  victim-specific, **425**
MCIT (mobile crisis intervention team), 290–291
MCMI-III (Millon Clinical Multiaxial Inventory–3), 63, 64, 65, 163
Medical disorders, 106, 196–205. *See also* Neurological disorders
  characteristics of aggression in, **186**
  delirium, 197, **197**
  in elderly persons, 386–388, 395–396
  hypoglycemia, 198
  medication side effects, 197–198
  misdiagnosis in elderly persons, 386–388
  psychosis and, 10
  rheumatic diseases, 198
  sleep disorders, 198
  toxin exposure, 197
  treatment of, 199–205
    assessment and quantification of aggressive episodes, 199
    behavioral strategies, 201, 204
    pharmacotherapy, 199–201
      for acute aggression and agitation, 199–200
      for chronic aggression, 200–201, **202–203**
Medical education in management of violent patients, 326
Medical history of elderly persons, 386–388
Medication side effects, 197–198
Medroxyprogesterone acetate, for paraphilias, 453, 454

Memantine, for Alzheimer's disease, 399, 402
Memory impairment in elderly persons, 381, 387
  assessment of, 390–392
  with dementia, 390
Mental handicap. *See* Intellectual disability
Mental health professionals. *See* Clinicians
Mental Health Triage Scale, 283
Mental retardation. *See* Intellectual disability
Mental status examination of elderly persons, 389–394
  attentional problems, 389–390
  cognitive and memory impairment, 390–392
  disorders of mood and affective regulation, 392–394
  thought processing, 392
Mercury exposure, 197
Metabolic syndrome, atypical antipsychotic–induced, 403
Metal detectors, 249
Methadone maintenance treatment, 154
Methamphetamine, 147
Michigan Alcoholism Screening Test, 445
Millon Clinical Multiaxial Inventory–3 (MCMI-III), 63, 64, 65, 163
Minimal brain dysfunction, 196
Mini-Mental State Examination (MMSE), 285, 390, 392, 402
Minimum Data Set, 397
Minnesota Multiphasic Personality Inventory–2 (MMPI-2), 28, 63–65, 67, 72, 163, 416, 491
  Clinical and Supplementary Scales of, 64
  for evaluation of test-taking style, 64
  Overcontrolled Hostility Scale of, 64–65
  profile most commonly associated with violence, 64
  Psychopathic Deviance Scale of, 65
Minor violence, defined, 108

Miscarriage, 41
MMSE (Mini-Mental State
  Examination), 285, 390, 392, 402
Mobile crisis intervention team
  (MCIT), 290–291
Modafinil, 150
Mode of death, 419
Monoamine oxidase-A, 364
Mood disorders, 77–94. *See also* Bipolar
    disorder; Depression; Mania
  in adolescents, 374
  biology of aggression in, 92–93
  in genesis of violence, 83–86
    among elderly persons, 392–394,
      399–400
    intermittent explosive disorder and,
      217
    substance abuse and, 84, 85
  violence in genesis of, 77–83
    community violence, war, and
      terrorism, 81
    direct abuse or neglect, 79–81
      adult assault, 80
      intimate partner violence, 80–
        81
      physical abuse, 79
      sexual abuse, 79–80
      verbal and emotional abuse, 79
    passive exposure, 77–79
      parental substance abuse, 78–
        79
      witness to domestic violence,
        77–78
    prevention of, 82
    treatment approaches for, 81–83
  and violence toward self, 86–92
    deliberate self-harm, 86–89
      bipolar disorder and, 88–89
      depression and, 86–88
    suicide, 89–92
      bipolar disorder and, 90–91
      depression and, 89–90
      homicide and, 91–92
Mood stabilizers, 84–85, **203**, 334. *See
    also* Anticonvulsants
  combination therapy with
    antipsychotics, 314–315

driving safety and, 522
for outpatients with impulsive
  aggression, 317
for violent youth, 374
Moral reasoning training, for students
  at risk for school violence, 550
Motivational enhancement therapy, for
  alcoholism, 155
Motivations for inpatient assault, 261–
  270
Movement disorders, 194–196
  Huntington's disease, 195, 204–205
  Parkinson's disease, 195
  Tourette's syndrome, 195–196
  Wilson's disease, 195
Multiple sclerosis, 196
Multisystem atrophy, 198
Multisystemic therapy, for delinquent
  adolescents, 374
Murder-suicide, 421–425
  definition of, 421
  extrafamilial, 424–425
    categories of mass killing, 424,
      425
    characteristics of perpetrators of,
      424–425
    school shootings, 543, 546
  gender and, 422
  motivators for, **422**
  of other family members, 423–424
    as altruistic, 423, 424
    familicide, 424
    filicide, 423
  prevalence of, 421–422
  spousal/consortial, 422–423
  time frame for, 421
  typology for, 422
  by vehicular crash, 526
Muslims, 35
  culturally appropriate assessment of
    interpersonal violence in, 47, 49

Nadolol, 316
Naidu v. Laird, 524
Nail biting, 225
Naltrexone, for alcoholism, 152–153
  in elderly persons, 399

Index

Narcissism, 252
Narcissistic personality disorder, 11
   purposeful, instrumental violence and, 168–169
   targeted, impulsive violence and, 172, 174
   violence related to chronic paranoia or related misconception and, 179
Narcolepsy and driving safety, 522, 531
NASH acronym for mode of death, 419
National Comorbidity Replication Study, 89
National Comorbidity Survey, 222
National Crime Victimization Survey, 415, 461
National Highway Traffic Safety Administration, 523
National Institute of Mental Health
   Clinical Antipsychotic Trials of Intervention Effectiveness, 107–108
   Epidemiologic Catchment Area study, 106, 148
National Institute of Occupational Safety and Health, 504
National Institute on Alcohol Abuse and Alcoholism, 151, 152, 155
National Institute on Drug Abuse, 151
National Research Council, 538, 549
National Triage Scale, 283
National Vietnam Veterans Readjustment Study (NVVRS), 125–126
National Violent Death Reporting System, 421
Native Americans, 35. *See also* Alaska Natives; American Indians
   substance abuse and suicidality among, 144
Natural History of Alcoholism, The, 155
Neglect of children. *See* Childhood abuse or neglect
Neonaticide, 423
Neurobiology
   of addiction, 149–150
   of aggression

   in mood disorders, 92–93
   neurochemistry, 92–93, 215–216
   of alcohol, 143
Neuroimaging
   of aggression in dementia, 187, 400, 402
   of brain regions associated with impulsivity and aggression, 214–215
Neuroleptics. *See* Antipsychotics
Neurological disorders, 185–196. *See also* Medical disorders
   central nervous system tumors, 194
   characteristics of aggression in, **186**
   congenital brain disorders and developmental disorders, 189–190, 219–221 (*See also* Intellectual disability)
   dementia, 185–187
   driving safety and, 522, 531
   encephalitis, 192–194
   epilepsy, 190–192
   among inpatients, **261**
   movement disorders, 194–196
      Huntington's disease, 195, 204–205
      Parkinson's disease, 195
      Tourette's syndrome, 195–196
      Wilson's disease, 195
   psychosis and, 10
   self-injurious behaviors, 225
   stroke, 188–189
   traumatic brain injury, 187–188, 204
   treatment of, 199–205
      assessment and quantification of aggressive episodes, 199
      behavioral strategies, 201, 204
      pharmacotherapy, 199–201
        for acute aggression and agitation, 199–200
        for chronic aggression, 200–201, **202–203**
Neurological soft signs, 196
Neuropsychological testing
   of persons with impulsive aggression, 213
   of violent offenders, 214

Neurotransmitters, 215–216
  definition of, 215
  norepinephrine, 215–216
  serotonin, 92–93, 215, 328
Nicotine patch, for elderly patients, 399, 400, 403
Nightmares, in posttraumatic stress disorder, 132, 133–136
Nitrous oxide exposure, 197
Noncompliance with medications, 11, 12, 114, 302–303, 335
Norepinephrine, aggression, impulsivity and, 215–216
Novaco Anger Scale, 67, 72
Nurses
  "cold" threats against, 268–269
  de-escalation techniques used by, 265, **266**
  inpatient assaults on, 259, 263–265
    debriefing after, 265
    psychological support for, 265
  prevalence of violence against, 461
  in psychiatric emergency room, 282
Nursing home placement, 186, 392
NVVRS (National Vietnam Veterans Readjustment Study), 125–126

Observation of patient
  agitated elderly persons, 394
  extended psychiatric observation services, 285–289
  during seclusion and restraint, 292, **342,** 344, 348–349
Obsessional stalkers, 411–412
Obsessive-compulsive disorder, 195
Obsessive-compulsive personality disorder
  nontargeted, impulsive violence incidental to emotional escape and, 176
  targeted, impulsive violence and, 172, 174
Occupational Safety and Health Act (OSHA), 507
OCF (Outline for Cultural Formulation), 43–44, **44,** 46, 54
O'Connor v. Donaldson, 438

ODD (oppositional defiant disorder), 363, 369
Office safety, 248–249, 332, 463–464, 465–466, 476–477
Olanzapine, 12, 311
  for aggressive elderly patients, 401
  anti-hostility effects of, 313
  for chronic aggression, **202**
  intramuscular, 303, **304,** 305, **306,** 309–310
    adverse effects of, 309
    dosage of, **304,** 309
    effectiveness of, 311
    indications for, 309
    transition to oral administration, 311
  long-term treatment with, 312–314
  valproate and, 314–315
  for violent psychotic inpatients, 114, 254
Olfactory aversion, for paraphilias, 453
Ondansetron, for alcoholism, 148
Opiate analgesics, 198
Opioid dependence, 147–148
  maintenance treatment of, 154
  withdrawal from, 147–148
Opportunistic rapists, 415
Oppositional defiant disorder (ODD), 363, 369
Organized and disorganized crime scenes, FBI profiling of, 417–418, **418**
OSHA (Occupational Safety and Health Act), 507
Osteopenia/osteoporosis, anti-androgen–induced, 454–455
Outline for Cultural Formulation (OCF), 43–44, **44,** 46, 54
Outpatient settings, violence risk assessment in, 237–255, 465–466
  actuarial assessment, 237–238
  assessing imminence of risk, 244–245
  Axis I diagnoses and, 250–252
  clinical assessment, 237–239
  conceptual framework and case example of, 239–243
  environmental variables and, 253

Index

gender and, 253
general principles for, 237–239
interview questions for, 238–239
legal aspects of potential violence, 246–247
in patients with past history of violence, 243–244
personality traits and, 252
preventive action to reduce risk, 245–246
risk of violence to clinician, 248–249, 254, 259, 332
screening questions for, 238
threats to patients, 247–248
treatment variables and, 253–254
use of HCR-20 for, 240–241
Overdose of drug
cocaine, 147
by suicidal patient, 295
Overt Aggression Scale, 7, **8**, 188, 199, 215
Oxcarbazepine, for aggression, 85, 253

PADs (Protective Aggression Devices), 352
PAI (Personality Assessment Inventory), 63, 64, 65, 163
Correctional Report of, 65
Pain, 41
Paint/paint thinner inhalation, 9
Paliperidone, 312
PANSS (Positive and Negative Syndrome Scale), 313, 314
Paraneoplastic encephalitis, 193
Paranoia, 168
assaultiveness and, 107
in bipolar disorder, 83
stimulant-induced, 9, 147
workplace violence and, 511
Paranoid defenders, 171
Paranoid delusions, 10, 12, 64, 118, 265–266, **267**, 284
Paranoid personality disorder, 11
nontargeted, impulsive violence incidental to emotional escape and, 175
purposeful, targeted, defensive violence and, 171–172
targeted, impulsive violence and, 172, 174
violence related to chronic paranoia or related misconception and, 179–181
Paranoid stalkers, 171, 179
Paraphilias, 327, 382, 441, 442
coercive, 446
cognitive distortions and, 453
treatment of, 452–455
algorithm for, 454
cognitive-behavioral therapy, 452–453
pharmacological, 453–455
relapse prevention, 453
Parasomnias, 198
Parasuicide, 222
Parent management training, 374
Parents
adolescent depression related to maternal depression, 78
children learning how to manage aggression from, 363
effects on children of passive exposure to violence between, 78
effects on children of substance abuse by, 78–79
murder of children by, 448
murder-suicide, 423–424
poor parenting by, 363
Parkinsonism, drug-induced, 402
Parkinson's disease, 195, 198
Paroxetine, for posttraumatic stress disorder, 132
Past history of violence or impulsive behaviors, 5, 7
in adolescents, 368–369
assessing potential future violence in patients with, 243–244
"dissecting" details of, 7
information to obtain about, 7
as risk factor for future violence, 7, 22, 23, 259–260
severity of, 7
Patriarchy theory of intimate partner violence, **486**
Paulhus Deception Scales (PDS), 69–70

PCL. *See* Psychopathy Checklist
PCL-R. *See* Psychopathy Checklist–Revised
PCL-YV (Psychopathy Checklist–Youth Version), 62, 369, 370
PCP (phencyclidine), 9, 148
PDS (Paulhus Deception Scales), 69–70
Pedicide, 423
Pedophile Index, 445, 449
Pedophilia, 329, 441, 442–445. *See also* Sexual abuse in childhood
   assessment of, 444–445
   child homicide and, 448–449
      measuring sexual arousal in perpetrators of, 449–450
   hormonal treatment of, 335
   treatment of, 445, 452–455
Peer effects and youth violence, 363, 364, 365, 375
Penile plethysmography (PPG), 70–71, 416, 445
Persecutory delusions, 10, 108, 266, **267**
Personality assessment, 63–65, 72
   Millon Clinical Multiaxial Inventory–3, 63, 64, 65, 163
   Minnesota Multiphasic Personality Inventory–2, 28, 63–65, 67, 72, 163
   Personality Assessment Inventory, 63, 64, 65, 163
   of specific characteristics, 67–69
      aggression, 68
      anger, 67–68
      hostility, 68
      impulsivity, 68–69
   of test-taking style, 63–64
Personality Assessment Inventory (PAI), 63, 64, 65, 67, 163
   Correctional Report of, 65
Personality changes
   in posttraumatic stress disorder, 124
   in Wilson's disease, 195
Personality disorders, 11, 13, 22, 27, 161–182, 301. *See also specific personality disorders*
   among adolescent offenders, 364
   anger attacks and, 252
   definition of, 161, 165
   in delinquent youth, 369
   kinds of violence associated with, 167–181
      nontargeted, impulsive violence incidental to emotional escape, 174–176
         case examples of, 175
      purposeful, instrumental violence, 167–169
         case examples of, 168
      purposeful, noninstrumental violence, 169–170
         case examples of, 170
      purposeful, targeted, defensive violence, 170–172
         case example of, 171
      random but purposeful violence, 176–177
         case example of, 177
      targeted, impulsive violence, 172–174
         case examples of, 172–174
      violence related to chronic paranoia or related misconception, 179–181
         case example of, 179–180
      violence related to perceived/feared loss or abandonment, 177–179
         case example of, 178
   prognosis for, 161
   self-injurious behaviors and, 225
   treatment and management of, 166–167
      pharmacotherapy, 317
   variations in diagnosis-related behavior in, 164–165
   violence and, 163–164
      intoxication and, 167, 171, 173, 178
      legal responsibility and, 165
Personality traits and violence, 252
Pervasive developmental disorder, 369. *See also* Autism spectrum disorder
Pervasively angry rapists, 416
Phallometry, 449

Index

Pharmacotherapy
  driving safety and, 522–523, 532–533
  for paraphilias, 453–455
  for posttraumatic stress disorder, 131–132, 133–136
  for sleep disturbances, 134
  for students at risk for school violence, 550
  for substance addiction, 152–154, 399
Pharmacotherapy for agitation/aggression, 84–85, 253–254, 301–318. *See also specific drugs and classes*
  during alcohol withdrawal, 302
  for chemical restraint, 351
  court-ordered, 114
  depot medications for, 11
  in elderly persons, 400–404
    acute/emergent management, 394–395
    cholinesterase inhibitors for Alzheimer's disease, 302, 303, 399, 402
  among inpatients, 113, 114
  long-term treatment, 312–316
  in medical or neurological illness, 199–201
    acute aggression and agitation, 199–200
    chronic aggression, 200–201, **202–203**
  noncompliance with, 11, 12, 114, 302–303, 335
  in psychiatric emergencies, 302, 303–311, **306–307**
    intramuscular medications for, 303–311, **304**
    with seclusion and restraint, 340, 343, 351–352
  psychotherapy and, 334–335
  refusal of, 302–303
  therapeutic alliance for, 114
  use on 72-hour extended observation unit, 287
  in violent youth, 374–375
Phencyclidine (PCP), 9, 148

Phenytoin, for impulsive aggression, 253
Physical abuse
  during childhood, mood disorders related to, 79
  by intimate partner, 483–495 (*See also* Intimate partner violence)
  psychiatric disorders in victims of, 80
  suicide risk and, 89
Physical distance from violent patient, 468
Physical space interventions, in inpatient settings, 114–115
Physicians. *See also* Clinicians
  violence against, 461–463
Physician's Guide to Assessing and Counseling Older Drivers, 528–530
Pibloktoq, 44, **45**
Poisoning of self, 225
Police
  interviewing of, 4
  racial stereotyping by, 46
  to subdue violent patient in emergency department, 13
Police reports, 5
Pornography on Internet, 444
Positive and Negative Syndrome Scale (PANSS), 313, 314
Positron emission tomography, 187, 402
Postictal aggression, 191
Posttraumatic stress disorder (PTSD), 123–137
  in combat veterans, 81, 123, 124–125
  diagnostic criteria for, 123
  "fight, flight, or freeze" responses in, 124
  history taking in, 133
  increased expectation of danger in, 124
  intimate partner violence and, 41, 80, 82, 485
  management of violent patients with, 81–83, 130–137
    case examples of, 133–137
    clinician safety and, 130–131
    cognitive-behavioral therapy, 132–133, 134

Posttraumatic stress disorder (*continued*)
  management of violent patients with (*continued*)
    in emergency department, 130–131
    marital/couples therapy, 134, 137
    pharmacological, 131–132, 133–134
    psychiatric comorbidity with, 124, 128, 129
    screening patients with trauma history for, 129
    suicide and, 128–129
    symptoms of, 123–124, 133–136
    terrorism and, 81
    violence and, 124–137
      assessment of, 129–130, **130**, **131**
      family violence, 127
      firearm-related, 128, 129, 133
      incarcerated men, 126–127
      risk factors for, 125–127, 133
  in violent youth, 369
Poverty, 11
Power-assertive rapists, **416**
Power-reassurance rapists, **416**
PPG (penile plethysmography), 70–71, 416, 445
Prazosin, for posttraumatic stress disorder, 132, 133–134, 135
Predatory stalkers, **413**
Predatory violence among adolescents, 370–372
Prednisone, 198
Pregnancy
  fetal substance exposure during, 213
  homicide during, 484
  intimate partner violence during, 41, 484
Premature labor, 41
Premeditated aggression, 212–213, 312
  by inpatients, 262
  psychopathy and, 213
Prenatal risk factors for impulsivity and aggression, 213–214
Prevalence of violence
  among adolescents, 359, 360–362

child sexual abuse, 443
toward clinicians, 461
intimate partner violence, 41, 80, 484
long-term pharmacotherapy for, 312
murder-suicide, 421–422
in persons with intellectual disability, 220
in psychiatric illness, 148–149, 250
  bipolar disorder, 107, 250
  depression, 106
  posttraumatic stress disorder, 126
  schizophrenia or psychosis, 106–107, 250–252
rape, 143
in substance-abusing patients, 107
symptoms of mental illness and, 107–109
in workplace, 505–507
Prevention
  Blueprints for Violence Prevention, 374
  de-escalation techniques for agitated inpatients, 265, **266**
  duty of clinicians to warn and protect potential victims, 246, 247, 269, 333–334, 373, 430–434, 524, 557–559, **560**
  legal duties of clinician to prevent vehicular crashes, 531–534
  of mood disorders in violence-exposed persons, 82
  of psychotic assaults by inpatients, 267
  to reduce violence risk in outpatient settings, 245–246
  of school violence, 549–550
  of short-term risk of violence, 3, 14
Private stranger stalkers, 412, **414**
Prodrome of violence, 467
Profiling
  by FBI of disorganized and organized crime scenes, 417–418, **418**
  of perpetrators of workplace violence, 509–510
  of school shooters, 547–548
Project Combine, 153

Index

Project MATCH, 155
Property destruction, 7, 27
   autism and, 222
   inpatient assaults and, 260
   intellectual disability and, 220
   intermittent explosive disorder and, 217
Propranolol, **203**, 204, 316
Protective Aggression Devices (PADs), 352
Psychiatric disorders and violence, 22, 162–163, 310. *See also specific disorders*
   actuarial risk assessment of, 4
   among adolescent offenders, 364
   association with symptoms of mental illness, 107–109
   Axis I diagnoses, 250–252
   in elderly persons, 398–400
      mood disorders, 392–394
   ethnicity and diagnosis of, 35
   among inpatients, **261**
   intermittent explosive disorder, 11, 13
   intimate partner violence, 41, 485
   mania, 10
   mood disorders, 77–94, 149
   personality disorders, 11, 161–182
   posttraumatic stress disorder, 123–137
   prevalence of, 148–149, 250
   psychotic disorders, 10, 105–119, 149
   public fear of, 148
   substance abuse and, 148–149
   suicide and, 89
   vehicular crashes, 521–523
   in workplace, 511
Psychiatric emergency services (PESs), 277–296. *See also* Emergency settings
   assessment issues in emergency setting, 291–295
      restraints, 292–293, 294–295
      safety, 291
      seclusion, 291–292, 293–294
      suicide risk, 294–295
   case examples of, 279–280, 284–285, 462–463
   in community, 289–291
   definition of psychiatric emergency, 277, 278
   description of, 277–278, 279
   extended psychiatric observation services, 285–289
      case example of, 287
   referral to on-call mental health specialist, 278
   safety in, 13, 14, 281, 282, 291, 462–463, 470
   service delivery models for, 278, 280–285
      psychiatric emergency room, 280–284
      design of, 281
      seclusion area of, 280, 350
      staff of, 282–283
      weapons search in, 46, 249, 462
Psychiatrists. *See* Clinicians
Psychological autopsy, 418–420
   indications for, 419
   of murder-suicide, 421–425
   of suicide by cop, 420–421, **421**
   techniques for, 419–420
Psychological testing, 59–73, 317
   actuarial assessment and, 59–60
   case example of, 60
   in civil vs. criminal settings, 61
   of a criminal defendant, 60
   instruments for violence risk assessment, 61–73
      defensiveness, 69–70
      general personality assessment, 63–65
      psychopathy, 61–63
      Rorschach test, 66–67
      sexual offenders, 60, 70–72
      specific personality characteristics, 67–69
      substance abuse, 69
   of special populations, 60
   time frame of concern for, 61
Psychologists. *See* Clinicians
Psychopathy
   assessment of, 62–63
   definition of, 61

Psychopathy (*continued*)
  instrumental assaults and, 110, 111
  premeditated-predatory aggression and, 213
Psychopathy Checklist (PCL), 62–63, 445
  cross-cultural validity of, 63
  in perpetrators of sexual violence, 445, 448, 451
  screening version of, 62
Psychopathy Checklist–Revised (PCL-R), 27, 62–63, 68, 213
Psychopathy Checklist–Youth Version (PCL-YV), 62, 369, 370
Psychosis, 10, 13, 105–119. *See also* Delusions; Hallucinations; Schizophrenia
  brain tumors and, 194
  driving safety and, 522, 523–524, 533
  in elderly persons, 399, 402
  ethnicity and diagnosis of, 35
  exacerbation by seclusion, 349
  inpatient assaults due to, 109, 110–111, 262–263, **264**, 266–267
    command hallucinations and, 108–109, **267**, 267–268
    indicators of impending assault, **267**
    strategies for prevention of, 267
  motivations for assault in patients with, 109, 113
  poststroke, 189
  prevalence of violence in, 106–107
  psychiatric disorders associated with, 10
  in rheumatological diseases, 198
  steroid-induced, 198
  violence associated with symptoms of, 107–109
  workplace violence and, 511
Psychosocial history of elderly persons, 389
Psychotherapy, 325–337
  for aggression, 317
  clinical inexperience of clinicians with violent patients, 326–327
  countertransference issues in, 332–333
  court-mandated, 327
  for depression and posttraumatic stress disorder resulting from violence exposure, 82
  deranged transferences in, 331–332
  determining feasibility of, 330–331
  for elderly patients, 399
  fears and liabilities in, 327
  goals and strategies of, 329–331
  for paraphilias, 452–453
  for personality disorders, 166, 169
  pharmacotherapy and, 334–335
  for posttraumatic stress disorder, 132–133
  problem of agency in, 327
  setting for, 332
  for substance addiction, 154–155
  supervision of, 335
  transference threats during, 472
  unstable treatment situations and, 335–336
  vectors of violence and, 328–329
  with victims, 333–334
  with violent youth, 374
Psychotic identification with victim, 10
PTSD. *See* Posttraumatic stress disorder
Public-figure stalkers, 412, **414**
Pupillary dilation, 6
Pyromania, 217–219, 227
  among arsonists, 218
  case example of, 217–218
  definition of, 218
  DSM classification of, 218
  gender and, 218
  helping patients recognize origins of, 329
  prevalence of, 218
  psychiatric comorbidity with, 219
  risk factors for, 218

QT interval prolongation, ziprasidone-induced, 308
Quetiapine
  for aggressive elderly patients, 382, 400, 401, 403
  for chronic aggression, **202**

Index

in emergency setting, 303
long-term treatment with, 312–314
Quiet patient, 6
Quinolone antibiotics, 198

Race. *See* Ethnicity/race
Racing thoughts, in intermittent explosive disorder, 217
Ramelteon, for sleep problems, 134
Rape. *See* Sexual assault/rape
Rapid eye movement behavior disorder, 198
Rapid Risk Assessment for Sexual Offender Recidivism (RRASOR), 29, 437
Rapists, 415–417. *See also* Sexual offenders
  assessment for future dangerousness, 416
  diagnostic classification of, 446
  factors associated with reoffense, 417
  recidivism risk for, 417, 450
  typology of, 415–416, **416**
Reactive assaults, 109–110
Reasoning abilities, assessing in elderly persons, 391
RECON stalker typology, 412, **414**
Rejected stalkers, **413**
Relationship instability, 11, 22
Religion. *See* Spirituality and religious beliefs
Reporting, of intimate partner violence, 492–494
Resentful stalkers, **413**
Resident physicians, violence against, 461–463
Resource theory of intimate partner violence, **486**
Restlessness
  antipsychotic-induced, 200
  after traumatic brain injury, 187, 188
Restraining orders
  in cases of intimate partner violence, 493–494
  against stalkers, 415
Restraint. *See* Seclusion and restraint
Rheumatic diseases, 198

Risk factors for suicide, 89
Risk factors for violence
  in adolescents, 364–365, **366,** 370
  available means to inflict harm, 6–7
  behavioral, 28
  on Classification of Violence Risk, 23
  clinician survey of relevance of, 28
  against clinicians, 465–466, **466**
  combining of, 21
  cultural, 35
  demographic factors, 11–12
  generating final risk estimate based on, 21
  on HCR-20, 22
  by intimate partner, 484
  intimate partner violence, 491
  minor violence, 108
  past history of violence, 7, 22, 23, 259–260
  personality disorders, 11
  in posttraumatic stress disorder, 125–126, 133
  protective factors and, 37
  psychosis, 10
  vs. risk markers, 37, 38
  in schools, 551
  selection and measurement of, 20
  serious violence, 108
  sexual violence, 70
  treatment noncompliance, 11
  on Violence Risk Appraisal Guide, 26–27
  in workplace, 508–512
Risperidone, 387
  for aggressive elderly patients, 391–392, 393, 401
  anti-hostility effects of, 313
  electroconvulsive therapy and, 316
  liquid, 311
  long-term treatment with, 312–314
  valproate and, 314–315
  for violent inpatients, 254
  for violent youth, 374
Rivastigmine, for Alzheimer's disease, 399
Robert Wood Johnson Foundation, 151
Rorschach Inkblot test, 29, 66–67, 72

RRASOR (Rapid Risk Assessment for Sexual Offender Recidivism), 29, 437

Sadism, 330. *See also* Sexual sadism
Safety
  of aggressive elderly persons and their caregivers, 395
  of clinician, 248–249, 254, 332, 461–478
  of clinician's office, 248–249, 332, 463–464, 465–466, 476–477
  vs. confidentiality, 241, 247
  driving, 521–535
  duty of clinicians to warn and protect potential victims, 246, 247, 269, 333–334, 373, 430–434, 524, 557–559, **560**
  in emergency settings, 13, 14, 281, 282, 291, 462–463, 470
  gun safety management, 6, 372, 373, 557, 562, **563**
  management of armed patient, 476
  of patient in restraints, 347
  protecting victims and reporting of intimate partner violence, 492–494
  seclusion room design for, 350
  weapons checks for, 46, 249, 332, 462
  of workplace, 507
Sarcoidosis, 198
SASSI (Substance Abuse Subtle Screening Inventory), 69, 72
Satiation (masturbatory), for paraphilias, 453
SAVD (School-Associated Violent Death) study, 539
SAVRY (Structured Assessment of Violence Risk in Youth), 370
Scheduling appointment for violence risk assessment, 466
Schizoaffective disorder, 12, 251, 302
Schizoid personality disorder
  purposeful, targeted, defensive violence and, 171
  targeted, impulsive violence and, 174

Schizophrenia, 4, 13, 27, 105–119, 301
  antisocial personality disorder and, 250–251
  availability of potential victim to patient with, 7
  causes of violence in, 10
  clinical violence risk assessment in, 12
  command hallucinations in, 108–109, **267**, 267–268
  conduct disorder and, 250–251
  delusions in, 10, 12, 265–266
  diagnosed in emergency setting, 279
  driving safety and, 523–524
  escalating pattern of violence in, 7
  inpatient management of violent patients, 113–118
    case examples of, 116–118
  intimate partner violence and, 485
  motivations for assault in patients with, 109, 113
  pharmacotherapy for aggression/agitation in, 113, 114, 302–303
  prevalence of violence in, 250–252
  psychosis in, 10
  pyromania and, 219
  reversible risk factors for violence in, 106
  self-injurious behaviors in, 225
  substance abuse and, 250
  violence and positive symptoms of, 252
  violence assessment in, 105–113
    association with symptoms of mental illness, 107–109
    classification of assaults, 109–111
    research on classification of assaults, 110–111
    videotape recording of inpatient assaults, 111–112
Schizotypal personality disorder, 174, 176, 179–180
Schneidman, E.S., 418–419
School threat assessments, 371–372
School violence, 79, 359, 365, 371, 537–552
  background of, 538
  bullying, 540–541

Index

criteria for, 538
current extent of, 538–540
homicides, 539–540
interventions for students at risk for, 550, 551
legal restrictions on administrators' response to, 541
prevention of, 549–550
risk factors for, 551
school size and, 539
shootings, 79, 359, 365, 371, 541–549, 551
   at Columbine High School, 543–544
   FBI report on myths about, 548
   at Jonesboro, Arkansas, 544–545
   managing threats or predictions of, 548–549
   National Research Council report on, 549
   notable cases of, 541–543
   operant styles of perpetrators of, 547
   profiles of perpetrators of, 547–548
   social causation model of, 541
   at Virginia Tech, 546–547
suicides, 539
unreliability of data on, 537
School-Associated Violent Death (SAVD) study, 539
Schuster v. Altenberg, 532
Seclusion and restraint, 339–354
of adolescents, 292
care of patient in, 349–350
case example of, 293–294
chemical restraint, 351
CMS requirements for, 341, 344–345, 351
committee to oversee use of, 353
contraindications to, 291, 352
controversy about, 339
danger and injury associated with, 352–353
debriefing after use of, 293, 348
definition of, 292
devices for, 346
unique restraints, 352
disallowance of standing orders for, 345
documentation of, 343, 345
of elderly persons, 395
emergency medication during, 340, 343, 351–352
emotional impact of, 349–350
explaining purpose to patient, 347
fluids for patient in, 349
forensic aspects of, 353
frequency of use, 340
inclusion in hospital policy manual, 345
indications for, 342–343
informing families about institutional policies and practices regarding, 346
initiation of, 343–345
   by licensed independent practitioner, 344
instructors for, 346
JCAHO regulations for, 339–340, 341, 344, 346, 351, 353
long-term use of, 345
meals for patient in, 349
of minority patients, 38
new governmental guidelines for use of, 341–342
observation and monitoring of patient during, 292, **342,** 344, 348–349
as part of patient's treatment plan, 346
patient positioning in restraint, 347–348
reasons for, 341
removal from, 350–351
seclusion room design, 280, 350
self-injurious behaviors during, 350, 352
staff certification for, 345–346
staff implementation of, 291, 292, 346–347
standard of care for, 339
studies of, 340–341
techniques for, 345–348

Seclusion and restraint (*continued*)
   time parameters for, 292, **342,** 344–345, 348
   toileting of patient during, 349
   use in emergency settings, 13, 280, 291–295, 340–341, 462–463
   of violent inpatients, 113–114, 259
Seizures
   during benzodiazepine withdrawal, 305
   driving safety and, 522, 531, 533
   epilepsy and violence, 190–192
   poststroke, 189
Selective serotonin reuptake inhibitors (SSRIs)
   for anger attacks in depressed outpatients, 254
   for chronic aggression, **202,** 316
   for paraphilias, 453–454
   for pedophilia, 445
   for posttraumatic stress disorder, 131–132, 134
Self-esteem
   childhood verbal and emotional abuse and, 79, 83
   intimate partner violence and, 491, 492
   self-injurious behaviors and, 226
Self-injurious behaviors (SIBs), 224–226, 228. *See also* Deliberate self-harm; Suicide
   among adolescents, 225–226
   autism and, 222
   case example of, 224–225
   childhood trauma exposure and, 214
   compulsive, 225
   definition of, 225
   diversity of, 225
   impulsivity and, 223, 225, 226
   intellectual disability and, 220
   in Klüver-Bucy syndrome, 193
   major, 225
   in posttraumatic stress disorder, 124
   prevalence of, 225–226
   psychiatric disorders associated with, 226
   psychological functions of, 226
   self-hitting, 225
   self-poisoning, 225
   skin burning, 225, 330
   skin cutting, 224–225, 226
   skin picking or scratching, 225
   stereotypic, 225
   substance abuse and, 226
   while in seclusion, 350, 352
Serial killing, 38
Serious violence, defined, 108
Serotonin, 92–93, 215, 328
Sertraline, 384
   for chronic aggression, **202**
   for paraphilias, 454
   for pedophilia, 445
   for posttraumatic stress disorder, 131–132, 134
Seventy-two–hour observation bed, psychiatric, 288–289
   admission criteria for, 288
   patient consent to treatment during, 288
   patient rights and, 288
   personnel who can place patient in, 288
Severity of violence, 7
Sexual abuse in childhood, 87, 214, 545
   among adult perpetrators of sexual violence, 442
   convictions for, 443
   deliberate self-harm and, 87
   impulsive aggression and, 214
   incest perpetrators, 450, 451–452
   Internet as tool for, 443–444
      case example of, 444–445
   mood disorders related to, 79–80
   prevalence of, 442–443
   programs for prevention of, 443
   verbal and emotional abuse and risk for sexual victimization as adult, 79, 82–83
Sexual acting out, 7
Sexual aggression
   against children, 333, 441
   definition of, 441
   by elderly persons, 382
   against women, 441

Index

Sexual arousal/interest assessment
  Abel Assessment of Sexual Interest, 71–72
  penile plethysmography, 70–71, 416, 445
  in perpetrators of sexual sadism and sexually motivated homicide, 449–450
  phallometry, 449
Sexual assault/rape, 237
  alcohol and, 143
  childhood sexual abuse and, 80, 82
  as crime of power and control, 448–449
  date rape, 143
  gender and, 415
  hormonal therapy for, 335
  by intimate partner, 484, 488
  legal elements of rape, 415
  number of victims of, 415
  prevalence of, 143
  robbery preceding, 363
  of stalking victims, 411
  typology of rapists, 415–416, **416**
Sexual deviations. *See* Paraphilias
Sexual Fantasy Checklist, 445
Sexual offenders, 164, 442
  bipolar disorder among, 84
  case example of, 327
  on Internet, 444–445
  recidivism risk for, 29, 416–417, 450–452
    factors associated with, 417, 451
    Rapid Risk Assessment for Sexual Offender Recidivism, 29, 437
    Static-99, 452
    structured violence risk assessment of, 29
    victim age and, 451–452
  treatment of, 452–455
    cognitive-behavioral therapy, 452–453
    pharmacological, 453–455
    relapse prevention, 453
  typology of rapists, 415–416, **416**
Sexual rapists, 416

Sexual sadism, 176, 441, 445–450
  brain abnormalities and, 446
  characteristics of, 446
  gender and, 446
  reliability of diagnosis of, 445–446
  sexually motivated homicide and, 442, 445–450
    child victims of, 448
    measuring sexual arousal in perpetrators of, 449–450
    XYY syndrome in perpetrators of, 447–448
Sexual violence, 441–456. *See also* Sexual abuse in childhood; Sexual assault/rape
  definition of, 441–442
  history of childhood sexual abuse among perpetrators of, 442
  intellectual disability and, 220
  Internet as tool for, 443–445
  recidivism risk for, 29, 416–417, 450–452
  sexual sadism and sexually motivated homicide, 442, 445–450
  suicide risk and, 89
  treatment for perpetrators of, 452–455
  women as perpetrators of, 80
Sexual violence risk assessment, 60, 70–72
  Abel Assessment of Sexual Interest, 71–72
  of Internet child pornographers, 444–445
  of known rapists, 415–417, **416**
  Pedophile Index, 445, 449
  penile plethysmography, 70–71, 416, 445
  in perpetrators of sexual sadism and sexually motivated homicide, 449–450
  Rapid Risk Assessment for Sexual Offender Recidivism, 29
  for recidivism, 29, 417, 450–452
  structured, 29
Sexually transmitted infections, 41

Sexually Violent Predator (SVP) commitment statutes, 70
Short-term violence risk
　clinical assessment for, 3–14
　psychological testing for assessment of, 61
　time frame for, 4, 18
SIBs. *See* Self-injurious behaviors
Single-photon emission computed tomography, 400
Situational threats, 472
Sjögren's syndrome, 198
Skilled nursing facilities, 396–397
Sleep apnea, driving safety and, 531
"Sleep attacks," driving safety and, 531
Sleep deprivation, 198
Sleep disturbances, 198
　driving safety and, 531
　pharmacotherapy for, 134
　in posttraumatic stress disorder, 133–136
Smoking
　cessation strategies for elderly persons, 399, 400, 403
　fetal tobacco exposure, 213, 214
Social learning theory of intimate partner violence, **486**
Social skills training, for students at risk for school violence, 550
Socioeconomic status, 11–12, 37, 38
Sodium amytal, 303, 305
Solvent exposure, 197
Somalis, culturally appropriate assessment of interpersonal violence in, 48–49
South African Truth and Reconciliation Commission, 82
Spirit possession, **45**
Spirituality and religious beliefs, 35
　about subservience of wives, 35
　as mitigating factors against violence, 252
　self-injurious behaviors and, 225
　support of African American women through, 81
Spousal abuse. *See* Intimate partner violence

Spousal/consortial murder-suicide, 422–423
　amorous-jealous subtype of, 423
　declining-health subtype of, 423
　psychiatric disorders and, 422
SSRIs. *See* Selective serotonin reuptake inhibitors
Stalking, 60, 247, 411–415
　assaults related to, 411
　circumstances of, 412
　clinical management of, 475
　of clinician, 474–475
　danger posed by stalker, 413
　definition of, 474–475
　duration of, 411
　elements of, 411
　false allegations of, 412
　gender and, 411
　interventions to reduce impact of, 413–415
　paranoid stalkers, 171, 179
　prevalence of, 411, 475
　psychological impact of, 475
　restraining orders against stalkers, 415
　stalker typologies, 411–412, **413**
　　according to relationship with victim and public-figure context, 412, **414**
　threats and, 475
　via electronic communication, 412–413
Standard Family Violence Index, 127
State/Trait Anger Expression Inventory, 67
Static-99, 437, 445, 452
Stimulant drugs. *See also* Amphetamine; Cocaine
　abuse of, 147
　agitation induced by, 9
　driving safety and, 522
　side effects of, 197–198
Strangulation, 446, 447
Stroke, 188–189, 196, 389
　antipsychotics and, 403
Structured Anchored Clinical Judgment–Minimum, 437

Index

Structured Assessment of Violence Risk in Youth (SAVRY), 370
Structured Guide for the Assessment of Violence, 285
Structured violence risk assessment, 3–4, 17–31. *See also* Actuarial violence risk assessment
    Classification of Violence Risk, 18, 23–26, 28, **28,** 30
    compared with clinical risk assessment, 3–4, 17–21, **28**
    comparison of tools for, **28,** 30
    components of, 20–21, 31
        combining risk factors, 21
        generating final risk estimate, 21
        selecting and measuring risk factors, 20
    continuum of, 18
    court and legislative openness to, 29, 31
    HCR-20, 21–23, **28,** 28–29, 30, 39, 46, 240–241
    predictive validity of, 30, 31
    psychological testing and, 59–60
    of sexual offenders, 29
    use in clinical practice, 27–29, 30–31, 59
    Violence Risk Appraisal Guide, 18, 26–27, **28,** 28–29, 30
Substance abuse disorders, 4, 7–9, 13, 22, 23, 39, 141–156. *See also* Alcohol use/abuse; *specific substances of abuse*
    addiction, 149–155
        definition of, 149
        as disease, 155
        identification of, 151–152
        media dramatization of, 151
        modafinil for patients with, 150
        neurobiology of, 149
        treatment of, 152–155
            in elderly persons, 399
            evidence-based strategies for relapse prevention, 152
            patient–treatment matching for, 155
            pharmacological, 152–154
            psychotherapy, 154–155
            12-Step facilitation therapy, 155
            12-Step programs, 152, 155
    alcohol, 7–9, 141–146
    among assault victims, 80, 82
    cannabis, 85, 86, 107, 148
    children of substance-abusing parents, 78–79
    cocaine, 9, 13, 39, 147
    ethnicity and, 35
    among female victims of intimate partner violence, 485, 488
    methamphetamine, 147
    opioids, 147–148
    phencyclidine, 9, 148
    prevalence of violence and, 250
    psychiatric comorbidity with, 148–149, 301
        bipolar disorder, 84, 85, 251
        intermittent explosive disorder, 217
        personality disorders, 167
        posttraumatic stress disorder, 129, 133
        psychosis, 10
        pyromania, 219
        schizophrenia, 250
    self-injurious behaviors and, 226
    signs of intoxication, 6
    suicide and, 89, 92, 143–144, 294
        among college students, 143
        risk factors for, 144
    workplace violence and, 510, 511
    youth violence and, 364, 369–370
Substance Abuse Subtle Screening Inventory (SASSI), 69, 72
Suicidal gestures, 222
Suicide, 7, 12, 211, 222–224, 227. *See also* Deliberate self-harm; Self-injurious behaviors
    antidepressants and risk for, 90, 92
    assessing potential for, 4, 6, 12
    to prevent death of child, 424
    assisted, 423
    borderline personality disorder and, 11

Suicide (*continued*)
  bullying and, 79
  childhood trauma and, 80, 214, 223
  cocaine and, 147
  drinking age and, 143
  emergency room management of suicidal patient, 294
    case example of, 294–295
  gender and, 89, 223
  homicide and, 91–92, 328–329
    clinician's anxiety about therapy with suicidal patients, 327–328
  hopelessness and, 87, 90
  impulsive, 222–224
    aggression as risk factor for, 224
    case example of, 222
    definition of, 223
    methods of, 224
  incidence of, 89
  intent for, 419
  intimate partner violence and, 80–81, 82, 485, 489
  mercy, 423
  mood disorders and, 85, 89–92, 223
  motive for, 419
  murder-suicide, 421–425
  national rate of, 294
  other deliberate self-harm and, 86, 92, 222
  past suicide attempts as predictor of, 89, 223
  posttraumatic stress disorder and, 128–129
  psychological autopsy of, 419
  in schools, 539
  serotonin level and, 92, 93, 215
  sociodemographic risk factors for, 89
  substance abuse and, 89, 92, 143–144, 294
    alcohol, 89, 146
    among college students, 143
    risk factors for, 144
Suicide attempts, 222–223
  definition of, 222
  impulsive, 223–224

  lethality of, 419
  as predictor of eventual death by suicide, 89, 223
  prevalence of, 222–223
  psychiatric comorbidity with, 223
  recurrence of, 223
  vehicular crashes as, 522, 524–526
"Suicide by cop," 180, 420–421
  behavioral clues to, 420–421
  characteristics of, 420, **421**
  definition of, 420
  of mass murderer, 425
  prevalence of, 420
  verbal clues to, 420
Supervision of therapy, 335
Supportive therapy, 82
Surgical history of elderly persons, 386–388
Suspiciousness
  assaultiveness and, 107–108
  cocaine-induced, 9
  in elderly persons, 381
SVP (Sexually Violent Predator) commitment statutes, 70
Syncope
  driving safety and, 531
  olanzapine-induced, 308
Systemic lupus erythematosus, 198

Tachycardia, olanzapine-induced, 308
Tarasoff v. Regents of the University of California, 246, 269, 328, 373, 430–434, 493, 524, 532, 557–558
TBI. *See* Traumatic brain injury
Telephone interview for violence risk assessment, 465
Telephone threats, 473
Temper tantrums
  in childhood, 216
  intellectual disability and, 220
Terrorism, 81, 501, 505
Testosterone, 92
  anti-androgens for suppression of, 453
Test-taking style, assessment of, 63–64
Thapar v. Zezulka, 433–434
Theft, in inpatient facilities, 115

Index

Therapeutic alliance
  duty to warn and, 557
  inpatient assaults and, 260
Therapists. *See* Clinicians
Thought insertion, 107
Threat assessment
  in schools, 371–372
  in workplace, 512–516
    crisis management teams for, 514
    difference from clinical evaluations, 512–513
    disclosure of information from, 513
    goal of, 512–513
    information used for, 513, 515
    mental illness and, 513
    process of, 514–516
"Threat book," 269
Threats
  to clinicians, 335, 463–465, 471–475
    (*See also* Violence toward clinicians)
    case example of, 464
  "cold," 268–269
  to inpatient staff, 268–269
  to patients, 247–248
  of school violence, 548–549
  by stalkers, 475
  in workplace, 502–503
Time frame for validity of risk assessment, 4, 18–19
Token economy, 201
Toluene exposure, 197
Topiramate, for aggression, 85
Tourette's syndrome, 195–196
  attention-deficit/hyperactivity disorder and, 195
  self-injurious behaviors in, 225
Toxin exposure, 197
Transference
  deranged, 331–332
    stalking due to, 475
  diluting of, 473
  monitoring of, 472–473
  psychotic, violence to clinician due to, 464–465
  racism and, 40

Transference threats, 472
Traumatic bonding theory of intimate partner violence, **487**
Traumatic brain injury (TBI), 187–188, 196
  alcohol response and, 149
  case example of, 204
  impulsivity, aggression and, 214–215
  relation of postinjury behavior to preexisting aggressive tendencies, 215
Trazodone
  for aggressive elderly patients, 403
  for sleep problems, 134
Treatment interventions, 253–254
  for elderly persons, 394–404
  electroconvulsive therapy, 316
  for intimate partner violence, 491–492
  involuntary hospitalization, 244–245
  involuntary outpatient treatment, 254
  lack of response to, 22
  noncompliance with, 11
  for pedophilia, 445
  pharmacotherapy, 301–318
  psychotherapy, 325–337
  racial differences in use of, 38–39
  seclusion and restraint, 339–354
  for violent inpatients, 113–118, 253–254
  for violent youth, 359–360, 372–374
    in schools, 550, 551
  for workplace violence risk, 515–516
Tremors, 6
Trichotillomania, 225
12-Step facilitation therapy, 155
12-Step programs for substance abusers, 152, 155
Twenty-three–hour observation bed, psychiatric, 286
Twin studies, 364

Unabomber, 546
Unstructured violence risk assessment. *See* Clinical violence risk assessment

U.S. Secret Service profiling of school shooters, 547–548
U.S. Surgeon General reports
 Mental Health: Culture, Race and Ethnicity, 36
 Report on Youth Violence, 36

Vaillant, George E., 155
Valproate, 12, 84–85, **203**, 303, 312, 387
 for aggressive elderly patients, 403
 for outpatients with impulsive aggression, 317
 with risperidone or olanzapine, 314–315
 for violent youth, 374
van Gogh, Vincent, 88–89
Vasculitis, 198
Vehicular crashes, 521–535
 dementia and, 527–531
 depression and, 524–526
 disturbances of consciousness and, 531
 intoxication and, 522
 legal duties of clinicians to prevent, 531–534
 medications and, 522–523, 532–533
 psychosis, schizophrenia and, 523–524
 suicidal drivers, 522, 524–526
Venlafaxine, 284, 393
Verbal abuse during childhood
 mood disorders related to, 79
 and risk of adult sexual victimization, 79, 82–83
Veterans
 depression in, 81
 head injury and aggression among, 215
 National Vietnam Veterans Readjustment Study, 125–126
 posttraumatic stress disorder in, 81, 123–137 (*See also* Posttraumatic stress disorder)
Victims
 of bullying, 540–541
 childhood abuse and, 79, 80
 of crime in schools, 539

duty of clinicians to warn and protect potential victims, 246, 247, 269, 333–334, 373, 430–434, 524, 557–559, **560**
 with intellectual disability, 220
 mental health professionals as, 248–249, 332, 461–478
 of patient with antisocial personality disorder, 11
 patients as, 247–248
 perpetrators' lack of empathy for, 61
 psychiatric disorders of, 80
 psychotherapy with, 333–334
 psychotic identification with, 10
Videotape recording of inpatient assaults, 111–112, 262
Vietnamese, 35
 culturally appropriate assessment of interpersonal violence in, 50–51
Vindictive rapists, 416
Violence. *See also* Aggression; Agitation
 Axis I diagnoses and, 250–252
 among children and adolescents, 359–376
 clinical inexperience with patients exhibiting, 326–327
 definition of, 237
 dynamics of, 467
 helping patients recognize origins of, 329
 heterogeneity of persons exhibiting, 325
 patients' disavowal of tendencies toward, 327
 prodrome of, 467
 serious, 237
 vectors of, 328–329
Violence Risk Appraisal Guide (VRAG), 18, 26–27, **28,** 30
 combining risk factors for, 27
 generating final risk estimate with, 27
 predictive validity of, 26
 Psychopathy Checklist–Revised and, 62
 selecting and measuring risk factors for, 26–27
 use in clinical practice, 28, 29

Index

Violence risk assessment, 465–466, **466**
   actuarial, 3–4, 17–31, 46, 59
   in adolescents, 365–372
   assessing imminence of risk, 244–245
   clinical, 3–14, 46
   components of, 20–21
   continuum of structure for, 18
   cultural competence in, 35–54
   exert testimony based on, 430, 434–437
   in inpatient settings, 259–272
   in outpatient settings, 237–255, 465–466
   in patient with past history of violence, 243–244
   of patients with posttraumatic stress disorder, 129–130, **130, 131**
   psychological testing in, 59–73
   reliability of assessments used for expert testimony, 437, 439
   for sexual violence, 60, 70–72
   structured, 3–4, 17–31
   in Texas criminal procedures, 438
   time frame for validity of, 4, 18–19
   for violence against clinician, 465–466, **466**
      clinician denial of risk and, 466
      components of, 465
      scheduling appointment for, 466
      setting for, 465–466
      telephone interview, 465
   in workplace, 512–516
Violence risk management, 555–564
   avoidant practices, 556
   case example of, 556–557
   documentation, 562
   duty to warn and protect potential victims, 246, 247, 269, 333–334, 373, 430–434, 524, 557–559, **560**
   goal of, 555
   gun safety management, 6, 372, 373, 557, 562, **563**
   patient discharge from inpatient facilities, 559–560, **561**
   preemptive practices, 555–556
   in schools, 550, 551
   in workplace, 515–516
Violence toward clinicians, 461–478
   additional management techniques for, 468–469
   affect management for, 463, 465, 467–468
   anticipation of, 466
   assessing risk for, 465–466, **466**
      components of, 465
      scheduling appointment for, 466
      setting for, 465–466
      telephone interview, 465
   dynamics of, 467
   in emergency settings, 462–463, 470
   on inpatient unit, 470
   limit setting and, 469–470
   managing the armed patient, 476
   office safety, 248–249, 332, 463–464, 465–466, 476–477
   prevalence of, 461
   prodrome of, 467
   psychiatrist's denial of risk for, 464, 465, 466
   as result of psychotic transference in outpatient setting, 464–465
   threats of, 335, 463–465, 471–475
      case example of, 464
      dynamics of, 471
      forms of, 471
      management of, 473–474
      monitoring of, 472–473
      settings for, 471
      situational, 472
      stalking, 474–475
      transference, 472
Violent ideation, 6
Virginia Tech shootings, 546–547
Visuospatial abilities, assessing in elderly persons, 391
Vitamin D, during anti-androgen therapy, 455
von Economo's disease, 192
Voyeurism, 441
VRAG. *See* Violence Risk Appraisal Guide

War exposure
  mood disorders and, 81
  posttraumatic stress disorder in
    combat veterans, 81, 123–137
"Warn" assaults, 112
Weapons checks, 46, 249, 332, 462
White matter disorders, 196
Whitman, Charles, 546
WHO (World Health Organization), 144
Wife abuse. *See* Intimate partner
    violence
Wilson's disease, 195
Women
  intimate partner violence
    perpetrated by, 491, 492
  murder-suicide of children by, 423
  religious beliefs about subservience
    of wives, 35
  sexual abuse perpetrated by, 80
  sexual assault of
    alcohol and, 143
    childhood sexual abuse and, 80
    date rape, 143
    prevalence of, 143
    use of Psychopathy Checklist–
      Revised in, 63
  as victims of intimate partner
    violence, 41–42, 80–81, 483–495
    alcohol-related, 82–83, 145–146
    culturally appropriate
      assessment of, 47–53
    during pregnancy, 41, 484
    treatment of, 82
  as victims of stalking, 411
  violence among, 253
Workplace violence, 501–516
  Americans with Disabilities Act
    and, 508
  case example of, 502–504
  common-law negligence claims
    related to, 508
  definition of, 504–505
  disaster plan for, 507
  homicide, 501, 505, 506, 509
  legal risks associated with, 507–508
  managing risk for, 515–516
  methodological problems in studies
    of, 508–509
  nonfatal assaults, 506
  prevalence of, 505–507
  profiles of perpetrators of, 509–510
  psychiatric disorders and, 511
  risk factors for, 508–512
    individual, 510–511
    organizational, 511–512
    profiling approach to, 509–510
    static vs. dynamic, 512
  threat assessment in, 512–516
  threats of, 502–503
  Types I to IV, 505–507
  types of, 501
  workers' compensation for injuries
    arising from, 508
  wrongful accusations of, 504, 508
World Health Organization (WHO), 144
Written threats, 473

XYY syndrome, 447–448

Youth violence. *See* Adolescents

Zar, 44, **45**
Ziprasidone
  for aggressive elderly patients, 401
  intramuscular, 295, 303, **304, 306,**
    308–309
    contraindications to, 308
    dosage of, **304,** 308
    effectiveness of, 311
    indications for, 308
    QT interval prolongation
      induced by, 308
    transition to oral administration,
      311
    use in renal disease, 308
  long-term treatment with, 312–314
Zolpidem, for sleep problems, 134